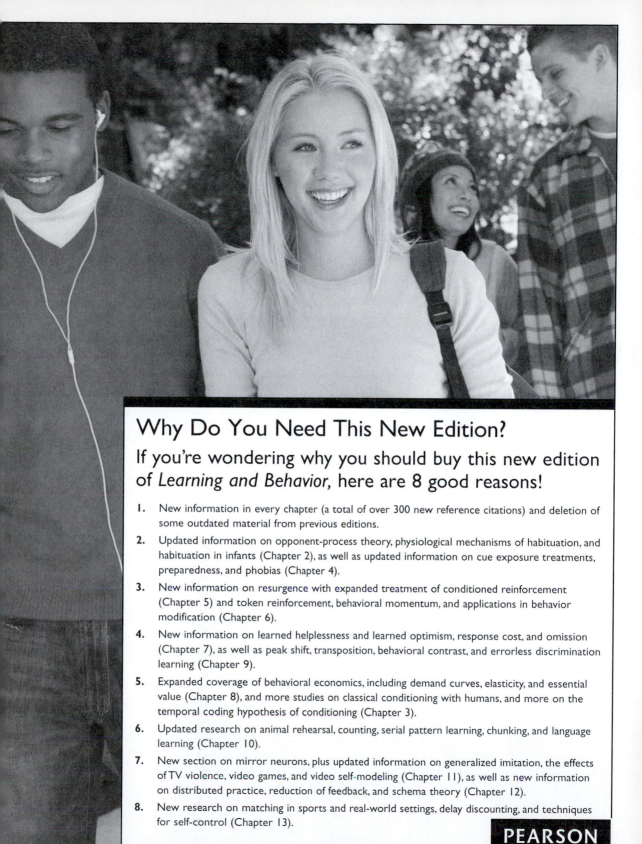

Why Do You Need This New Edition?

If you're wondering why you should buy this new edition of *Learning and Behavior,* here are 8 good reasons!

1. New information in every chapter (a total of over 300 new reference citations) and deletion of some outdated material from previous editions.

2. Updated information on opponent-process theory, physiological mechanisms of habituation, and habituation in infants (Chapter 2), as well as updated information on cue exposure treatments, preparedness, and phobias (Chapter 4).

3. New information on resurgence with expanded treatment of conditioned reinforcement (Chapter 5) and token reinforcement, behavioral momentum, and applications in behavior modification (Chapter 6).

4. New information on learned helplessness and learned optimism, response cost, and omission (Chapter 7), as well as peak shift, transposition, behavioral contrast, and errorless discrimination learning (Chapter 9).

5. Expanded coverage of behavioral economics, including demand curves, elasticity, and essential value (Chapter 8), and more studies on classical conditioning with humans, and more on the temporal coding hypothesis of conditioning (Chapter 3).

6. Updated research on animal rehearsal, counting, serial pattern learning, chunking, and language learning (Chapter 10).

7. New section on mirror neurons, plus updated information on generalized imitation, the effects of TV violence, video games, and video self-modeling (Chapter 11), as well as new information on distributed practice, reduction of feedback, and schema theory (Chapter 12).

8. New research on matching in sports and real-world settings, delay discounting, and techniques for self-control (Chapter 13).

PEARSON

Seventh Edition

LEARNING AND BEHAVIOR

James E. Mazur
Southern Connecticut State University

PEARSON

Boston   Columbus   Indianapolis   New York   San Francisco   Upper Saddle River
Amsterdam   Cape Town   Dubai   London   Madrid   Milan   Munich   Paris   Montreal   Toronto
Delhi   Mexico City   São Paulo   Sydney   Hong Kong   Seoul   Singapore   Taipei   Tokyo

Editorial Director: Craig Campanella
Editor in Chief: Jessica Mosher
Executive Acquisitions Editor: Susan Hartman
Editorial Assistant: Shiva Ramachandran
Vice President, Director of Marketing: Brandy Dawson
Executive Marketing Manager: Wendy Albert
Marketing Assistant: Frank Alarcon
Production Project Manager: Liz Napolitano
Manager, Central Design: Jayne Conte
Cover Designer: Suzanne Behnke
Cover Image: © Brian Finestone/Fotolia

Image Permission Coordinator: Martha Shethar
Visual Research: Stephen Merland/ PreMediaGlobal
Director of Digital Media: Brian Hyland
Senior Media Editor: Peter Sabatini
Full-Service Project Management: Murugesh Namasivayam/ PreMediaGlobal
Composition: PreMediaGlobal
Printer/Binder: Courier Corp./Westford
Cover Printer: Lehigh-Phoenix Color/ Hagerstown
Text Font: Minion Pro

Credits and acknowledgments borrowed from other sources and reproduced, with permission, in this textbook appear on the appropriate page within text and on pages 395–396.

Library of Congress Cataloging-in-Publication Data
Mazur, James E.
    Learning and behavior / James E. Mazur. —7th ed.
        p. cm.
    Includes bibliographical references and index.
    ISBN-13: 978-0-205-24644-1 (alk. paper)
    ISBN-10: 0-205-24644-3 (alk. paper)
    1. Learning, Psychology of.   2. Conditioned response.   3. Behavior modification.
    4. Psychology, Comparative.   I. Title.

    BF318.M38 2013
    153.1'5—dc23

                                                            2011036784

10 9 8 7 6 5 4 3 2 1   V013

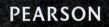

ISBN 10:   0-205-24654-0
ISBN 13: 978-0-205-24654-0

In memory of my parents, Ann and Lou Mazur, who responded to my early interests in science with encouragement, understanding, and patience.

CONTENTS

PREFACE

The purpose of this book is to introduce the reader to the branch of psychology that deals with how people and animals learn and how their behaviors are later changed as a result of this learning. This is a broad topic, for nearly all of our behaviors are influenced by prior learning experiences in some way. Because examples of learning and learned behaviors are so numerous, the goal of most psychologists in this field has been to discover general principles that are applicable to many different species and many different learning situations. What continues to impress and inspire me after many years in this field is that it is indeed possible to make such general statements about learning and behavior. This book describes some of the most important principles, theories, controversies, and experiments that have been produced by this branch of psychology in its first century.

This text is designed to be suitable for introductory or intermediate-level courses in learning, conditioning, or the experimental analysis of behavior. No prior knowledge of psychology is assumed, but the reading may be a bit easier for those who have had a course in introductory psychology. Many of the concepts and theories in this field are fairly abstract, and to make them more concrete (and more relevant), I have included many real-world examples and analogies. In addition, most of the chapters include sections that describe how the theories and principles have been used in the applied field of behavior modification.

Roughly speaking, the book proceeds from the simple to the complex, with respect to both the difficulty of the material and the types of learning that are discussed. Chapter 1 discusses the behavioral approach to learning and contrasts it with the cognitive approach. It also describes some of the earliest theories about the learning process; then it presents some basic findings about the physiological mechanisms of learning. Chapter 2 discusses innate behaviors and the simplest type of learning, habituation. Many of the terms and ideas introduced here reappear in later chapters on classical conditioning, operant conditioning, and motor-skills learning.

The next two chapters deal with classical conditioning. Chapter 3 begins with basic principles and ends with some therapeutic applications. Chapter 4 describes more recent theoretical developments and experimental findings in this area. The next three chapters discuss the various facets of operant conditioning: Chapter 5 covers the basic principles and terminology of positive reinforcement, Chapter 6 covers schedules of reinforcement and applications, and Chapter 7 covers negative reinforcement and punishment. Chapters 8 and 9 have a more theoretical orientation. Chapter 8 presents differing views on such fundamental questions as what constitutes a reinforcer and what conditions are necessary for learning to occur. Chapter 9 takes a more thorough look at generalization and discrimination, and it also examines research on concept learning.

Chapter 10 surveys a wide range of findings in the rapidly growing area of comparative cognition. Chapters 11 and 12 discuss two types of learning that are given little or no emphasis in many texts on learning—observational learning and motor-skills learning. These chapters are included because a substantial portion of human learning involves either observation or the development of new motor skills. Readers might well be puzzled or disappointed (with some justification) with a text on learning that includes no mention of these topics. Finally, Chapter 13 presents an overview of behavioral research on choice.

In this seventh edition, two introductory chapters from previous editions have been condensed and combined into one. The remaining 12 chapters retain the same overall structure as in previous editions, but each chapter has been updated with new studies and new references that reflect recent developments in the field. As in the previous edition, the book includes a number of learning aids for students, including a list of learning objectives at the beginning of each chapter, practice quizzes and review questions, and a glossary for all important terms.

SUPPLEMENTS

Pearson Education is pleased to offer the following supplements to qualified adopters.

Instructor's Manual and Test Bank (0205254012)

Written by the author of the text, James E. Mazur, the instructor's manual is a wonderful tool for classroom preparation and management. Corresponding to the chapters in the text, each of the manual's 13 chapters contains a brief overview of the chapter with suggestions on how to present the material, sample lecture outlines, classrooms activities and discussion topics, ideas for in-class and out-of-class projects, recommended outside readings and related films and videos.

The test bank contains over 1,300 multiple-choice, short-answer, and essay questions, each referencing the relevant page in the text.

Pearson MyTest Computerized Test Bank PEARSON mytest ☑ (0205254004) (www.pearsonmytest.com):

The Test Bank comes with Pearson MyTest, a powerful assessment-generation program that helps instructors easily create and print quizzes and exams. You can do this online, allowing flexibility and the ability to efficiently manage assessments at any time. You can easily access existing questions and edit, create, and store questions using the simple drag-and-drop and Word-like controls. Each question comes with information on its level of difficulty and related page number in the text. For more information, go to www.pearsonmytest.com.

PowerPoint Presentation (0205253997)

Written by Professor Anne Foreman, the PowerPoint Presentation is an exciting interactive tool for use in the classroom. Each chapter pairs key concepts with images from the textbook to reinforce student learning.

MySearchLab (0205864813) MySearchLab®

Provided with this edition, **MySearchLab** offers engaging experiences that personalize, stimulate, and measure student learning. Pearson's **MyLabs** deliver proven results from a trusted partner in helping students succeed. Features available with this text include:

- **A complete eText**—just like the printed text, you can highlight and add notes, listen to audio files, and more!
- **Assessment**—chapter quizzes, topic-specific assessment and flashcards offer and report directly to your grade book.
- **Chapter-specific learning applications**—ranging from videos to case studies, and more.
- **Writing and research assistance**—a wide range of writing, grammar and research topics including access to a variety of databases that contain academic journals, census data, Associated Press newsfeeds, and discipline specific readings.

MySearchLab can be packaged with this text at no additional cost—just order using the MySearchLab ISBN shown on the back cover. Instructors can request access to preview MySearchLab by contacting their local Pearson representative or by visiting www.mysearchlab.com.

ACKNOWLEDGMENTS

I owe thanks to many people for the help they have given me as I wrote this book. Many of my thoughts about learning and about psychology in general were shaped by my discussions with the late Richard Herrnstein—my teacher, advisor, and friend.

I am also grateful to several others who read portions of the book and gave me valuable feedback. Thanks go to the reviewers of this edition: Matthew C. Bell, Santa Clara University; Thomas Brown, Utica College; Maureen Bullock; April Fugett, Marshall University; Melinda Leonard, University of Louisville; Harold L. Miller, Jr., Brigham Young University; Erin Rasmussen, Idaho State University; Steve Weinert, Cuyamaca College; and to reviewers of previous editions: Mark Branch, University of Florida; Gary Brosvic, Rider University; Valerie Farmer-Dougan, Illinois State University; Adam Goodie, University of Georgia; Kenneth P. Hillner, South Dakota State University; Peter Holland, Duke University; Ann Kelley, Harvard University; Kathleen McCartney, University of New Hampshire; David Mostofsky, Boston University; Thomas Moye, Coe College; Jack Nation, Texas A&M University; David Schaal, West Virginia University; James R. Sutterer, Syracuse University; E. A. Wasserman, University of Iowa; and Joseph Wister, Chatham College. In addition, I thank Marge Averill, Stan Averill, John Bailey, Chris Berry, Paul Carroll, David Coe, David Cook, Susan Herrnstein, Margaret Makepeace, Margaret Nygren, Steven Pratt, and James Roach for their competent and cheerful help on different editions of this book. I am also grateful for the assistance and advice provided by Susan Hartman of Pearson Education. Finally, I thank my wife, Laurie Averill, for her help on this and previous editions.

J. E. M.

1

History, Background, and Basic Concepts

LEARNING OBJECTIVES

After reading this chapter, you should be able to

- describe the early theories of memory proposed by the Associationists and the early memory studies of Hermann Ebbinghaus

- explain the behavioral and cognitive approaches to studying learning and how they differ

- explain the advantages and disadvantages of using animals in psychological research

- discuss intervening variables, and the debate over whether they should be used in psychology

- explain how our sensory receptors respond to "simple sensations" and how feature detectors in the visual system respond to more complex patterns

- list three main types of changes that can take place in the brain as a result of a learning experience, and present evidence for each type

If you know nothing about the branch of psychology called *learning,* you may have some misconceptions about the scope of this field. I can recall browsing through the course catalog as a college freshman and coming across a course offered by the Department of Psychology with the succinct title "Learning." Without bothering to read the course description, I wondered about the contents of this course. Learning, I reasoned, is primarily the occupation of students. Would this course teach students better study habits, better reading, and better note-taking skills? Or did the course examine learning in children, covering such topics as the best ways to teach a child to read, to write, to do arithmetic? Did it deal with children who have learning disabilities? It was difficult to imagine spending an entire semester on these topics, which sounded fairly narrow and specialized for an introductory-level course.

My conception of the psychology of learning was wrong in several respects. First, a psychology course emphasizing learning in the classroom would probably have a title such as "Educational Psychology" rather than "Learning." My second error was the assumption that the psychology of learning is a narrow field. A moment's reflection reveals that students do not have a monopoly on learning. Children learn a great deal before ever entering a classroom, and adults must continue to adapt to an ever-changing environment. Because learning occurs at all ages, the psychological discipline of learning places no special emphasis on the subset of learning that occurs in the classroom. Furthermore, since the human being is only one of thousands of species on this planet that have the capacity to learn, the psychological discipline of learning is by no means restricted to the study of human beings. For reasons to be explained, a large percentage of all psychological experiments on learning have used nonhuman subjects. Though they may have their faults, psychologists in the field of learning are not chauvinistic about the human species.

Although even specialists have difficulty defining the term *learning* precisely, most would agree that it is a process of change that occurs as a result of an individual's experience. Psychologists who study learning are interested in this process wherever it occurs—in adults, in school children, in other mammals, in reptiles, and in insects. This may sound like a large subject matter, but the field of learning is even broader than this, because researchers in this area study not only the *process* of learning but also the *product* of learning—the long-term changes in an individual's behavior that result from a learning experience.

An example may help to clarify the distinction between process and product. Suppose you glance out the window and see a raccoon near some garbage cans in the backyard. As you watch, the raccoon gradually manages to knock over a garbage can, remove the lid, and tear open the garbage bag inside. Imagine that the smell of food attracted the raccoon to the garbage cans, but that it has never encountered such objects before. If we were interested in studying this particular type of behavior, many different questions would probably come to mind. Some questions might deal with the learning process itself: Did the animal open the can purely by accident, or was it guided by some "plan of action"? What factors determine how long the raccoon will persist in manipulating the garbage can if it is not immediately successful in obtaining something to eat? Such questions deal with what might be called the **acquisition phase**, or the period in which the animal is acquiring a new skill.

Once the raccoon has had considerable experience in dealing with garbage cans, it may encounter few surprises in its expeditions through the neighborhood. Although the acquisition process is essentially over as far as garbage cans are concerned, we can continue to examine the raccoon's behavior, asking somewhat different questions that deal with the *performance* of learned behaviors. The raccoon will have only intermittent success in obtaining food from garbage cans—sometimes a can will be empty and sometimes it will contain nothing edible. How frequently will the raccoon visit a given backyard, and how will the animal's success rate affect the frequency of its visits? Will its visits occur at the most advantageous times of the day or week? Such questions concern the end product of the learning process, the raccoon's new behavior patterns. This text is entitled *Learning and Behavior,* rather than simply *Learning,* to reflect the fact that the psychology of learning encompasses both the acquisition process and the long-term behavior that results.

THE SEARCH FOR GENERAL PRINCIPLES OF LEARNING

Because the psychology of learning deals with all types of learning and learned behaviors in all types of creatures, its scope is broad indeed. Think, for a moment, of the different behaviors you performed in the first hour or two after rising this morning. How many of those behaviors would not have been possible without prior learning? In most cases, the decision is easy to make. Getting dressed, washing your face, making your bed, and going to the dining room for breakfast are all examples of behaviors that depend mostly or entirely on previous learning experiences. The behavior of eating breakfast depends on several different types of learning, including the selection of appropriate types and quantities of food, the proper use of utensils, and the development of coordinated hand, eye, and mouth movements. Except for behaviors that must occur continuously for a person to survive, such as breathing and the beating of the heart, it is difficult to think of many human behaviors that do not depend on prior learning.

Considering all of the behaviors of humans and other creatures that involve learning, the scope of this branch of psychology may seem hopelessly broad. How can any single discipline hope to make any useful statements about all these different instances of learning? It would make no sense to study, one by one, every different example of learning that one might come across, and this is not the approach of most researchers who study learning. Instead, their strategy has been to select a relatively small number of learning situations, study them in detail, and then try to generalize from these situations to other instances of learning. Therefore, the goal of much of the research on learning has been to develop general principles that are applicable across a wide range of species and learning situations.

B. F. Skinner, one of the most influential figures in the history of psychology, made his belief in this strategy explicit in his first major work, *The Behavior of Organisms* (1938). In his initial studies, Skinner chose white rats as subjects and lever pressing as a response. An individual rat would be placed in a small experimental chamber containing little more than a lever and a tray into which food was occasionally presented after the rat pressed the lever. A modern version of such a chamber is shown in Figure 1-1. In studying the behavior of rats in such a sparse environment, Skinner felt that he could discover principles that govern the behavior of many animals, including human beings, in the more complex environments found outside the psychological laboratory. The work of Skinner and his students will be examined in depth beginning in Chapter 5, so you will have the opportunity to

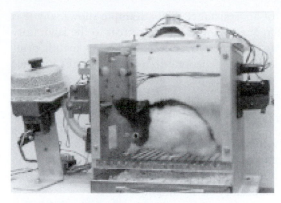

FIGURE 1-1 An experimental chamber in which a rat can receive food pellets by pressing a lever. The pellets are delivered into the square opening below the lever. This chamber is also equipped with lights and a speaker so that visual and auditory signals can be presented. (Photo courtesy of James E. Mazur).

decide for yourself whether Skinner's strategy has proven to be successful.

This strategy of searching for general principles is certainly not unique to the psychology of learning. Attempts to discover principles or laws with wide applicability are a part of most scientific endeavors. For example, a general principle in physics is the law of gravity, which predicts, among other things, the distance a freely falling object will drop in a given period of time. If an object starts from a stationary position and falls for t seconds, the equation $d = 16t^2$ predicts the distance (in feet) that the object will fall. The law of gravity is certainly a general principle, because in theory it applies to any falling object, whether a rock, a baseball, or a skydiver. Nevertheless, the law of gravity has its limitations. As with most scientific principles, it is applicable only when certain criteria are met. Two restrictions on the equation are that it applies (1) only to objects close to the earth's surface, and (2) only as long as no other force, such as air resistance, plays a role. If we chose to ignore these criteria, it would be easy to "disprove" the law of gravity. We could simply drop a rock and a leaf and show that the leaf falls much more slowly. But once the restrictions on the law of gravity are acknowledged, our experiment proves nothing, because we did not eliminate the influence of air resistance. This example shows why it is frequently necessary to retreat to the laboratory to perform a meaningful test of a scientific principle. In the laboratory, the role of air resistance can be minimized through the use of a vacuum chamber. The leaf and the rock will fall at the same rate in this artificial environment, thereby verifying the law of gravity. For similar reasons, orderly principles of learning and behavior that might be obscured by many extraneous factors in the natural environment may be uncovered in a laboratory environment.

Once the restrictions on the law of gravity are specified, a naive reader might conclude that the law has no practical use, because the natural environment provides no vacuums near the earth's surface. However, this conclusion is correct only if extremely precise measurements are demanded, because for many solid objects with a roughly spherical shape, the role of air resistance is so negligible that the law of gravity makes reasonably accurate predictions. Similarly, it would be naive to assume that a psychological principle has no relevance to the natural environment simply because that principle is most clearly demonstrated in the laboratory. Every chapter in this book will introduce several new principles of learning and behavior, nearly all of which have been investigated in laboratory settings. To demonstrate that these principles have applicability to more natural settings, each chapter will also describe real-world situations in which these principles play an important role.

Within the field of psychology, researchers have studied the topic of learning in several different ways. The remainder of this chapter gives an overview of these different approaches, plus a brief history of the field and some background information that will help you to understand the topics covered in later chapters. We will begin with some of the earliest recorded thoughts about learning and memory, developed by philosophers called Associationists and later tested by the psychologist Hermann Ebbinghaus. We will then examine and compare two modern approaches to learning—the behavioral and cognitive approaches—and how they differ. Finally, this chapter will introduce a third approach to studying learning—the physiological approach—which examines what happens in the brain and in individual nerve cells when we learn.

THE ASSOCIATIONISTS

Aristotle

The Greek philosopher Aristotle (c. 350 B.C.) is generally acknowledged to be the first **Associationist**. He proposed three principles of association that can be viewed as an elementary theory of memory. Aristotle suggested that these principles describe how one thought leads to another. Before reading about Aristotle's principles, you can try something Aristotle never did: You can conduct a simple experiment to test these principles. This experiment, which should take only a minute or two, can be called a study of free association. Get a piece of paper and a pencil, and write numbers 1 through 12 in a column down the left side of the paper. Figure 1-2 contains a list of words also numbered 1 through 12. Reading one word at a time, write down the first two or three words that come to mind. Do not spend much time on any one word—your first few responses will be the most informative.

Once you have your list of responses to the 12 words, look over your answers and try to formulate some rules that describe the types of responses you made. Can you guess any of Aristotle's three principles? Aristotle's first principle of association was **contiguity**: The more closely together (contiguous) in space or time two items occur, the more likely will the thought of one item lead to the thought of the other. For example, the response *chair* to the word *table*

1. apple	7. girl
2. night	8. dentist
3. thunder	9. quiet
4. bread	10. sunset
5. chair	11. elephant
6. bat	12. blue

FIGURE 1-2 Words for the free-association experiment.

illustrates association by spatial contiguity, since the two items are often found close together. The response *lightning* to the word *thunder* is an example of association by temporal contiguity. Other examples of association by contiguity are *bread-butter* and *dentist-pain*.

Aristotle's other two principles of association were **similarity** and **contrast**. He stated that the thought of one concept often leads to the thought of similar concepts. Examples of association by similarity are the responses *orange* or *pear* to the prompt *apple,* or the responses *yellow* or *green* to the prompt *blue*. By *contrast*, Aristotle meant that an item often leads to the thought of its opposite (e.g., *night-day, girl-boy, sunset-sunrise*). Most people who try this simple free-association experiment conclude that Aristotle's principles of association have both strengths and weaknesses. On the negative side, the list of principles seems incomplete; other factors that affect the train of thought may have already occurred to you. On the positive side, Aristotle's principles have some intuitive validity for most people, and they seem to be a reasonable first step in the development of a theory about the relationship between experience and memory.

The British Associationists: Simple and Complex Ideas

For Aristotle, the principles of association were simply hypotheses about how one thought leads to another. For many of the philosophers who wrote about Associationism several centuries later, this topic assumed a much greater significance: Associationism was seen as a theory of all knowledge. The **British Associationists** included Thomas Hobbes (1651), John Locke (1690), James Mill (1829), and John Stuart Mill (1843). These writers are also called the British Empiricists because of their belief that every person acquires all knowledge empirically, that is, through experience. This viewpoint is typified by John Locke's statement that the mind of a newborn child is a tabula rasa (a blank slate) on which experience makes its mark. The Empiricists believed that every memory, every idea, and every concept a person has is based on one or more previous experiences.

The opposite of Empiricism is **Nativism**, or the position that some ideas are innate and do not depend on an individual's past experience. For instance, the Nativist Immanuel Kant (1781) believed that the concepts of space and time are inborn and that through experience new concepts are built on the foundation of these original, innate concepts. The Empiricist position is the more extreme of the two because it allows for no counterexamples—it takes just one example of an innate concept to refute the Empiricist position. As we will see many times throughout this book, modern research has uncovered numerous examples that contradict the extreme Empiricist position.

Fortunately, Associationism is not logically tied to extreme Empiricism. We can grant that some concepts are innate but many concepts are developed through experience. The British Empiricists offered some hypotheses both about how old concepts become associated in memory and about how new concepts are formed. According to the Associationists, there is a direct correspondence between experience and memory. Experience consists of sensations, and memory consists of ideas. Furthermore, any sensory experience can be broken down into simple sensations. For instance, if a person observes a red box-shaped object, this sensation might be broken down into two simple sensations: *red* and *rectangular*. At some later time, the person's memory of this experience would consist of the two corresponding simple ideas of *red* and *rectangular*. Thus, as illustrated in Figure 1-3a, there is a one-to-one correspondence between simple sensations and simple ideas. A simple idea was said to be a sort of faint replica of the simple sensation from which it arose.

Now suppose that the person repeatedly encounters such a red box-shaped object. Through the principles of contiguity, an association should develop between the ideas of *red* and *rectangle,* as shown in Figure 1-3b. Once such an association is formed, if the person experiences the color red, this will not only invoke the idea of *red,* but by

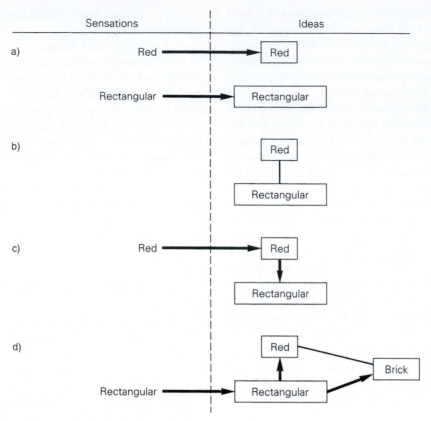

FIGURE 1-3   Some principles of Associationism. (a) One-to-one correspondence between simple sensations and simple ideas. (b) After repeated pairings of the two sensations, an association forms between their respective ideas. (c) Once an association is formed, presenting one stimulus will activate the ideas of both. (d) With enough pairings of two simple ideas, a complex idea encompassing both simple ideas is formed. The complex idea may now be evoked if either of the simple stimuli is presented.

virtue of the association the idea *rectangular* will be invoked as well (Figure 1-3c).

It should be obvious how this sort of hypothesis can explain at least some of the results of a free-association experiment. For instance, the idea of *thunder* will "excite" the idea of *lightning* because of the association between them, an association developed according to the principle of contiguity. But many of our concepts are more complex than the simple ideas of *red, rectangular, thunder,* and *lightning.* In an attempt to come to grips with the full range of memories and knowledge of the world that all people have, several Associationists speculated about the formation of complex ideas. James Mill (1829) proposed

that if two or more simple sensations are repeatedly presented together, a product of their union may be a **complex idea**. For instance, if the sensations *red* and *rectangular* occur together repeatedly, a new, complex idea of *brick* may form. Figure 1-3d shows one way to depict Mill's hypothesis graphically. Once such a complex idea is formed, it can also be evoked by the process of association when the sensation of either red or rectangle occurs. Mill went on to say that complex ideas could themselves combine to form **duplex ideas**. In short, Mill suggested that all complex ideas (1) can be decomposed into two or more simple ideas, and (2) are always formed through the repeated pairing of these simple ideas.

In the following passage, Mill (1829) describes the formation of a hierarchy of ideas of increasing complexity:

> Some of the most familiar objects with which we are acquainted furnish instances of these unions of complex and duplex ideas. Brick is one complex idea, mortar is another complex idea; these ideas, with ideas of position and quantity, compose my idea of a wall. . . . In the same manner my complex idea of glass, and wood, and others, compose my duplex idea of a window; and these duplex ideas, united together, compose my idea of a house, which is made up of various duplex ideas. (pp. 114–116)

This, then, was the view that all ideas, no matter how complex, are the product of simple ideas, which are in turn the product of simple sensations. As with Aristotle's principles of association, there are both strengths and weaknesses in this hypothesis. Some complex concepts are taught to children only after they have become familiar with the simpler ideas that compose them. For instance, it is only after a child understands the concepts of *addition* and *repetition* that the more complex concept of *multiplication* is presented, and it is often introduced as a procedure for performing repeated additions. For older students who know how to calculate the area of a rectangle, *integration* may be initially presented as a technique for calculating the total area of a series of very thin rectangles. In both of these examples, a complex idea is formed only after the mastery of simpler ideas, and it is difficult to imagine learning these concepts in the opposite order. However, other concepts do not seem to follow as nicely from Mill's theory, including his own example of the concept of *house*. A 2-year-old may know the word *house* and use it appropriately without knowing the "simpler" concepts of *mortar, ceiling,* or *rafter*. With *house* and many other complex concepts, people seem to develop at least a crude idea of the entire concept before learning all of the components of the concept, although according to Mill's theory this

should not be possible. Thus, although it appears to have validity in some cases, Mill's theory is at best incomplete. More recent theories about concepts and how they are learned will be presented in Chapter 9.

As already mentioned, Aristotle's three principles of association (contiguity, similarity, and contrast) seem incomplete. Another Associationist, Thomas Brown (1820), tried to supplement Aristotle's list by adding some additional principles. For example, he proposed that the *length of time* two sensations coexist determines the strength of the association, and the *liveliness* or vividness of the sensations also affects the strength of the association. According to Brown, intense stimuli or emotional events will be more easily associated and better remembered. He also proposed that a stronger association will also occur if the two sensations have been paired *frequently,* or if they have been paired *recently*.

The ideas of Aristotle and the British Associationists can be called the earliest theories of learning, for they attempted to explain how people change as a result of their experiences. However, the Associationists never conducted any experiments to test their ideas. In retrospect, it is remarkable that despite an interest in principles of learning spanning some 2,000 years, no systematic experiments on learning were conducted until the end of the nineteenth century. This absence of research of learning was not a result of technological deficiencies, because the first experiments on learning were so simple that they could have been performed centuries earlier.

EBBINGHAUS'S EXPERIMENTS ON MEMORY

Hermann Ebbinghaus (1885) was the first to put the Associationists' principles to an experimental test. In his memory experiments, Ebbinghaus served as his own subject. This arrangement is not acceptable by modern standards, because the experimenter's behavior could easily be biased by his or her expectations. Furthermore, any single subject might be somehow atypical and unrepresentative of people in general. Despite these potential pitfalls, Ebbinghaus's results have withstood the test of time: All of his major findings have been replicated by later researchers using the multiple-subject procedures that are standard in modern research.

To avoid using stimuli that had preexisting associations (such as *coffee-hot*), Ebbinghaus invented the **nonsense syllable**—a meaningless syllable consisting of two consonants separated by a vowel (e.g., HAQ, PIF, ZOD). He would read a list of nonsense syllables out loud at a steady pace, over and over. Periodically, he would test his memory by trying to recite the list by heart, and he would record the number of repetitions needed for one perfect recitation.

In a typical scientific experiment, the researcher manipulates an **independent variable** and observes its effect on a **dependent variable**. The term *independent variable* refers to the fact that the researcher is "free" to vary it as he or she desires. For example, after learning a list, Ebbinghaus might allow different amounts of time to pass (20 minutes, 1 hour, or 24 hours), so the amount of time elapsed would be his independent variable. Then he would relearn the list to perfection, again counting how many repetitions were necessary. The number of repetitions needed to relearn the list was therefore Ebbinghaus's dependent variable. He could then calculate his **savings**—the decrease in the number of repetitions needed to relearn the list. For example, if he needed 20 repetitions to learn a list the first time, but only 15 repetitions to relearn the list at a later time, this was a savings of 5 repetitions, or 25%.

The following three examples from Ebbinghaus's research show how he was able to use these simple experimental methods to test some of the principles proposed by the Associationists.

The Effects of Repetition

One of Thomas Brown's principles of association stated that the frequency of pairings affects the strength of an association. This principle is obviously supported by the simple fact that a list that is not memorized after a small number of repetitions will eventually be learned after more repetitions. However, one of Ebbinghaus's findings offers some additional support for the frequency principle. If he continued to study a list beyond the point of one perfect recitation (e.g., for an additional 10 or 20 repetitions), his savings after 24 hours increased substantially. In other words, even after he appeared to have perfectly mastered a list, additional study produced improved performance in a delayed test. Continuing to practice after performance is apparently perfect is called **overlearning**, and Ebbinghaus demonstrated that Brown's principle of frequency applies to periods of overlearning as well as to periods in which there is visible improvement during practice.

The Effects of Time

Another of Thomas Brown's principles was recency: The more recently two items have been paired, the stronger will be the association between them. Ebbinghaus tested this principle by varying the length of time that elapsed between his study and test periods. As shown in Figure 1-4, he examined intervals as short as 20 minutes and as long as 1 month. The graph in Figure 1-4 is an example of a **forgetting curve**, for it shows how the passage of time has a detrimental effect on performance in a memory task. The curve shows that forgetting is rapid immediately after a study period, but the rate of additional forgetting slows as more time passes. The shape of this curve is similar to the forgetting curves obtained by later researchers in numerous experiments with both human and animal subjects (Blough, 1959; Peterson & Peterson, 1959), although the time scale on the x-axis varies greatly, depending on the nature of the task and the species of the subjects. Forgetting curves of this type provide strong confirmation of Brown's principle of recency.

The Role of Contiguity

The Associationists' principle of contiguity states that the more closely together two items are presented, the better will the thought of one item lead to the thought of the other. Ebbinghaus reasoned that if the contiguity principle is correct, the strongest associations in his lists should be between adjacent syllables, but there should also

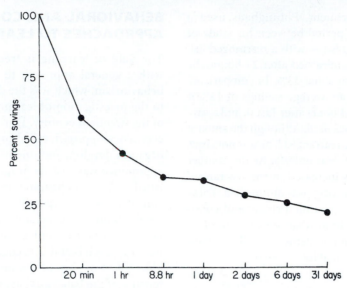

FIGURE 1-4 Ebbinghaus's forgetting curve. The percentage savings is shown for various time intervals between his initial learning and relearning of lists of nonsense syllables. (After Ebbinghaus, 1885)

be measurable (though weaker) associations between nonadjacent items. He devised an ingenious method for testing this idea, which involved rearranging the items in a list after it was memorized, and then learning the rearranged list.

His technique for rearranging lists is illustrated in Figure 1-5. The designations I1 through I16 refer to the 16 items as they were ordered in the original list (List 0). Once this list is memorized, there should be a strong association between I1 and I2, a somewhat weaker association between I1 and I3 (since these were separated by one item in the original list), a still weaker association between I1 and I4, and so on. There should be similar gradations in strength of association between every other item and its neighbors.

The rearranged list, called List 1 in Figure 1-5, was used to test for associations between items one syllable apart. Observe that every adjacent item in List 1 was separated by one syllable in the original list. If there is any association between I1 and I3, between I3 and I5, and so on, then List 1 should be easier to learn than a totally new list (there should be some savings that are carried over from List 0 to List 1). In a similar fashion, List 2 tests for associations between items that were two syllables apart in the original list.

List 0 (Original list)	List 1 (1 item skipped)	List 2 (2 items skipped)
I1	I1	I1
I2	I3	I4
I3	I5	I7
I4	I7	I10
I5	I9	I13
I6	I11	I16
I7	I13	I2
I8	I15	I5
I9	I2	I8
I10	I4	I11
I11	I6	I14
I12	I8	I3
I13	I10	I6
I14	I12	I9
I15	I14	I12
I16	I16	I15

FIGURE 1-5 Ebbinghaus's rearranged list experiment. An original list of 16 syllables (represented here by the symbols I1 through I16) was rearranged to test for possible associations between items separated by one syllable (List 1) or associations between items separated by two syllables (List 2).

In this experiment, Ebbinghaus used a 24-hour forgetting period between his study of an original list and his test with a rearranged list. If List 0 was simply relearned after 24 hours, the savings amounted to about 33%. In comparison, Ebbinghaus found an average savings of 11% if List 1 was studied 24 hours after List 0, and a savings of 7% if List 2 was used. Although the amount of savings with these rearranged lists was not large, the pattern of results was orderly: As the number of skipped syllables increased in the rearranged lists, the amount of savings was diminished. These results therefore support the principle of contiguity, because they imply that the strength of an association between two items depends on their proximity in the original list.

The Influence of the Associationists and Ebbinghaus

Several themes from the Associationists and Ebbinghaus can still be seen in the work of present-day psychologists. During the twentieth century, two major approaches to the study of learning arose—the behavioral and cognitive approaches. Many researchers from both the behavioral and cognitive traditions have adopted the idea that learning involves the formation of associations, as the next several chapters will show. Both behavioral and cognitive psychologists continue to be interested in how factors such as contiguity, similarity among stimuli, repetition, and the passage of time affect what we learn and what we remember. They continue to investigate how people (and animals) learn complex concepts and novel ideas. Although some of Ebbinghaus's methods are not used by modern researchers (such as serving as his own research subject), his research designs were otherwise quite sound. Ebbinghaus's efforts to vary his independent variables systematically and to record his dependent variables accurately and objectively are goals that modern learning researchers also strive for in their experiments. Now that we have surveyed the contributions of these early thinkers, we can turn to the modern-day learning researchers who followed them.

BEHAVIORAL AND COGNITIVE APPROACHES TO LEARNING

The field of learning is frequently associated with a general approach to psychology called **behaviorism**, which was the dominant approach to the investigation of learning for the first half of the twentieth century. During the 1960s, however, a new approach called **cognitive psychology** began to develop, and one of the reasons for its appearance was that its proponents were dissatisfied with the behavioral approach. This book considers both perspectives, but it places more emphasis on the behavioral approach, so it is important for you to understand what the behavioral approach is and why cognitive psychologists objected to it. Two of the most notable characteristics of the behavioral approach are (1) heavy reliance on animal subjects and (2) emphasis on external events (environmental stimuli and overt behaviors) and a reluctance to speculate about processes inside the organism. Let us examine each of these characteristics in turn and see why cognitive psychologists objected to them.

The Use of Animal Subjects

ADVANTAGES AND DISADVANTAGES.   A large proportion of the studies described in this text used animals as subjects, especially pigeons, rats, and rabbits. Researchers in this field frequently choose to conduct their experiments with non-human subjects for a number of reasons. First, in research with humans, **subject effects** can sometimes pose serious problems. A subject effect occurs when those who are participating in an experiment change their behavior because they know they are being observed. Whereas people may change the way they behave when they know a psychologist is watching, subject effects are unlikely to occur with animal subjects. Most studies with animal subjects are conducted in such a way that the animal does not know its behavior is being monitored and recorded. Furthermore, it is unlikely that an animal subject will be motivated to either please or displease the experimenter, a motive that can ruin a study with human subjects.

A second reason for using animal subjects is convenience. The species most commonly used are easy and inexpensive to care for, and animals of a specific age and sex can be obtained in the quantities the experimenter needs. Once animal subjects are obtained, their participation is as regular as the experimenter's: Animal subjects never fail to show up for their appointments, which is unfortunately not the case with human subjects.

Probably the biggest advantage of domesticated animal subjects is that their environment can be controlled to a much greater extent than is possible with either wild animals or human subjects. This is especially important in experiments on learning, where previous experience can have a large effect on a subject's performance in a new learning situation. When a person tries to solve a brain teaser as part of a learning experiment, the experimenter cannot be sure how many similar problems the subject has encountered in his or her lifetime. When animals are bred and raised in the laboratory, however, their environments can be constructed to ensure they have no contact with objects or events similar to those they will encounter in the experiment.

A final reason for using animal subjects is that of comparative simplicity. Just as a child trying to learn about electricity is better off starting with a flashlight than a cell phone, researchers may have a better chance of discovering the basic principles of learning by examining creatures that are less intelligent and less complex than human beings. The assumption here is that although human beings differ from other animals in some respects, they are also similar in some respects, and it is these similarities that can be investigated with animal subjects.

Criticisms of the use of animal subjects seem to boil down to three major arguments. First, it is argued that many important skills, such as the use of language, reading, and solving complex problems, cannot be studied with animals. Although cognitive skills such as language and problem solving have been studied with animals (see Chapter 10), most behavioral psychologists would agree that some complex abilities are unique to human beings. The difference between behavioral psychologists and cognitive psychologists seems to be only that cognitive psychologists are especially interested in those complex abilities that only human beings possess, whereas behavioral psychologists are typically more interested in learning abilities that are shared by many species. This is nothing more than a difference in interests, and it is pointless to argue about it.

The second argument against the use of animal subjects is that human beings are so different from all other animals that it is not possible to generalize from the behavior of animals to human behavior. This is not an issue that can be settled by debate; it can only be decided by collecting the appropriate data. As will be shown throughout this book, there is abundant evidence that research on learning with animal subjects produces findings that are also applicable to human behavior.

The third argument against the use of animals as research subjects involves ethical concerns, as discussed in the next section.

ETHICAL ISSUES AND ANIMAL RESEARCH. In recent years there has been considerable debate about the use of animals as research subjects. Viewpoints on this matter vary tremendously. At one extreme, some of the most radical animal rights advocates believe that animals should have the same rights as people, and that no animals should be used in any type of research whatsoever (Regan, 1983). Some animal rights organizations are trying to promote legislation that would ban all medical and scientific research with animals. Others, both animal welfare advocates and members of the general public, take less extreme positions but believe that steps should be taken to minimize and eventually phase out the use of animals in research (see Bowd & Shapiro, 1993; Compton, Dietrich, & Johnson, 1995).

In response to such criticisms of animal research, some scientists have emphasized that the many advances in medicine, including vaccines, surgical techniques, and prescription drugs would not have been possible without research on animals. They warn that if research with animals were to stop, it would severely impede progress in medical research and hamper efforts to improve the health of the world population (Conn & Parker, 2008; Paul & Paul, 2001).

In the realm of psychological research, N. E. Miller (1985) documented the many benefits that have resulted from psychological research with animals, including ". . . behavior therapy and behavior medicine; rehabilitation of neuromuscular disorders; understanding and alleviating effects of stress and pain; discovery and testing of drugs for treatment of anxiety, psychosis, and Parkinson's disease; new knowledge about the mechanisms of drug addiction, relapse, and damage to the fetus; . . . and understanding the mechanisms and probable future alleviation of some deficits of memory that occur with aging" (p. 423).

Others have agreed that the benefits of psychological research with animals have been substantial, and that progress in dealing with mental health problems would be jeopardized if animals were no longer used as subjects in psychological research (Baldwin, 1993). For those interested in learning more about the complex issues related to the use of animals in scientific research, a thought-provoking book by Petrinovich (1999) provides a comprehensive review of this topic from historical, legal, and ethical perspectives.

One trend that has resulted from the debate over animal research is the development of alternatives to the use of animals in experiments. For example, the cosmetics industry has made progress in devising methods to test the safety of its products that do not involve animals. However, such alternatives to animal experimentation are seldom possible in psychological research (Cuthill, 2007). If you want to study the behavior of an animal, you must observe the animal, not a culture in a test tube or a computer simulation.

Although it may not be possible to eliminate the use of animals in psychological and biomedical research, many new regulations have been put in place in an effort to improve the well-being of animal subjects. In the United States, most colleges, universities, and research centers that use animal subjects are required to have an Institutional Animal Care and Use Committee (IACUC) to oversee all research projects involving animals. The IACUC must review each project with animal subjects, before it begins, to ensure that all governmental regulations are met and that the animals are well cared for. Any pain or discomfort to the animals must be minimized to the extent possible. For example, if an animal undergoes surgery, appropriate anesthesia must be used. Regulations also require that all research animals have adequate food and water, a clean and well-maintained living environment with appropriate temperature, humidity, and lighting conditions, and the continual availability of veterinary care. (It is unfortunate that there are no similar regulations guaranteeing adequate food, a warm place to live, and health care for the human members of our society.)

For the animal experiments described in this book, the year of publication offers a good indication of what types of regulations governed the research. Studies conducted since about 1980 have been governed by increasingly strict regulations designed to ensure the humane treatment of animal subjects. Older studies were conducted during times when there were fewer regulations about animal research. Nevertheless, it is probably safe to say that even before the advent of tighter regulations, the vast majority of the experiments were done by researchers who took very good care of their animals, because they realized that one of the best ways to obtain good research results is to have subjects that are healthy and well treated.

The Emphasis on External Events

The term *behaviorism* was coined by John B. Watson, who is often called the first behaviorist. His book *Psychology from the Standpoint of a Behaviorist* (1919) was very influential. In this book, Watson criticizes the research techniques that prevailed in the field of psychology at that time. A popular research method was introspection, which involves reflecting on, reporting, and analyzing one's own mental processes. Thus, a psychologist might attempt to examine and describe his thoughts and emotions while looking at a picture or performing some other specific task. A problem with introspection was that it required considerable practice to master this skill, and even then, two experienced psychologists might report different thoughts and emotions when performing the same task. Watson (1919) recognized this weakness, and he argued that verbal reports of private events (e.g., sensations, feelings, states of consciousness) should have no place in the field of psychology.

Watson's logic can be summarized as follows: (1) We want psychology to be a science; (2) sciences deal only with events everyone can observe; therefore, (3) psychology must deal only with observable events. According to Watson, the observable events in psychology are the *stimuli* that a person senses and the *responses* a person makes; they are certainly not the subjective reports of trained introspectionists.

Whereas Watson argued against the use of unobservable events as psychological *data,* B. F. Skinner has repeatedly criticized the use of unobservable events in psychological *theories.* Skinner (1950, 1985) asserted that it is both dangerous and unnecessary to point to some unobservable event, or intervening variable, as the cause of behavior. Consider an experiment in which a rat is kept without water for a certain number of hours and is then placed in a chamber where it can obtain water by pressing a lever. We would probably find an orderly relationship between the independent variable, the number of hours of water deprivation, and the dependent variable, the rate of lever pressing. The rule that described this relationship is represented by the arrow in Figure 1-6a.

Skinner has pointed out that many psychologists would prefer to go further, however, and postulate an **intervening variable** such as *thirst,* which is presumably controlled by the hours of deprivation and which in turn controls the rate of lever pressing (see Figure 1-6b). According to Skinner, this intervening variable is unnecessary because it does not improve our ability to predict the rat's behavior—we can do just as well simply by knowing the hours of deprivation. The addition of the intervening variable needlessly complicates our theory. Now our theory must describe two relationships: the relationship between hours of deprivation and thirst, and that between thirst and lever pressing. Scientists from all disciplines tend to agree that, if all else is equal, a simpler theory is preferable to a more complex theory. In this example, because both theories are equally predictive (i.e., both end up predicting how lever pressing changes with different amounts of water deprivation), by the criterion of simplicity, the theory without the intervening variable (Figure 1-6a) is preferable.

Skinner also argued that the use of an intervening variable such as thirst is dangerous because we can easily fool ourselves into thinking we have found the cause of a behavior when we are actually talking about a hypothetical and unobservable entity. Some other intervening variables that can find their way into a psychological theory are *anger, intelligence, stubbornness,* and *laziness.* To illustrate how an intervening variable can be treated as the cause of a behavior, suppose we ask a father why his 10-year-old son does not always do his homework. The father's answer might be, "Because he is lazy." In this case,

a) Hours of deprivation ⟶ Rate of lever pressing for water

b) Hours of deprivation ⟶ Thirst ⟶ Rate of lever pressing for water

FIGURE 1-6 (a) A schematic diagram of a simple theory of behavior with no intervening variables. (b) The same theory with an intervening variable added. In this example, the intervening variable, thirst, is unnecessary, for it only complicates the theory. (After Miller, 1959).

laziness, an unobservable entity, is offered as an explanation, and accepting this explanation could prematurely curtail any efforts to improve the problem behavior. After all, if the cause of a behavior is inside the person, how can we control it? However, Skinner proposes that the causes of many behaviors can be traced back to the external environment, and that by changing the environment, we can change the behavior. Perhaps the boy does not do his homework because he plays video games all afternoon, eats dinner with the family at a fairly late hour, and then is too tired to do his assignments. If so, a simple change in the boy's environment might improve his behavior. As just two possibilities, either the family dinner hour could be made earlier or the boy could be required to complete his homework before he is allowed to play any video games. In short, the potential for controlling a behavior may be recognized if an intervening variable such as laziness is rejected and an external cause of the behavior is sought.

N. E. Miller (1959), another psychologist with a behavioral orientation, took issue with Skinner's position that intervening variables are always undesirable. Miller suggested that intervening variables are often useful when several independent and dependent variables are involved. Starting with the example shown in Figure 1-6, he noted that the number of hours without water is only one factor that might influence a rat's rate of lever pressing for water. The rat's rate of pressing might also increase if it were fed dry food, or if it were given an injection of a saline solution. Furthermore, the rate of lever pressing is only one of many dependent variables that might be affected by hours of deprivation, dry food, or a saline injection. Two other dependent variables are the volume of water consumed and the amount of quinine (which would give the water a bitter taste) that would have to be added to make the rat stop drinking.

As shown in Figure 1-7a, Miller proposed that each of these three dependent variables would be influenced by each of the three independent variables. Once all of these variables are added, a theory without intervening variables would need to have a separate rule for describing each of the nine cause-and-effect relationships, as symbolized by the nine crossing arrows in Figure 1-7a. This fairly complicated theory could be simplified by including the intervening variable, thirst. We can assume that each of the three independent variables affects an animal's thirst, and thirst controls each of the three dependent variables. Figure 1-7b shows that once the intervening variable, thirst, is included in this way, only six cause-and-effect relationships (represented by the six arrows in the figure) have to be described. In this case, the criterion of simplicity favors the theory with the intervening variable. Miller showed that the potential advantage of including intervening variables increases as a theory is expanded to deal with more and more independent and dependent variables.

Miller's argument has not ended the debate over intervening variables. In reply to the sort of logic presented by Miller, Skinner's (1956a) position is that if so many variables affect thirst, and if thirst controls so many different behavior patterns, then whatever thirst is, it must be quite complicated, and the simpler theory depicted in Figure 1-7b does not do justice to this complexity. On the other side, those who favor the use of intervening variables also use another line of argument: They point out that intervening variables are commonplace in other, firmly established sciences. As already noted, many familiar concepts from physics (e.g., gravity) are intervening variables, since they are not directly observable. Some psychologists have therefore reasoned that progress in psychology would be needlessly restricted if the use of intervening variables were disallowed (Nicholas, 1984).

As Miller's position shows, it is not correct to say that all behaviorists avoid using intervening variables. As we will see, the theories of many psychologists of the behavioral tradition include intervening variables. The difference between theorists of the behavioral and cognitive approaches is only one of degree. As a general rule, cognitive psychologists tend to use intervening variables more freely and more prolifically than do behavioral psychologists. The theories of cognitive psychologists include a wide range of concepts that are not directly observable, such as short-term

a)

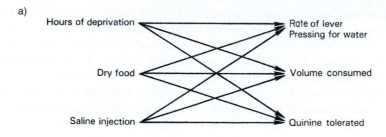

b)

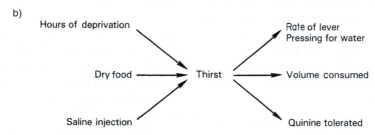

FIGURE 1-7   (a) The arrows represent the nine relationships between independent and dependent variables that must be defined by a theory without intervening variables. (b) The arrows represent the six relationships the theory must define if it includes the intervening variable of thirst. N. E. Miller argued that the second theory is superior because it is more parsimonious. (After Miller, 1959).

SOURCE: From N.E. Miller, "Liberalization of Basic S-R Concepts", in S. Koch PSYCHOLOGY A STUDY OF SCIENCE Vol 2, copyright © 1959 The McGraw-Hill Companies, Inc. Reprinted by permission.

memory, long-term memory, sensory information storage, attention, and rehearsal. Behavioral psychologists tend to use intervening variables more sparingly and more cautiously.

The debate over the use of intervening variables has gone on for decades, and we will not settle it here. My own position (though hardly original) is that the ultimate test of a psychological theory is its ability to predict behavior. If a theory can make accurate predictions about behaviors that were previously unpredictable, then the theory is useful, regardless of whether it contains any intervening variables. In this book, we will encounter many useful theories of each type.

THE PHYSIOLOGICAL APPROACH: BRAIN AND BEHAVIOR

What happens in the nervous system when the stimuli *red* and *rectangular* are repeatedly paired and the animal begins to associate the two? How does a creature's sensory systems allow it to recognize more complex stimuli, such as bricks, automobiles, or people's faces? Physiological psychologists have attempted to answer these questions and many others like them, with varying degrees of progress so far. This section provides a brief overview of some of this research. This material should give you a different way to think about sensations, ideas, and associations, and it will provide a useful foundation for topics discussed in later chapters. To understand this material, it is necessary to have some understanding of how nerve cells or neurons function. The section on The Basic Characteristics of Neurons provides a short summary; for more information, you may want to read the section on neurons that can be found in nearly every textbook on introductory psychology.

The Basic Characteristics of Neurons

Despite large differences in their overall structures, the nervous systems of all creatures are composed of specialized cells called neurons, whose major function is to transmit information. The human brain contains many billions of neurons, and there are many additional neurons throughout the rest of the body. Whereas neurons vary greatly in size and shape, the basic components of all neurons, and the functions of those components, are quite similar. Figure 1-8 shows the structure of a typical neuron.

The three major components of a neuron are the **cell body**, the **dendrites**, and the **axons**.

The cell body contains the nucleus, which regulates the basic metabolic functions of the cell, such as the intake of oxygen and the release of carbon dioxide. In the transmission of information, the dendrites and the cell body are on the receptive side; that is, they are sensitive to certain chemicals called **transmitters** that are released by other neurons. When its dendrites and cell body receive sufficient stimulation, a neuron is said to "fire"—it exhibits a sudden change in electrical potential lasting only a few milliseconds (thousandths of a second). The more stimulation a neuron receives, the more rapidly it fires: It may fire only a few dozen times a second with low stimulation but several hundred times a second with high stimulation. The axons are involved on the transmission side. Each time a neuron fires, enlarged structures at the ends of the axons, the axon terminals, release a transmitter that may stimulate the dendrites of other neurons. Thus, within a single neuron, the flow of activity typically begins with the dendrites, travels down the axons, and ends with release of transmitter by the axon terminals.

The term **synapse** refers to a small gap between the axon terminal of one neuron (called the *presynaptic neuron*) and the dendrite of another neuron (called the *postsynaptic neuron*). As Figure 1-9 shows, the presynaptic neuron releases its transmitter into the synapse. This transmitter can affect the postsynaptic neuron in one of two ways. In an *excitatory synapse,* the release of transmitter makes the postsynaptic neuron more

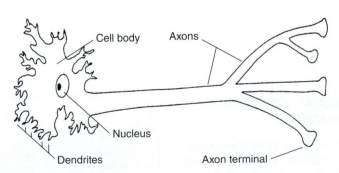

FIGURE 1-8   A schematic diagram of a neuron.

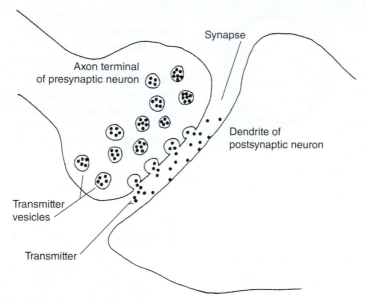

FIGURE 1-9 A schematic diagram of a synapse between two neurons. The chemical transmitter released by the axon terminal of the presynaptic neuron causes changes in the dendrite of the postsynaptic neuron that makes the neuron more likely to fire (in an excitatory synapse) or less likely to fire (in an inhibitory synapse).

likely to fire. In an *inhibitory synapse,* the release of transmitter makes the postsynaptic neuron less likely to fire. A single neuron may receive inputs, some excitatory and some inhibitory, from thousands of other neurons. At any moment, a neuron's firing rate reflects the combined influence of all its excitatory and inhibitory inputs.

Physiological Research on Simple Sensations

One theme of the Associationists that has been uniformly supported by subsequent physiological findings is the hypothesis that our sensory systems analyze the complex stimulus environment that surrounds us by breaking it down into "simple sensations." Quite a bit is now known about the traditional "five senses" (sight, hearing, touch, taste, and smell) and about several internal senses (which monitor the body's balance, muscle tensions, position of the limbs, etc.). The evidence consistently shows that each of these sensory systems begins by detecting fairly basic characteristics of incoming stimuli. A few examples will help to illustrate how this is accomplished.

The nervous system's only contact with the stimuli of the external environment comes through a variety of specialized neurons called **receptors**. Instead of dendrites that are sensitive to the transmitters of other neurons, receptors have structures that are sensitive to specific types of external stimuli. In the visual system, for example, the effective stimulus modality is, of course, light, and receptors sensitive to light are located on the retina. As shown in Figure 1-10, light entering the eye is focused by the cornea and lens, passes through a gelatinous substance called the vitreous humor, and finally reaches the retina. If we make an analogy between the eye and a camera, then the retina is the counterpart of photographic film. It is on the retina, which lines the inside surface of the eyeball, that a miniature inverted image of the visual world is focused. Some of the receptors on the retina are called cones (because of their shape), and different cones are especially sensitive to different colors in the spectrum of visible light. In the normal human eye, there are three classes of cones, which are most effectively stimulated by light in the red, green,

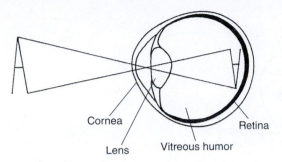

Cornea

Retina

Lens   Vitreous humor

FIGURE 1-10   How light from an object in the environment enters the eye and is focused on the retina as an inverted image.

and blue regions of the spectrum, respectively. A red-sensitive cone, for example, is most responsive to red light, but it will also exhibit a weaker response when stimulated by other colors in the red region of the spectrum, such as orange, violet, and yellow. Similarly, a green-sensitive cone is most effectively stimulated by green light, but it is also stimulated to some extent by blue and yellow light. Although we have only three types of cones, our ability to distinguish among a large number of subtle differences in color stems from the fact that different colors will produce different patterns of activity in the three types of cones. A particular shade of yellow, for example, will produce a unique pattern of activity: The red and green cones may be activated to approximately the same extent, and the blue cones will exhibit very little activity. Since no other color will produce exactly the same pattern of activity in the cones, this pattern is the visual system's method of encoding the presence of a particular shade of yellow.

We can think of the cones in the eye as neurons that decompose the complex visual world into what the Associationists called "simple sensations." Notice that no matter how intricate a visual stimulus may be, a single red-sensitive cone can communicate only two primitive pieces of information to the rest of the nervous system: its color and its location in the visual field (which determines where the light hits the retina).

All the other sensory systems have specialized receptors that are activated by simple features of their respective sensory modalities. The skin contains a variety of tactile receptors, some sensitive to pressure, some to pain, some to warmth, and some to cold. In the auditory system, single neurons are tuned to particular sound frequencies, so that one neuron might be most sensitive to a tone with a frequency of 1,000 cycles/second. Such a neuron would be less sensitive to equally intense tones of higher or lower pitches. Regarding the sense of taste, most experts believe that all gustatory sensations can be decomposed into four simple tastes: sour, salty, bitter, and sweet. Some very exacting experiments by Bekesy (1964, 1966) showed that individual taste receptors on the tongue are responsive to one and only one of these four simple tastes. In summary, the evidence from sensory physiology is unambiguous: All sensory systems begin by breaking down incoming stimuli into simple sensations.

Physiological Research on Feature Detectors

Whereas our visual systems start by detecting the basic features of a stimulus—color, brightness, position, and so on—each of us can recognize complex visual patterns, such as the face of a friend or a written word. The same is true of our other senses. We do not simply hear sounds of different pitches and intensities; we can perceive spoken sentences, automobile engines, and symphonies. When we eat, we do not just detect the four basic tastes; we perceive the complex tastes of a pepperoni pizza or a strawberry sundae. How do our nervous systems start with simple sensations and arrive at these much more complex perceptions?

In their ground-breaking research, Hubel and Wiesel (1965, 1979) found neurons in the brain that can be called **feature detectors**, because each neuron responded to a specific visual stimulus. Using an anesthetized monkey or cat, Hubel and Wiesel would isolate a single neuron somewhere in the visual system and record its electrical activity while presenting a wide range of visual stimuli (varying in color, size, shape, and location in the visual field) to the animal.

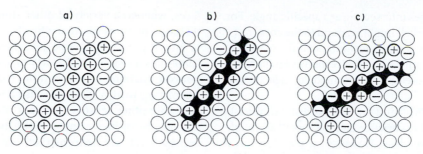

FIGURE 1-11 (a) A schematic diagram of a portion of the retina illustrating the possible connections between receptors on the retina and a simple cell in the visual cortex. The plus signs mark receptors with excitatory inputs to the cortical cell, and the minus signs mark receptors with inhibitory inputs to the cortical cell. (b) If a line of 45 degrees is projected onto this portion of the retina, the cortical cell becomes highly active because of the many excitatory inputs. (c) A line of less than 45 degrees stimulates some receptors that inhibit the cortical cell and fewer receptors that excite the cortical cell, so as a result, the cortical cell fires less rapidly.

The question Hubel and Wiesel wished to answer was simple: What type of feature detector is this neuron? That is, what type of visual stimuli would make the neuron fire most rapidly?

Hubel and Wiesel found several different types of feature detectors in the **visual cortex**, an area in the back of the head, just beneath the skull. Recall that individual cells on the retina can be activated by a simple point of light: If the point of light strikes the receptor, it will respond. In the visual cortex, however, Hubel and Wiesel found individual neurons that responded to more complex shapes. One class of cells, which they called **simple cells**, fired most rapidly when the visual stimulus was a line of a specific orientation, presented in a specific part of the visual field. For example, one simple cell might fire most rapidly in response to a line at a 45-degree angle from the horizontal, projected on a specific part of the retina. If the orientation of the line were changed to 30 or 60 degrees, the cell would fire less rapidly, and with further deviations from 45 degrees, the cell would respond less and less.

What sort of neural connections from the retina to the visual cortex might explain why a simple cell is most responsive to a line of a specific orientation? Imagine that a simple cell in the cortex receives (through a chain of intervening neurons) excitatory inputs from individual receptors that are positioned in a row on the surface of the retina, as illustrated in Figure 1-11. Furthermore, suppose that receptors on either side of this row have inhibitory connections to the simple cell (as represented by the minus signs in Figure 1-11). Because each receptor becomes active when light falls on it, and because the simple cell's activity level is increased by excitatory inputs and decreased by inhibitory inputs, you should be able to see that this simple cell will be maximally excited by a line of 45 degrees. You should also see why lines of somewhat different orientations will produce some lesser degrees of activity in the simple cell.

It should be emphasized that this discussion of the neural connections between the retina and the visual cortex is speculative, because no one has yet managed to trace the "wiring diagram" for a simple cell. Nevertheless, since all receptors on the retina are responsive to single points of light, it seems logically inescapable that some such integration of information must occur between the retina and the line-detecting cells in the visual cortex. However, a line of a specific orientation is still quite simple compared to some of the complex ideas about which James Mill wrote—bricks, mortar, walls, and windows. Unfortunately, relatively little is known about how the visual system reacts to such complex stimuli. However, Hubel and Wiesel did find some cells a bit more sophisticated than their simple cells. Some cells in the visual cortex were maximally excited by stimuli, with two edges intersecting at a specific angle. For instance, one cell might respond to the corner of a rectangle—two edges forming a 90-degree angle. Another cell might be most responsive to part of a triangle—two edges that formed an angle of, say, 45 degrees.

James Mill and the other British Empiricists believed that experience is at the root of all simple and complex ideas. However, when Hubel and Wiesel (1963) examined cells in the visual cortex of newborn kittens with no previous visual experience, they found feature detectors similar to those found in adult cats (though the neurons of kittens were more sluggish in their responsiveness to visual stimuli). This shows that individual cells in a kitten's visual cortex are prewired to respond to specific visual features (lines, angles) before the kitten has seen any visual patterns whatsoever. Yet although feature detectors are present at birth, experience plays an important role in two ways. First, visual experience keeps the feature detectors functioning well. Hubel and Wiesel (1970) found that if kittens were deprived of visual stimulation during certain critical periods of their young lives, the feature detectors of these kittens would deteriorate and become nonfunctional. Second, the response characteristics of such feature detectors can be modified depending on the type of visual stimulation a kitten receives. Blakemore and Cooper (1970) raised some kittens in an environment with large vertical stripes on the walls and other kittens in an environment with horizontal stripes. The feature detectors of kittens raised with vertical stimuli responded primarily to edges of approximately vertical orientation, and few cells responded to horizontal lines. The opposite was found for kittens raised with horizontal stimulation. These studies with young kittens show that both heredity and environment contribute to the types of visual feature detectors found in the adult animal.

Among the most complex visual detectors ever reported are cortical neurons in macaque monkeys that could be called "hand detectors" and "face detectors" (Desimone, Albright, Gross, & Bruce, 1984). For instance, the face detectors responded vigorously to human or monkey

faces, whereas a variety of other stimuli (shapes, textures, pictures of other objects) evoked little or no response. This type of evidence has led some sensory psychologists to propose the **single neuron doctrine of perception** (Barlow, 1972). According to this view, the visual system (and probably other sensory systems) is arranged in a hierarchy of increasing complexity, and at the highest levels are neurons that respond to very specific features. Are there single neurons that are activated by such complex stimuli as the face of a friend or a 2010 Porsche? Current research suggests that the human brain does not have individual neurons for every complex stimulus we can recognize. For instance, in research on human perception of faces, there is evidence from both infants and adults that large parts of the visual cortex are activated when people perceive human faces, and it is the entire pattern of brain activity that allows us to recognize a face (Nichols, Betts, & Wilson, 2010; Scott, Shannon, & Nelson, 2006). And although human face perception may be different in some ways from other types of object perception, many different areas of the brain are involved when we perceive other objects as well (Konen & Kastner, 2008). Yet even with modern brain-imaging technology and extensive research on this topic, there is much that neuroscientists still do not understand about what takes place in the brain when a person recognizes a familiar object (Peissig & Tarr, 2007).

Physiological Research on Learning

For many decades, psychologists and neuroscientists have tried to discover the physiological changes that take place during learning. A survey of this research could fill many volumes, so this section provides only a very brief summary of a few important theories and research findings. There are several possible ways in which the brain might change during learning. One possibility is that learning involves chemical changes at the level of individual synapses that alter flow of communication among neurons. A second possibility is that neurons may grow new axons and/or new dendrites as a result of a learning experience, so that new synaptic connections are formed. A third possibility is that completely new neurons are grown during a learning experience. Let us examine each of these possibilities.

CHEMICAL CHANGES. There is now plenty of evidence that some changes in the brain do not depend on the growth of new synapses, but rather on chemical changes in already existing synapses. For example, say the neurons in a slice of rat brain tissue are given a brief burst of electrical stimulation; this action can produce long-lasting increases in the strength of existing connections between neurons. The increase in the strength of excitatory synapses as a result of electrical stimulation is called **long-term potentiation**, and the effect can last for weeks or months (Bliss & Lomo, 1973). Long-term potentiation has also been observed in human brain tissue removed during the course of surgical procedures (Chen et al., 1996) and even in the intact brains of humans (Heidegger, Krakow, & Ziemann, 2010).

Long-term potentiation has been demonstrated in brain areas that are implicated in the storage of long-term memories, such as the hippocampus and the cerebral cortex. For this reason, some investigators believe that long-term potentiation may be a basic process through which the brain can change as a result of a learning experience. There is growing evidence that it may play a role in the learning of new associations (Wang & Morris, 2010; Wixted, 2004).

What type of chemical changes could cause an increase in the strength of a synaptic connection? One possibility is that as a result of a learning experience, the axon terminal of the presynaptic neuron develops the capacity to release more transmitter. Another possibility is that the cell membrane of the postsynaptic neuron becomes more sensitive to the transmitter, so that although the amount of transmitter in the synapses may be the same, the response of the postsynaptic neuron will be greater. In experiments on long-term potentiation, researchers have found evidence that both presynaptic and postsynaptic changes may be involved (Davies, Lester, Reymann, & Collingridge, 1989). It seems

that the mammalian brain has at its disposal a number of different chemical mechanisms for altering the strengths of the connections between neurons. Some examples of how simple learning experiences can produce chemical changes in individual synapses will be presented in later chapters.

GROWTH OF NEW SYNAPSES. There is now abundant evidence that learning experiences can lead to the growth of new synaptic connections between neurons. Some of the earliest evidence for the hypothesis that new synapses are developed as a result of experience came from studies in which animals were exposed to enriched living environments. Rosenzweig and colleagues (Rosenzweig, 1966; Rosenzweig, Mollgaard, Diamond, & Bennet, 1972) placed young rats in two different environments to determine how early experience influences the development of the brain. Some rats were placed in an environment rich in stimuli and in possible learning experiences. These animals lived in groups of 10 to 12, and their cages contained many objects to play with and explore—ladders, wheels, platforms, mazes, and the like. Other rats were raised in a much more impoverished environment. Each animal lived in a separate, empty cage, and it could not see or touch other rats. These rats certainly had far fewer sensory and learning experiences. After the rats spent 80 days in these environments, Rosenzweig and colleagues found that the brains of the enriched rats were significantly heavier than those of impoverished rats. Differences in weight were especially pronounced in the cerebral cortex, which is thought to play an important role in the learning process. Many recent studies have found evidence that growth in specific parts of the cerebral cortex and other brain areas can result from a variety of different learning experiences, ranging from rats learning mazes (Lerch et al., 2011) to people learning to juggle (Draganski et al., 2004). It seems clear that learning experiences can produce growth in brain tissue.

What types of changes at the cellular level accompany these differences in overall brain size? Microscopic examinations have revealed a variety of changes in the brain tissue of rats exposed to enriched environments, including more branching of dendrites (indicative of more synaptic connections between axons and dendrites) and synapses with larger surface areas (Gelfo, De Bartolo, Giovine, Petrosini, & Leggio, 2009; Rosenzweig, 1984). Other studies have found that more structured types of learning experiences can produce cellular changes in more localized areas of the brain. Spinelli, Jensen, and DiPrisco (1980) trained young kittens on a task in which they had to flex one foreleg to avoid a shock to that leg. After a few brief sessions with this procedure, each kitten's cortex was examined. The experimenters found that (1) a larger region of the cortex was responsive to stimulation of the foreleg involved in the avoidance training (compared to the cortical region responsive to the other, untrained foreleg) and (2) there was a marked increase in the number of dendritic branches in this specific area of the cortex. These and other studies provide compelling evidence that relatively brief learning experiences can produce significant increases in the number, size, and complexity of synaptic connections.

Many neuroscientists believe that the growth of new dendrites and synaptic connections underlies the formation of long-term memories (Kolb & Gibb, 2008). In humans, studies have shown that dramatic **arborization**, or the branching of dendrites, occurs in the months before birth and in the first year of life. At the same time, other connections between neurons disappear. It is not clear how much of this change is due to maturation and how much to the infant's learning experiences. It appears, however, that as a child grows and learns, numerous new synaptic connections are formed and other unneeded connections are eliminated. These neural changes continue at least until the adolescent years (Huttenlocher, 1990).

GROWTH OF NEW NEURONS. Until fairly recently, it was generally believed that except before birth and possibly during early infancy, no new neurons can grow in the brains of animals. According to this view, all learning takes the form of changes in existing neurons (through chemical changes or synaptic growth), and any neurons

that are lost due to illness or injury cannot be replaced. Today, however, there is convincing evidence that this traditional view of neural growth is incorrect, and that new neurons continue to appear in the brains of adult mammals (Leuner & Gould, 2010). For example, research with adult macaque monkeys has found new neurons developing in several areas of the cerebral cortex (Gould, Reeves, Graziano, & Gross, 1999). The growth of new neurons, called **neurogenesis**, has also been observed in other species, and in some cases this growth appears to be related to learning experiences. For instance, in one experiment, some rats learned tasks that are known to involve the hippocampus, and other rats learned tasks that do not involve the hippocampus. For the first group of rats, after the learning period, new neurons were found in a nearby area of the brain that receives inputs from the hippocampus. For the second group of rats, no new neurons were found in this area. These results suggest that new neurons can grow during a learning experience, and that exactly where they grow may depend on the specific type of learning that is involved (Gould, Beylin, Tanapat, Reeves, & Shors, 1999).

Studies of adult humans have shown that their brains, like those of other mammals, continue to produce new neurons, and several types of evidence suggest that neurogenesis may play an important part in the functioning of the adult brain. If a person's level of neurogenesis is unusually low, this may be related to various types of psychological disorders, such as clinical depression (Jacobs, 2002). After a brain injury, neurogenesis may help restore some level of brain functioning in the damaged area. Some researchers have found evidence that after such an injury, new brain cells grow through mitosis (cell division), and they appear to develop some of the same physical characteristics and neural connections as the neurons that were damaged (Kokaia & Lindvall, 2003).

WHERE ARE "COMPLEX IDEAS" STORED IN THE BRAIN? Before concluding this brief survey of the physiological approach to learning, let us take one final look at James Mill's concept of complex ideas. What happens at the physiological level when a child learns the concept *house* or when a kitten learns to recognize and respond appropriately to a snake? Although the answer to this question is not yet known, a number of different possibilities have been proposed.

One hypothesis is that every learning experience produces neural changes that are distributed diffusely over many sections of the brain. That is, the physical or chemical changes described in the preceding sections do not occur in just a few neurons in one part of the brain, but in many neurons in many different brain areas. This hypothesis was supported by some classic experiments by Karl Lashley (1950). After training rats to run through a maze, Lashley removed sections of the cerebral cortex (different sections for different rats) to see whether he could remove the memories of the maze. If he could, this would show where the memories about the maze were stored. However, Lashley's efforts to find the location of these memories were unsuccessful. When a small section of cortex was removed, this had no effect on a rat's maze performance, no matter which section was removed. When a larger section of cortex was removed, this caused a rat's performance in the maze to deteriorate, no matter which section was removed. Lashley concluded that memories are stored diffusely throughout the brain and that removing small sections of the brain will not remove the memory. Many later studies have also provided support for the view that large sections of the brain undergo change during simple learning experiences (John, 1967; Tomie, Grimes, & Pohorecky, 2008).

A very different hypothesis is that the information about individual concepts or ideas is *localized,* or stored in small, specific sections of the brain. For example, some psychologists have suggested that, in addition to innate feature detectors like those found by Hubel and Wiesel, the cerebral cortex may contain many unused or dormant neurons, perhaps with weak inputs from various feature detectors. As a result of an animal's learning experiences, one (or a small set) of these dormant neurons might come to

respond selectively to a particular complex object (Konorski, 1967; Wickelgren, 1979). To take a simple example, after an animal has had sufficient exposure to the complex object we call an *apple,* some cortical neuron might develop excitatory inputs from detectors responsive to the apple's red color, roughly spherical shape, specific odor, and other characteristics. In this way, an animal that at birth had no complex idea of an apple might develop the ability to recognize apples as a result of its experience.

The hypothesis that specific memories and ideas are stored in small sections of the brain also has evidence to support it. One type of evidence came from the pioneering research of Penfield (1959), who electrically stimulated areas of the cerebral cortex of human patients during brain surgery. When Penfield stimulated small areas of the cortex, his patients, who were anesthetized but awake, reported a variety of vivid sensations, such as hearing a specific piece of music or experiencing the sights and sounds of a circus. Although it might be tempting to conclude that the electrical stimulation had triggered a site where specific memories of the past were stored, Penfield's findings can be interpreted in many ways, and their significance is not clear.

Better evidence for localized memories comes from reports of people who suffered damage to small sections of the brain as a result of an accident or stroke. Brain injury can, of course, produce a wide range of psychological or physical problems, but in a few individuals the result was a loss of very specific information. For example, one man had difficulty naming any fruit or vegetable, whereas he had no trouble identifying any other types of objects (Hart, Berndt, & Caramazza, 1985). Another person could not name objects typically found in a room, such as furniture and walls (Yamadori & Albert, 1973). Another could no longer remember the names of well-known celebrities, but he had no problem with the names of other famous people, such as historical and literary figures (Lucchelli, Muggia, & Spinnler, 1997). There are also findings from brain-imaging studies, indicating that specific but different areas of the brain are activated when people look at pictures of animals versus pictures of tools (Chouinard & Goodale, 2010). These findings suggest that specific concepts are stored in specific areas of the brain, and that concepts belonging to a single category are stored close together.

The debate over whether the neural representation of complex ideas is localized or distributed has gone on for many years, and it has not yet been resolved. It is possible that both hypotheses are partially correct, with some types of learning producing changes in fairly specific parts of the brain, and others producing changes over large portions of the brain. Modern-day neuroscientists continue to investigate the question asked by James Mill over a century and a half ago: What are complex ideas, and how does the human brain acquire them and retain them? We still do not have a very good answer to this question, but we know much more than Mill did, and we are learning more every year. If and when neuroscientists eventually discover exactly how the brain stores information about complex concepts and ideas, this will be a milestone in the psychology of learning.

PRACTICE QUIZ (2)

1. In communication between neurons, a chemical transmitter is released by the _____ of one neuron and received by the _____ of another neuron.
2. There are three types of cones in the human retina, which respond to three different types of stimuli: _____, _____, and _____.
3. The "simple cells" in the visual cortex found by Hubel and Wiesel respond specifically to _____.
4. Three main types of changes that can occur in the brain as a result of a learning experience are _____, _____, and _____.
5. By removing different parts of the brains of rats after they learned a maze, Lashley concluded that memories are stored _____.

Answers

1. axon terminals, dendrites 2. red, green, and blue 3. lines of specific orientations 4. chemical changes, growth of new synapses, growth of new neurons 5. diffusely throughout the brain

---

Summary

The field of learning is concerned with both how people and animals learn and how their long-term behavior changes as a result of this learning. The earliest ideas about learning were developed by the Associationists, who proposed principles about how the brain forms associations between different thoughts and ideas. Aristotle proposed the principles of contiguity, similarity, and contrast. James Mill developed a theory of how two or more simple ideas can be combined to form more complex ideas. Hermann Ebbinghaus conducted some of the first studies on learning and memory, using lists of nonsense syllables as his stimuli and repeating the lists to himself until he memorized them. By letting some time pass, relearning the list, and measuring his "savings," Ebbinghaus demonstrated several basic principles of learning, including contiguity, recency, and overlearning.

Two main approaches to studying learning are the behavioral and cognitive approaches. Behavioral psychologists have often used animal subjects because they are interested in general principles of learning that are shared by many species, because animals are less complex than human subjects, and because animal environments can be controlled to a greater degree. Critics of animal research have questioned whether we can generalize from animals to people, and they have raised ethical concerns about the use of animal subjects.

Behaviorists have argued that psychology should deal only with observable events, whereas cognitive psychologists regularly use intervening variables such as hunger, memory, and attention. B. F. Skinner argued that intervening variables make scientific theories more complex than necessary. However, N. E. Miller showed that if a theory includes many independent variables and many dependent variables, then using intervening variables can actually simplify a theory.

Specialized sensory neurons in the eyes, ears, and other sense organs respond to very simple sensory properties, much as the Associationists suggested. Neurons in the eye respond to specific colors, and neurons in the ear respond to specific pitches of sound. In the brain, the inputs from many sensory neurons are often combined, so that individual neurons may respond to features such as edges, angles, and corners of a visual stimulus. How the nervous system combines all this information so that we can perceive and identify objects in our environments is still not well understood, but there is evidence that object recognition involves patterns of brain activity across large sections of the brain.

Physiologists assume that whenever an individual learns something new, there is a physical change somewhere in the brain or nervous system. Some axon terminals may begin to produce neurotransmitters in greater quantities, some dendrites may become more sensitive to existing neurotransmitters, new synapses may form between neurons, and completely new neurons may grow. Brain researchers have obtained good evidence for each of these different types of changes. Lashley's early research with rats suggested that many different sections of the brain are changed during a simple learning experience. However, research on humans with brain injuries suggests that some types of information may be stored in fairly small, specific areas of the brain.

Review Questions

1. Describe Aristotle's three principles of association and some of the additional principles proposed by Brown. Illustrate these principles by giving some examples from your own life of words or concepts that you tend to associate.

2. What procedure did Ebbinghaus use to study memory? How did his results offer evidence for the principles of frequency, recency, and contiguity?

3. What are some of the advantages and disadvantages to using animals as subjects in research on learning?

4. Why did B. F. Skinner believe that intervening variables should not be used in psychological theories? In your opinion, what is the biggest disadvantage of using intervening variables? What do you consider the biggest advantage?

5. How did Hubel and Wiesel study the properties of individual neurons in the visual cortex of animals, and what types of feature detectors they find? Do you think there are single neurons in the brain that respond to more specific and more complex stimuli, such as the face of your best friend? Why or why not?

6. Describe some research results that provide evidence that learning can result in (1) chemical changes in the brain, (2) the growth of new synaptic connections, and (3) the growth of new neurons.

2

Innate Behavior Patterns and Habituation

LEARNING OBJECTIVES

After reading this chapter, you should be able to

- describe the major concepts of control systems theory, and apply the concepts to both living and nonliving examples of goal-directed behavior

- describe four different types of innate behavior patterns, and explain how they differ

- describe some human abilities and predispositions that may be inborn

- define habituation, and list the general principles of habituation that are found in all animal species

- discuss what is known about the physiological mechanisms of habituation

- describe opponent-process theory, and diagram the typical pattern of an emotional response to a new stimulus and to a stimulus that has been repeated many times

When any animal is born, it is already endowed with a variety of complex abilities. Its immediate survival depends on the ability to breathe and to pump blood through its veins. If it is a mammal, it has the ability to regulate its temperature within narrow limits. If its survival depends on the ability to flee from predators, it may start to walk and run within minutes after birth. Newborn animals are also equipped with a range of sensory capacities. As Hubel and Wiesel (1963) have shown, kittens have inborn visual cells responsive to colors, edges, and probably other aspects of the visual world. Such innate sensory structures are by no means limited to kittens, nor to the visual system.

One major purpose of this chapter is to provide examples of the types of behavioral abilities that an animal may already possess as it enters the world. There are good reasons for examining innate behavior patterns in a book about learning. First, many learned behaviors are derivatives, extensions, or variations of innate behaviors. Second, many of the features of learned behaviors (e.g., their control by environmental stimuli, their mechanisms of temporal sequencing) have parallels in inborn behavior patterns. Another purpose of this chapter is to examine the phenomenon of habituation, which is often said to be the simplest type of learning.

Most of the examples of innate behavior patterns described in this chapter are based on the work of **ethologists**—scientists who study how animals behave in their natural environments. Although both ethologists and psychologists in the field of learning study animal behavior, their purposes and strategies are different. The testing environments of learning psychologists tend to be barren and artificial, for their goal is to discover general principles of learning that do not depend on specific types of stimuli. Ethologists usually conduct their experiments in the animal's natural habitat or in a seminaturalistic setting, because their purpose is to determine how an animal's behavior helps it to survive in its environment. Ethologists are interested in both learned and innate behaviors, and many of the behavior patterns they have studied in detail are species specific (unique to a single species).

One characteristic that is common to many behaviors, both learned and unlearned, is that they appear to be purposive, or goal directed. As we will see, this is true of some of our most primitive reflexes as well as our most complex skills. For this reason, it will be useful to begin this chapter with some concepts from **control systems theory**, a branch of science that deals with goal-directed behaviors in both living creatures and inanimate objects.

CHARACTERISTICS OF GOAL-DIRECTED SYSTEMS

Control systems theory provides a general framework for analyzing a wide range of goal-directed systems. The terminology used here is based on the work of McFarland (1971). A relatively simple example of an inanimate goal-directed system is a house's heating system. The goal of the heating system is to keep the house temperature above some minimum level, say 65°F. If the house temperature drops below 65°F, the heating system "spontaneously" springs into action, starting the furnace. Once the temperature goal is reached, the activity of the heating system ceases. Of course, we know there is nothing magical about this process. The activity of the heating system is controlled by the thermostat, which relies on the fact that metals expand when heated and contract when cooled. The cooling of the metals in the thermostat causes them to bend and close an electrical switch, thus starting the furnace. Heating of the metals opens the switch and stops the furnace.

The thermostat is an example of a fundamental concept in control systems theory, the **comparator**. As shown in Figure 2-1, a comparator receives two types of input, called the **reference input** and the **actual input**. The reference input is often not a physical entity but a conceptual one (the temperature that, when reached, will be just enough to open the switch and stop the furnace). On the other hand, the actual input measures some actual physical characteristic of

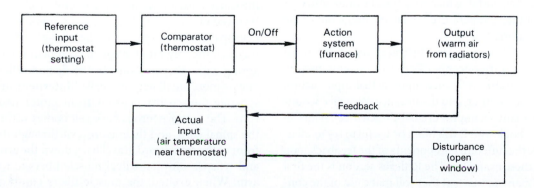

FIGURE 2-1   Concepts of control systems theory as applied to a house's heating system.

the present environment, in this case, the air temperature in the vicinity of the thermostat.

Any comparator has rules that it follows to determine, based on the current actual input and reference input, what its output will be. In the case of a thermostat, the output is an on/off command to the furnace, which is an example of an *action system*. The rules that the thermostat follows might be these: (1) If the furnace is off and the air temperature becomes one degree lower than the reference input, turn on the furnace; (2) if the furnace is on and the air temperature becomes one degree higher than the reference input, turn off the furnace. With a setting of 65°F, these rules would keep the air temperature between 64°F and 66°F.

The product of the action system is simply called the *output*—the entry of warm air from the radiators in this example. As Figure 2-1 shows, the output of the action system feeds back and affects the actual input to the comparator. For this reason, such a goal-directed system is frequently called a *feedback system* or a *closed-loop system*. The output of the action system (warm air) and the actual input to the comparator (air temperature) seem closely related, and you may wonder why two separate terms are needed to describe them. The reason is that a close relationship does not always exist between the output of the action system and the actual input; other factors can affect the actual input. One example is the *disturbance* depicted in Figure 2-1. A window open on a cold day will also affect the air temperature near the thermostat, which may then be quite different from the temperature of the air coming out of the radiators.

This example illustrates six of the most important concepts of control systems theory: comparator, reference input, actual input, action system, output, and disturbance. We will encounter many examples of goal-directed behaviors in this book, and it will often be useful to try to identify the different components of the feedback loop in these examples. The Reflexes section is the first of many in this text that will make use of the concepts of control systems theory.

REFLEXES

A **reflex** is a stereotyped pattern of movement of a part of the body that can be reliably elicited by presenting the appropriate stimulus. You are probably familiar with the patellar (knee-jerk) reflex: If a person's leg is supported so that the foot is off the ground and the lower leg can swing freely, a light tap of a hammer just below the kneecap will evoke a small kicking motion from the leg. As with all reflexes, the patellar reflex involves an innate connection between a stimulus and a response. The stimulus in this example is the tapping of the tendon below the kneecap, and the response is the kicking motion.

A normal newborn child displays a variety of reflexes. A nipple placed in the child's mouth will elicit a sucking response. If the sole of the foot is pricked with a pin, the child's knees will flex, pulling the feet away from the painful stimulus. If an adult places a finger in the child's palm, the child's fingers will close around it in a grasping reflex. Some of the newborn's reflexes disappear with age. Others, such as the constriction of the pupils and the closing of the eyes in response to a bright light, or coughing in response to a throat irritation, persist throughout life.

If you ever accidentally placed your hand on a hot stove, you probably exhibited a flexion reflex—a rapid withdrawal of the hand caused by a bending of the arm at the elbow. The response is very rapid because the association between sensory and motor neurons occurs directly in the spinal cord. Figure 2-2 depicts a cross section of the spinal cord and some of the neural machinery involved in this reflex. The hand contains sensory neurons sensitive to pain, and their lengthy axons travel all the way into the spinal cord before synapsing with other neurons. In the flexion reflex, one or more small neurons, called **interneurons**, separate the sensory neurons from motor neurons. The motor neurons have cell bodies within the spinal cord, and their axons exit through the front of the spinal cord, travel back down the arm, and synapse with individual muscle fibers in the arm. When excited, the muscle fibers contract, thereby producing the response. The physiology

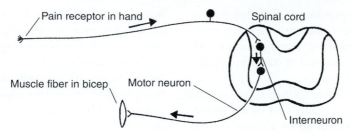

FIGURE 2-2 A cross section of the spinal cord, along with the components of the spinal withdrawal reflex.

of this reflex is sometimes called the **spinal reflex arc**, after the shape of the path of neural excitation shown in Figure 2-2. Not one but many of such sensory neurons, interneurons, and motor neurons are involved in producing the reflexive response.

This description of the chain of connections in the spinal reflex arc is consistent with the standard definition of a reflex, that is, a stimulus elicits a response. There is more to the story of the spinal reflex arc, however, so now let us see how this reflex can be viewed as a feedback system. Within the muscles of the arm are structures called *stretch receptors,* which serve as the comparators of the feedback system. We will not go into detail about how this happens, but the stretch receptors compare (1) the goal or reference input—the commands sent from the motor neurons to the muscle fibers telling them to contract, and (2) the actual amount that the muscles have contracted. Notice that just because some motor neurons have sent their commands to the muscle, this does not guarantee that the arm is safely withdrawn from the dangerous object. There might be a disturbance—an obstruction that impedes the movement of the arm. Or the muscles may be in a state of fatigue and therefore fail to respond sufficiently to the commands of the motor neurons. If the muscles have not contracted sufficiently for any such reason, the stretch receptors begin to stimulate the motor neurons (which in turn stimulate the muscle fibers more vigorously), and this stimulation continues until the contraction is completed. In short, the comparators (the stretch receptors) continue to stimulate the action system

(the motor neurons and muscle fibers) until the goal (a successful muscle contraction) is achieved. This analysis of the spinal reflex arc shows that feedback can play a crucial role in even the simplest reflexive behaviors.

TROPISMS AND ORIENTATION

Whereas a reflex is the stereotyped movement of a part of the body, a **tropism** is a movement or change in orientation of the entire animal. The first to study tropisms was Jacques Loeb (1900), who called tropisms *forced movements* to suggest that no intelligence, will, or choice was involved. Later researchers (e.g., Fraenkel & Gunn, 1940) grouped tropisms into two major categories: kineses (plural of **kinesis**) and taxes (plural of **taxis**).

Kineses

A frequently cited example of a kinesis is the humidity-seeking behavior of the wood louse. This creature, though actually a small crustacean, resembles an insect, and it spends most of its time under a rock or a log in the forest. The wood louse must remain in humid areas in order to survive; if the air is too dry, it will die of dehydration in a matter of hours. Fortunately for the wood louse, nature has provided it with a simple yet effective technique for finding and remaining in moist areas. To study the wood louse's strategy, Fraenkel and Gunn (1940) placed several wood lice in the center of a chamber in which the air was moist at one end and dry at the other. They found that the wood lice usually kept walking when they were in the dry end of the chamber, but they frequently stopped for long periods of time in the moist end. As a result, wood lice tended to congregate in the moist end of the chamber.

What distinguishes a kinesis from a taxis is that in a kinesis the *direction* of the movement is random in relation to a stimulus. The wood louse does not head directly toward a moist area or away from a dry one, because it has no means of sensing the humidity of a distant location—it can only sense the humidity of its present location. Nevertheless, its tendency to keep moving when in a dry area and stop when in a moist area is generally successful in keeping the creature alive. Kineses can also help to keep creatures away from predators. For instance, one species of slugs displays rapid movement when exposed to a chemical produced by a predatory beetle, and less movement when the chemical is not present (Armsworth, Bohan, Powers, Glen, & Symondson, 2005).

The wood louse's humidity-seeking behavior is another example of a feedback system. Although we do not know exactly how the wood louse measures humidity, its behavior tells us that it must have a comparator that can detect the actual input (current humidity) and compare it to the reference input (the goal of high humidity). The action system in this case is the creature's locomotion system, that is, the motor neurons, muscles, and legs that allow it to move about. Locomotion is, of course, the output of this action system, but there is no guarantee that locomotion will lead to the goal of high humidity. The wood louse may move about incessantly if it finds itself in a dry location, but if there are no humid areas nearby, the goal of high humidity will not be reached.

Taxes

Unlike kineses, in a taxis, the direction of movement bears some relationship to the location of the stimulus. One example of a taxis is a maggot's movement away from any bright light source. If a bright light is turned on to the maggot's right, it will promptly turn to the left and move in a fairly straight line away from the light. The maggot accomplishes this directional movement by using a light-sensitive receptor at its head end. As the maggot moves, its head repeatedly swings left and right, and this oscillating movement allows it to compare the brightness of light in various directions and to move toward the direction where the light is less intense.

The maggot's taxis is primitive, for it can only point the organism in a single direction—away from the light. A more sophisticated taxis is exhibited by the ant, which can use the sun as a navigational aid when traveling to or from its home. On a journey away from home, the ant travels in a straight path by keeping the sun at a constant angle to its direction of motion. To return home, the ant changes the angle by 180 degrees. The ant's reliance on the sun can be demonstrated by providing it with an artificial sun that the experimenter can control. If this light source is gradually moved, the ant's direction of travel will change to keep its orientation constant with respect to the light (Schneirla, 1933).

SEQUENCES OF BEHAVIOR

So far we have discussed innate behaviors that consist of either a brief movement or a continuous series of adjustments. The innate behavior patterns we will now examine are more complex, for they consist of a series of different movements performed in an orderly sequence.

Fixed Action Patterns

The ethological term **fixed action pattern** has been used to describe some behavioral sequences. Although some ethologists (Eibl-Eibesfeldt, 1975) include simple reflexes in the broader category of fixed action patterns, this category also encompasses more elaborate sequences of behavior. A fixed action pattern has the following characteristics: (1) It is a part of the repertoire of all members of a species, and it may be unique to that species; (2) suitable experiments have confirmed that the animal's ability to perform the behavior is not a result of prior learning experiences; and (3) in a sequence of behaviors, the behaviors occur in a rigid order regardless of whether they are appropriate in a particular context; that is, once a fixed action pattern is initiated, it will continue to completion without further support from environmental stimuli.

As an example of a fixed action pattern, Eibl-Eibesfeldt (1975) described the nut-burying behavior of a particular species of squirrel:

> The squirrel *Sciurus vulgaris L.* buries nuts in the ground each fall, employing a quite stereotyped sequence of movement. It picks a nut, climbs down to the ground, and searches for a place at the bottom of a tree trunk or a large boulder. At the base of such a conspicuous landmark it will scratch a hole by means of alternating movements of the forelimbs and place the nut in it. Then the nut is rammed into place with rapid thrusts of its snout, covered with dirt by sweeping motions and tamped down with the forepaws. (p. 23)

Although all members of the species exhibit this behavior pattern, this does not prove that the behavior is innate. Each squirrel may learn how to bury nuts by watching its parents early in life. To determine whether the behavior pattern is innate, Eibl-Eibesfeldt conducted a deprivation experiment in which all possible means of learning the behavior were removed. A squirrel was separated from its parents at birth and raised in isolation so that it had no opportunity to observe other squirrels burying nuts (or doing anything else, for that matter). In addition, the squirrel received only liquid food and it lived on a solid floor, so it had no experience in handling food or in digging or burying objects in the ground. The animal was kept well fed so that it had little chance of discovering that storing away food for a time of need is a good strategy. When the squirrel was full-grown, Eibl-Eibesfeldt finally gave it some nuts, one at a time. At first the squirrel ate the nuts until apparently satiated. When given additional nuts, it

did not drop them but carried them around in its mouth as it searched about the cage. It seemed to be attracted by vertical objects, such as a corner of the cage, where it might drop the nut. Obviously, it could not dig a hole in the floor, but it would scratch at the floor with its forepaws, push the nut into the corner with its snout, and make the same covering and tamping-down motions seen in the burying sequence of a wild squirrel. This careful experiment demonstrates conclusively that the squirrel's nut-burying repertoire is innate. The caged squirrel's scratching, covering, and tamping-down motions in the absence of dirt show how the components of a fixed action pattern will occur in their usual place in the sequence even when they serve no function.

As with simple reflexes, it usually takes a fairly specific stimulus, which ethologists call a **sign stimulus**, to initiate a fixed action pattern. In the case of the squirrel, the sign stimulus is clearly the nut, but without further experiments we cannot tell which features—its size, shape, color, and so on—are essential ingredients for eliciting the response. For other fixed action patterns, systematic investigation has revealed which features of a stimulus are important and which are irrelevant. In humans, Provine (1989) has found evidence that contagious yawning (the tendency to yawn when someone else yawns) is a fixed action pattern that may occur if we see the entire face of a yawning person. Seeing only the yawner's eyes or only the mouth is not enough to elicit contagious yawning.

Another example of a fixed action pattern is the territorial defense response of the male three-spined stickleback (Tinbergen, 1951). During the mating season, this fish will fiercely defend its territory against intrusion by other male sticklebacks (female sticklebacks are allowed to enter). The male's stereotyped threat behaviors are elicited by the sight of a red patch on the underside of the intruding male. If the intruding male stickleback does not have a red patch (which can only happen if the spot has been painted over by a devious experimenter), it will not be attacked. On the other hand, the defending male will attack pie-shaped or cigar-shaped pieces of wood that are placed in its territory if the objects have a red patch on the bottom. This example shows that the sign stimulus is often a simple specific detail; as a result, a seemingly poor imitation of the natural sign stimulus can elicit a fixed action pattern.

A more surprising finding is that sometimes an unrealistic model can elicit a stronger response than the actual sign stimulus itself. One example is provided by the oyster catcher, a bird that lays white eggs with brown spots. If one of its eggs rolls out of its nest, the bird will retrieve it with stereotyped head and neck movements. However, if given a choice between one of its own eggs and a replica that is four times as large, it prefers this supernormal stimulus to the normal one and strains to bring this "egg" to its nest (Figure 2-3). In a similar way, Rowland (1989) found that female sticklebacks were strongly attracted to models of male sticklebacks that were larger than any males they had ever seen.

Reaction Chains

Ethologists distinguish between fixed action patterns and what are sometimes called **reaction chains**. Whereas fixed action patterns continue until completion once started, in a reaction chain the progression from one behavior to the next depends on the presence of the appropriate external

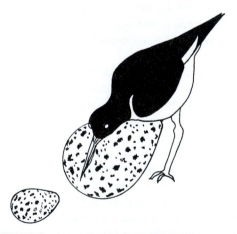

FIGURE 2-3   An oyster catcher attempts to roll a supernormal egg back to its nest. (After Tinbergen, 1951)

stimulus. If the stimulus is not present, the chain of behaviors will be interrupted. On the other hand, if a stimulus for a behavior in the middle of a chain is presented at the outset, the earlier behaviors will be omitted.

An interesting example of such a sequence of behaviors, all innate, is provided by the hermit crab. The hermit crab has no shell of its own; instead, it lives in the empty shells of gastropods (mollusks). Frequently during its life, the hermit crab grows too large for its present shell and must find a larger one. Reese (1963) identified at least eight separate fixed action patterns that usually occur in a sequence as this creature searches for and selects a new shell. A crab with no shell or with an inadequate shell exhibits a high level of locomotion. Eventually during its travels, the crab spots a shell visually, at which point it approaches the shell and touches it. The crab grasps the shell with its two front legs, then climbs on top of it. Its cheliped (claw) is used to feel the texture of the surface—a rough texture is preferred. The crab then climbs down and rotates the shell in its legs, exploring the external surface. When the aperture of the shell is located, this too is explored by inserting the cheliped as far as possible. If there is sand or other debris in the aperture, it is removed. Once the aperture is clear, the crab turns around and inserts its abdomen deeply into the shell and then withdraws it, evidently to determine whether the size of the interior is acceptable. If the shell is suitable, the crab turns the shell upright, enters it once again, and then goes on its way.

The behaviors in this sequence and the stimuli that prompt them are diagrammed in Figure 2-4, which helps to emphasize the distinguishing characteristic of reaction chains, namely, the performance of one behavior usually produces the stimulus that elicits the next behavior in the chain. For instance, the first behavior of the chain, locomotion, eventually results in visual contact with a shell, which is the stimulus for the second response, approach. The response of approach brings the crab into close proximity with the shell, which is the stimulus for the third response, lifting, and so on. Unlike the behaviors of a fixed action pattern, those of a reaction chain

Stimuli | Responses

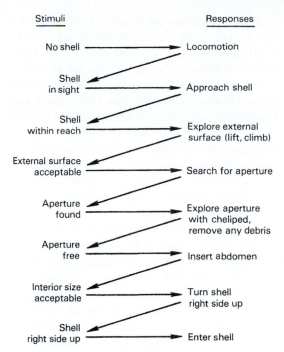

FIGURE 2-4 The hermit crab's reaction chain of shell searching and selecting behaviors. The behaviors form a chain because each successive behavior usually leads to the stimulus for the next behavior in the chain.

do not always occur in this complete sequence. The sequence can stop at any point if the stimulus required for the next step is not forthcoming. For example, Reese (1963) found that shells filled with plastic were similar enough to usable shells to elicit the first six behaviors shown in Figure 2-4. However, since the aperture was not open, the seventh behavior did not occur, and the crab would eventually walk away. On the other hand, the initial steps of the sequence may be omitted if the stimulus for a behavior in the middle of the sequence occurs. When crabs were presented with a suitable shell with the aperture directly in front of them, they would often omit the first five behaviors and proceed with the last four behaviors of the sequence. This dependence on external stimulus support makes the behaviors of a reaction chain more variable, but at the same time more adaptable, than those of a fixed action pattern.

INNATE HUMAN ABILITIES AND PREDISPOSITIONS

Although human beings have a variety of reflexes, plus a few fixed action patterns and other inborn behaviors, these innate responses certainly constitute a very small portion of what we do. As noted in Chapter 1, almost all of our daily behaviors are products of our learning experiences. Because learning plays such a large role in human behavior, some philosophers, such as the British Empiricists, have maintained that all human behavior is based on prior learning. (Recall John Locke's statement that the mind of a child at birth is a tabula rasa, or blank slate.) This viewpoint about the all-important role of experience was shared by many psychologists, including the behaviorist John B. Watson (1925), whose bold statement about the importance of upbringing is often quoted:

> Give me a dozen healthy infants, well-formed, and my own specified world to bring them up in and I'll guarantee to take any one at random and train him to become any type of specialist I might select— doctor, lawyer, artist, merchant-chief, and yes, even beggar-man and thief, regardless of his talents, penchants, tendencies, abilities, vocations, and race of his ancestors. I am going beyond the facts and I admit it, but so have advocates of the contrary, and they have been doing it for thousands of years. (p. 82)

Watson believed that the environment could play such a dominant role in determining what type of adult a child will become because he thought heredity had little or nothing to do with how people behave. In *The Blank Slate,* Steven Pinker (2002) argues that this point of view, though widely held in modern society, is incorrect, and that heredity plays a much larger role than is commonly assumed. Pinker reviews evidence from various areas of scientific research, including neurophysiology, genetics, psychology, and anthropology, to support his contention that all human beings have in common a large set of inborn abilities, tendencies, and predispositions, which collectively might be called "human nature." He argues that the human brain is not simply a batch of uniform, undifferentiated neurons that are waiting to be shaped by whatever the environment presents. He reviews evidence that neurons in different parts of the brain are specialized to perform certain functions or to respond to the environment in certain preestablished ways.

We have already seen a bit of this evidence. Chapter 1 showed that our sensory receptors are specialized neurons that respond to specific colors, tastes, sounds, smells, and so on. This sort of specialization does not end with sensory neurons. For example, it is well known that certain parts of the human brain play a critical role in our ability to use language. A section of the cerebral cortex called Wernicke's area is essential for language comprehension: If this area is damaged through accident or illness, a person cannot understand spoken language. Another area of the cerebral cortex, Broca's area, is necessary for speech production, and if this area is damaged, a person loses the ability to speak in coherent sentences. Pinker maintains that the presence of neurons specifically designed to respond to human speech is what allows young children to learn language so easily. As will be shown in Chapter 10, chimpanzees, dolphins, and a few other species can be taught to use human-like language to a certain degree, but no other species comes close to what young children can do.

A strategy used by Pinker (and by other scientists) to support the claim that a particular characteristic of human beings is innate is to demonstrate that this characteristic is found in people everywhere on earth. We cannot conduct deprivation experiments with people as Eibl-Eibesfeldt (1975) did with a squirrel, but we can demonstrate that people living in vastly different cultures and environments all exhibit a particular characteristic. There are many different languages on earth, but all human societies have verbal language, and all human languages have nouns, verbs, adjectives, and adverbs. Although different languages use different word orders, there are certain commonalities

in the way sentences are structured (Baker, 2001). Children of all cultures babble before they learn to speak, and even deaf children babble at an early age (Lenneberg, 1967), although the nature of their babbling is different from that of children with normal hearing (Oller & Eilers, 1988). These and other cross-cultural universals have been used as evidence for an innate human ability to acquire language. However, some researchers have argued that upon closer inspection, the similarities across human languages are not really as universal as they may appear (Evans & Levinson, 2009), and this issue has not been settled.

Another aspect of human behavior that may be innate is the range of emotions people experience, how emotions are reflected in their facial expressions, and how others interpret these facial expressions. Charles Darwin (1872) first proposed that different emotions may have evolved because they helped creatures survive, and that gestures and facial expressions of emotion are important means of social communication among members of a species. Since the 1970s, the psychologist Paul Ekman (1973, 2003) has conducted research showing that facial expressions can be understood by people from cultures around the world. For instance, Ekman showed people from many different cultures photographs of faces that depicted six different emotions (happiness, disgust, surprise, sadness, anger, and fear) and asked them to classify the emotion of the person in the photograph. Regardless of where they lived, people showed a high degree of accuracy in classifying the emotions shown in the photographs. Ekman and his colleagues have also suggested that there is a cross-cultural ability to recognize basic emotions through a person's vocalizations, such as screams or laughs (Sauter, Eisner, Ekman, & Scott, 2010). Some of Ekman's hypotheses remain controversial, but many psychologists now agree that there is cross-cultural uniformity in how people express emotions and interpret facial expressions. However, learning is also involved, because some types of facial expressions are culture specific. For example, in China, sticking out your tongue is a way of showing surprise, and this is not so in Western societies.

The anthropologist Donald E. Brown (1991) has compiled a list of **human universals**—abilities or behaviors that are found in all known human cultures. The list contains about 400 items, and it includes some very specific behaviors such as dance, music, death rituals, hygienic care, jokes, and folklore, as well as some major characteristics of human life, such as marriage, inheritance rules, tool making and tool use, government, sanctions for crimes, and division of labor. Learning and experience clearly affect just about every item on Brown's list: Dance, music, and folklore vary tremendously from culture to culture, so do a society's type of government, what is considered a crime and how people are punished, what types of tools people make, and how labor is divided among individuals. However, Brown's point is that every human society has *some* type of dance, *some* type of government, *some* type of division of labor, and so on. He maintains that because these characteristics of human existence are found in all cultures, even those that are completely isolated from the modern world, they most likely reflect innate human tendencies.

Deciding that a particular behavioral tendency or characteristic is innate is not an easy matter. The fact that a behavioral characteristic is found in all human cultures does not, by itself, constitute proof that the characteristic is innate. Another possibility is that the behavior is seen in people everywhere because the environment places similar constraints on people everywhere. For example, one could argue that division of labor is advantageous in all environments because it is more efficient for an individual to become an expert in one line of work than to try to master dozens of different skills. Perhaps future research on human genetics will help sort out which of these universal human characteristics are hereditary, which are the products of similar environments, and which are a combination of the two. Whatever the case may be, Brown's list of human universals is interesting to contemplate because it shows, in a world full of people with vastly different lifestyles, interests, beliefs, and personalities, how much the human species has in common.

PRACTICE QUIZ (1)

1. In control systems theory, the comparator compares the _____ and the _____, and if they do not match, the comparator signals the _____.
2. In the flexion reflex, pain receptors in the hand have synaptic connections with _____, which in turn have synapses with _____.
3. A kinesis is a _____ movement in response to a stimulus, and a taxis is a _____ movement in response to a stimulus.
4. The main difference between fixed action patterns and reaction chains is that _____.
5. Abilities or behaviors that are found in all known human cultures are called _____.

Answers

1. actual input, reference input, action system
2. interneurons, motor neurons 3. random, directional
4. the behavior sequence occurs in a rigid order in fixed action patterns, but it is more flexible in reaction chains 5. human universals

---

HABITUATION

Habituation is defined as a decrease in the strength of a response after repeated presentation of a stimulus that elicits the response. In principle, any elicited response can exhibit habituation, but in practice, habituation is most evident in the body's automatic responses to new and sudden stimuli. Here is a typical example. For his vacation, Dick has rented a cottage on a picturesque lake deep in the woods. The owner of the cottage has advised Dick that although the area is usually very quiet, members of the fish and game club just down the shore often engage in target practice for a few hours during the evening. Despite this forewarning, the first loud rifle shot elicits a startle reaction from Dick—he practically jumps out of his chair, his heart beats rapidly, and he breathes heavily for several seconds. After about half a minute, Dick has fully recovered and is just returning to his novel when he is again startled by a second gunshot. This time, the startle reaction is not as great as the first one: Dick's body does not jerk quite as dramatically, and there is not so large an increase in heart rate. With additional gunshots, Dick's startle response decreases until it has disappeared completely, that is, the noise no longer disrupts his concentration on his novel.

Another behavior that often displays habituation is the **orienting response**. If a new sight or sound is presented to a dog or other animal, the animal may stop its current activity, lift its ears and its head, and turn in the direction of the stimulus. If the stimulus is presented repeatedly but is of no consequence, the orienting response will disappear. Similarly, if an infant is played a tape recording of an adult's voice, the infant will turn its head in the direction of the sound. If, however, the same word is played over and over, the infant will soon stop turning toward the sound. Therefore, both animals and humans will typically exhibit an orienting response to a novel stimulus, and they will both exhibit habituation of the orienting response if the same stimulus is presented many times.

An important characteristic of habituation (which distinguishes it from both sensory adaptation and muscular fatigue) is that it is *stimulus specific*. Thus, after Dick's startle reaction to the sound of gunfire has habituated, he should still exhibit such a reaction if the back door slams. An infant who has stopped turning his or her head toward a speaker playing the same syllable over and over will again turn toward the speaker if a different syllable is played. In this way, psychologists can tell that even infants just a few months old can distinguish subtle differences in human speech sounds (Polka, Rvachew, & Molnar, 2008).

The function that habituation serves for the individual should be clear. In its everyday activities, a creature encounters many stimuli, some potentially beneficial, some potentially dangerous, and many neither helpful nor harmful. It is to the creature's advantage to be able to ignore the many insignificant stimuli it repeatedly encounters. Being continually startled or distracted by such stimuli would be a waste of the creature's time and energy.

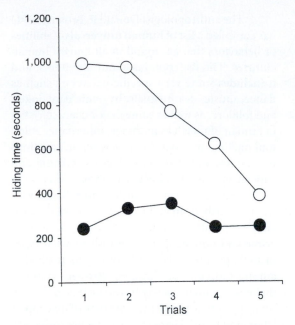

FIGURE 2-5   The amount of time rats spent hiding when exposed to a cat collar with cat odor exhibits habituation over successive days of exposure. The filled circles are from a control group of rats exposed to a cat collar that had no cat odor.

SOURCE: From Dieienberg, R.A. and McGregor, I.S., 1999, "Habituation of the hiding response to cat odor in rats," *Journal of Comparative Psychology, 113*(4), December 1999, 376–387, © American Psychological Association. Adapted with permission.

A study by Dielenberg and McGregor (1999) shows how animals can habituate to a fear-provoking stimulus if the stimulus repeatedly proves to be insignificant. Rats were presented with a cat collar that contained a cat's odor, and the response of the rats was to run into a hiding place and remain there for quite a while. However, Figure 2-5 shows that after several presentations of the cat collar, the rats' hiding times decreased and came close to those of the control group (rats that were exposed to a cat collar that had no cat odor on it).

A creature that was unable to habituate to insignificant stimuli would probably have a difficult time attending to more important stimuli. In fact, there is some evidence that the rate of habituation in human infants and children is correlated with mental abilities later in life. Laucht, Esser, and Schmidt (1994) found that infants who displayed faster habituation to repetitive stimuli at 3 months of age obtained, on average, slightly higher scores on intelligence tests when they were 4½ years old. Even before birth, the human fetus exhibits habituation to such stimuli as vibration or sounds, and one study found that a fetus's rate of habituation was related to performance on tests of cognitive functioning 6 months after birth (Gaultney & Gingras, 2005). Another study found that adolescents who showed very slow habituation to repetitive stimuli had a higher risk of developing the severe psychiatric disorder schizophrenia later in life (Hollister, Mednick, Brennan, & Cannon, 1994). These are correlational studies, not experiments, so it would be a mistake to try to draw any conclusions about cause and effect from them. Nevertheless, this research does suggest that the ability to habituate to repetitive, unimportant stimuli early in life may be one predictor of later mental abilities and mental health.

The usefulness of habituation is witnessed by its universality throughout the animal kingdom. Habituation can be seen in hydra, whose diffuse networks of neurons are among the most primitive nervous systems found on our planet (Rushford, Burnett, & Maynard, 1963). There have even been reports of habituation in protozoa (one-celled organisms). In one study, Wood (1973) found a decline in the contraction response of the protozoan *Stentor coeruleus* with repeated presentations of a tactile stimulus. At the same time, the responsiveness of *S. coeruleus* to another stimulus, a light, was undiminished.

General Principles of Habituation

Anyone who questions the feasibility of discovering general principles of learning applicable to a wide range of species should read the extensive literature on habituation. We have seen that habituation occurs in species as different as *S. coeruleus* and *Homo sapiens*. Furthermore, it is not just the existence of habituation that is shared by such diverse species. In a frequently cited article, Thompson and Spencer (1966) listed some of the most salient properties of habituation, properties that have been observed in human beings, other mammals, and invertebrates. Several of Thompson and Spencer's principles are described next.

1. *Course of Habituation.* Habituation of a response occurs whenever a stimulus is repeatedly presented. The decrements in responding from trial to trial are large at first but get progressively smaller as habituation proceeds.

2. *Effects of Time.* If after habituation the stimulus is withheld for some period of time, the response will recover. The amount of recovery depends on the amount of time that elapses. To draw a parallel to Ebbinghaus's findings, we might say that habituation is "forgotten" as time passes. Suppose that after Dick's startle response to the gunshots has habituated, there are no more gunshots for 30 minutes, but then they begin again. Dick is likely to exhibit a weak startle reaction to the first sound of gunshot after the break. (Thus, there is some savings over time, but also some forgetting.) In comparison, if there were no further shooting until the following evening, Dick's startle reaction after this longer time interval would be larger.

3. *Relearning Effects.* Whereas habituation may disappear over a long time interval, it should proceed more rapidly in a second series of stimulus presentations. In further series of stimulus presentations, habituation should occur progressively more quickly. To use Ebbinghaus's term, there are savings from the previous periods of habituation. For example, although Dick's initial startle response to the sound of gunfire on the second evening of his vacation might be almost as large as on the first evening, the response should disappear more quickly the second time.

4. *Effects of Stimulus Intensity.* We have already seen that a reflexive response is frequently stronger with a more intense stimulus. Such a response is also more resistant to habituation. Habituation proceeds more rapidly with weak stimuli, and if a stimulus is very intense, there may be no habituation at all.

5. *Effects of Overlearning.* As in Ebbinghaus's experiments, further learning can occur at

a time when there is no longer any change in observable behavior. Thompson and Spencer called this *below-zero habituation* because it occurs at a time when there is no observable response to the stimulus. Suppose that after 20 gunshots, Dick's startle response has completely disappeared. After a 24-hour interval, however, he might show little savings from the previous day's experience. If there were 100 gunshots on the first evening, Dick would probably show less of a startle response on the second evening. In other words, although the additional 80 gunshots produced no additional changes in Dick's behavior at the time, they did increase his long-term retention of the habituation.

6. *Stimulus Generalization.*   The transfer of habituation from one stimulus to new but similar stimuli is called **generalization**. For example, if on the third evening the sounds of the gunshots are somewhat different (perhaps because different types of guns are being used), Dick may have little difficulty ignoring these sounds. The amount of generalization depends on the degree of similarity between the stimuli, and it is always the subject, not the experimenter, who is the ultimate judge of similarity. For this reason, psychologists can use habituation as a tool to determine exactly which stimuli an individual finds similar. For

example, Johnson and Aslin (1995) presented 2-month-old infants with a display that featured a dark rod moving from side to side behind a white box (Figure 2-6). At first, the infants would look at this display for many seconds, but after repeated presentations, this orienting response habituated. Then, the infants were tested with two new stimuli: a solid rod moving back and forth with no box in front and a broken rod moving back and forth. Which new stimulus would the infants find more similar to the original display? Evidently, they found the solid rod more similar, because they spent less time looking at the solid rod than at the broken rod. In other words, the infants showed more generalization of habituation to the solid rod than to the broken rod. Based on this finding, Johnson and Aslin inferred that these young infants treated the original stimulus as a solid rod (not a broken rod) moving behind the box, even though the middle part of the rod could not be seen.

Many experiments have used similar procedures to examine a wide range of skills in human infants, including their ability to perceive faces (Easterbrook, Kisilevsky, Muir, & Laplante, 1999), to use perspective cues to perceive depth in two-dimensional images (Durand, Lecuyer, &

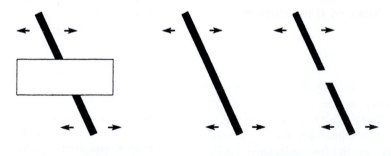

Habituation Stimulus   Test Stimuli

FIGURE 2-6   In the study of Johnson and Aslin (1995), infants were repeatedly shown the stimulus on the left until their orienting responses to the stimulus habituated. They were then tested for generalization, using each of the two stimuli on the right.

Frichtel, 2003), and to analyze cause and effect in a chain of events (Kosugi, Ishida, Murai, & Fujita, 2009). This strategy of using habituation to measure surprise or changes in attention has proven to be a valuable technique for studying the perceptual and mental abilities of infants, even those less than a month old.

Physiological Mechanisms of Habituation

RESEARCH WITH A SIMPLE CREATURE. Because the principles of habituation are common to a wide range of creatures, simple and complex, some psychologists have speculated that the physiological mechanisms of habituation may

also be similar in different species. The strategy of studying fairly primitive creatures, which have nervous systems that are smaller and less complex, is known as the **simple systems approach**. A good example is the work of Eric Kandel.

Kandel and his colleagues (Antonov, Kandel, & Hawkins, 2010; Castellucci, Pinsker, Kupfermann, & Kandel, 1970; Hawkins, Cohen, & Kandel, 2006) have spent several decades studying both the behavior and the nervous system of *Aplysia*, a large marine snail (see Figure 2-7a). They chose to study this animal because its nervous system is relatively simple—it contains only a few thousand neurons, compared to the billions in a mammal's nervous system. Kandel and his co-workers investigated the process

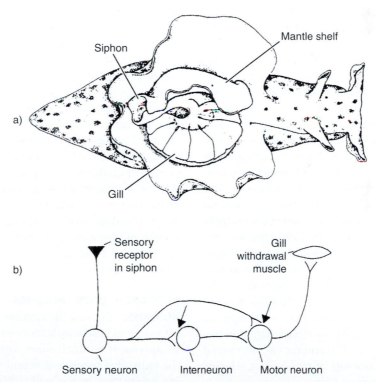

FIGURE 2-7 (a) The marine snail *Aplysia*. (b) A small portion of the neural circuitry involved in the gill-withdrawal reflex. The sensory receptors in the siphon synapse directly either with a gill motor neuron or with an interneuron. In either case, Kandel and his associates found that habituation occurs in the first synapse of the chain, as indicated by the arrows. (From Kandel, 1979).

SOURCE: Reprinted by permission of Patricia J. Wynne, www.patriciawynne.com.

of habituation in one of *Aplysia*'s reflexes, the gill-withdrawal reflex. If the creature's siphon (described as a "fleshy spout") is touched lightly, its gill contracts and is drawn inside the mantle for a few seconds. The neural mechanisms that control this reflex are well understood. The siphon contains 24 sensory neurons that respond to tactile stimulation. Six motor neurons control the gill-withdrawal response. Each of the 24 sensory neurons has a *monosynaptic* connection (i.e., a direct connection that involves just one synapse) with each of the six motor neurons. In addition, other axons from the sensory neurons are involved in *polysynaptic* connections (indirect connections mediated by one or more interneurons) with these same motor neurons. Figure 2-7b depicts a small portion of this neural circuitry.

If the siphon is stimulated about once every minute for 10 or 15 trials, the gill-withdrawal reflex habituates. Complete habituation lasts for about an hour, and partial habituation may be observed for as long as 24 hours. If such trials are given on three or four successive days, long-term habituation (lasting several weeks) can be observed. What changes at the physiological level are responsible for this habituation? Through a series of elaborate tests, Kandel's group was able to determine that during habituation, a decrease in excitatory conduction always occurred at the synapses involving the axons of the sensory neurons (the points marked by arrows in Figure 2-7b). These researchers also found that there was no change in the postsynaptic neuron's sensitivity to the transmitter. What had changed was the amount of transmitter released by the presynaptic (sensory) neurons: With repeated stimulus presentations, less transmitter was released into the synapse. Kandel (1979) noted that this mechanism of habituation is not unique to *Aplysia*. Physiological investigations of habituation in two other species (the crayfish and the cat) also found decreases in the amount of transmitter released by the sensory neurons.

Having determined exactly which neurons underwent changes during the habituation of the gill-withdrawal reflex, Kandel proceeded to ask questions at a deeper level: What chemical mechanisms are responsible for the depressed transmitter release of the sensory neurons? Each time a neuron fires, there is an influx of calcium ions into the axon terminals, and this calcium current is thought to cause the release of transmitter into the synapse. Perhaps this calcium current into the axon terminals becomes progressively weaker with repeated stimulation of the sensory neuron. Kandel's studies supported this idea: The calcium current grew weaker during habituation, and in the recovery period after habituation, both the calcium current and the response of the postsynaptic (motor) neuron increased at the same rate (Klein, Shapiro, & Kandel, 1980). The experimenters concluded that a decrease in the calcium current causes a decrease in the amount of transmitter released into the synapse, which in turn decreases the excitation of the motor neuron, producing a weakened gill-withdrawal response.

The work of Kandel and associates nicely illustrates the potential advantages of the simple systems strategy in physiological research on learning. Because of the comparative simplicity of *Aplysia*'s neural networks, researchers have been able to pinpoint the neural changes responsible for habituation and to begin examining the chemical processes involved as well. This research shows that, at least in some cases, learning depends on changes at very specific neural locations, not on widespread changes in many parts of the nervous system. Furthermore, this learning involved no anatomical changes, such as the growth of new axons, but merely changes in the effectiveness of already established connections between neurons.

RESEARCH WITH MAMMALS, INCLUDING HUMANS. Because the nervous system of a typical mammal is so much more complex than that of *Aplysia,* it is much more difficult to identify the individual neurons that undergo change during habituation to a stimulus. Nevertheless, substantial progress has been made in locating the brain locations involved in habituation, at least in certain specific cases. Michael Davis (1989) has conducted extensive research on one such specific case: a rat's startle response to a sudden loud noise. The startle response is measured by testing a rat in a chamber that sits on springs, so that the rat's movement when it is startled shakes the chamber slightly, and this movement is measured by a sensor. As with humans, the rat's startle reaction will habituate if the same loud noise is presented many times. Davis wanted to know what parts of the rat's nervous system were responsible for this habituation.

To begin, Davis had to determine which parts of the nervous system were involved in the startle reaction in the first place. Through many careful studies, Davis and colleagues were able to trace the entire circuit through the nervous system (Davis, Gendelman, Tischler, & Gendelman, 1982). The circuit began in the auditory nerve, then worked its way through auditory pathways to the brainstem, then went to motor pathways that controlled the muscles involved in the startle response. Further research indicated that the changes during habituation took place in the early portions of this circuit (i.e., in the auditory pathways). Although the exact neurons responsible for the habituation have not been identified, Davis's findings are similar to those from *Aplysia* in two respects. First, the neurons that undergo change during habituation are on the sensory side of the circuit. Second, the changes take place within the reflex circuit itself, rather than being the result of new inputs from neurons elsewhere in the nervous system.

Other studies with mammals extend but also complicate the physiological picture of habituation. In some cases of habituation, higher sections of the brain seem to be involved, including the auditory cortex, which is located on both sides of the brain, in the area of the temples. Using guinea pigs, Condon and Weinberger (1991) found that if the same tone was presented repeatedly, individual cells in the auditory cortex "habituated"; that is, they decreased their sensitivity to this tone, but not to tones of higher or lower pitch.

With modern brain-imaging techniques, such as **positron emission tomography (PET)** and **functional magnetic resonance imaging (fMRI)**, it has become possible to identify brain areas that are involved in habituation in humans. With fMRI, researchers can measure the activity of different parts of the brain in real time, as a person performs some task or is presented with some stimulus. For instance, one study using fMRI found habituation in many different parts of the brain, including the cerebral cortex and the hippocampus, when people were repeatedly shown the same pictures of human faces (Fischer et al., 2003). Other brain areas show habituation when people are presented with repeated speech sounds (Joanisse, Zevin, & McCandliss, 2007). PET scans have displayed changes in the cerebellum as a person's startle response to a loud noise habituates (Timmann et al., 1998). There is growing evidence that many different areas of the brain and nervous system display habituation (a decrease in responsiveness) when the same stimulus is repeatedly presented.

Neurophysiologists use the term **plasticity** to refer to the nervous system's ability to change as a result of experience or stimulation. All in all, the physiological studies of habituation demonstrate that plasticity is possible in many different levels of the nervous system and that this plasticity sometimes results from chemical changes in existing synapses rather than from the growth of new synapses.

Habituation in Emotional Responses: The Opponent-Process Theory

Richard Solomon and John Corbit (1974) proposed a theory of emotion that has attracted a good deal of attention. The theory is meant to apply to a wide range of emotional reactions. The type of learning they propose is quite similar to the examples of habituation we have already examined: In both types of learning, a subject's response to a stimulus changes simply as a result of repeated presentations of that stimulus. However, according to the opponent-process theory of Solomon and Corbit, with stimulus repetition, some emotional reactions weaken while others are strengthened.

THE TEMPORAL PATTERN OF AN EMOTIONAL RESPONSE. Imagine that you are a premedical student taking a course in organic chemistry. You received a C+ on the midterm, and your performance in laboratory exercises was fair. You studied hard for the final exam, but there were some parts of the exam that you could not answer. While leaving the examination room, you overheard a number of students say that it was a difficult test. A few weeks later you receive your grades for the semester, and you learn to your surprise that your grade in organic chemistry was an A–! You are instantly ecstatic and you tell the good news to everyone you see. You are too excited to do any serious work, but as you run some errands, none of the minor irritations of a typical day (long lines, impolite salespeople) bother you. By evening, however, your excitement has settled down, and you experience a state of contentment. The next morning you receive a call from the registrar's office. There has been a clerical error in reporting the grades, and it turns out

that your actual grade in organic chemistry was B–. This news provokes immediate feelings of dejection and despair. You reevaluate your plans about where you will apply to medical school, and you wonder whether you will go at all. Over the course of a few hours, however, your emotional state gradually recovers and returns to normal.

This example illustrates all of the major features of a typical emotional episode as proposed by opponent-process theory. Figure 2-8 presents a graph of your emotional states during this imaginary episode. The solid bar at the bottom marks the time during which some emotion-eliciting stimulus is present. In this example, it refers to the time when you believed your grade was an A–. The y-axis depicts the strength of an individual's emotional reactions both while the stimulus is present and afterward. (Solomon and Corbit always plot the response to the stimulus itself in the positive direction, regardless of whether we would call the emotion "pleasant" or "unpleasant.") According to the theory, the onset of such

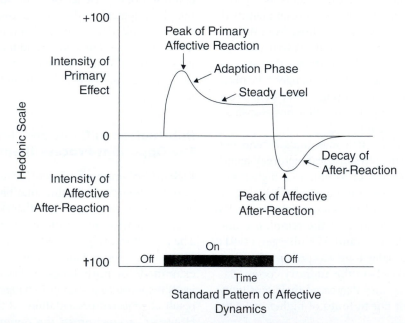

FIGURE 2-8 The typical pattern of an emotional response according to the opponent-process theory. The solid bar shows the time during which an emotion-eliciting stimulus is present.

SOURCE: Solomon, R.L., and Corbit, J.D., 1974, "An opponent-process theory of motivation: I. Temporal dynamics of affect," *Psychological Review, 81*(2), March 1974, 119–145, © American Psychological Association. Reprinted with permission.

a stimulus produces the sudden appearance of an emotional reaction, which quickly reaches a peak of intensity (the initial ecstasy in this example). This response then gradually declines to a somewhat lower level, or plateau (your contentment during the evening). With the offset of the stimulus (the telephone call), there is a sudden switch to an emotional after-reaction that is in some sense the opposite of the initial emotion (the dejection and despair). This after-reaction gradually declines, and the individual's emotional state returns to a neutral state.

To strengthen their arguments, Solomon and Corbit reviewed some experimental data from a situation where the initial emotional response was decidedly negative, but where heart rate was used as an objective measure of a subject's emotional reaction. In this experiment (Church, LoLordo, Overmier, Solomon, & Turner, 1966), dogs were restrained in harnesses and received a series of shocks. During the first few shocks, a dog's overt responses were typically those of terror—it might shriek, pull on the harness, urinate or defecate, and its hair might stand on end. At the termination of the shock, a typical dog's behavior was characterized as "stealthy, hesitant, and unfriendly" (1966, p. 121). Intuitively, we might not feel that these after-reactions are the opposite of terror, but they are certainly different from the initial reaction. After a short time, the stealthiness would disappear and the dog's disposition would return to normal—"active, alert, and socially responsive" (1966, p. 121). Heart-rate measures provided more compelling support for the pattern in Figure 2-8: During the shock, heart rate rose rapidly from a resting state of about 120 beats/minute to a maximum of about 200 beats/minute and then began to decline. At shock termination, a rebound effect occurred in which heart rate dropped to about 90 beats/minute and then returned to normal after 30 or 60 seconds.

THE A-PROCESS AND B-PROCESS. Solomon and Corbit proposed that many emotional reactions exhibit the pattern shown in Figure 2-8. They theorized that this pattern is the result of two antagonistic internal processes that they call the **a-process** and the **b-process**. The a-process is largely responsible for the initial emotional response, and the b-process is totally responsible for the after-reaction. The left half of Figure 2-9 shows how these two processes supposedly combine to produce the pattern in Figure 2-8. Solomon and Corbit describe the a-process as a fast-acting response to a stimulus that rises to a maximum and remains there as long as the stimulus is present. When the stimulus ends, the a-process decays very quickly (see the middle left graph in Figure 2-9). In the heart-rate study, the a-process would be some hypothetical internal mechanism (perhaps the flow of adrenaline) that produces, among other responses, an increase in heart rate. The antagonistic b-process is supposedly activated only in response to the activity of the a-process, and it is supposedly more sluggish both to rise and to decay. The middle left graph in Figure 2-9 also shows the more gradual increase and decrease in the b-process. In the heart-rate example, the b-process would be some internal mechanism causing a decrease in heart rate.

Note in Figure 2-9 that the b-process begins to rise while the stimulus (the shock) is still present. Solomon and Corbit propose that when both the a- and b-processes are active to some degree, the resulting emotional response can be predicted by simple subtraction. That is, the action of the a-process will be countered to some extent by the action of the b-process, and the emotional response will be weaker. According to the theory, it is the rise in the b-process that causes the drop in the initial emotional reaction from the peak to the plateau. When the stimulus ends and the a-process quickly decays, all that remains is the b-process, which produces the emotional after-reaction. You should see how the two processes in the middle left graph of Figure 2-9 combine to produce the pattern in the upper left graph.

THE EFFECTS OF REPEATED STIMULATION. Up to now the discussion has been restricted to an individual's first encounter with a new

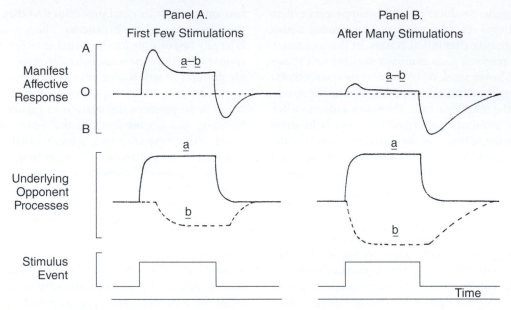

FIGURE 2-9   According to opponent-process theory, a person's emotional reaction (or "manifest affective response") is jointly determined by the underlying a- and b-processes. The proposed time course of these processes during the first few presentations of an emotion-eliciting stimulus is shown on the left. The right side shows the predicted patterns after many repetitions of the same stimulus.

SOURCE: Solomon, R.L., and Corbit, J.D., 1974, "An opponent-process theory of motivation: I. Temporal dynamics of affect," *Psychological Review, 81*(2), March 1974, 119–145, © American Psychological Association. Reprinted with permission.

stimulus. However, a crucial feature of the opponent-process theory is its predictions about how the pattern of an emotional response changes with repeated presentations of the same stimulus. To put it simply, the theory states that with repeated exposures to a stimulus, the primary emotional response exhibits a sort of habituation—it becomes progressively smaller—while at the same time there is a marked increase in the size and duration of the after-reaction. The top right graph in Figure 2-9 shows the predicted pattern of an emotional response after many stimulations. The middle right graph shows that, according to the theory, this change is the result of an increase in the size of the b-process. Solomon and Corbit propose that whereas the a-process does not change, the b-process is strengthened with use and weakened with disuse. With repeated stimulations, the b-process rises more quickly, reaches a higher maximum, and is slower to decay after the stimulus is terminated.

Solomon and Corbit supported these predictions by describing the pattern of responding after dogs received a number of shocks in the study by Church and colleagues (1966). After several sessions, there was little, if any, increase in heart rate during the shock. However, after shock termination, heart rate decreased by as much as 60 beats/minute, and it took from 2 to 5 minutes (instead of 1 minute or less) for heart rate to return to normal. The dogs' overt behaviors also exhibited changes with experience:

During shocks, the signs of terror disappeared. Instead, the dog appeared pained, annoyed, anxious, but not terrified. For example, it whined rather than shrieked, and showed no further urination, defecation, or struggling. Then, when released suddenly at the end of the session, the dog rushed about, jumped up on people, wagged its tail, in what we called at the time "a fit of joy." Finally, several minutes later, the dog was its normal self: friendly, but not racing about. (Solomon & Corbit, 1974, p. 122)

In short, with extended experience the dog's overt behaviors paralleled its heart-rate response: The reaction to the shock was smaller than before, but the after-reaction was larger and of longer duration.

OTHER EXAMPLES OF EMOTIONAL REACTIONS. Solomon and Corbit (1974) claim that opponent-process theory describes the temporal dynamics of many different types of emotional experiences, and a few more of their examples will give some indication of the generality of the theory. They discuss the emotional responses of parachutists on their initial jumps and on later jumps, as reported by S. M. Epstein (1967). Overall, the emotional experiences of parachutists resemble those of the dogs in the heart-rate study. Novice parachutists appear terrified during a jump; after the jump, they look stunned for a few minutes and then return to normal. Experienced parachutists appear only moderately anxious during a jump, but afterward they report feelings of exhilaration and euphoria that can last for hours. They claim that this feeling of euphoria is one of the main reasons they continue to jump.

A graphic example involving a pleasurable initial reaction followed by an aversive after-reaction deals with the use of opiates. After a person's first opiate injection, an intense feeling of pleasure (a "rush") is experienced. This peak of emotion declines to a less intense state of pleasure. As the effect of the drug wears off, however, the aversive after-reactions set in—nausea, insomnia, irritability, anxiety, inability to eat, and other physical problems, along with feelings of craving for the drug. The withdrawal symptoms can last for hours or a few days.

For an experienced opiate user, the pattern changes. The injection no longer brings an initial rush, but only mild feelings of pleasure, if any. This decrease in the effects of a drug with repeated use is called **tolerance**, and it is observed with many drugs besides opiates. Some theorists

have suggested that drug tolerance is a good example of habituation (Baker & Tiffany, 1985). According to the opponent-process theory, however, tolerance is the product of a strengthened b-process. The stronger b-process also explains why, with repeated opiate use, the withdrawal symptoms become more severe, and they may last for weeks or longer. At this stage, the individual does not take the opiate for pleasure but for temporary relief from the withdrawal symptoms. In terms of the opponent-process theory, each injection reinstates the a-process, which counteracts the withdrawal symptoms produced by the b-process. Unfortunately, each injection also further strengthens the b-process, so the individual is caught in a vicious cycle. Solomon and Corbit propose that their theory provides a framework for understanding not only opiate use, but all addictive behaviors (such as smoking, alcoholism, and the use of barbiturates and amphetamines). We will see in Chapter 4, however, that other researchers who study drug use disagree with the details of the opponent-process theory.

Why is it that many emotional reactions include both an a-process and an antagonistic b-process? Solomon and Corbit suggest that the b-process is the body's mechanism, albeit imperfect, of avoiding prolonged, intense emotions. Extremes of emotion, whether positive or negative, tax the body's resources, so when any a-process persists for some time, the corresponding b-process is evoked to counteract it, at least in part. If this is indeed the function of the b-process, then the examples of addictive behaviors clearly demonstrate that this mechanism is imperfect.

A BRIEF EVALUATION. Two characteristics of good scientific theories are that they make testable predictions and that these predictions are found to be consistent with experimental results. Opponent-process theory does make specific predictions about the pattern of emotional responses that have been tested in numerous experiments. In many cases, the theory's predictions have been supported (e.g., Glover, 1992; Vargas-Perez, Ting-A-Kee, Heinmiller, Sturgess, & van der Kooy, 2007), but in some cases they have not (Newton,

Kalechstein, Tervo, & Ling, 2003). Another characteristic of good theories is fruitfulness—the ability to stimulate new ideas and new research. Opponent-process theory can definitely be classified as a fruitful theory. It has been followed by a number of related theories that use the basic opponent-process idea in somewhat different ways (some of which are discussed in Chapter 4). It has been applied to a diverse range of human behaviors, including the effects of exercise (Lochbaum, 1999), leisure travel by retired persons (Staats & Pierfelice, 2003), and how people experience the sensations of pain followed by relief when the pain ends (Leknes, Brooks, Wiech, & Tracey, 2008).

Recent research on the brain mechanisms of drug addiction supports the assumptions of opponent-process theory about the weakening of the a-process (the pleasures derived from a drug dose) and the strengthening of the b-process (the withdrawal symptoms, Koob & Le Moal, 2006, 2008). One study with rats has identified a section of the brain (the *nucleus accumbens*) that appears to be involved in both the initial positive reaction to opiates and the negative after-reactions (Koob, Caine, Parsons, Markou, & Weiss, 1997). Research on brain changes in drug addiction is consistent with the idea of Solomon and Corbit that addicts are motivated to keep using drugs not so much because they continue to provide pleasure but rather because they provide temporary relief from the unpleasant withdrawal symptoms (Baker, Piper, McCarthy, Majeskie, & Fiore, 2004).

Critics of opponent-process theory have pointed out that the different examples used by Solomon and Corbit exhibit vastly different time courses. In the heart-rate studies with dogs, the b-process lasts only seconds or a few minutes. In an addiction, the b-process may continue for months. Is it likely that the same physiological mechanisms are involved in emotional events whose durations differ by a factor of 10,000 or more? The critics have argued that there may be nothing more than a superficial resemblance among the different examples Solomon and Corbit present.

In defense of opponent-process theory, we might assert that as long as emotional responses conform to the predictions of the theory, it does not matter whether these patterns are based on a single physiological mechanism or on a dozen different ones. On a strictly descriptive level, the major characteristics of emotional episodes emphasized by opponent-process theory (the peak, the plateau, the after-effect, the changes with repeated stimulation) appear to be fairly well documented by case histories, systematic observations, and experiments. Whether or not these patterns share a common physiological mechanism, the data suggest that the theory captures some characteristics of emotional responses that are quite general. Though it has been called a weakness, the theory's ambitious attempt to unite diverse emotional situations in a single framework may actually be its greatest virtue. The broad viewpoint provided by opponent-process theory allows us to see commonalities among our emotions that would probably go unnoticed in a more myopic analysis of individual emotional responses.

PRACTICE QUIZ (2)

1. The second time a stimulus undergoes habituation, the time course of habituation is ——————.
2. More intense stimuli habituate —————— than weaker stimuli.
3. Research with *Aplysia* has found that habituation involves —————— changes in the —————— neurons.
4. In opponent-process theory, with repeated stimulation, the —————— does not change, but the —————— starts earlier, becomes stronger, and lasts longer.
5. In drug addiction, the b-process appears as ——————, whereas in parachute jumping, the b-process appears as ——————.

Answers

1. more rapid 2. more slowly 3. chemical, sensory 4. a-process, b-process 5. cravings and withdrawal symptoms, euphoria

Summary

One of the simplest types of innate behaviors is the reflex, which is a simple response to a specific stimulus, such as blinking when a bright light is shined in the eye. Kineses are random movements in response to a specific stimulus, whereas taxes are directed movements (such as an ant using the sun as a compass). Fixed action patterns are sequences of behavior that always occur in a rigid order, whereas reaction chains are more flexible sequences that can be adapted to current circumstances. The concepts of control systems theory, which describe a comparison between the actual state of the world and a goal state, are helpful in analyzing these innate behavior patterns. Few innate behavior patterns have been found in humans, but there is evidence that humans may have quite a few innate abilities and predispositions, including language skills, how emotions are displayed in facial expressions, and a variety of other social behaviors.

Habituation is the decline and eventual disappearance of a reflexive response when the same stimulus is repeatedly presented. Habituation gives a creature the ability to ignore unimportant, repetitive events. In both simple and complex creatures, habituation exhibits the same set of properties, such as forgetting, overlearning, and stimulus generalization. Research with simple creatures such as the snail *Aplysia,* as well as with mammals, has traced the physiological and chemical changes that occur in the brain during habituation and specific brain structures involved in habituation in a few cases.

The opponent-process theory of Solomon and Corbit states that many emotional reactions consist of an initial response called the a-process and a later, opposing response called the b-process. Repeated presentations of the same stimulus strengthen the b-process, so that the initial reaction grows weaker and the after-reaction grows stronger and lasts longer. This theory has been applied to a wide variety of emotional reactions, including drug addiction, the emotions involved in parachute jumping, and responses to painful or aversive stimuli.

Review Questions

1. Describe an example of each of the following innate behavior patterns: reflex, kinesis, taxis, fixed action pattern, and reaction chain. Select one of these examples and show how it can be analyzed using the concepts of control systems theory.

2. What types of evidence do scientists use to support claims that human beings are born with certain abilities and predispositions? Which examples of innate human predispositions do you find most convincing, and which do you find less convincing? Explain your reasoning.

3. If you bought a clock for your room that made a loud ticking sound, you would probably soon habituate to the sound. Use this example to illustrate the general principles of habituation. Why is this simple type of learning useful?

4. How can habituation be studied in human infants?

5. Why have researchers devoted so much study to habituation in the snail *Aplysia*? What has been learned about the neural and chemical mechanisms of habituation in the gill-withdrawal reflex in this creature?

6. Draw a diagram that shows the pattern of a typical emotional response to a new stimulus, according to opponent-process theory. Now diagram the changed pattern that occurs in response to a stimulus that has been frequently repeated. Use a specific example, such as drug addiction or smoking, to explain the diagrams.

3

Basic Principles of Classical Conditioning

LEARNING OBJECTIVES

After reading this chapter, you should be able to

- describe the procedure of classical conditioning and some of the most common ways it is studied in the laboratory

- explain Pavlov's stimulus substitution theory, and describe its strengths and weaknesses

- describe the basic principles of classical conditioning, including acquisition, extinction, spontaneous recovery, conditioned inhibition, generalization, and discrimination

- explain how the timing of the stimuli in a classical conditioning procedure affects the results

- give examples of classical conditioning that are found in everyday life

- describe some of the main behavior therapies that are based on classical conditioning, and evaluate their effectiveness

PAVLOV'S DISCOVERY AND ITS IMPACT

Although he eventually became one of the most famous figures in the history of psychology, the Russian scientist Ivan Pavlov was trained as a physiologist, not as a psychologist. Pavlov studied the physiology of the digestive system, and in 1904 he was awarded the Nobel Prize in Physiology or Medicine for this work. Pavlov was interested in the various substances secreted by an animal's digestive system to break down the food eaten. One of the digestive juices Pavlov studied was saliva, which is the first secretion to make contact with any ingested food. The subjects in Pavlov's studies were dogs, and he developed a surgical technique that enabled him to redirect the saliva from one of the dog's salivary ducts through a tube and out of the mouth, so that it could be measured. Figure 3-1 pictures Pavlov's experimental apparatus, which included a harness to restrain the subject and the devices for recording each drop of saliva.

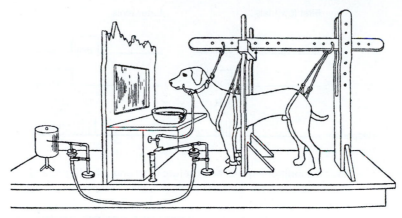

FIGURE 3-1   Pavlov's salivary conditioning situation. A tube redirects drops of saliva out of the dog's mouth so they can be recorded automatically. (From Yerkes & Morgulis, 1909)

In Pavlov's research, a single dog might receive several test sessions on successive days. In each session the animal would be given food, and its salivation would be recorded as it ate. Pavlov's important observation came when studying dogs that had been through the testing procedure several times. Unlike a new subject, an experienced dog would begin to salivate even before the food was presented. Pavlov reasoned that some stimuli that had regularly preceded the presentation of food in previous sessions, such as the sight of the experimenter, had now acquired the capacity to elicit the response of salivation. Pavlov recognized the significance of this unexpected result, and he spent the rest of his life studying this phenomenon, which is now known as **classical conditioning**. He concluded that his animals were exhibiting a simple type of learning: Salivation, which began as a reflexive response to the stimulus of food in the dog's mouth, was now elicited by a new (and initially ineffective) stimulus. Pavlov speculated that many of an animal's learned behaviors might be traced back to its innate reflexes, just as a dog's learned behavior of salivating when the experimenter appeared developed from the initial food-salivation reflex. If so, then we might be able to discover a good deal about an animal's learning mechanisms by studying the development of learned reflexes, or **conditioned reflexes**, in the laboratory. With this goal in mind, Pavlov developed a set of procedures for studying classical conditioning that are still in use today.

The Standard Paradigm of Classical Conditioning

To conduct a typical experiment in classical conditioning, an experimenter first selects some stimulus that reliably elicits a characteristic response. The stimulus of this pair is called the **unconditioned stimulus** (US), and the response is called the **unconditioned response** (UR). The term *unconditioned* is used to signify that the connection between the stimulus and response is unlearned (innate). In Pavlov's experiments on the salivary response, the US was the presence of food in the dog's mouth, and the UR was the secretion of saliva. The third element of the classical-conditioning paradigm is the **conditioned stimulus** (CS), which can be any stimulus that does not initially evoke the UR (e.g., a bell). The term *conditioned stimulus* indicates that it is only after conditioning has taken place that the bell will elicit the response of salivation.

Figure 3-2 is a diagram of the sequence of events of a single trial of classical conditioning. In its simplest form, a classical-conditioning trial involves the presentation of the CS (e.g., a bell) followed by the US (e.g., the food). On the initial trials, only the US will elicit the response of

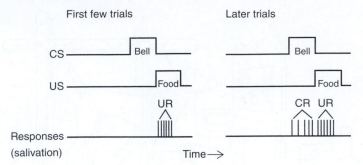

FIGURE 3-2   Events of a classical-conditioning trial both before (left) and after (right) a CR is established.

salivation. However, as the conditioning trials continue, the dog will begin to salivate as soon as the CS is presented. Any salivation that occurs during the CS but before the US is referred to as a **conditioned response** (CR), since it is only because of the conditioning procedure that the bell now elicits salivation.

The abbreviations for the four basic elements of the classical-conditioning paradigm will appear repeatedly in this and later chapters, so be sure that you have no confusion about what each term represents. The two components of the initial stimulus–response pair are the US and the UR. Through the procedures of classical conditioning, a new stimulus, the CS, begins to elicit responses of its own, and these responses to the CS are called CRs (since they are learned, or conditioned, responses).

The Variety of Conditioned Responses

Classical conditioning has been observed in many reflexes, including the knee-jerk reflex and the eyeblink. It is also possible to classically condition various organs such as the heart, the stomach, the liver, and the kidneys. Although classical conditioning can be obtained with many different responses, much of the research on this type of learning has been conducted with a small number of conditioning *preparations* (i.e., conditioning situations using a particular US, UR, and species of subject) that can be studied easily and efficiently. The following conditioning preparations are among the most commonly used.

EYEBLINK CONDITIONING.   Conditioning of the eyeblink reflex has been studied with humans, rabbits, rats, and other animals. Figure 3-3 shows a modern apparatus for eyeblink conditioning with humans. The US is a puff of air directed at the eye, and the UR is of course an eyeblink. Eyeblinks are recorded by a photocell that measures movement

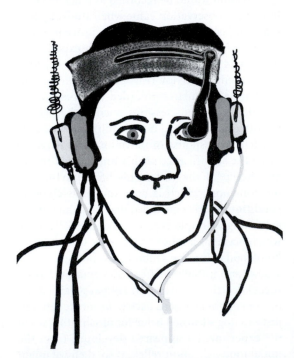

FIGURE 3-3   An eyeblink conditioning arrangement. The participant wears a headset that has a tube to direct a puff of air to the eye, a photocell to measure movement of the eyelid, and earphones for the presentation of auditory stimuli.

of the eyelid. In eyelid-conditioning research with rabbits, the US can be an air puff or a mild electric shock delivered to the skin in the vicinity of the eye, which also reliably elicits an eyeblink as a UR. The CS may be a light, a tone, or some tactile stimulus such as a vibration of the experimental chamber, and the duration of the CS is typically about 1 second. Like the UR, the CR is an eyeblink, but its form may be different. Whereas the unconditioned eyeblink is a large and rapid eyelid closure, the CR is often a smaller and more gradual eyelid movement. Eyeblink conditioning often requires a large number of CS–US pairings. For example, it may take well over 100 pairings before a CR is observed on 50% of the trials.

Research in eyeblink conditioning has helped scientists to map the brain areas and chemical mechanisms involved in conditioning, to diagnose psychological disorders, to study the effects of aging, and in other ways (Steinmetz, 1999; Woodruff-Pak & Disterhoft, 2008). For instance, one study with young rats found that exposure to alcohol led to long-term impairments in the ability to learn a conditioned eyeblink response (Brown, Calizo, & Stanton, 2008). This type of research provides insights into the damaging effects of alcohol on specific parts of the brain.

CONDITIONED SUPPRESSION. In the conditioned suppression procedure, which is also called the **conditioned emotional response** (CER) procedure, the subjects are usually rats, and the US is an aversive event such as a brief electric shock delivered through the metal bars that form the floor of the experimental chamber. The UR to shock may include several different behaviors; for example, the animal may jump or flinch and temporarily stop what it was doing before the shock occurred. The measure of conditioning in this situation is the suppression of ongoing behavior when the CS (which signals that a shock is forthcoming) is presented. The rat is given a separate task in which it can earn occasional food pellets by pressing a lever, so that its "ongoing behavior" can be measured. It is fairly easy to schedule the delivery of food pellets in such a way that the animal will press the lever slowly but steadily for an hour or more, now and then earning a bit of food.

As in eyeblink conditioning, the CS may be visual, auditory, or tactile, but the duration of the CS is generally much longer in the conditioned suppression procedure—CSs of 1 minute or more are typical. When the CS is first presented, it may have little effect on the rat's lever-pressing behavior. However, after a few pairings of the CS and shock (in which the shock arrives at the end of the 1-minute CS and lasts for perhaps 1 second), the rat's rate of lever pressing suddenly decreases as soon as the CS is presented, and it may make only a few lever presses during the minute that the CS is present. The amount of suppression of lever pressing is used as a measure of the strength of conditioning. For example, if a rat was pressing the lever at a rate of 40 responses per minute before the CS and this rate dropped to 10 responses per minute in the presence of the CS, this would constitute a suppression of 75%.

Conditioning takes place in far fewer trials in the conditioned suppression procedure than in the eyeblink procedure, perhaps partly because the shock is more intense than the air puffs or mild shocks used in eyeblink conditioning. Whatever the reasons, strong conditioned suppression can often be observed in fewer than 10 trials, and in some cases significant suppression to the CS is found after just one CS–US pairing.

THE SKIN CONDUCTANCE RESPONSE. The conditioning preparation called **skin conductance response** (SCR) is also referred to as the *electrodermal response,* and in the past it was known as the *galvanic skin response.* In this preparation, the subjects are usually human. The SCR is a change in the electrical conductivity of the skin. To measure a person's SCR, two coin-shaped electrodes are attached to the palm, and the electrodes are connected to a device that measures momentary fluctuations in the conductivity of the skin (caused by small changes in perspiration). The conductivity of the skin is altered by emotions such as fear or surprise, which is why the SCR is often one measure used in lie detector tests. One stimulus that reliably produces a large increase in skin conductivity is electric shock, and a similar increase in conductivity can be conditioned to any CS that is paired with shock. For instance, the CS might be a tone, the US a shock to the left wrist, and the response an increase in conductivity of the right palm. One reason for the interest in the SCR is that since it provides a response that can be quickly and reliably conditioned with human subjects, many complex stimuli (such as spoken or written words) can be examined as CSs.

TASTE-AVERSION LEARNING.   Beginning in the 1960s, the conditioning procedure called taste-aversion learning has been extensively investigated (Reilly & Schachtman, 2009). Rats are frequently the subjects in this research, but other species (pigeons, quail, guinea pigs) have also been used. The CS in this procedure is the taste of something the subject eats or drinks. In many cases, the food is one that the subject has never tasted before. After eating or drinking, the animal is given an injection of a poison (the US) that makes it ill. Several days later, after the animal has fully recovered from its illness, it is again given the opportunity to consume the substance that served as the CS. The usual result is that the animal consumes little or none of this food. Thus, the measure of conditioning is the degree to which the animal avoids the food.

There are a number of reasons why taste-aversion learning has received so much attention in recent years. First, as you will see in Chapter 4, some psychologists have suggested that taste-aversion learning is not an ordinary example of classical conditioning, but that it violates some of the general principles that apply to most examples of classical conditioning. Second, a taste aversion often develops after just one conditioning trial, and this rapidity of conditioning is advantageous for certain theoretical questions. Third, a taste aversion is something that many people experience at least once in their lives. Perhaps there is some type of food that you refuse to eat because you once became ill after eating it. You may find the very thought of eating this food a bit nauseating, even though most people enjoy the food. If you have such a taste aversion, you are not unusual—one study found that more than half of the college students surveyed had at least one taste aversion (Logue, Ophir, & Strauss, 1981). A taste aversion may develop even if the individual is certain that the food was not the cause of the subsequent illness. I once attended a large dinner party where the main course was chicken tarragon. Besides passing food around the table, we evidently passed around an intestinal virus, because many of the guests became quite ill that evening. For some, the illness lasted for over a week. The result of this accidental pairing of food and illness was that several years later some of these guests still refused to eat chicken tarragon or any food with tarragon spicing. Taste aversion can be strong and long lasting!

Pavlov's Stimulus Substitution Theory

THE THEORY.   Pavlov was the first to propose the theory of classical conditioning that is now called the **stimulus substitution theory**. On a behavioral level, the theory simply predicts the changes that supposedly take place among the observable events of conditioning—the stimuli and responses. The theory states that through repeated pairings between CS and US, the CS becomes a substitute for the US, so that the response initially elicited only by the US is now also elicited by the CS. At first glance, this theory seems to provide a perfectly satisfactory description of what takes place in many common examples of classical conditioning. In salivary conditioning, initially only food elicits salivation, but later the CS also elicits salivation. In eyeblink conditioning, both the UR and the CR are eyelid closures. In SCR conditioning, an increase in skin conductance is first elicited by a shock, and after conditioning, a similar increase in skin conductance occurs in response to some initially neutral stimulus.

PROBLEMS WITH THE THEORY.   Despite these apparent confirmations of the stimulus substitution theory, today very few conditioning researchers believe the theory to be correct. The theory has several problems. First, the CR is almost never an exact replica of the UR. For instance, it was already noted that whereas an eyeblink UR to an air puff is a large, rapid eyelid closure, the CR that develops is a smaller and more gradual eyelid closure. That is, both the size and the temporal pattern of the CR differ from those of the UR. Second, not all parts of the UR to a stimulus become part of the CR. For example, Zener (1937) noted that when a dog is presented with food as a US, many responses, such as chewing and swallowing the food, occur in addition to salivation. Yet, although a well-trained CS such as a bell will elicit salivation, it will generally not elicit the chewing and swallowing responses. Therefore, not all of the components of the UR are present in the CR. Conversely, a CR may include some responses that are *not* part of the UR. For instance, using a bell as a CS, Zener found that many dogs would turn their heads and look at the bell when it was rung. Sometimes a dog would move its entire body closer to the ringing bell. Obviously, these behaviors were not a normal part of the dog's UR to food. Because of such results, it was clear that stimulus substitution theory had to be modified if it were to remain a viable theory of classical conditioning.

Hilgard (1936) suggested two ways in which the theory might be amended. First, it should be acknowledged that only some components of the UR are transferred to the CR. Some components of the UR may depend on the physical characteristics of the US, and they will not be transferred to a CS with very different physical characteristics. Thus, although a dog will chew and swallow food when it is presented, it cannot chew and swallow food that is not there (when the bell is rung). Second, it should be recognized that a CS such as a bell frequently elicits URs of its own, and these may become part of the CR. For instance, when it first hears a bell, a dog may exhibit an orienting response: The dog may raise its ears, look in the direction of the bell, and possibly approach the bell. Although such orienting responses usually habituate if the bell is inconsequential, they persist or increase if the bell is paired with food. A different theory of classical conditioning, called the **sign-tracking theory** (Costa & Boakes, 2009; Hearst & Jenkins, 1974), emphasizes precisely this aspect of an animal's response to a CS. It states that animals tend to orient themselves toward, approach, and explore any stimuli that are good predictors of important events, such as the delivery of food. It is not surprising that some components of the orienting response to the CS are retained as part of the CR. In short, the form of the CR may reflect both the UR to the US and the UR to the CS itself.

Possibly the strongest argument against stimulus substitution theory arises from the finding that in some cases the direction of the CR is opposite to that of the UR. For instance, one response to an electric shock is an increase in heart rate, but in studies with guinea pigs, Black (1965) observed conditioned heart rate decreases to a CS paired with shock. Another example involves studies in which animals (usually rats) are given a morphine injection as the US. One of the URs to morphine is hyperthermia, or an increase in body temperature. In experiments where some CS is repeatedly paired with morphine, two types of CRs have been observed. Sometimes the CR is an increase in body temperature, as predicted by stimulus substitution theory, but in other cases the CR is a decrease in body temperature. Conditioned responses that are the opposite of the UR have been called **conditioned compensatory responses** (Siegel, 1982).

In summary, one of the most widely held beliefs about classical conditioning—that it involves the simple transfer of a response from one stimulus to another—is not consistent with the following facts:

1. The sizes and temporal patterns of the CR and UR may differ.
2. Not all components of the UR become part of the CR.
3. The CR may include response components that are not part of the UR.
4. The CR is sometimes opposite in direction to the UR (or at least to the most obvious part of the UR).

For these reasons, it is often difficult to predict in advance what the CR will look like in a specific instance. It may resemble the UR, or it may be very different.

WHAT IS LEARNED IN CLASSICAL CONDITIONING? Having surveyed the arguments for and against stimulus substitution theory, let us now turn to Pavlov's speculations about what changes might take place in the brain during classical conditioning. He proposed that there is a specific part of the brain that becomes active whenever a US (such as food) is presented, and we can call this part of the brain the *US center.* Similarly, for every different CS (a tone, a light), there is a separate *CS center,* which becomes active whenever that particular CS is presented. From what we know about the physiology of the sensory systems (Chapter 1), these assumptions seem quite reasonable, especially since the exact nature of CS centers and US centers is not important to Pavlov's theory. Pavlov also assumed that for every UR (say, salivation) there is part of the brain that can be called a *response center,* and it is the activation of this response center that initiates the neural commands that ultimately produce the observed response. Furthermore, since the US elicits the UR without any prior training, Pavlov assumed that there is an innate connection between the US center and the response center (see Figure 3-4). Finally, Pavlov proposed that somehow an association develops during the course of classical conditioning, so that now the CS produces activity in the response center (and a CR is observed).

As Figure 3-4 suggests, there are at least two types of new associations that would give the CS the capacity to elicit a CR. On one hand, a direct association between the CS center and the response center might develop during conditioning. Since this association is between a stimulus and a response, it is sometimes called an **S-R association**. On the other hand, the connection between the CS and response centers might be less direct. Perhaps an association between the CS center and the US center is formed during conditioning. Later, when the CS is presented, the CS center is activated, which activates the US center (through the newly formed association), which in turn activates the response center (through the innate association). This hypothesis constitutes the position that an **S-S association** is formed during classical conditioning. Pavlov tended to favor the S-S position, but he had little empirical support for this view. Later, however, experimenters devised some clever techniques to try to distinguish between these two alternatives. The S-S or S-R Connections? section describes one such procedure.

S-S or S-R Connections?

If we do not know what neural changes take place during classical conditioning, how can we possibly distinguish between the S-S and S-R positions? Rescorla (1973) used the following reasoning: If the S-S position is correct, then after conditioning, the occurrence of a CR depends on the continued strength of two associations: the learned association between the CS center and the

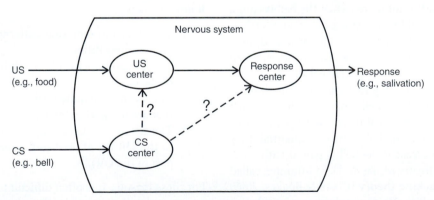

FIGURE 3-4 Two possible versions of Pavlov's stimulus substitution theory. During classical conditioning, an association might develop from the CS center to the US center, or from the CS center directly to the response center.

US center, and the innate association between the US center and the response center (see Figure 3-4). If the US-response connection is somehow weakened, this should cause a reduction in the strength of the CR, since the occurrence of the CR depends on this connection. However, if the S-R position is correct, the strength of the CR does not depend on the continued integrity of the US-response association, but only on the direct association between the CS center and the response center. But how can a reflexive US-response association be weakened? Rescorla's solution was to rely on habituation.

Rescorla used a conditioned suppression procedure with rats, with a loud noise as the US. Rescorla's previous work had indicated that a conditioned suppression of lever pressing would develop to any CS paired with the noise, but also that the noise was susceptible to habituation if it was repeatedly presented. The design of the experiment is shown in Figure 3-5. In Phase 1, two groups of rats received identical classical conditioning with a light as the CS and the noise as the US. In Phase 2, the habituation group received many presentations of the noise by itself, in order to habituate the rats' fear of the noise. The technique of decreasing the effectiveness of the US after an excitatory CS has been created is called *US devaluation*. The control rats spent equal amounts of time in the experimental chamber in Phase 2, but no stimuli were presented, so there was no opportunity for the noise to habituate in this group. In the test phase of the experiment, both groups were presented with the light by itself for a number of trials, and their levels of suppression of lever pressing were recorded. Rescorla found high levels of suppression to the light in the control group, but significantly lower levels of

suppression in the habituation group. He concluded that the strength of the CR depends on the continued strength of the US-response association, as predicted by the S-S position but not the S-R position.

Similar studies on *US revaluation* have been conducted with human subjects, and the results have been similar. For example, in experiments using the SCR, a CS (e.g., a picture of some common object) is paired with an aversive US (either shock or loud noise); then the intensity of the US is changed. If the US intensity is decreased, SCRs to the CS decrease as well (Davey & McKenna, 1983). Conversely, if the intensity of US is increased, SCRs to the CS also increase (White & Davey, 1989). This pattern of results supports the S-S position, because it shows that the response to the CS changes depending on the current size of the response to the US. Other research on the associations formed during classical conditioning will be described in Chapter 4. For now, it is important to understand how questions about the workings of the nervous system can be addressed in a meaningful way without actually tracing any specific neural connections.

BASIC CONDITIONING PHENOMENA

Acquisition

In most classical conditioning experiments, several pairings of the CS and the US are necessary before the CR becomes fully developed. The part of a conditioning experiment in which the subject first experiences a series of CS–US pairings, and during which the CR gradually appears and increases in strength, is called the **acquisition phase**. Figure 3-6 shows the results

Group	Phase 1	Phase 2	Test
Habituation	Light→Noise	Noise (habituation)	Light
Control	Light→Noise	No stimuli	Light

FIGURE 3-5 Design of Rescorla's (1973) experiment on S-S versus S-R connections.

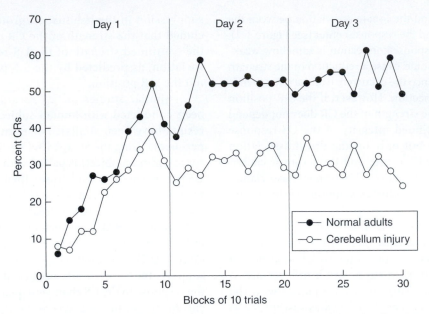

FIGURE 3-6 The acquisition of eyeblink CRs by normal adults and by those who had suffered strokes that caused damage to the cerebellum.

SOURCE: Reprinted from *Behavioural Brain Research, 212*(2), Gerwig, M. et. al. "Evaluation of multiple-session delay eyeblink conditioning comparing patients with focal cerebellar lesions and cerebellar degeneration," pages 143–151, copyright © 2010, with permission from Elsevier.

of an acquisition phase in an experiment on eyeblink conditioning with human participants (Gerwig et al., 2010). The measure of conditioning is the percentage of trials on which a conditioned eyeblink response was recorded. The participants received three sessions of 100 trials per day, in which a brief tone was followed by an air puff directed at the eye. For the normal adults, the percentage of trials with a CR gradually increased until it leveled off at about 55%. This value—the maximum level of conditioned responding that is gradually approached as conditioning proceeds—is called the *asymptote*. Figure 3-6 also shows the results from a group of adults who had suffered strokes that caused damage to the cerebellum, a part of the brain that plays an important role in eyeblink conditioning. These participants showed weaker levels of conditioned responding, which reached an asymptote of about 30%.

One factor that has a major influence on the asymptote of conditioning is the size or intensity of the US. In general, if a stronger stimulus is used

as a US (a stronger puff of air, a larger amount of food), the asymptote of conditioning will be higher (a higher percentage of conditioned eyeblinks, more salivation). Strong USs also usually result in faster conditioning; that is, it may take fewer trials for a CR to appear with a strong US than with a weak one. The same is true about the intensity of the CS. Imagine one conditioning experiment in which a faint tone was used as a CS, and another with a very loud tone as a CS. It should come as no surprise that conditioning will occur more rapidly with the loud tone.

Extinction

The mere passage of time has relatively little effect on the strength of a CR. Suppose we conducted an experiment in salivary conditioning, repeatedly pairing a bell and food until our subject reliably salivated as soon as the bell was rung. We could then remove the animal from the experimental chamber and allow a week, a month, or even a year to pass before returning the subject to the chamber. At this later time, upon ringing the bell, we would most likely still observe a CR of salivation (though probably not as much salivation as on the last trial of the initial training session). The point is that the simple passage of time will not cause an animal to "forget" to produce the CR once the CS is presented again.

This does not mean, however, that a CR, once acquired, is permanent. A simple technique for producing a reduction and eventual disappearance of the CR is the procedure of **extinction**, which involves repeatedly presenting the CS *without* the US. Suppose we followed the acquisition phase with an extinction phase in which the bell was presented for many trials but no food was delivered. The first two panels in Figure 3-7 show, in an idealized form, the likely results of our hypothetical experiment. As the bell is presented trial after trial without food, the amount of salivation gradually decreases, and eventually it disappears altogether.

When the extinction phase is completed, we have a dog that behaves like a dog that is just beginning the experiment—the bell is presented and no salivation occurs. We might conclude that the procedure of extinction simply reverses the effects of the previous acquisition phase. That is, if the animal has formed an association between the CS and the US during the acquisition phase, perhaps this association is gradually destroyed during the extinction phase. The simplicity of this hypothesis is appealing, but it is almost certainly wrong. At least three different phenomena show that whatever association was formed during acquisition is not erased during extinction. These phenomena are spontaneous recovery, disinhibition, and rapid reacquisition.

Spontaneous Recovery, Disinhibition, and Rapid Reacquisition

Suppose that after an acquisition phase on Day 1 and an extinction phase on Day 2, we return our subject to the experimental chamber on Day 3 and conduct another series of extinction trials with the bell. Figure 3-7 shows that on the first several trials of Day 3, we are likely to see some conditioned responding to the bell, even though no CRs were observed at the end of Day 2. Pavlov called this reappearance of conditioned responding **spontaneous recovery**, and he treated it as proof that the CS–US association is not permanently destroyed in an extinction procedure. Pavlov's conclusion was obviously correct: If extinction serves to undo or erase the learning that occurred in acquisition, why would CRs spontaneously reappear without further conditioning trials? Whatever happens during extinction, it is not a simple erasure of the previous learning. Furthermore, if more time elapses between the first and second extinction sessions, more spontaneous recovery is observed (Brooks & Bouton, 1993).

Several different theories about spontaneous recovery have been proposed. One popular theory, which we can call the *inhibition theory,* states that after extinction is complete, the subject is left with two counteracting associations (Konorski, 1948). The CS–US association formed during acquisition is called an *excitatory association* because through this association the CS now

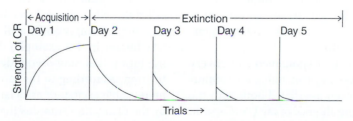

FIGURE 3-7 Idealized changes in the strength of a CR across one acquisition day followed by 4 days of extinction.

excites, or activates, the US center. According to this theory, a parallel but *inhibitory associa-tion* develops during extinction. When extinc-tion is complete, the effects of the excitatory and inhibitory associations cancel out, so that the US center is no longer activated by the presentation of the CS. Referring to Figure 3-7, at the end of Day 2, the inhibitory CS–US association is strong enough to counteract completely the excitatory association, so no CRs are observed. However, Pavlov proposed that inhibitory associations (at least newly formed ones) are more fragile than excitatory associations, and they are more severely weakened by the passage of time. Therefore, at the beginning of Day 3, the weak-ened inhibitory association can no longer fully counteract the excitatory association, and so some CRs are observed. Further extinction trials on Day 3 strengthen the inhibitory association, and so conditioned responding once again disappears.

If we were to conduct further extinction sessions on Days 4, 5, 6, and so on, we might again observe some spontaneous recovery, but typi-cally the amount of spontaneous recovery would become smaller and smaller until it no longer occurred (see Figure 3-7). According to the inhi-bition theory, this happens because the inhibitory association becomes progressively stronger with repeated extinction sessions.

The inhibition theory is just one of several theories about why spontaneous recovery occurs. Some experiments by Robbins (1990) supported a theory that, during extinction, the subject stops "processing" or "paying attention to" the CS. Conditioned responses then disappear, because when the animal stops paying attention to the CS, it stops responding to the CS. Later, when the ani-mal is brought back to the conditioning chamber after some time has passed, the animal's attention to the CS is revived for a while, leading to a spon-taneous recovery of CRs.

Another theory of spontaneous recovery states that the CS becomes an ambiguous stimu-lus because it has been associated both with the US and then with the absence of the US (Capaldi, 1966). Referring again to Figure 3-7, after Day 2, the dog has experienced one session in which

the bell was followed by food and one session in which it was not. At the start of Day 3, the dog cannot know whether this session will be like that of Day 1 or like that of Day 2, and its behavior (some weak CRs at the start of the session) may be a reflection of this uncertainty. As Bouton (2000) has put it, the CS "is ambiguous, and like an ambiguous word, its current meaning—or the behavior it currently evokes—is determined by the context. . . . Instability, lapse, and relapse are to be expected from a modern understand-ing of behavioral change" (pp. 57–58). Consistent with this theory, rats in one experiment dis-played less spontaneous recovery of a taste aver-sion when a specific stimulus (a buzzer) was presented throughout every extinction session. The rats may have learned that the CS presented in a quiet environment was followed by the US, but the CS presented with the buzzer was not (Brooks, Palmatier, Garcia, & Johnson, 1999). In other words, the presence of the buzzer may have helped to reduce the ambiguity of the CS.

If these different theories of spontaneous recovery seem confusing to you, it may be reas-suring to know that there is confusion and dis-agreement among the experts about this topic. Surprisingly, psychologists still do not fully un-derstand the causes of extinction and spontane-ous recovery, two of the most basic phenomena of classical conditioning.

More evidence that extinction is not the complete erasure of previous learning comes from the phenomenon of **disinhibition**. Suppose that an extinction phase has progressed to the point where the CS (a bell) no longer evokes any saliva-tion. Now, if a novel stimulus such as a buzzer is presented a few seconds before the bell, the bell may once again elicit a CR of salivation. Pavlov called this effect *disinhibition* because he believed that the presentation of a distracting stimulus (the buzzer in this example) disrupts the fragile inhibition that supposedly develops during ex-tinction. According to the inhibition theory, the more stable excitatory association is less affected by the distracting stimulus than is the inhibitory association, and the result is a reappearance of the conditioned salivary response.

The phenomenon of **rapid reacquisition** is a third piece of evidence that extinction does not completely eliminate what was learned in the acquisition phase. Rapid reacquisition is similar to the "savings" that are found in experiments on list learning (Chapter 1) or habituation (Chapter 2). In classical conditioning, if a subject receives an acquisition phase, an extinction phase, and then another acquisition phase with the same CS and the same US, the rate of learning is substantially faster in the second acquisition phase—the reacquisition phase (Bouton, Woods, & Pineño, 2004). In addition, the rate of learning tends to get faster and faster if a subject is given repeated cycles of extinction followed by reacquisition (Hoehler, Kirschenbaum, & Leonard, 1973).

As with spontaneous recovery and disinhibition, we do not yet have a complete explanation for the phenomenon of rapid reacquisition. Nevertheless, these three phenomena make it abundantly clear that there is no simple way to get a subject to "unlearn" a CR, and that no amount of extinction training can completely wipe out all the effects of a classical conditioning experience. Extinction can cause a CR to disappear, and after repeated extinction sessions, spontaneous recovery may disappear, but the subject will never be exactly the same as before the conditioning began.

Conditioned Inhibition

Although there is still disagreement about whether inhibition plays an important role during extinction, there is general agreement that a CS can develop inhibitory properties as a result of certain conditioning procedures (see Miller & Spear, 1985; Urcelay & Miller, 2008). If it can be shown that a CS prevents the occurrence of a CR, or that it reduces the size of the CR from what it would otherwise be, then this CS is called an *inhibitory* CS or a **conditioned inhibitor** (sometimes designated as a CS⁻). Pavlov discovered a fairly simple and effective procedure for changing a neutral stimulus into a conditioned inhibitor. This procedure involves the use of two different CSs, such as a buzzer and a light. Suppose that in the first phase of an experiment, we repeatedly pair the sound of the buzzer with the presentation of food until the dog always salivates at the sound of the buzzer. The buzzer can now be called an **excitatory CS** (or CS⁺), because it regularly elicits a CR. In the second phase of the experiment, the dog receives two types of trials. Some trials are exactly like those of phase one (buzzer plus food). However, on occasional trials both the buzzer and the light are presented simultaneously, but no food is delivered. The simultaneous presentation of two or more CSs, such as the buzzer and the light, is called a **compound CS**. At first, the dog may salivate both on trials with the buzzer and on trials with the compound CS. As Phase 2 continues, however, the dog will eventually salivate on trials with the buzzer alone, but not on trials with both the buzzer and the light.

One way to give a convincing demonstration that the light has become a conditioned inhibitor is to show that it can prevent salivation to some other CS, not just to the buzzer with which it was trained. Suppose that a third stimulus, a fan blowing air into the chamber, is paired with food until it reliably elicits salivation. Now suppose that, for the first time, the animal receives a trial with a compound CS consisting of the fan and the light. This procedure of testing the combined effects of a known excitatory CS and a possible inhibitory CS is called a *summation test*. If the light is truly a conditioned inhibitor, it should have the capacity to reduce the salivation produced by any CS, not just by the buzzer with which it was originally presented. In this test, we would find that the light reduced or eliminated the CR to the fan, even though these two stimuli were never presented together before. This type of result indicates that the light is a general conditioned inhibitor, because it evidently has the ability to block or diminish the salivation elicited by any excitatory CS.

A second method for determining whether a stimulus is inhibitory is to measure how long it takes to turn the stimulus into an excitatory CS. Suppose that one group of dogs, the experimental group, has received the training with the buzzer and light described earlier, so we believe the light is a conditioned inhibitor. A second group of dogs, the control group, has not been exposed to the light before, so it is presumably a neutral stimulus for this group. Now suppose that both groups receive a series of trials with the light paired with food. Since the light is supposedly a conditioned inhibitor in the experimental group, this group should be slower to develop a CR of salivation to the light. This is because the training with the light and food must first offset the inhibitory properties of the light before a CR is observed. This technique of testing for conditioned inhibition is called a *retardation test* (Rescorla, 1969) because acquisition should be retarded with a CS that is initially inhibitory. The retardation test and the summation test are two of the most common techniques for showing that a CS is a conditioned inhibitor, and they have been used effectively with human participants as well as with animals (Campolattaro, Schnitker, & Freeman, 2008; Urcelay, Perelmuter, & Miller, 2008).

Why does a stimulus become a conditioned inhibitor in this procedure? The following rule of thumb may make this phenomenon easier to understand: A stimulus will become a conditioned inhibitor if it reliably signals the absence of the US in a context where the US would otherwise be expected to occur. In our example, the buzzer was normally followed by food, but not when the light was also presented. Because the light signaled the absence of an otherwise imminent US, it became an inhibitory CS.

Generalization and Discrimination

After classical conditioning with one CS, other, similar stimuli will also elicit CRs, although these other stimuli have never been paired with the US. This transfer of the effects of conditioning to similar stimuli is called **generalization**, which is illustrated in Figure 3-8. In this experiment on eyeblink conditioning, rabbits received a few hundred trials with a 1,200-Hz tone as the CS and a shock near the eye as a US (Liu, 1971). The data shown in Figure 3-8 were collected on a test day when tones of five different frequencies were repeatedly presented in a random sequence, but no US occurred on any trial. In other words, these tests were conducted under extinction conditions. As can be seen, the 1,200-Hz tone elicited the highest percentage of CRs. The two tones closest in frequency to the 1,200-Hz tone elicited an intermediate level of responding, and the more distant tones elicited the fewest responses. The function in Figure 3-8 is a typical **generalization gradient**, in which the *x*-axis plots some

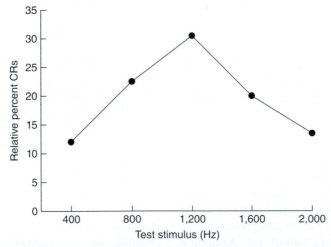

FIGURE 3-8 A typical generalization gradient. Rabbits in an eyeblink conditioning experiment received several hundred pairings of a 1,200-Hz tone and a shock. The graph shows the results from a subsequent generalization test in which the 1,200-Hz tone and four others were presented but never followed by the US. (Adapted from Liu, 1971). Copyright 1971 by the American Psychological Association. Adapted by permission.

SOURCE: Reprinted from *Journal of Comparative and Physiological Psychology*, 77, Liu, S., "Differential conditioning and stimulus generalization of the rabbit's nictating membrane response," pages 136–142, copyright ©1971, with permission from Elsevier.

dimension along which the test stimuli are varied and the *y*-axis shows the strength of conditioned responding to the different stimuli. In general, the more similar a stimulus is to the training stimulus, the greater will be its capacity to elicit CRs.

Generalization can be used by advertisers to help them sell their products. Till and Priluck (2000) found that if consumers have a favorable attitude toward a particular brand name of a product, this favorable attitude generalizes to other brands that have similar names, and to other products with the same brand name. This can help to explain why many products you see in supermarkets and department stores have names and package designs similar to those of well-known brands.

The opposite of generalization is **discrimination**, in which a subject learns to respond to one stimulus but not to a similar stimulus. We have seen that if a rabbit's eyeblink is conditioned to a 1,200-Hz tone, there will be substantial generalization to an 800-Hz tone. However, if the 800-Hz tone is never followed by food, but the 1,200-Hz tone is always followed by food, the animal will eventually learn a discrimination in which the 1,200-Hz tone elicits an eyeblink and the 800-Hz tone does not. This type of discrimination learning is important in many real-world situations. For instance, impala and other species of prey on the African plains can learn to discriminate between wild dogs that have just eaten (and will not attack again) and wild dogs on the hunt (which are very dangerous). The latter will elicit an obvious fear reaction in the prey, whereas the former will not.

THE IMPORTANCE OF TIMING IN CLASSICAL CONDITIONING

In all types of classical conditioning, the precise timing of the CS and the US can have a major effect, in several different ways. The timing of events can affect (1) how *strong* the conditioning will be, (2) whether a CS will become *excitatory* or *inhibitory,* and (3) exactly *when* the CR occurs.

All of the experiments discussed so far used **short-delay conditioning** (Figure 3-9) in which the CS begins a second or so before the

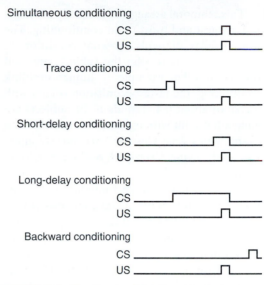

FIGURE 3-9 The temporal relationships between CS and US in five types of classical conditioning.

PRACTICE QUIZ (1)

1. In eyeblink conditioning, a tone could be used as the —————, and an air puff as the —————; an eyeblink is the —————.

2. A problem with Pavlov's stimulus substitution theory is that the ————— does not always resemble the —————.

3. Rescorla's (1973) experiment supported the theory of S-S associations because after responding to the US (loud noise) was reduced through habituation, responding to the CS —————.

4. Three phenomena that show that extinction is not the complete elimination of a learned association are —————, —————, and —————.

5. After classical conditioning with one CS, the appearance of CRs to new but similar stimuli is called —————.

Answers

US. This temporal arrangement usually produces the strongest and most rapid conditioning. The optimal delay depends on what conditioning preparation is used, who the subjects are, and other factors. For example, in human eyeblink conditioning, the fastest acquisition occurs with a delay of about 0.4 seconds if the subjects are young adults, but with older adults, conditioning is faster with a delay closer to 1 second (Solomon, Blanchard, Levine, Velazquez, & Groccia-Ellison, 1991).

Studies have shown that the early onset of the CS is important: In **simultaneous conditioning**, where the CS and US begin at the same moment (see Figure 3-9), conditioned responding is much weaker than in short-delay conditioning (Smith & Gormezano, 1965). This may be so for a number of reasons. For one thing, if the US begins at the same moment as the CS, the subject may respond to the US but fail to notice the CS. Furthermore, if the CS does not precede the US, it cannot serve to signal or predict the arrival of the US. As we will see again and again, the predictiveness of a CS is an important determinant of the degree of conditioning the CS undergoes and of whether this conditioning is excitatory or inhibitory. The following rules of thumb, though not perfect, are usually helpful in predicting the outcome of a conditioning arrangement:

- To the extent that a CS is a good predictor of the presence of the US, it will tend to become excitatory.
- To the extent that a CS is a good predictor of the absence of the US, it will tend to become inhibitory.

Keep these rules in mind when examining the other conditioning arrangements discussed in this section.

As shown in Figure 3-9, **trace conditioning** refers to the case in which the CS and US are separated by some time interval in which neither stimulus is present. The term a *trace conditioning* is derived from the notion that since the CS is no longer physically present when the US occurs, the subject must rely on a "memory trace" of the CS if conditioning is to occur. In a number of studies, the amount of time elapsing between CS and US presentations, or the **CS–US interval**, was systematically varied. That is, one group of subjects might receive a series of conditioning trials with a 2-second CS–US interval, another group with a 5-second CS–US interval, and so on. The results of such studies showed that as the CS–US interval is increased, the level of conditioning declines systematically (Ellison, 1964; Lucas, Deich, & Wasserman, 1981).

A similar pattern emerges in **long-delay conditioning**, where the onset of the CS precedes that of the US by at least several seconds, but the CS continues until the US is presented (see Figure 3-9). In long-delay conditioning, CS–US interval refers to the delay between the onsets of the CS and US. Here, too, the strength of the conditioned responding decreases as the CS–US interval increases, but the effects of delay are usually not as pronounced as in trace conditioning (which is understandable, since in long-delay conditioning, the subject does not have to rely on its memory of the CS).

In long-delay conditioning, Pavlov noted that the timing of the CRs changed over trials. Early in training, a dog would salivate as soon as the CS was presented, although the CS–US interval might be 10 seconds. As conditioning trials continued, however, these early CRs would gradually disappear, and the dog would salivate shortly before the food was presented (8 or 9 seconds after CS onset). This pattern indicates, first of all, that the dog had learned to estimate the duration of the CS quite accurately. In addition, it is consistent with the rule that the stimulus that is the best predictor of the US will be the most strongly conditioned. In this example, what stimulus is a better predictor of the US than CS onset? It is the compound stimulus—CS onset plus the passage of about 10 seconds. Therefore, it is this latter stimulus that ultimately elicits the most vigorous CRs.

The bottom of Figure 3-9 shows an example of **backward conditioning** in which the CS is presented after the US. Even if the CS is presented immediately after the US, the level of conditioning is markedly lower than in simultaneous or short-delay conditioning. From the perspective of the contiguity principle, this does not make sense: If the CS and US are equally contiguous in short-delay conditioning and in backward conditioning, the contiguity principle predicts that equally strong CRs should develop. The weakness of backward conditioning points to a limitation of the contiguity principle; that is, besides their temporal proximity, the order of the stimuli is important. Although backward conditioning may result in a weak excitatory association (Ayres, Haddad, & Albert, 1987; Champion & Jones, 1961), there is evidence that after a sufficient number of trials, a backward CS becomes inhibitory (Siegel & Domjan, 1971). Once again the predictiveness rule can serve as a useful guide: In backward conditioning, the onset of the CS signals a period of time in which the US will be absent; that is, as long as the backward CS is present, the subject can be certain that no US will occur.

One hypothesis about classical conditioning that addresses the timing of events is the **temporal coding hypothesis** (Arcediano, Escobar, & Miller, 2005; Matzel, Held, & Miller, 1988). This hypothesis states that in classical conditioning, more is learned than a simple association between CS and US—the individual also learns about the timing of these two events, and this learning affects when the CR occurs. This hypothesis can explain why the CR may occur just before the onset of the US in long-delay conditioning—the subject has learned that a delay of a certain duration separates the onset of the CS and the onset of the US.

A set of experiments by Williams, Johns, and Brindas (2008) nicely demonstrated the role of temporal coding in both excitatory and inhibitory conditioning. The subjects were rats, the USs were food pellets, and the excitatory CSs were 30-second tones. The CRs were head entries into a receptacle where the food pellets were delivered. In one conditioning arrangement, one food pellet was delivered 10 seconds after the onset of each tone, and a second food pellet was delivered 30 seconds after the onset of each tone. After training, there was a sharp increase of head entries into the food receptacle about 10 seconds after tone onset and another peak at around 30 seconds. In other words, the rats' head entries anticipated the timing of the food pellets, just as the temporal coding hypothesis would predict. In addition, this experiment included two different lights as inhibitory CSs, each of which was sometimes presented for 30 seconds along with the tone. For instance, when an overhead light was presented, the 10-second food pellet was omitted, and when a wall light was presented, the 30-second food pellet was omitted. After training, the rats' head entries showed that these two lights had become inhibitory CSs: On trials with the tone and overhead light, there was no increase in head entries around the 10-second mark, whereas on trials with the tone and the wall light, there was no increase in head entries near the 30-second mark. In other words, the inhibitory effects of the lights were restricted to the times when the usual food delivery was omitted. These and other experiments on the timing of CRs make it very clear that animals learn about temporal relations between CS and US, not just CS–US associations (Denniston & Miller, 2007; Kirkpatrick & Church, 2004).

CS–US Correlations

In each of the conditioning arrangements discussed so far, the temporal pattern of stimulus presentations is exactly the same on every trial. For example, in long-delay conditioning the US always follows the onset of the CS by the same amount of time, and the US never occurs at any other time. We can describe this perfect correlation between CS and US with two probabilities: When the CS is presented, the probability that the US will follow is 100% (i.e., the US is certain to occur); when the CS is not present, the probability that the US will follow is 0%. In the real world, however, the relationships between stimuli are seldom so regular. A rabbit in the forest must learn to recognize stimuli that could indicate that a predator is nearby. The rustling of leaves could be a predator, or it could be simply a breeze. On some occasions the sound of a snapped twig may mean a hunter is nearby; on other occasions it may not. At other times a predator's attack may occur without any warning signal. Although the relationships among stimuli are variable and uncertain in the real world, it is important for an animal to know which stimuli are the most dependable signals of possible danger. In the laboratory, classical conditioning procedures can be used to evaluate an animal's ability to detect imperfect correlations between stimuli.

A series of experiments by Rescorla (1966, 1968) showed how the probability of the US in the presence of the CS and in its absence combine to determine the size of the CR. In a conditioned suppression procedure with rats, the CS was a 2-minute tone that was presented at random intervals. For one group of rats, there was a 40% chance that a shock would occur during a 2-minute tone presentation, and there was a 20% chance that a shock would occur in any 2-minute period when the tone was off. The shock might occur at any moment during the presence or absence of the tone. Notice that neither the presence of the tone nor its absence was a definite signal that a shock would occur, and neither provided any information about the timing (since a shock could occur at any time). The only information the tone provided was whether the probability of shock was high or low.

The results can be summarized as follows. Whenever the probability of shock was greater when the tone was on than when it was off, the tone became an excitatory CS (i.e., the rats' lever pressing for food was suppressed when the tone was on). In other conditions, the probability of shock was the same in the presence and absence of the tone (e.g., a 40% chance of shock both when the tone was on and when it was off). In these conditions, the rats showed no suppression at all to the tone. In another experiment, Rescorla included a group in which the chance of shock was *lower* when the tone was on than when it was off (so the tone signaled a relative level of safety from shock), and in this case the tone became an inhibitory CS.

Based on these results, Rescorla concluded that the traditional view of classical conditioning, which states that the *contiguity* of CS and US is what causes an association to develop, is incorrect. Notice that in the groups with equal probabilities of shock in the presence and absence of the tone, there were many pairings of the tone and shock, yet there was no conditioning to the tone. Rescorla therefore proposed that the important variable in classical conditioning is not the contiguity of CS and US but rather the *correlation* between CS and US. If the correlation is positive (i.e., if the CS predicts a higher-than-normal probability of the US), the CS will become excitatory. If there is no correlation between CS and US (if the probability of the US is the same whether or not the CS is present), the CS will remain neutral. If the correlation between CS and US is negative (if the CS signals a lower-than-normal probability of the US), the CS will become inhibitory.

These results provide another instance where the predictiveness rule is a useful guide: If a CS predicts that the US is likely to occur, the CS will become excitatory; if the CS predicts that the US is not likely to occur, the CS will become inhibitory. This rule is not perfect, but it works well in most cases.

HIGHER ORDER CONDITIONING

So far we have examined only procedures in which a CS is paired with (or correlated with) a US. However, this is not the only way a CS can acquire the ability to elicit a CR. In **second-order conditioning**, a CR is transferred from one CS to another. Pavlov described the following experiment to illustrate this process. First, the ticking of a metronome was firmly established as a CS in salivary conditioning by pairing the metronome with food. Because it was paired with the US, the metronome is called a **first-order CS**. Then another stimulus, a black square, was presented and immediately followed by the metronome on a number of occasions, but no food was presented on these trials. After a few trials of this type, the black square began to elicit salivation on its own, despite the fact that this stimulus was *never paired directly with the food* (but only with the metronome, a CS that was frequently paired with the food). In this example, the black square is called a **second-order CS** because it acquired its ability to elicit a CR by being paired with a first-order CS, the metronome.

Pavlov also reported that although it was quite difficult to obtain, he sometimes found evidence of third-order conditioning (the transfer of a CR from a second-order CS to yet another stimulus). He believed that these examples of second- and higher order conditioning were important because they broadened the scope of classical conditioning. The following example illustrates how higher order conditioning can play an important role in an animal's ability to avoid dangerous situations in its environment. Although wolves are among the major predators of deer, the sight of a wolf does not elicit an unconditioned fear reaction in a young whitetail deer. Instead, the sight of a wolf must become a CS for fear as a result of a young deer's experience. This conditioning might occur in at least two ways. The sight of a wolf might be followed by an attack and injury to the young deer. More likely, however, the sight of wolves is simply paired with visible signs of fear in other deer. (Presumably, seeing the fear reactions of other deer elicits a fear reaction in the young deer.) Eventually, the sight of wolves becomes a first-order CS for a fear response in the young deer. Once this happens, higher order conditioning can occur whenever some initially neutral stimulus is paired with the sight of wolves. Perhaps certain sounds or odors frequently precede the appearance of wolves, and through second-order conditioning, these may come to elicit fear. Or perhaps wolves are usually encountered in certain parts of the forest, and so the deer becomes fearful and cautious when traveling through these places. Although these examples are hypothetical, they show how an initially neutral stimulus (the sight of wolves) can first develop the capacity to elicit a fear response and can then transfer this response to other stimuli.

Second-order conditioning has also been demonstrated with humans. For example, in a procedure called **evaluative conditioning**, subjects are asked to evaluate different stimuli—to rate how much they like them using a scale that ranges from "very disliked" to "very liked." The first-order CSs are typically words that people consistently rate as being positive (e.g., *honest* or *friendly*) or negative (e.g., *cruel* or *arrogant*). These words are first-order CSs, not unconditioned stimuli, because they would certainly have no value to someone who did not know the English language. For English speakers, these words presumably attained their positive or negative values because they have been associated with good or bad experiences in the past. In some studies, the second-order CSs are nonsense syllables, and if a nonsense syllable is repeatedly paired with a positive (or negative) word, subjects later give the nonsense syllable itself a positive (or negative) rating (Cicero & Tryon, 1989).

In one interesting study, pictures of people's faces were the second-order stimuli, and while looking at some of these faces, subjects heard either positive or negative adjectives (Figure 3-10). The subjects later rated the faces as being "liked" if they had been paired with positive adjectives and "disliked" if they had been paired with negative adjectives. These positive

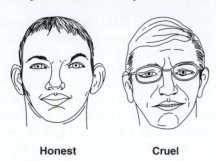

Honest   **Cruel**

FIGURE 3-10 In evaluative conditioning, initially neutral stimuli such as pictures of faces are paired with positive or negative adjectives. After conditioning, people will have positive or negative reactions to the faces as well.

or negative ratings of the faces occurred even if the subjects could not remember the adjectives that had been paired with individual faces. In other words, subjects knew they liked some faces and disliked others, but they could not say exactly why (Baeyens, Eelen, Van den Bergh, & Crombez, 1992).

This type of evaluative conditioning has long been used in advertising. A commercial may present a certain brand of cola along with stimuli that most viewers will evaluate positively, such as young, attractive people having a good time. Advertisers hope that viewers will be attracted to the people and that this positive reaction will become conditioned to the product being sold. So if the conditioning is successful, you may later have a positive reaction when you see the product in a store, regardless of whether you remember the commercial.

CLASSICAL CONDITIONING OUTSIDE THE LABORATORY

Although experiments on salivation, eyeblinks, and the SCR may seem far removed from the world outside the laboratory, we should not underestimate the importance of classical conditioning in everyday life. Classical conditioning is important outside the laboratory in at least

two ways. First, it gives us a way of understanding "involuntary" behaviors, those that are automatically elicited by certain stimuli whether we want them to occur or not. As discussed in the Classical Conditioning and Emotional Responses section, many emotional reactions seem to fall into this category. Second, research on classical conditioning has led to several major treatment procedures for behavior disorders. These procedures can be used to strengthen desired "involuntary" responses or to weaken undesired responses. The remainder of this chapter examines the role of classical conditioning in these nonlaboratory settings.

Classical Conditioning and Emotional Responses

Everyday emotional responses such as feelings of pleasure, happiness, anxiety, or excitement are frequently triggered by specific stimuli. In many cases, the response-eliciting properties of a stimulus are not inborn but acquired through experience. Suppose you open your mailbox and find a card with the return address of a close friend. This stimulus may immediately evoke a pleasant and complex emotional reaction that you might loosely call affection, warmth, or fondness. Whatever you call the emotional reaction, there is no doubt that this particular stimulus—a person's handwritten address on an envelope— would not elicit the response from you shortly after your birth, nor would it elicit the response now if you did not know the person who sent you the letter. The envelope is a CS that elicits a pleasant emotional response only because the address has been associated with your friend. Other stimuli can elicit less pleasant emotional reactions. For many college students, examination periods can be a time of high anxiety. This anxiety can be conditioned to stimuli associated with the examination process—the textbooks on one's desk, a calendar with the date of the exam circled, or the sight of the building where the exam will be held.

Classical conditioning can also affect our emotional reactions to other people. In one study using evaluative conditioning, participants were asked to look at photographs of people's faces, and each photograph was paired with either a pleasant, neutral, or unpleasant odor. When they later had to evaluate their preferences for the people in the photographs (with no odors present), they gave the highest ratings to faces previously paired with pleasant odors and the lowest ratings to those paired with unpleasant odors (Todrank, Byrnes, Wrzesniewski, & Rozin, 1995). This research surely encourages companies that sell mouthwash, deodorant, and perfume.

A personal example shows that CERs are not under voluntary control, and that they are not necessarily guided by logic or by a knowledge of one's environment. Before my wife, Laurie, and I were married, our jobs required us to live more than 200 miles apart. We visited each other on weekends, about twice a month. Laurie owned a very distinctive winter coat—a white coat with broad horizontal stripes of red, yellow, and green. It is easy to find her in a crowd when she is wearing that coat. One day when Laurie was at her job and I was at mine, I was walking across the campus when I saw, ahead of me, someone wearing a coat just like Laurie's. My immediate reaction was a good example of a CR: My heart started pounding rapidly, as when a person is startled by a loud noise. This response persisted for 10 or 20 seconds. What is noteworthy about the response is that it did not make sense, because I knew Laurie was several hundreds of miles away and the person wearing the coat could not possibly be her. In addition, whereas Laurie has a full-length coat, the coat I saw was short, and the person wearing it was a man with a beard. Yet none of these discrepancies was enough to prevent my conditioned heart-rate response.

Classical Conditioning and the Immune System

As you probably know, the body's immune system is designed to fight off infections. Whenever bacteria, viruses, or foreign cells enter a person's body, the immune system produces antibodies that attack and kill these invaders. For a long time, scientists tended to think of the immune system as a fairly independent system that had little communication with other bodily functions. This viewpoint has changed, however, and there is now abundant evidence for complex interactions between the immune system and the nervous system. To put it another way, there is abundant evidence that psychological factors can affect the workings of the immune system (Ader, 2001). For example, it is known that intense or prolonged psychological stress can weaken the immune system, making the individual more susceptible to illnesses ranging from the common cold to cancer.

There is also convincing evidence that the immune system can be influenced by classical conditioning. Ader and Cohen (1975) conducted a landmark study in this area. They gave rats a single conditioning trial in which the CS was saccharin-flavored water and the US was an injection of cyclophosphamide, a drug that suppresses the activity of the immune system. A few days later, the rats were injected with a small quantity of foreign cells (red blood cells from sheep) that their immune systems would normally attack vigorously. One group of rats was then given saccharin-flavored water once again, whereas a control group received plain water. Ader and Cohen found that for rats in the saccharin-water group, the response of the immune system was weaker than for rats in the plain-water group; that is, fewer antibodies were produced by rats in the saccharin-water group. In other words, it appeared that the saccharin, which normally has no effect on the immune system, now produced a CR, a weakening of the immune system. Later studies replicated this effect and, by ruling out other possible explanations, demonstrated that it is indeed due to classical conditioning (Ader, Felten, & Cohen, 1990).

On the other side of the coin, there is evidence that immune system activity can also be increased through classical conditioning.

Solvason, Ghanata, and Hiramoto (1988) reported a particularly clear example of a conditioned increase in immune activity. Mice exposed to the odor of camphor as a CS were then injected with the drug interferon as the US. Interferon normally causes an increase in the activity of natural killer cells in the bloodstream—cells that are involved in combating viruses and the growth of tumors. After a few pairings of the camphor odor and interferon, presenting the camphor odor by itself was enough to produce an increase in activity of the natural killer cells. A similar study with healthy human adults also obtained increases in natural killer cells through classical conditioning (Buske-Kirschbaum, Kirschbaum, Stierle, Jabaij, & Hellhammer, 1994). In one study, rats received just a single pairing of saccharin-flavored water and ovalbumin, a substance that stimulates the production of antibodies by the immune system. When presented by itself, ovalbumin produces an increase in antibodies that lasts for more than 40 days. Thirty days after the pairing of saccharin and ovalbumin, the rats were given saccharin-flavored water but no ovalbumin. The immune reaction to the saccharin was similar to the response produced by the ovalbumin. Through classical conditioning, the saccharin acquired the ability to produce a strong and long-lasting immune response (Chen et al., 2004).

Researchers have recognized the potential importance of this phenomenon, and they have begun to understand the brain mechanisms that make conditioning of the immune system possible (Schedlowski & Pacheco-López, 2010). For people whose immune systems have been temporarily weakened through illness or fatigue, developing psychological techniques to strengthen immune activity could be beneficial. In other cases, decreasing the activity of the immune system may be what is needed. For example, common allergies are the product of an overactive immune system. In one study, people who were allergic to dust mites were given five trials in which flavored water was paired with an antihistamine (a drug that reduces the allergic reaction). Later, when they received a trial with the flavored water but no drug, they showed the same signs of relief from their allergy symptoms as when they actually received the drug (Goebel, Meykadeh, Kou, Schedlowski, & Hengge, 2008). Human research on classical conditioning and the immune system is still fairly limited, but this type of research may eventually produce ways to better control immune system activity for the benefit of the patient.

Applications in Behavior Therapy

SYSTEMATIC DESENSITIZATION FOR PHOBIAS.   One of the most widely used procedures of behavior therapy is **systematic desensitization**, a treatment for phobias that arose directly out of laboratory research on classical conditioning. A phobia is an excessive and irrational fear of an object, place, or situation. Phobias come in numerous forms, for example, fear of closed spaces, of open spaces, of heights, of water, of crowds, of speaking before a group, of taking an examination, of insects, of snakes, of dogs, and of birds. Some of these phobias may sound almost amusing, but they are no joke to those who suffer from them, and they are frequently quite debilitating. A fear of insects or snakes may preclude going to a picnic or taking a walk in the woods. A fear of crowds may make it impossible for a person to go to the supermarket, to a movie, or to ride on a bus or train.

How do phobias arise? After Pavlov's discovery, classical conditioning was seen as one possible source of irrational fears. This hypothesis was bolstered by a famous (or, more accurately, infamous) experiment by John B. Watson and Rosalie Rayner (1921). Watson and Rayner used classical conditioning to develop a phobia in a normal 11-month-old infant named Albert. Before the experiment, few things frightened Albert, but one that did was the loud noise of a hammer hitting a steel bar. Upon hearing the noise, Albert would start to cry. Since this stimulus elicited a reliable response from Albert, it was used as the US in a series of conditioning trials. The CS was a live white rat, which initially produced no signs of fear in Albert. On the first conditioning trial, the noise was presented just as Albert was reaching out to touch the rat, and as a result Albert began to cry. Albert subsequently received seven more conditioning trials of this type. After this experience, Albert's behavior indicated that he had been classically conditioned: He cried when he was presented with the white rat by itself. This fear also generalized to a white rabbit and to other white furry objects, including a ball of cotton and a Santa Claus mask.

If this experiment sounds cruel and unethical, rest assured that modern legal safeguards for the protection of human subjects would make it difficult or impossible for a psychologist to conduct such a study today. But based on this study, Watson and Rayner concluded that a long-lasting fear of an initially neutral stimulus can result from the pairing of that stimulus with some fearful event. If this analysis is correct, then the principles of classical conditioning should also describe how a phobia can be cured. To be specific, if the CS (the phobic object or event) is repeatedly presented without the US, the phobia should extinguish.

Systematic desensitization is a procedure in which the patient is exposed to the phobic object gradually, so that fear and discomfort are kept to a minimum and extinction is allowed to occur. The treatment has three parts: the construction of a fear hierarchy, training in relaxation, and the gradual presentation of items in the fear hierarchy to the patient. The *fear hierarchy* is a list of fearful situations of progressively increasing intensity. At the bottom of the list is an item that evokes only a very mild fear response in the patient, and at the top is the most highly feared situation. After the fear hierarchy is constructed, the patient is given training in **progressive relaxation**, or deep muscle relaxation. This technique, developed by Wolpe (1958), is a way to produce a state of bodily calm and relaxation by having the person alternately tense and relax specific groups of muscles.

The procedure takes about 20 minutes, and when it is completed patients usually report that they feel very relaxed. At this point the extinction of the phobia can begin.

The therapist begins with the weakest item in the hierarchy, describes the scene to the patient, and asks the patient to imagine this scene as vividly as possible. For example, in the treatment of a teenager who developed a fear of driving after an automobile accident, the first instruction was to imagine "looking at his car as it was before the accident" (Kushner, 1968). Because the patient is in a relaxed state, and because the lowest item did not evoke much fear to begin with, it usually can be imagined with little or no fear. The patient is instructed to continue to imagine the scene for about 20 seconds. After a short pause in which the patient is told to relax, the first item is again presented. If the patient reports that the item produces no fear, the therapist moves on to the second item on the list, and the procedure is repeated. The therapist slowly progresses up the list, being certain that the fear of one item is completely gone before going on to the next item. A typical fear hierarchy contains 10 or 15 items, but there have been cases in which lists of over 100 items were constructed.

G. L. Paul (1969) reviewed about 75 published reports on the use of systematic desensitization that together involved thousands of patients. In most of these reports, about 80 to 90% of the patients were cured of their phobias—a very high success rate for any type of therapy in the realm of mental health. There were only a few reports of relapses and no evidence of symptom substitution (the appearance of a new psychological disorder after the original problem disappears). This mass of evidence suggests that systematic desensitization is an effective and efficient treatment for phobias.

The basic systematic desensitization procedure has been adapted and modified in many ways for use in different circumstances. In some cases, real stimuli are used instead of relying on the patient's imagination. Sturges and Sturges (1998) treated an 11-year-old girl with a fear of elevators by systematically exposing her to an elevator (beginning by having her just stand near an elevator, and ending with her riding alone on the elevator). In another variation of systematic desensitization, humor was used in place of relaxation training, based on the reasoning that humor would also counteract anxiety. Individuals with an extreme fear of spiders were asked to create jokes about spiders, and they were presented with humorous scenes involving spiders. This treatment proved to be just about as effective as the more traditional relaxation training in reducing spider phobias (Ventis, Higbee, & Murdock, 2001).

In the aftermath of the terrorist attacks of September 11, 2001, many employees of the Pentagon building in Washington, DC, were not emotionally prepared to reenter the building where so many of their friends and co-workers were killed or injured. To help them recover, health specialists used mass desensitization in which groups of about 50 employees were gradually reexposed to their workplace environment. They began with a bus ride to a hill overlooking the Pentagon, then proceeded to some of the damaged offices, and finally to the Pentagon's "ground zero," the site where the plane hit the building. Each step of the way the workers were encouraged to discuss their memories and their emotions, and they were assisted by stress management counselors. Although we must be careful in drawing conclusions because this was not a controlled experiment, all but one worker (who had physical injuries) were later able to return to work (Waldrep & Waits, 2002).

A technique that relies on modern computer technology is **virtual reality therapy**, in which the patient wears a headset that displays realistic visual images that change with every head movement, simulating a three-dimensional environment. For instance, a man with a fear of flying was exposed to more and more challenging simulations of riding in a helicopter, and eventually his fear of flying diminished.

Virtual reality therapy has been successfully used for fears of animals, heights, public speaking, and so on (North, North, & Coble, 2002). This technique has several advantages over traditional systematic desensitization: The stimuli are very realistic, they can be controlled precisely, and they can be tailored to the needs of each individual patient. The procedure does not rely on the patient's ability to imagine the objects or situations. Because of these advantages, it seems likely that the use of computer-generated stimuli will become more widespread in the future.

AVERSIVE COUNTERCONDITIONING. The goal of **aversive counterconditioning** is to develop an aversive CR to stimuli associated with the undesirable behavior. For instance, if a person is an alcoholic, the procedure may involve conditioning the responses of nausea and queasiness of the stomach to the sight, smell, and taste of alcohol. The term *counterconditioning* is used because the technique is designed to replace a positive emotional response to certain stimuli (such as alcohol) with a negative one. In the 1940s, Voegtlin and his associates conducted extensive research on the use of aversive counterconditioning as a treatment for alcoholism (Lemere, Voegtlin, Broz, O'Hallaren, & Tupper, 1942; Voegtlin, 1940). Over the years, more than 4,000 alcoholics volunteered to participate in Voegtlin's distinctly unpleasant therapy. Over a 10-day period, a patient received about a half dozen treatment sessions in which alcoholic beverages were paired with an emetic (a drug that produces nausea). Conditioning sessions took place in a quiet, darkened room in which a collection of liquor bottles was illuminated to enhance their salience. First, the patient received an emetic, and soon the first signs of nausea would begin. The patient was then given a large glass of whiskey and was instructed to look at, smell, taste, and swallow the whiskey until vomiting occurred (which was usually no more than a few minutes). In later conditioning sessions, the whiskey was replaced with a variety of other liquors to ensure that the aversion was not limited to one type of liquor. It is hard to imagine a more unpleasant therapy, and the patients' willingness to participate gives an indication both of their commitment to overcome their alcoholism and of their inability to do so on their own.

Because a number of different treatments for alcoholism are known to promote short-term abstinence, the real test of a treatment's effectiveness is its long-term success rate. Figure 3-11 shows the percentages of former patients who were totally abstinent for various lengths of time after the therapy. As can be seen, the percentage of individuals who were totally abstinent declined over time. The diminishing percentages may reflect the process of extinction: If over the years a person repeatedly encounters the sight or smell of alcohol (at weddings, at parties, on television) in the absence of the US (the emetic), the CR of nausea should eventually wear off. At least two types of evidence support the role of extinction. First, patients who received "booster sessions" (further conditioning sessions a few months after the original treatment) were, on the average, abstinent for longer periods of time. Such reconditioning sessions probably

counteracted the effects of extinction. Second, those who continued to associate with old drinking friends (and were thereby exposed to alcohol) were the most likely to fail.

If the declining percentages in Figure 3-11 seem discouraging, it is important to realize a similar pattern of increasing relapses over time occurs with other treatments for alcoholism; in fact, Voegtlin's success rates are quite high compared to other treatments. Furthermore, Voegtlin used a very strict criterion for success—total abstinence. Individuals who drank with moderation after the treatment were counted as failures, as were those who suffered a relapse, received reconditioning sessions, and were once again abstinent. Figure 3-11 therefore presents the most pessimistic view possible regarding the effectiveness of this treatment. Despite the evidence for its effectiveness, the use of aversive counterconditioning in the treatment for alcoholism has declined since the 1980s (Revusky, 2009). When used, aversive counterconditioning is often included as one component of multifaceted treatment programs that also involve family counseling, self-control training, and other techniques (Smith & Frawley, 1990).

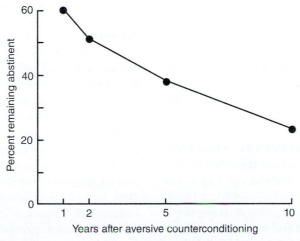

FIGURE 3-11 The percentages of Voegtlin's clients who remained completely abstinent for various amounts of time following aversive counterconditioning for alcoholism. (Based on Lemere & Voegtlin, 1950).

Aversive counterconditioning has also been applied to other behavioral problems, including drug use, cigarette smoking, overeating, and sexual deviations. Different aversive stimuli have been used, including electric shock, unpleasant odors, or disgusting mental images. One method that has been used to help people quit smoking cigarettes is called "rapid smoking": The smoker inhales cigarette smoke at a rapid pace, which makes it a sickening experience. This technique has had a respectable success rate (Gifford & Shoenberger, 2009).

In a case study involving a sexual deviation, Marshall (2006) used an unpleasant odor, the smell of ammonia, as a US to treat an exhibitionist—a male who found pleasure in exposing himself to females. The smell of ammonia was presented when the client had urges to expose himself, and as a result these urges decreased and his acts of exhibitionism stopped. The man was then able to develop a more normal social life. Aversive counterconditioning has also been successful in treating fetishes and other sexual deviations (Marks & Gelder, 1967).

In summary, aversive counterconditioning is a procedure that attempts to decrease unwanted behaviors by conditioning aversive reactions to stimuli associated with the behaviors. Its effectiveness is variable. It appears to be a useful procedure for eliminating certain sexual deviations. When used as a treatment for alcoholism or smoking, some clients have had relapses, but others have remained abstinent for years. The success rates are significantly higher than when individuals try to stop drinking or smoking without professional help.

TREATMENT OF NOCTURNAL ENURESIS. Children usually learn to use the toilet instead of wetting their pants by about age 3 or 4. For most children, the control of nighttime elimination occurs shortly afterward. However, a substantial portion of children continue to wet their beds at ages 5 and older, and this behavior becomes an increasing problem for both children and parents. Fortunately, most cases of nocturnal enuresis (bedwetting) can be cured by a straightforward procedure developed by Mowrer and Mowrer (1938), called the bell-and-pad method. The pad, a water-detecting device, is placed beneath the child's sheets; a single drop of urine will activate the device and ring the bell to wake up the child. The child is instructed in advance to turn off the alarm, go to the toilet and urinate, and then go back to sleep. The bell and pad are used every night until the problem disappears.

In this procedure, the bell is a US that elicits two responses in the child: (1) awakening and (2) the tightening of those muscles necessary to prevent further urination (responses that occur because the child has no difficulty retaining urine when awake). The goal of the procedure is to transfer either or both of these responses to an internal CS—the sensations associated with having a full bladder. For simplicity, let us call the CS a full bladder. By repeatedly pairing a full bladder with the bell, the response of awakening and/or tightening the muscles so as to retain one's urine should eventually be elicited by the full bladder alone, before the bell sounds.

Various studies have found success rates of about 80% for the bell-and-pad method, and in some of the "unsuccessful" cases, the symptoms, though not completely gone, were improved. Relapses are a frequent problem, however, with perhaps 25% of the children eventually experiencing a return of bedwetting. These relapses can be readily treated with a period of reconditioning, but Young and Morgan (1972) tried a modified procedure in an effort to minimize relapses. With the alarm system active, children were given a type of overlearning in which they drank two pints of liquid just before going to bed (thus making the task of remaining dry more difficult). Only 10% of the children trained with this procedure had relapses, compared to 20% without the overlearning procedure. The bell-and-pad method is more effective than the medications that are commonly prescribed to treat enuresis, and more doctors are now recommending this treatment method to parents (Bennett, 2005; Houts, 2003).

Summary of the Classical Conditioning Therapies. Behavior therapies based on principles of classical conditioning have been used to strengthen, eliminate, or replace behaviors. The bell-and-pad treatment for nocturnal enuresis is an example of a procedure designed to strengthen a behavior (i.e., nighttime retention). Systematic desensitization is used to eliminate the emotional responses of fear and anxiety. Aversive counterconditioning is designed to replace pleasant emotional responses to such stimuli as alcohol and cigarette smoke with aversion. Each of these procedures has its share of failures and relapses, but each can also boast of long-term successes for a significant percentage of those who receive treatment.

PRACTICE QUIZ (2)

1. When the CS and US are separated by some time interval, this is called _____.
2. In an evaluative conditioning procedure in which pictures of people are paired with either positive or negative adjectives, the adjectives are _____ and the pictures of people are _____.
3. If a rat drinks sweetened water and then receives a drug that suppresses the immune system, giving sweetened water at a later time can _____.
4. When the effectiveness of aversive counterconditioning for alcoholism weakens over time, this could be an example of the conditioning principle of _____.
5. In the classical conditioning treatment for bedwetting, the US is _____.

Answers

1. trace conditioning   2. first-order CSs, second-order CSs   3. suppress the immune system   4. extinction   5. an alarm that wakes up the child

---

Summary

In its simplest form, classical conditioning involves the repeated pairing of a CS with a US that naturally elicits a UR. After repeated pairings, the CS starts to elicit a CR. Pavlov used the salivation response of dogs to study classical conditioning, but in modern research, some common conditioning preparations are eyeblink conditioning, conditioned suppression, the SCR, and taste-aversion learning.

According to Pavlov's stimulus substitution theory, the CS should produce the same response that the US originally did. In reality, however, sometimes the CR is different in form, and sometimes it is actually the opposite of the UR. At the physiological level, stimulus substitution theory states that neural centers for the CS become connected to either the center for the US (an S-S connection) or directly to the center for the response (an S-R connection). Some experiments on US devaluation or revaluation favor the S-S view.

Throughout the animal kingdom, instances of classical conditioning exhibit the same basic principles, including acquisition, extinction, spontaneous recovery, disinhibition, conditioned inhibition, generalization, and discrimination. The most effective temporal arrangement for conditioning occurs in short-delay conditioning; weaker conditioning usually occurs in simultaneous, long-delay, or trace conditioning. In backward conditioning, the CS may become a conditioned inhibitor. In other conditioning arrangements, such as second-order conditioning a CR is transferred, not from US to CS, but from one CS to another.

In everyday life, classically CRs can be seen in our emotional reactions to many different stimuli. In behavior therapy, systematic desensitization is used to extinguish phobias by gradually presenting more and more intense fear-provoking stimuli while the patient is in a relaxed state. Aversive counterconditioning is used to replace positive responses to certain stimuli (e.g., alcohol, cigarettes) with negative responses. The bell-and-pad method is used to train children to avoid bedwetting.

Review Questions

1. Define CS, US, UR, and CR. Use the examples of salivary conditioning and conditioning of the SCR to illustrate these four concepts.

2. What is Pavlov's stimulus substitution theory? What are its strengths and weaknesses? How do experiments on US devaluation or revaluation help to decide whether S-S or S-R associations are formed during classical conditioning?

3. What three different types of evidence show that extinction does not simply erase the association that was formed during classical conditioning?

4. Describe one temporal arrangement between CS and US that produces strong excitatory conditioning, one that produces weak excitatory conditioning, and one that can produce inhibitory conditioning. Give a reasonable explanation of why each different procedure produces the results that it does.

5. Explain how television advertisers can use classical conditioning to give viewers a positive feeling about their product. How could they use classical conditioning to give viewers a negative reaction to other brands? Can you think of actual commercials that use these techniques?

6. Explain how systematic desensitization is used to treat phobias. Explain how extinction and generalization are important parts of the procedure. Why don't phobias extinguish by themselves, without the need for treatment?

7. Describe how aversive counterconditioning can be used to treat alcoholism. Does the fact that some patients have relapses, especially many years after treatment, indicate that there is something incorrect about the principles of classical conditioning? Why or why not?

CHAPTER 4

Theories and Research on Classical Conditioning

LEARNING OBJECTIVES

After reading this chapter, you should be able to

- explain the blocking effect and why it is important
- describe the basic concepts of the Rescorla–Wagner model and how it accounts for conditioning phenomena such as acquisition, extinction, blocking, and conditioned inhibition
- describe the different types of associations that can form during classical conditioning

- explain how heredity can influence what animals and people learn through classical conditioning
- discuss the role that classical conditioning plays in drug tolerance and addiction
- describe research on the physiological mechanisms of classical conditioning in primitive animals, mammals, and humans

Chapter 3 described some of the most basic terms and concepts of classical conditioning and some of the ways it can affect our daily lives. Most of the concepts presented in that chapter either were developed by Pavlov or can be traced back to some of his ideas. This chapter describes how psychologists' conceptions of classical conditioning have changed over the years. Perhaps the clearest theme emerging from modern research on classical conditioning is that although it is one of the simplest types of learning, it is more complicated than was once believed.

This chapter surveys some current themes and issues in the field of classical conditioning. The chapter is divided into five sections, each of which addresses different questions. The first section is concerned with the conditioning process and the question of *when* conditioning takes place: Under what conditions will a stimulus become an excitatory conditioned stimulus (CS), or become an inhibitory CS, or remain neutral? What factors determine whether the stimulus will become a strong CS or a weak CS? These are certainly very basic questions, and this section describes a few well-known theories that attempt to answer them. The second section deals with the products of conditioning: *What types of associations* are developed in different conditioning situations? We will see that a CS–US (unconditioned stimulus) association is only one of many possible associative products of the classical conditioning process. The third section, on biological constraints, examines *what types of stimuli* are easily associated in classical conditioning and what types are not. The answer to this question is not simple, and it depends on the specific CS–US combination used and on the species of the subject.

The fourth section of this chapter presents modern theories that try to predict *what form* a conditioned response (CR) will take. Will the CR be similar to the unconditioned response (UR), the opposite of the UR, or something entirely different? Besides its theoretical importance, this issue has significant practical consequences; for example, a stimulus that has been associated with a drug might later elicit a response that either mimics or opposes the reaction to the drug itself. The final section of this chapter examines both the process and products of classical conditioning from a neurophysiological perspective. This section describes research that examines how classical conditioning alters the functioning of individual neurons as well as studies that investigate what areas of the brain are involved.

THEORIES OF ASSOCIATIVE LEARNING

One of the oldest principles of associative learning is the principle of frequency: The more frequently two stimuli are paired, the more strongly will an individual associate the two. Thomas Brown (1820) first proposed this principle, and we have seen data from Ebbinghaus and from classical conditioning experiments that support this principle. The principle was also the cornerstone of several influential theories of learning (Bush & Mosteller, 1955; Estes, 1950; Hull, 1943). Because

of this widespread acceptance of the frequency principle, an experiment by Kamin (1968) that contradicted this principle attracted considerable attention. We will examine Kamin's experiment in The Blocking Effect section. We will then go on to consider several different theories of classical conditioning that have been developed in an effort to avoid the limitations of the frequency principle and provide a more adequate analysis of the processes of associative learning.

The Blocking Effect

To make the description of Kamin's experiment and others in this chapter easier to understand, some notational conventions will be adopted. Because these experiments included not one but several CSs, we will use capital letters to represent different CSs (e.g., T will represent a tone, and L will represent a light). Usually only one US is involved, but it may be present on some trials and absent on others, so the superscripts $+$ and $\circ$ will represent, respectively, the presence and absence of the US. For example, T^+ will denote a trial on which one CS, a tone, was presented by itself and was followed by the US. The notation TL° will refer to a trial on which two CSs, the tone and the light, were presented simultaneously, but were not followed by the US.

Kamin's original experiment used rats in a conditioned suppression procedure. Figure 4-1 outlines the design of the experiment. There were two groups of rats, a **blocking group** and a **control group**. In Phase I of the experiment, rats in the blocking group received a series of L^+ trials, and by the end of this phase, L elicited a strong CR. In Phase 2, the blocking group received a series of LT^+ trials. These trials were exactly the

Group	Phase 1	Phase 2	Test Phase	Results
Blocking	L+	LT+	T	T → no fear
Control	–	LT+	T	T → fear

FIGURE 4-1 Design of Kamin's blocking experiment.

same as Phase 1 trials except that a second CS, T, occurred along with L. In the test phase, T was presented by itself (with no shock) for several trials so as to measure the strength of conditioning to this CS.

There was only one difference in the procedure for the control group: In Phase 1 no stimuli were presented at all. Therefore, the first time these rats were exposed to L, T, and the US was in Phase 2. The important point is that both groups received *exactly the same number of pairings of T and shock,* so the frequency principle predicts that *conditioning to T should be equally strong* in the two groups. However, this is not what Kamin found: Whereas he observed a strong fear response (conditioned suppression) to T in the control group, there was almost no fear response at all to T in the blocking group. Kamin concluded that the prior conditioning with L somehow "blocked" the later conditioning of T. Since Kamin's pioneering work, the blocking effect has been demonstrated in numerous experiments using a variety of conditioning situations, with subjects ranging from humans to snails (e.g., Acebes, Solar, Carnero, & Loy, 2009; Mitchell, Lovibond, Minard, & Lavis, 2006).

An intuitive explanation of the blocking effect is not difficult to construct: To put it simply, T was redundant in the blocking group; it supplied no new information. By the end of Phase 1, rats in the blocking group had learned that L was a reliable predictor of the US—the US always occurred after L and never at any other time. Adding T to the situation in Phase 2 added nothing to the rat's ability to predict the US. This experiment suggests that conditioning will not occur if a CS adds no new information about the US.

This experiment demonstrates that conditioning is not an automatic result when a CS and a US are paired. Conditioning will occur only if the CS is informative, only if it predicts something important, such as an upcoming shock. This view seems to imply that the subject has a more active role in the conditioning process than was previously thought; that is, the subject is a selective learner, learning about informative stimuli and ignoring uninformative stimuli. For

two psychologists, Robert Rescorla and Allan Wagner (1972), the blocking effect and related findings underscored the need for a new theory of classical conditioning, one that could deal with these loose notions of informativeness and predictiveness in a more rigorous, objective way. The Rescorla–Wagner model has become one of the most famous theories of classical conditioning.

The Rescorla–Wagner Model

The **Rescorla–Wagner model** is a mathematical model about classical conditioning, and for some people the math makes the model difficult to understand. However, the basic ideas behind the theory are quite simple and reasonable, and they can be explained without the math. This section is designed to give you a good understanding of the concepts behind the model without using any equations.

Classical conditioning can be viewed as a means of learning about signals (CSs) for important events (USs). The Rescorla–Wagner model is designed to predict the outcome of classical conditioning procedures on a trial-by-trial basis. For any trial in which one or more CSs are presented, the model assumes that there can be excitatory conditioning, inhibitory conditioning, or no conditioning at all. According to the model, two factors determine which of these three possibilities actually occurs: (1) the strength of the subject's expectation of what will occur and (2) the strength of the US that is actually presented. The model is a mathematical expression of the concept of *surprise:* It states that learning will occur only when the subject is surprised, that is, when what actually happens is different from what the subject expected to happen.

You should be able to grasp the general idea of the model if you learn and understand the following six rules:

1. If the strength of the actual US is greater than the strength of the subject's expectation, all CSs that were paired with the US will receive excitatory conditioning.

2. If the strength of the actual US is less than the strength of the subject's expectation, all the CSs that were paired with the US will receive some inhibitory conditioning.
3. If the strength of the actual US is equal to the strength of the subject's expectation, there will be no conditioning.
4. The larger the discrepancy between the strength of the expectation and the strength of the US, the greater the conditioning (either excitatory or inhibitory) that occurs.
5. More salient (more noticeable) CSs will condition faster than less salient (less noticeable) CSs.
6. If two or more CSs are presented together, the subject's expectation will be equal to their total strength (with excitatory and inhibitory stimuli tending to cancel each other out).

We will now examine several different examples to illustrate how each of these six rules applies in specific cases. For all of the examples, imagine that a rat receives a conditioning procedure in which a CS (a light, a tone, or some other signal) is followed by food as a US. In this conditioning situation, the CR is activity, as measured by the rat's movement around the conditioning chamber (which can be automatically recorded by movement detectors). In actual experiments using this procedure, the typical result is that as conditioning proceeds, the rat becomes more and more active when the CS is presented, so its movement can be used as a measure of the amount of excitatory conditioning.

ACQUISITION.   Consider a case in which a light (L) is paired with one food pellet (Figure 4-2). On the very first conditioning trial, the rat has no expectation of what will follow L, so the strength of the US (the food pellet) is much greater than the strength of the rat's expectation (which is zero). Therefore, this trial produces some excitatory conditioning (Rule 1). But conditioning is rarely complete after just one trial. The second time L is presented, it will elicit a weak expectation, but it is still not as strong as the actual US, so Rule 1 applies again, and more excitatory conditioning occurs. For the same reason, further excitatory conditioning should take place on trials 3, 4, and so on. However, with each conditioning trial, the rat's expectation of the food pellet should get stronger, and so the difference between the strength of the expectation and the strength of the US gets smaller. Therefore, the fastest growth in excitatory conditioning occurs on the first trial, and there is less and less additional conditioning as the trials proceed (Rule 4). Eventually, when L elicits an expectation of food that is as strong as the actual food pellet itself, the asymptote of learning is reached, and no further excitatory conditioning will occur with any additional L and food pairings.

BLOCKING.   Continuing with this same example, now suppose that after the asymptote of conditioning is reached for L, a compound CS of L and tone (T) are presented together and are followed by one food pellet (Figure 4-3). According to Rule 6, when two CSs are presented, the subject's expectation is based on the total expectations from the two. T is a new stimulus, so it has no expectations associated

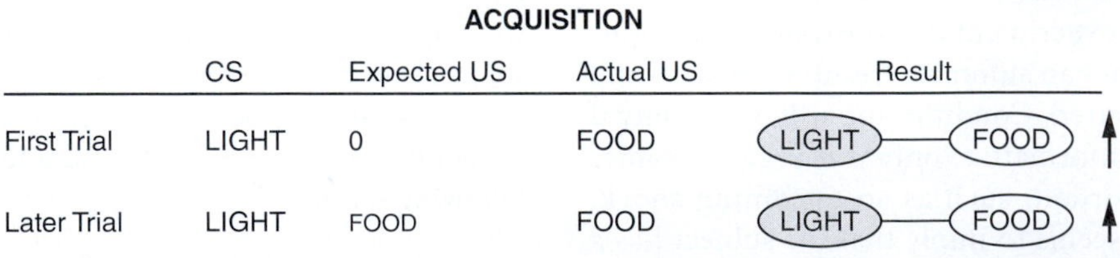

ACQUISITION

	CS	Expected US	Actual US	Result	
First Trial	LIGHT	0	FOOD	(LIGHT)——(FOOD)	↑
Later Trial	LIGHT	FOOD	FOOD	(LIGHT)——(FOOD)	↑

FIGURE 4-2 According to the Rescorla–Wagner model, during acquisition, the actual US is greater than the expected US, so there is excitatory conditioning (an increase in the strength of the CS–US association). The strength of the expected US is greater on later acquisition trials, so the amount of conditioning is not as great as on the first trial.

BLOCKING AFTER LIGHT HAS BEEN CONDITIONED

CS	Expected US	Actual US	Result
LIGHT and TONE	FOOD	FOOD	No change

FIGURE 4-3 According to the Rescorla–Wagner model, the blocking effect occurs because there is no learning on a conditioning trial if the expected US is equal to the actual US.

EXTINCTION

CS	Expected US	Actual US	Result
LIGHT	FOOD	0	LIGHT — FOOD ↓

FIGURE 4-4 According to the Rescorla–Wagner model, during extinction, the expected US is greater than the actual US, so there is inhibitory conditioning (a decrease in the strength of the CS–US association).

with it, but L produces an expectation of one food pellet. One food pellet is in fact what the animal receives, so the expected US matches the actual US, and no additional conditioning occurs (Rule 3); that is, L retains its excitatory strength, and T retains zero strength.

This, in short, is how the Rescorla–Wagner model explains the blocking effect: No conditioning occurs to the added CS because there is no surprise—the strength of the subject's expectation matches the strength of the US.

How could the blocking effect be prevented? According to the Rescorla–Wagner model, one way would be to increase the size of the US when L and T are presented together in Phase 2 (e.g., by delivering two food pellets instead of one). If the animal is expecting one food pellet but receives two, this increase in the strength of the US should lead to excitatory conditioning of both L and T. Studies have shown that increasing the size of the US in Phase 2 does indeed lead to "unblocking" (Bradfield & McNally, 2008).

EXTINCTION AND CONDITIONED INHIBITION. Suppose that after conditioning with L, a rat receives extinction trials in which L is presented without food (Figure 4-4). The expected US is food, but the actual US is nothing (i.e., no food is presented). This is a case where the strength of the expected US is greater than that of the actual US, so according to Rule 2, there will be a decrease in the association between L and food. Further extinction trials will cause more and more decline in the association between L and food.

Now think about a slightly different example. Suppose that after conditioning with L has reached its asymptote, the rat receives trials in which L and T are presented together, but no food pellet is delivered on these trials. This is another case where Rule 2 applies: The strength of the expected US will be greater than the strength of the actual US. According to Rule 2, both CSs, L and T, will acquire some inhibitory conditioning on these extinction trials.

Let us be clear about how this inhibitory conditioning will affect L and T. Because L starts with a strong excitatory strength, the trials without food (and the inhibitory conditioning they produce) will begin to counteract the excitatory strength. This is just another example of extinction. In contrast, T begins the extinction phase with zero strength, because it has not been presented before. Therefore, the trials without food (and the inhibitory conditioning they produce) will cause T's strength to decrease below zero—it will become a conditioned inhibitor.

OVERSHADOWING. In a conditioning experiment with a compound CS consisting of one intense stimulus and one weak one, Pavlov discovered

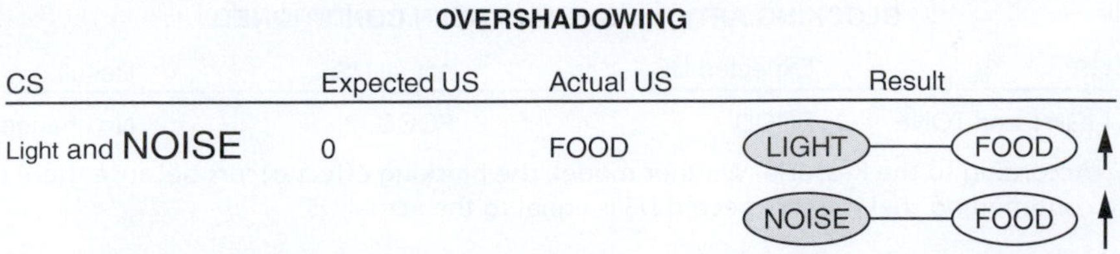

OVERSHADOWING

CS	Expected US	Actual US	Result

Light and NOISE   0   FOOD

FIGURE 4-5   According to the Rescorla–Wagner model, overshadowing occurs because the amount of conditioning depends on the salience of a stimulus. Here, the noise is more salient, so there is a larger increase in the noise–food association than in the light–food association.

a phenomenon he called **overshadowing**. After a number of conditioning trials, the intense CS would produce a strong CR if presented by itself, but the weak CS by itself would elicit little, if any, conditioned responding. It was not the case that the weak CS was simply too small to become an effective CS, because if it were paired with the US by itself, it would soon elicit CRs on its own. However, when presented in conjunction with a more intense CS, the intense CS seemed to mask, or overshadow, the weaker CS. Overshadowing has been observed in experiments with both animal and human subjects (Spetch, 1995).

The Rescorla–Wagner model's explanation of overshadowing is straightforward (Figure 4-5). According to Rule 5, more salient stimuli will condition faster than less salient stimuli. If, for example, a dim light and a loud noise are presented together and followed by a food pellet, the noise will acquire excitatory strength faster than the light. When the total expectation based on both the noise and the light equals the strength of the actual US, food, conditioning will stop. Because the noise is more salient, it will have developed much more excitatory strength than the light. If the dim light is presented by itself, it should elicit only a weak CR.

THE OVEREXPECTATION EFFECT.   One characteristic of a good theory is the ability to stimulate new research by making new predictions that have not been previously tested. The Rescorla–Wagner model deserves good grades on this count, because hundreds of experiments have been conducted to test the model's predictions. Its prediction of a phenomenon known as the **overexpectation effect** is a good case in point.

Figure 4-6 presents the design of an experiment that tests the overexpectation effect. Two CSs, L and T, are involved. For Phase 1, the notation L^+, T^+ means that on some trials L is presented by itself and followed by a food pellet, and on other trials T is presented by itself and followed by a food pellet. The two types of trials, L^+ and T^+, are randomly intermixed in Phase 1. Consider what should happen on each type of trial. On L^+ trials, the strength of the expectation based on L will continue to increase and eventually approach the strength of one food pellet. Similarly, on T^+ trials, the strength of the expectation based on T will grow and also approach the strength of one food pellet. Note that because L and T are never presented together, the conditioned strengths of both stimuli can individually approach the strength of one food pellet. To put it simply, at

Group	Phase 1	Phase 2	Test Phase	Results
Overexpectation	L^+, T^+	LT^+	L, T	moderate CRs
Control	L^+, T^+	no stimuli	L, T	strong CRs

FIGURE 4-6   Design of an experiment on the overexpectation effect.

the end of Phase 1, the rat expects one food pellet when L is presented, and it also expects one food pellet when T is presented.

In Phase 2, rats in the control group receive no stimuli, so no expectations are changed. Therefore, in the test phase, these rats should exhibit a strong CR to both L and T on the first several test trials (which are extinction trials).

The results should be quite different for rats in the overexpectation group. In Phase 2, these rats receive a series of trials with the compound stimulus, LT, followed by one food pellet. On the first trial of Phase 2, a rat's total expectation, based on the sums of the strengths of L and T, should be roughly equal to the strength of two food pellets (because each stimulus has a strength of about one food pellet). Loosely speaking, we might say that the rat expects a larger US on the compound trial because two strong CSs are presented, but all it gets is a single food pellet (Figure 4-7). Thus, compared to what it actually receives, the animal has an overexpectation about the size of the US, and Rule 2 states that under these conditions, both CSs will experience some inhibitory conditioning (they will lose some of their associative strength).

With further trials in Phase 2 for the overexpectation group, the strengths of L and T should continue to decrease, as long as the total expectation from the two CSs is greater than the strength of one food pellet. When tested in the next phase, the individual stimuli L and T should exhibit weaker CRs in the overexpectation group because their strengths were weakened in Phase 2. Experiments have confirmed this prediction that CRs will be weaker in the overexpectation group than in the control group (Khallad & Moore, 1996; Kremer, 1978).

The model's accurate prediction of the overexpectation effect is especially impressive because the prediction is counterintuitive. If you knew nothing about the Rescorla–Wagner model when you examined Figure 4-7, what result would you predict for this experiment? Notice that subjects in the overexpectation group actually receive more pairings of L and T with the US, so the frequency principle would predict stronger CRs in the overexpectation group. Based on the frequency principle, the last thing we would expect from more CS–US pairings is a weakening of the CS–US associations. Yet this result is predicted by the Rescorla–Wagner model, and the prediction turns out to be correct.

SUMMARY. The Rescorla–Wagner model might be called a theory about *US effectiveness*: It states that an unpredicted US is effective in promoting learning, whereas a well-predicted US is ineffective. As the first formal theory that attempted to predict when a US will promote associative learning and when it will not, it is guaranteed a prominent place in the history of psychology. The model has been successfully applied to many conditioning phenomena, but it is not perfect. Some research findings are difficult for the model to explain. In the Other Theories

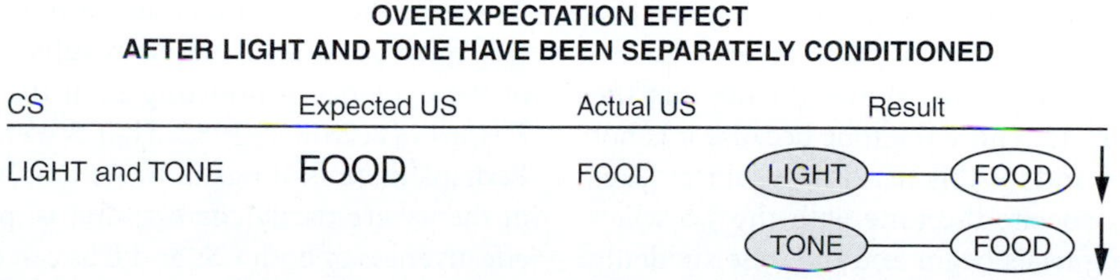

OVEREXPECTATION EFFECT
AFTER LIGHT AND TONE HAVE BEEN SEPARATELY CONDITIONED

CS	Expected US	Actual US	Result
LIGHT and TONE	FOOD	FOOD	LIGHT — FOOD ↓
			TONE — FOOD ↓

FIGURE 4-7 According to the Rescorla–Wagner model, the overexpectation effect occurs because when two separately conditioned stimuli are presented together, the expected US is greater than the actual US, so there is inhibitory conditioning (a decrease in the strength of each CS–food association).

section, we will take a brief look at some of these findings, and at alternative theories of classical conditioning that are based on fairly different assumptions about the learning process.

Other Theories

THEORIES OF ATTENTION.   Some theories of classical conditioning focus on how much attention the learner pays to the CS (e.g., Mackintosh, 1975; Pearce & Hall, 1980). One common feature of these theories is the assumption that the learner will pay attention to informative CSs but not to uninformative CSs. If the learner does not pay attention to a CS, there will be no conditioning of that CS. These theories might also be called *theories of CS effectiveness,* because they assume that the conditionability of a CS, not the effectiveness of the US, changes from one situation to another. A phenomenon called the **CS preexposure effect** provides one compelling piece of evidence for this assumption.

The **CS preexposure effect** is the finding that classical conditioning proceeds more slowly if a CS is repeatedly presented by itself before it is paired with the US. Imagine a simple conditioning experiment with two groups of rats. The control group receives simple pairings of a tone (the CS) and food (the US). The only difference in the CS preexposure group is that before the conditioning trials, the tone is presented by itself a number of times. With both animal and human subjects, conditioning proceeds more rapidly in the control group than in the CS preexposure group (Lubow & Moore, 1959; Zalstein-Orda & Lubow, 1995). A commonsense explanation is that because the tone is presented repeatedly but initially predicts nothing during CS preexposure, the subject gradually pays less and less attention to this stimulus. We might say that the subject learns to ignore the tone because it is not informative, and for this reason the subject takes longer to associate the tone with the US when conditioning trials begin and the tone suddenly becomes informative.

The problem for the Rescorla–Wagner model is that it does not predict the CS preexposure effect.

It is easy to see why. When a new CS is presented by itself, the expected US is zero, and the actual US is zero. Because the expected US equals the actual US, according to the Rescola–Wagner model there should be no learning of any kind. But evidently, subjects do learn something on CS preexposure trials, and what they learn hinders their ability to develop a CS–US association when the two stimuli are paired in at a later time.

Unlike the Rescorla–Wagner model, attentional theories such as those of Mackintosh (1975) and Pearce and Hall (1980) can easily explain the CS preexposure effect: Because the CS predicts nothing during the preexposure period, attention to the CS decreases, and so conditioning is slower when the CS is first paired with the US at the beginning of the conditioning phase. The attentional theories can also account for other basic conditioning phenomena. As one example, we can examine how Mackintosh's (1975) theory explains Kamin's blocking effect. Mackintosh assumes that attention to a CS changes with experience in the following way. If we have two stimuli, L and T, and L is a better predictor of the US than T, then attention to L will increase and attention to T will decrease and eventually reach zero. In other words, the subject will attend to the more informative stimulus, L, but not to T. Now consider what this theory predicts for the second phase of a blocking experiment, as diagrammed in Figure 4-1. In the blocking group, L will be more informative than T because of the conditioning that took place in Phase 1. T predicts nothing new for the animals in the blocking group, so attention to T drops to zero, and if this drop is rapid, there will be little learning about T in Phase 2.

Experiments designed to compare the Rescorla–Wagner model and attentional theories have produced mixed results, with some of the evidence supporting each theory (Balaz, Kasprow, & Miller, 1982; Hall & Pearce, 1983). Perhaps these findings indicate that both classes of theory are partly correct; that is, perhaps the effectiveness of both CSs and USs can change as a result of a subject's experience. If a US is well predicted, it may promote no conditioning (which is the basic premise of the Rescorla–Wagner model). Likewise, if nothing surprising follows a CS, it may become ineffective (the basic premise of the attentional theories).

COMPARATOR THEORIES OF CONDITIONING. Other theories of classical conditioning, called **comparator theories**, assume that the animal compares the likelihood that the US will occur in the presence of the CS with the likelihood that the US will occur in the absence of the CS (Miller & Schachtman, 1985; Stout & Miller, 2007). This idea may sound familiar because it is fairly similar to Rescorla's (1968, 1969) analysis of CS–US correlations, discussed in Chapter 3.

Comparator theories differ from those we have already examined in two ways. First, comparator theories do not make predictions on a trial-by-trial basis, because they assume that what is important is not the events of individual trials but rather the overall, long-term correlation between a CS and a US. Second, comparator theories propose that the correlation between CS and US does not affect the learning of a CR but rather its performance. As a simple example, suppose that the probability of a US is 50% in the presence of some CS, but its probability is also 50% in the absence of this CS. The comparator theories predict that this CS will elicit no CR, which is what Rescorla (1968) found, but not because the CS has acquired no excitatory strength. Instead, the theories assume that both the CS and **contextual stimuli**—the sights, sounds, and smells of the experimental chamber—have acquired equal excitatory strengths, because both have been paired with the US 50% of the time. Comparator theories also assume that a CS will not elicit a CR unless it has greater excitatory strength than the contextual stimuli. Unlike the Rescorla–Wagner model, however, comparator theories assume that an animal in this situation has indeed learned something about the CS—that the US sometimes occurs in its presence—but the animal will not respond to the CS unless it is a better predictor of the US than the context.

To test comparator theories, one common research strategy is to change the strength of one stimulus and try to show that the conditioned responding changes to another stimulus. For example, suppose that after conditioning, an animal exhibits only a weak CR to a light because both the light and the contextual stimuli have some excitatory strength. According to comparator theories, one way to increase the response to the light would be to extinguish the excitatory strength of the context by keeping the subject in the context and never presenting the US. If the response to the light depends on a comparison of the light and the context, extinction of the context should increase the response to the light. Experiments of this type have shown that extinction of the context does increase responding to the CS (Matzel, Brown, & Miller, 1987).

In a related experiment by Cole, Barnet, and Miller (1995), one CS was followed by a US every time it was presented, whereas a second CS was followed by a US only 50% of the time. At first, the second CS did not elicit much conditioned responding. However, after responding to the first CS was extinguished, CRs to the second CS increased dramatically. The Rescorla–Wagner model does not predict these effects, because it states that the conditioned strength of one CS cannot change if that CS itself is not presented. According to comparator theories, however, subjects may learn an association between a CS and a US that cannot initially be seen in their performance, but this learning can be unmasked if the strength of a competing CS is weakened.

Research designed to test comparator theories has provided mixed results. Some studies have provided support for this approach (e.g., Leader, Loughnane, McMoreland, & Reed, 2009; Yin, Barnet, & Miller, 1994), whereas other studies have supported the predictions of traditional associative learning theories such as the Rescorla–Wagner model (Ayres, Bombace, Shurtleff, & Vigorito, 1985; Dopson, Pearce, & Haselgrove, 2009; Rauhut, McPhee, DiPietro, & Ayres, 2000). Because there is evidence supporting both types of theories, it may be that future theories of classical conditioning will need to take into account both learning and performance variables to accommodate the diverse findings that researchers have obtained.

Summary

In this section we have examined the Rescorla–Wagner model, attentional theories, and comparator theories. In recent years, other theories about classical conditioning have been proposed, including those that emphasize the temporal relationships between CS and US (Balsam & Gallistel, 2009; Gallistel & Gibbon, 2002) or the storage and retrieval of information in a complex neural network (Schmajuk, 2010; Schmajuk & Larrauri, 2006). Describing all of these different theories and their strengths and weaknesses is well beyond the scope of this chapter, and there is currently no agreement among researchers about which theory is best.

Although many questions remain unanswered, substantial progress has been made toward the goal of understanding the processes of classical conditioning. The theories that we have examined differ in many ways, but they share one common theme that is important to remember: The predictiveness or informativeness of a stimulus is a critical determinant of whether a CR will occur. And the predictiveness or informativeness of a stimulus cannot be judged in isolation: It must be compared to the predictiveness of other stimuli also present in the learner's environment.

TYPES OF ASSOCIATIONS

Associations in First-Order Conditioning

Chapter 3 considered the question of whether an S-S or an S-R association is formed during simple first-order conditioning. As explained in that chapter, experiments using US devaluation (in which the ability of the US to evoke a UR is diminished in one way or another after the CS has been conditioned) tended to support the S-S position. That is, any change that decreases the ability of the US to evoke a response also decreases the ability of the CS to evoke this response. These results favor the S-S position and the more indirect route from CS center to response center in Figure 3-4, because the response-eliciting capacity of the CS seems to be tied to the response-eliciting capacity of the US.

Associations in Second-Order Conditioning

Compared to the findings on first-order conditioning, studies on the associations formed during second-order conditioning have painted a more complex and confusing picture. Imagine an experiment with rats in which a light is paired with food and the CR to the light is an increase in activity. Food is the US, and light is CS1 (the first-order conditioned stimulus). Next, a tone (the second-order conditioned stimulus, CS2) is repeatedly paired with the light, and second-order conditioning is eventually demonstrated—the tone now also elicits an increase in activity. What sorts of associations make the CR to the tone possible? Based on the evidence for S-S associations in first-order conditioning, you might guess that an S-S-S association was involved in second-order conditioning (i.e., the tone is associated with the light, which is associated with the food, which leads to the increased activity). This is a sensible guess, but it is wrong. When Holland and Rescorla (1975) conducted this experiment, they found evidence for a direct S-R association between the tone center and the response center. Their method involved devaluing the US by satiating the rats and then retesting their responses to the tone. Activity responses in the presence of the tone were not diminished, even though the animals showed little interest in eating the food. Holland and Rescorla concluded that S-S associations are formed in first-order conditioning, but that S-R associations are formed in second-order conditioning.

Other experiments, however, have found evidence for second-order S-S associations (Rashotte, Griffin, & Sisk, 1977; Rescorla, 1982). Why S-S associations are found in some cases of second-order conditioning and S-R associations are found in others is still not fully understood, but certain procedural differences (such as whether CS2 and CS1 are paired by presenting them simultaneously or one after the other) can make a big difference (Holland, 1986; Rescorla, 1982). In any case, one general conclusion we can draw about associations in second-order conditioning is that they do not fall into any single category: Both S-S and S-R associations can and do occur.

Associations with Contextual Stimuli

No experiment on classical conditioning takes place in a vacuum. As discussed earlier in this chapter, an experimental chamber inevitably contains a variety of distinctive sights, sounds, and smells that are collectively called contextual stimuli. When a stimulus is repeatedly presented in one experimental chamber, an association can develop between the contextual stimuli and that stimulus. For instance, if a light is occasionally presented in the chamber, the animal may form a *context–CS association* (an association between the context and the light), and we might say the animal learns to "expect" the light when it is placed in the chamber. This might help explain the CS preexposure effect: Because the light is no longer a surprising stimulus, it becomes harder to condition if it is now paired with a US. But it should be possible to reverse the CS preexposure effect by repeatedly placing the animal in the context without presenting the light. When this is done, the effects of CS preexposure are reversed, and the CS again becomes easier to condition when paired with a US (Wagner, 1978).

Other studies have provided parallel evidence for the existence of *context–US associations* when a US is repeatedly presented in a given context (Domjan & Best, 1980). Rescorla, Durlach, and Grau (1985) demonstrated several standard conditioning phenomena with context–US associations: acquisition, extinction, discrimination, and discrimination reversal (in which the roles of CS^+ and CS^- are reversed). It has also been shown that if an animal first learns a context–US association, this can interfere with the acquisition of a CS–US association (Williams, MacKenzie, & Johns, 2010). In many ways, associations involving contextual stimuli behave similarly to associations involving CSs and USs.

CS–CS Associations

Besides learning associations between a CS and a US, animals can also acquire associations between two CSs. In **sensory preconditioning**, two CSs are repeatedly paired *before* the US is introduced. For example, in the first phase of an experiment,

rabbits could be given trials in which a light and tone are presented together. In the second phase of the experiment, they receive trials in which the light is followed by an air puff, and the rabbits eventually start to blink when the light is presented. In the final phase of the experiment (the test phase), the tone is now presented by itself, and if the rabbit blinks to the tone, this is a successful demonstration of sensory preconditioning. Experiments of this type have demonstrated that sensory preconditioning does occur (Batsell, Trost, Cochran, Blankenship, & Batson, 2003; Brogden, 1939; Pfautz, Donegan, & Wagner, 1978). These results provide further evidence for the existence of S-S associations, and they show that these associations can form between two "neutral" stimuli as well as between a CS and a US.

Occasion Setting

An excitatory CS tends to elicit a CR, and an inhibitory CS tends to prevent the occurrence of a CR. However, these are not the only ways a CS can affect an animal's behavior. Experiments by Holland (1991; Ross & Holland, 1981) suggest a third possibility. Holland has found that under certain circumstances a stimulus can control a CR in an indirect way: It can determine whether the subject will respond to another CS. For instance, in one experiment with rats, Ross and Holland (1981) arranged two types of trials. On half of the trials, a light was presented for a few seconds, followed by a tone for a few seconds, followed by food. On the other trials, the tone was presented by itself, and there was no food. Thus, the presence of the light meant that the tone would be followed by food. From previous research, the experimenters knew that when a tone is paired with food, it elicits a distinctive "head-jerk" CR in rats; that is, the animal repeatedly moves its head from side to side (as though it is looking for the source of the sound). In this experiment, Ross and Holland found that the tone elicited this head-jerk response when it was preceded by the light, but not otherwise. In other words, the light seemed to regulate the CR to the tone. Ross and Holland called the light an **occasion setter**, because it signaled those occasions on which the

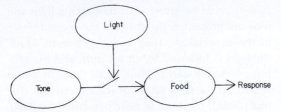

FIGURE 4-8   One theory of how a light can act as an occasion setter for a tone. The light might act like a switch that completes the tone–food connection.

tone would be paired with food (and those occasions on which the tone would elicit a CR).

Holland favored the hypothesis that an occasion setter regulates a CS–US association. The idea is that an occasion setter (the light) acts as a sort of switch that must be turned on to complete the connection between tone and food (Figure 4-8). However, additional research has shown that occasion setters have some interesting and unusual properties that make them more complex than a simple switching mechanism (Bonardi & Jennings, 2009; Maes & Vossen, 1993). Although the nature of occasion setters is still being studied, we can be confident about one conclusion: Occasion setters are certainly different from ordinary excitatory or inhibitory CSs.

Summary

Some of the types of associations we have examined are summarized in Figure 4-9, which depicts the possible consequences of repeatedly pairing a compound CS (a light and a tone) with a food US.

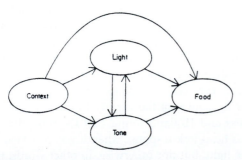

FIGURE 4-9   The associations that may form when a compound stimulus composed of a light and a tone is paired with food.

PRACTICE QUIZ (1)

1. According to the Rescorla–Wagner model, excitatory conditioning occurs when the _____ is greater than the _____.
2. According to the Rescorla–Wagner model, extinction is a case where the _____ is greater than the _____, so _____ conditioning occurs.
3. Comparator theories state that a CS will produce a CR if it is a better predictor of the US than the _____.
4. If two different tastes are paired, and then one is associated with illness, an animal may show an aversion to the other taste as well. This is an example of a _____ association.
5. If a tone elicits a fear response when it is preceded by a light, but not otherwise, the light can be called _____.

Answers

1. actual US, expected US 2. expected US, actual US, inhibitory 3. contextual stimuli 4. CS–CS 5. an occasion setter

In addition to the light–food and tone–food associations, CS–CS associations can form between the light and the tone, and each of these three stimuli can become associated with the context. Still other associations can develop in second-order conditioning and occasion-setting situations. In addition, each type of association can be either excitatory or inhibitory. Therefore, although classical conditioning might be loosely described as a procedure in which the subject learns to associate a CS and a US, in reality a rich array of associations can develop in any classical conditioning situation.

BIOLOGICAL CONSTRAINTS ON CLASSICAL CONDITIONING

As discussed in Chapter 1, probably the most fundamental assumption underlying research on animal learning is that it is possible to discover general principles of learning that are not dependent in any important way on an animal's biological makeup. According to this line of reasoning, the same general principles of learning will be discovered regardless of what species of subject, what response, and what stimuli one chooses to study. If this assumption turned out to be wrong, the extensive research on the arbitrary responses (e.g., eyeblink conditioning, conditioned suppression) of a small number of species (rabbits, rats) in artificial environments would make little sense. Why would psychologists care, for example, about how different CS–US relationships affect a rat's responding in a conditioned suppression procedure if completely different patterns were likely with different mammals, or with different CSs or USs?

During the 1960s, researchers began to report findings that questioned the validity of the general-principle approach to learning. For the most part, these findings took the form of alleged exceptions to some of the best-known general principles of learning. As this type of evidence began to accumulate, some psychologists started to question whether the goal of discovering general principles of learning was realistic (Lockard, 1971; Rozin & Kalat, 1971; Seligman, 1970). They reasoned, if we find too many exceptions to a rule, what good is the rule?

This section will examine the evidence against the general-principle approach in the area of classical conditioning, and it will attempt to come to some conclusions about its significance for the psychology of learning. Biological constraints on other types of learning will be discussed in later chapters.

The Contiguity Principle and Taste-Aversion Learning

As discussed in Chapter 1, the principle of contiguity is the oldest and most persistent principle of association, having been first proposed by Aristotle. We have seen that CS–US contiguity is an important independent variable in classical conditioning: In trace conditioning, the separation of CS and US by only a few seconds can produce large decreases in both the rate and asymptote of conditioning. A popular textbook from the

early 1960s summarized the opinion about the importance of contiguity that prevailed at that time: "At the present time it seems unlikely that learning can take place at all with delays of more than a few seconds" (Kimble, 1961, p. 165).

Given this opinion about the importance of contiguity, it is easy to see why the work of John Garcia and colleagues on long-delay learning attracted considerable attention. Garcia's research involved a classical conditioning procedure in which poison was the US and some novel taste was the CS. In one study (Garcia, Ervin, & Koelling, 1966), rats were given the opportunity to drink saccharin-flavored water (which they had never tasted before), and they later received an injection of a drug that produces nausea in a matter of minutes. For different rats the interval between drinking and the drug injection varied from 5 to 22 minutes. Although these durations were perhaps a hundred times longer than those over which classical conditioning was generally thought to be effective, all subjects developed aversions to water flavored with saccharin. A second experiment found that rats developed aversions to the taste of saccharin when the drug was delayed more than an hour. Later, Etscorn and Stephens (1973) found aversions to saccharin when a full 24 hours separated the CS from the poison US.

Many experiments on taste-aversion learning have been conducted since the initial research by Garcia, and it has been found that taste aversions can be acquired by many different species when the CS–US interval is several hours long. This learning ability is certainly adaptive: If an animal in the wild eats a poisonous food, it may not become ill until many hours later. Creatures that have the ability to associate their illness with what they have previously eaten will be able to avoid that food in the future and thereby have a better chance of survival. However, because the effective CS–US intervals are many times longer than in traditional experiments on classical conditioning, some psychologists proposed that taste-aversion learning is a special type of learning, one that does not obey the principle of contiguity. Taste-aversion learning was seen by some as an exception to one of the most basic principles of association. As the Biological Preparedness in Taste-Aversion Learning section shows, taste-aversion learning was also involved in another line of attack on the general-principle approach.

Biological Preparedness in Taste-Aversion Learning

A crucial assumption underlying most research on classical conditioning is that the experimenter's choice of stimuli, responses, and species of subject is relatively unimportant. Suppose, for example, that an experimenter wishes to test some hypothesis about learning using the salivary conditioning preparation. The subjects will be dogs, and the US will be food powder, but what stimulus should be used as the CS? According to what Seligman and Hager (1972) called the **equipotentiality premise**, it does not matter what stimulus is used; the decision is entirely arbitrary. The following quotation from Pavlov (1928) documents his belief in the equipotentiality premise: "Any natural phenomenon chosen at will may be converted into a conditional stimulus . . . any visual stimulus, any desired sound, any odor, and the stimulation of any part of the skin" (p. 86).

The equipotentiality premise does not state that all stimuli and all responses will result in equally rapid learning. Pavlov himself recognized that different CSs will condition at different rates: A bright light will acquire a CR more rapidly than a dim light. Yet although stimuli (and responses) certainly differ in their conditionability, the equipotentiality premise states that a stimulus (or a response) that is difficult to condition in one context should also be difficult to condition in other contexts. For example, if a dim light is a poor CS in a salivary conditioning experiment, it should also be a poor CS in an eyeblink conditioning experiment. In short, the equipotentiality premise states that a given stimulus will be an equally good (or equally bad) CS in all contexts.

The simplicity of the equipotentiality premise might seem appealing, but plenty of evidence has shown that it is wrong. Garcia and Koelling (1966) conducted an important experiment showing that

the same two stimuli can be differentially effective in different contexts. Two groups of rats were each presented with a compound stimulus consisting of both taste and audiovisual components. Each rat received water that had a distinctive flavor, and whenever the rat drank the water, it was presented with flashing lights and a clicking noise. For one group, the procedure consisted of typical taste-aversion learning: After drinking the water, a rat was injected with a poison, and it soon became ill. For the second group, there was no poison; instead, a rat's paws were shocked whenever it drank. In summary, both groups of rats received pairings of both taste and audiovisual stimuli with an aversive event, but the aversive event was illness for one group and shock for the other.

Garcia and Koelling wanted to determine how strongly the two types of stimuli (taste and audiovisual) were associated with the two different aversive consequences. To do so, they conducted extinction tests (no shock or poison present) in which the taste and audiovisual stimuli were presented separately. The results were very different for the two groups. The group that received poison showed a greater aversion to the saccharin taste than to the lights and noises. However, exactly the opposite pattern was observed for the group that received the shock. These animals consumed almost as much of the saccharine-flavored water as in baseline, but when drinking was accompanied by the lights and noises, they drank very little.

What can we conclude about the stimuli used in this experiment? Which was the better stimulus, taste or the audiovisual stimuli? What was the more effective aversive event, shock or illness? There is no simple answer to these questions. Taste was a more effective stimulus when the aversive event was poison, but the audiovisual stimulus was more effective when the aversive event was shock. Figure 4-10 summarizes the results of this experiment, using thick arrows to represent strong associations and thin arrows to represent weak associations. Garcia and his colleagues concluded that before we can predict the strength of a CR, we must know something about the *relationship* between the CS and the US.

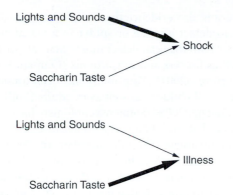

FIGURE 4-10 The results of the Garcia and Koelling (1966) experiment are summarized by using thick arrows to represent strong associations and thin arrows to represent weak associations. The rats that had shock as the US acquired a strong association between the lights and noises and shock, but only a weak association between the taste of saccharin and shock. The opposite was found for rats that experienced illness from a poison after exposure to the saccharin, lights, and noises.

They suggested that because of a rat's biological makeup, it has an innate tendency to associate illness with the taste of the food it had previously eaten. The rat is much less likely to associate illness with visual or auditory stimuli that are present when a food is eaten. On the other hand, the rat is more likely to associate a painful event like shock with external auditory and visual stimuli than with a taste stimulus.

Seligman (1970) suggested that some CS–US associations might be called **prepared associations** because the animal has an innate propensity to form such associations quickly and easily (e.g., a taste–illness association). Other potential associations might be called *contraprepared associations,* because even after many pairings, a subject may have difficulty forming an association between the two stimuli (such as taste and shock). In between are *unprepared associations*—those for which the creature has no special predisposition, but which can nevertheless be formed after a moderate number of pairings.

It should be clear that Seligman's concept of preparedness is at odds with the equipotentiality premise. It implies that to predict how effective a particular CS will be, it is not enough to know how effective this CS has been in other contexts. We must also know what US will be used and whether this CS–US pair is an example of a prepared, unprepared, or contraprepared association. To complicate matters further, the predisposition to associate two stimuli can vary across different species. Although rats may be predisposed to associate taste stimuli with illness, other animals may not be. Wilcoxon, Dragoin, and Kral (1971) compared the behaviors of rats and bobwhite quail that became ill after drinking water that had a distinctive (sour) taste, or water with a distinctive (dark blue) color, or water that both tasted sour and was dark blue. As we would expect, rats displayed aversions to the sour taste but not to the blue color. In contrast, quail developed aversions both to the sour water and the blue water, and the blue color was actually the more effective stimulus for these animals.

Wilcoxon and his colleagues hypothesized that the differences between rats and quail are related to their methods of obtaining food in the natural environment. Rats have excellent senses of taste and smell but relatively poor vision, and they normally forage for food at night. Quail are daytime feeders, and they have excellent vision, which they use in searching for food. It makes sense that those stimuli that are most important for a given species at the time of ingestion are also those that are most readily associated with illness. Therefore, an analysis of a creature's lifestyle in its natural environment may provide clues about which associations are prepared, unprepared, and contraprepared for that creature. These findings show that attempting to generalize about preparedness or ease of learning from one species to another can be a dangerous strategy.

Biological Preparedness in Human Learning

People can also develop a strong aversion to a food that is followed by illness, even if the illness follows ingestion of the food by several hours. Logue, Ophir, and Strauss (1981) used questionnaires to ask several hundred college students about any food aversions they might have that developed as a result of an illness that occurred after they ate the food. Of the 65% who reported at least one aversion, 83% claimed that the taste of the food was now aversive to them. Smaller percentages claimed they found other sensory characteristics of the food aversive: The smell of the food was aversive for 51%, the texture of the food for 32%, and the sight of the food for only 26%. These percentages suggest that people are more similar to rats than to quail when it comes to the acquisition of food aversions following illness. In many cases, people develop an aversion to some food even though they know that their illness was caused by something completely unrelated to the food, such as the flu or chemotherapy treatment (Bernstein, Webster, & Bernstein, 1982; Scalera & Bavieri, 2009).

The other major area of research on possible preparedness in human conditioning involves the development of fears, or phobias. Öhman and colleagues have proposed that human beings have a predisposition to develop fears of things that have been dangerous to our species throughout our evolutionary history, such as snakes, spiders, and thunder (Öhman & Mineka, 2001). Quite a few experiments have tested this hypothesis. In one procedure, the CR is a person's skin conductance response (SCR, see Chapter 3), with pictures of snakes and spiders as CSs and a shock as the US. Subjects in one group learn a conditional discrimination in which pictures of snakes are followed by shock and pictures of spiders are not. In a second group, the roles of snakes and spiders are reversed. For the subjects in two control groups, pictures of flowers are followed by shock and pictures of mushrooms are not, or vice versa. The usual result of this type of study is that subjects learn the discrimination and exhibit a strong SCR to the stimulus paired with shock but not to the other stimulus. Although the acquisition of the SCR is typically just as fast with flowers and mushrooms as it is with snakes and spiders, some studies have found greater resistance to extinction in the spider/snake groups compared to the flower/mushroom groups (Öhman, Dimberg, & Ost, 1985; Schell, Dawson, & Marinkovic, 1991).

There is also evidence that people have the ability to detect a snake or spider in a visual array faster than they can detect more "neutral" stimuli such as flowers and mushrooms (Öhman, Flykt, & Esteves, 2001). This ability has been found in preschool children as well as in adults (LoBue & DeLoache, 2008). Some psychologists have suggested that this ability evolved because of its survival advantage. Overall, however, the evidence for human preparedness involving snakes and spiders is not conclusive, and there are other ways to interpret the data that do not involve biological preparedness. For example, it is possible that fear conditioning with snakes and spiders may be different than fear conditioning with other stimuli because of prior learning experiences in which we have been taught to fear these creatures, not because of a biological predisposition (Purkis & Lipp, 2009).

Dimberg and Öhman (1996) proposed that people are also predisposed to associate angry faces with aversive consequences. Their reasoning is that throughout our evolutionary history, when one person stared with an angry expression toward another person, the angry person often followed this expression with some attempt to hurt or intimidate the other person. As a result, human beings have become prepared to produce a fearful or defensive reaction to an angry face. This hypothesis has been tested with discrimination procedures similar to those used for spiders and snakes, except that angry faces are used in one group and happy or neutral faces are used in a control group. Once again, the results have been mixed; some studies found support for the preparedness hypothesis (Dimberg & Öhman, 1983), and others found none (Packer, Clark, Bond, & Siddle, 1991). Overall, the evidence for preparedness in human phobias remains inconclusive. Further research may help clarify this issue.

Biological Constraints and the General-Principle Approach

No doubt the findings of Garcia and his colleagues were a surprise to traditional learning theorists—few would have predicted that associative learning could occur with such long delays between stimuli, at least with animal subjects. In retrospect, the findings have not proven to be damaging to the general-principle approach to learning. It is true that taste-aversion learning can occur with long delays between CS and US, but long-delay learning is not found only in taste-aversion paradigms. In a series of experiments, Lett (1973, 1979) inserted delays of various lengths between a rat's choice response in a T-maze and the delivery of food (if the response was correct). During the delay, a rat was returned to its home cage so that no cues in the end of the maze could be used to bridge the delay between choice response and the food. Lett found that rats' choices of the correct arm of the maze increased over trials even when the delay interval was 60 minutes. Other studies have found learning when stimuli are separated by as much as 24 hours (Capaldi, 1966). Studies like these show that, at least in certain circumstances, animals can associate events separated by long delays in situations that do not involve taste aversions.

Besides showing that long-delay learning is not unique to taste aversions, we can also dispute the claim that taste-aversion learning violates the principle of contiguity. In essence, this principle states that individuals will more readily associate two events the more closely the events occur in time. Figure 4-11a shows the results from an experiment in which rats obtained food by pressing a lever and shocks were used to suppress the rats' responding (Baron, Kaufman, & Fazzini, 1969). As the delay between a response and shock increased, there was less and less suppression of responding, as compared to the rats' baseline response rates.

Figure 4-11b shows the results from a study on taste-aversion learning in which different groups of rats experienced different delays between their initial exposure to a saccharin solution and a poison injection (Andrews & Braveman, 1975). The graph shows the amount of saccharin consumed in a later test. Observe the similarity in the shapes of the two functions (Figure 4-11b). Both sets of results are consistent with the principle of contiguity—the shorter the interval between a response and an aversive event, the stronger the conditioning. The only major difference between the two experiments is the scale on the *x*-axis (seconds in Figure 4-11a, hours in Figure 4-11b). Taste aversions were conditioned with considerably longer delays, but this is merely a quantitative difference, not a qualitative one. That is, the results in Figure 4-11b do not require the postulation of a different law to

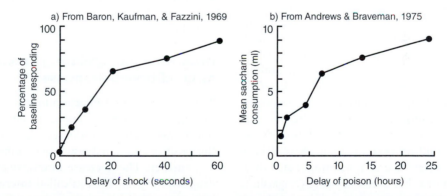

FIGURE 4-11 (a) The effects of delay between a lever press and shock in an experiment on punishment (Baron, Kaufman, & Fazzini, 1969). With increasing delays, the punishment caused less suppression of lever pressing. (b) The effect of delay between saccharin consumption and poison administration in an experiment on taste-aversion learning (Andrews & Braveman, 1975). With increasing delays, the poisoning caused less suppression of saccharin consumption.

SOURCE: An adaptation of Figure 1 from Andrews and Braveman, "The combined effects of dosage level and interstimulus interval on the formation of one-trial poison-based aversions in rats," *Animal Learning & Behavior, 3*(4), 1975. Reprinted with kind permission from Springer Science + Business Media B.V.

replace the principle of contiguity; they merely require the use of different numbers in describing the relationship between contiguity and learning.

In the 1960s and 1970s, the evidence for biological preparedness in taste-aversion learning (and in other learning situations) was also seen as a problem for the general-principle approach. This research clearly showed that some associations are more easily formed than others. Furthermore, an association that is difficult for one species to learn (e.g., between the visual appearance of a food and illness) may be easy for another species. Notice, however, that Seligman's continuum of preparedness deals with differences in the speed of learning or the amount of learning, not in the kind of learning that takes place. It is not impossible for rats to develop an association between a visual stimulus and illness; it simply requires more conditioning trials than does a taste–illness association. The same can be said for a taste–shock association. Once again, this alleged evidence against general principles of learning merely amounts to a quantitative difference, not a qualitative one. A description of the learning of prepared, unprepared, and contraprepared associations would require different numbers but not necessarily different laws.

Seligman and Hager (1972) had proposed that taste-aversion learning is a unique type of learning that does not obey the laws of traditional learning theory. However, in a review of the findings on this topic, Logue (1979) described considerable evidence that there is actually nothing unique about taste-aversion learning. She noted that many of the most familiar phenomena of classical conditioning, including generalization gradients, extinction, conditioned inhibition, blocking, and second-order conditioning, have all been observed in taste-aversion learning. Later studies have shown that overshadowing (Nagaishi & Nakajima, 2010), sensory preconditioning (Loy & Hall, 2002), and stimulus preexposure effects (Lubow, 2009) can all be observed in taste-aversion learning. Logue (1979) concluded that taste-aversion learning violates no traditional principles of learning and requires no new principles of learning, and this viewpoint is shared

by many researchers on classical conditioning (Domjan, 1983; Shettleworth, 1983). In fact, taste-aversion learning has joined the conditioned suppression and eyeblink paradigms as a commonly used procedure for investigating the general principles of classical conditioning procedure (e.g., Gottlieb & Rescorla, 2010; Schachtman, Ramsey, & Pineño, 2009). This fact, perhaps more than any other, should put to rest the notion that taste-aversion learning is inconsistent with the general-principle approach to learning theory.

THE FORM OF THE CONDITIONED RESPONSE

As we have already seen, predicting the form of a CR is often difficult. In some cases, the CR is quite similar to the UR, and in others it is the opposite of the UR. When a CR is the opposite of the UR, it is sometimes called a *compensatory CR,* because it tends to compensate for, or counteract, the UR (just as the b-process in opponent-process theory is thought to counteract the a-process). In this section, we will first investigate how classical conditioning can affect an individual's reaction to a drug. In this area of research, both mimicking and compensatory CRs have been observed. We will then examine some theories that try to explain why CRs assume the variety of forms that they do.

Drug Tolerance and Drug Cravings as Conditioned Responses

A heroin user's first injection produces a highly pleasurable response of euphoria, but with later injections of the same dosage, the intensity of this positive emotional response becomes smaller and smaller. The decrease in effectiveness of a drug with repeated use is called **tolerance**, and it occurs with many drugs. Several hypotheses about why tolerance occurs have been proposed. Typical pharmacological explanations attribute tolerance to possible physiological changes, such as a change in metabolism that allows the drug to pass through the body more quickly. According to the Solomon and Corbit theory (Chapter 2), drug tolerance is the result of an automatic strengthening of the b-process over trials. Both the pharmacological explanations and the Solomon and Corbit theory, therefore, attribute drug tolerance to a change in the individual's body that alters the way the body reacts to the drug. However, from his research on morphine and other drugs, Shepard Siegel (1975, 2005) has proposed a very different explanation of tolerance, one based on classical conditioning. In short, Siegel claims that drug tolerance is due, at least in part, to a compensatory CR that is elicited by CSs that regularly precede a drug administration. These CSs may include the contextual stimuli (environmental surroundings), the stimuli associated with drug administration (needles, drug paraphernalia, etc.), and even the early bodily sensations that occur when the drug starts to produce its effects in the body (Sokolowska, Siegel, & Kim, 2002). A description of a few of Siegel's experiments will illustrate how he came to these conclusions.

One of the URs produced by morphine is *analgesia,* or a decreased sensitivity to pain. In one experiment, Siegel (1975) found that a decrease in analgesia over successive morphine injections (i.e., tolerance of the analgesic response) was controlled by contextual stimuli. Siegel's subjects were rats, and he tested their sensitivity to pain by placing them on a metal plate that was heated to an uncomfortably warm temperature of about 54°C. When a rat's paws become painfully hot, the rat makes an easily measurable response—it lifts its forepaws and licks them. By measuring the latency of this paw-lick response, Siegel had a measure of the animal's sensitivity to pain.

Rats in a control group received four test trials (separated by 48 hours) on which they were brought into a special experimental room, given an injection of a saline solution (as a placebo), and later placed on the metal surface. The paw-lick latencies for these control subjects were short and roughly the same on all four trials, which shows that pain sensitivity for the control group did not change over trials. The procedure for one experimental group was exactly the same, except that these rats received four morphine injections,

not saline injections. On the first trial, the average paw-lick latency for this group was nearly double that of the control group. This result shows that the morphine had its expected analgesic effect. However, the latencies for this group decreased over the next three trials, and on the fourth trial, their latencies were about the same as those of the control group. Therefore, in four trials these rats had developed a tolerance to the morphine; that is, it no longer had an analgesic effect.

According to Siegel's hypothesis, this tolerance occurred because the contextual stimuli that accompanied each morphine injection (the sights, sounds, and smells of the experimental room) acquired the capacity to elicit a compensatory CR of *hyperalgesia,* or an increased sensitivity to pain. By trial 4, this compensatory CR of hyperalgesia completely counteracted the UR of analgesia, so the net effect was no change in pain sensitivity. If this hypothesis is correct, it should be possible to eliminate the tolerance simply by changing the contextual stimuli on the final trial. Therefore, a third group of rats received their first three morphine injections in their home cages, but on their fourth trial, they received their morphine injections in the experimental room for the first time. Since this context was completely novel, it should elicit no compensatory CRs. Indeed, these animals showed a strong analgesic response, and their paw-lick latencies were just as long on their fourth trial as they were for the other morphine group on their first trial. They looked like rats that had never received a morphine injection before. This big difference between the two morphine groups was obtained simply by *changing the room* in which the morphine was injected.

If a rat's tolerance to a drug such as morphine is indeed a CR, it should be possible to extinguish this response by presenting the CS (the context) without the US (morphine). In another study, Siegel, Sherman, and Mitchell (1980) demonstrated such an extinction effect. Rats first received three daily injections of morphine, during which they developed tolerance to its analgesic effects. They then received nine extinction trials in which they were transported to the experimental room and were given an injection as usual, except that they received saline instead of morphine. These can be called extinction trials because the CS (the experimental room and injection routine) was presented without the morphine. The extinction trials were followed by one final test with morphine. The experimenters found that the morphine again produced a modest analgesic response; that is, the rats' tolerance to morphine had been partially extinguished as a result of the saline trials.

Some of the most convincing evidence for the compensatory-CR theory has come from studies in which the CS is presented without the drug US, and a compensatory CR has been observed directly. For instance, Rozin, Reff, Mack, and Schull (1984) showed that for regular coffee drinkers, the smell and taste of coffee can serve as a CS that elicits a compensatory CR counteracting the effects of caffeine. In addition to its effects on arousal and alertness, caffeine normally causes an increase in salivation. However, for regular coffee drinkers, this increase in salivation is minimal (a tolerance effect). Rozin and colleagues had their subjects drink a cup of coffee that either did or did not contain caffeine (and the subjects were not told which). After they drank coffee with caffeine, subjects showed only a small increase in salivation, as would be expected of habitual coffee drinkers. However, after they drank coffee without caffeine, these subjects showed a substantial *decrease* in salivation. The experimenters concluded that this decrease was a compensatory CR elicited by the stimuli that were usually paired with caffeine (the smell and taste of coffee). In addition, when these subjects drank a cup of hot apple juice containing caffeine, they showed substantial increases in salivation, which shows that they had not developed a general tolerance to the salivation-increasing effects of caffeine—their tolerance was found only when the caffeine was paired with the usual CS, coffee.

In summary, Rozin and co-workers demonstrated that coffee can come to elicit a compensatory CR, a decrease in salivation, after it has been repeatedly paired with caffeine. Similar evidence for compensatory CRs has been obtained with morphine (Paletta & Wagner, 1986) and

with many other pharmacological agents, including adrenalin (Russek & Pina, 1962) and alcohol (Crowell, Hinson, & Siegel, 1981).

If it is generally true that classical conditioning contributes to the phenomenon of drug tolerance, it should be possible to find evidence for this effect in nonlaboratory settings. Siegel, Hinson, Krank, and McCully (1982) presented some evidence from regular heroin users who died, or nearly died, after a heroin injection. Of course, an overdose of heroin can be fatal, but in some cases the dosage that caused a death was one the user had tolerated on the previous day. Siegel proposes that in some cases of this type, the user may have taken the heroin in an unusual stimulus environment, where the user's previously acquired compensatory CRs to the heroin injection would be decreased. He states that survivors of nearly fatal injections frequently report that the circumstances of the drug administration were different from those under which they normally injected the drug.

Another implication of the research on conditioned drug responses is that stimuli in the individual's environment can produce drug cravings and withdrawal symptoms, which make it difficult for a recovering addict to remain abstinent. As Siegel and Ramos (2002) have noted, there is abundant evidence that stimuli previously associated with an addictive substance can elicit cravings, and this has been known for a long time. Well before Pavlov studied classical conditioning, Macnish (1859) described how environmental stimuli can affect an alcoholic:

> Man is very much the creature of habit. By drinking regularly at certain times he feels the longing for liquor at the stated return of these periods—as after dinner, or immediately before going to bed, or whatever the period may be. He even finds it in certain companies, or in a particular tavern at which he is in the habit of taking his libations. (p. 151)

Because conditioned stimuli can elicit cravings for a drug, some drug treatment programs have included **cue exposure treatment** in which clients are exposed to stimuli normally associated with a drug (without the drug), so that conditioned drug cravings can be extinguished (Drummond, Tiffany, Glautier, & Remington, 1995). For example, in a smoking-cessation program, the smoker might be presented with cigarettes to look at, handle, and light up (but not smoke), so that the cravings associated with these cues can gradually extinguish. Smoking-related stimuli can also be presented using computer-generated images in virtual environments, and this has been shown to decrease cravings for cigarettes. In one study, Moon and Lee (2009) used functional magnetic resonance imaging (fMRI) to show that areas of the brain that are normally active when a person has nicotine cravings were less active after smokers were given computer-generated stimuli. Cue exposure treatment has also been used in the treatment of opiate addictions (de Quirós Aragón, Labrador, & de Arce, 2005), alcoholism (Stasiewicz, Brandon, & Bradizza, 2007), and even chocolate cravings (Van Gucht et al., 2008). The success of this approach has been mixed, however. Siegel and Ramos (2002) recommend several ways to make it more effective. One way is to give cue exposure treatment in several different contexts, making them as similar as possible to various real-life situations. (Otherwise, a person who normally smoked a lot at work might well have a relapse when he returned to the work environment.) Also, because spontaneous recovery is a property of classical conditioning, several cue exposure sessions, given over a period of time, may be necessary.

In summary, Siegel has found evidence that drug tolerance is due, at least in part, to the acquisition of compensatory CRs that tend to counteract the effects of the drug itself. He has shown that stimuli associated with the drug can elicit these compensatory CRs, which are commonly called cravings or withdrawal symptoms. His findings suggest that many cases of drug overdose reactions may occur when a habitual drug user takes the drug in a new or unfamiliar setting. The findings also suggest that some of the biggest obstacles to remaining abstinent after drug treatment are the cravings CSs in the individual's environment,

and that drug treatment programs need to focus on ways to minimize these conditioned reactions.

Conditioned Opponent Theories

Schull (1979) proposed an interesting theory about compensatory CRs. He called his theory a **conditioned opponent theory** because he accepted most of the assumptions of the Solomon and Corbit theory but made one important change. Whereas Solomon and Corbit proposed that the b-process is increased by a nonassociative strengthening mechanism, Schull proposed that any increase in the size of the b-process is based on classical conditioning. His theory may be easier to understand if we consider a specific example. As discussed in Chapter 2 in the section on the Solomon and Corbit theory, a person's response to an initial heroin injection is a very pleasurable sensation followed by unpleasant withdrawal symptoms. The initial pleasure is the a-process, and the unpleasant aftereffect is the b-process. Now, according to Schull, only the b-process is conditionable. Let us assume the stimuli that accompany the heroin injection—the needle, the room, and so on—serve as CSs that, after a few pairings with heroin, begin to elicit the withdrawal symptoms by themselves. These CSs have several effects. First, they tend to counteract the a-process, so a heroin injection no longer produces much of a pleasurable sensation. Second, they combine with the b-process to produce more severe and longer lasting withdrawal symptoms. Third, when no heroin is available, the presence of these stimuli can still produce withdrawal symptoms and cravings for the drug. Thus, Schull proposed that classically conditioned stimuli may contribute to many of the debilitating characteristics of drug addiction.

Schull's conditioned opponent theory deals exclusively with the conditioning of b-processes, but A. R. Wagner and his associates (Donegan & Wagner, 1987; Wagner, 1981) proposed a general theory that is meant to apply to all CRs, whether or not we would want to call them "b-processes." Wagner calls this theory a **sometimes opponent process (SOP)** theory because it predicts that in some cases a CR will be the opposite of the UR, but in other cases a CR will mimic the UR. How can we predict what type of CR we will see in a particular conditioning situation? According to SOP, the CR will mimic the UR if the UR is *monophasic,* but it will be the opposite of the UR if the UR is *biphasic.* In essence, the terms *monophasic* and *biphasic* concern whether a b-process can be observed in the UR. For example, the heart-rate UR to shock is biphasic because it consists of an increase in heart rate when the shock is on, followed by a decrease in heart rate *below baseline* when the shock is terminated. Because the UR exhibits such a "rebound effect," SOP predicts that the CR will be the opposite of the UR, and Black's (1965) research has demonstrated that this is the case. On the other hand, the UR of an eyeblink to a puff of air is monophasic: The eye closes, then opens, but there is no rebound—the eye does not open wider than it was initially. For this reason, SOP predicts that the CR will mimic the UR in eyeblink conditioning, which is of course the case. A number of studies have found support for the predictions of SOP (e.g., Albert, Ricker, Bevins, & Ayres, 1993; McNally & Westbrook, 2006). Although these conditioned opponent theories are complex, one basic message is clear: Many factors can affect the type of CR that is elicited by any particular CS, so the size and form of the CR may be difficult to predict in advance.

PHYSIOLOGICAL RESEARCH ON CLASSICAL CONDITIONING

The final topic of this chapter complements each of the previous ones. Regardless of their theoretical perspectives, just about all researchers who study classical conditioning agree that our understanding of this type of learning would be greatly enhanced if we knew what changes take place in the nervous system during the acquisition and subsequent performance of a new CR. This topic has been the focus of intense research efforts in recent years. Much has been learned about the physiological mechanisms of classical conditioning, and the following discussion can provide only a brief survey of some of the major developments in this area.

Some of the research on the neural mechanisms of habituation has been done with primitive creatures. Kandel's research on habituation in the mollusk *Aplysia* was discussed in Chapter 2. He has also been able to study classical conditioning in the gill-withdrawal reflex of *Aplysia*. In this research, the US was a shock to the tail, and the UR was the gill-withdrawal response (see Figure 2-7). The CS was weak stimulation of the siphon, which initially produced only a minor gill-withdrawal response. After several pairings of the CS and US, however, the CS began to elicit a full gill-withdrawal response (Carew, Hawkins, & Kandel, 1983). As in classical conditioning with mammals, the precise temporal arrangement of CS and US was crucial. Optimal learning occurred with short-delay conditioning (with the CS preceding the US by 0.5 seconds), and there was no evidence of conditioning with a delay of 2 seconds (Hawkins, Carew, & Kandel, 1983). Other studies on the gill-withdrawal reflex have demonstrated more complex conditioning phenomena, such as discrimination learning and second-order conditioning (Hawkins, Greene, & Kandel, 1998).

Kandel and his associates have been able to trace the neural circuitry involved in gill-withdrawal conditioning. They found that the CR in this procedure (the increased response to siphon stimulation) was due to an increase in the amount of transmitter released by the sensory neurons of the siphon. Note that precisely the opposite neural change (decreased transmitter release by the sensory neurons) was found to be responsible for habituation of the gill-withdrawal response (see Chapter 2). However, other changes have been observed in *Aplysia*'s nervous system during classical conditioning as well. Glanzman (1995) found that the dendrites of the postsynaptic neurons in the circuit develop enhanced sensitivity, so they exhibit stronger responses to chemical stimulation. In addition to these chemical changes, repeated classical conditioning trials can produce more permanent, structural changes in *Aplysia*'s nervous system—the growth of new synapses between the sensory neurons in the siphon and motor neurons

(Bailey & Kandel, 2004, 2009). These are important findings because they show that even in the simple nervous system of *Aplysia,* a variety of chemical and structural changes can take place during a simple learning episode. Classical conditioning has also been studied in other primitive creatures, including two other species of mollusk, *Hermissenda* and *Limax* (Jin, Tian, & Crow, 2009; Watanabe, Kirino, & Gelperin, 2008).

Turning to higher animals such as mammals, the task of uncovering the physiological mechanisms of classical conditioning becomes extremely difficult because of the staggering complexity of their nervous systems. Nevertheless, substantial progress has been made, and research on this topic is proceeding in several different directions. Some studies have examined human participants with damage in specific areas of the brain due to accident or illness; these individuals are trained in a classical conditioning paradigm, such as eyeblink conditioning. Another strategy is to condition people without brain damage while using modern imaging technologies to measure activity in different parts of the brain. With nonhuman subjects, researchers have examined chemical mechanisms and the effects of lesions to different brain areas.

Our brief review of this topic will focus on five main points.

1. *The neural pathways involved in the CR are often different from those involved in the UR.* This can be shown through procedures that eliminate one of these responses but not the other. For example, in baboons, a certain part of the hypothalamus appears to be intimately involved in the conditioned heart-rate changes elicited by CSs paired with shock. If this part of the hypothalamus is destroyed, heart-rate CRs disappear, whereas unconditioned heart-rate responses are unaffected (Smith, Astley, DeVito, Stein, & Walsh, 1980).

For another common classical conditioning preparation, rabbit eyeblink conditioning, the neural circuitry has been studied extensively, and the brain locations involved are fairly well understood. The **cerebellum**, a part of the brain that is important for many skilled movements, plays a critical role in eyeblink conditioning (Canli & Donegan, 1995; Christian & Thompson, 2003). As in heart-rate conditioning, different neural pathways are involved in eyeblink URs and CRs. The eyeblink UR to an air puff directed at the eye seems to be controlled by two distinct pathways—a fairly direct pathway in the brainstem and a more indirect pathway passing through the cerebellum. Considerable evidence shows that the eyeblink CR is controlled by this second, indirect pathway. If sections of this pathway in the cerebellum are destroyed, eyeblink CRs disappear and cannot be relearned (Knowlton & Thompson, 1992). If neurons in this same part of the cerebellum are electrically stimulated, eyeblink responses similar to the CR are produced (Thompson, McCormick, & Lavond, 1986). If this divergence of UR and CR pathways is found in other response systems, it would help to explain why the forms of the UR and CR are often different.

2. *Many different brain structures may be involved in the production of a simple CR.* For example, although the cerebellum is important in rabbit eyeblink conditioning, many other brain areas are involved as well. When human subjects undergo eyeblink conditioning, brain-imaging techniques such as positron emission tomography (PET) reveal increased blood flow in one side of the cerebellum (corresponding to the side of the eye involved in conditioning), but there is increased blood flow in many other parts of the brain as well (Molchan, Sunderland, McIntosh, Herscovitch, & Schreurs, 1994).

In other species, a number of different brain sites have been implicated in heart-rate conditioning, including parts of the amygdala, hypothalamus, and cingulate cortex (Schneiderman et al., 1987). With humans, fMRI techniques have been used to obtain detailed maps of brain activity when people receive classical conditioning. During classical conditioning with the SCR, fMRIs show complex patterns of activity involving many parts of the brain, which again supports the idea that multiple brain structures are involved in classical conditioning (Knight, Waters, King, & Bandettini, 2010). In one study, pictures of faces were used as CSs, and both pleasant and unpleasant odors were used as USs. Particularly interesting was the finding that even within the same conditioning preparation (pairing faces with odors), the areas of activation were different for pleasant odors and unpleasant odors (Gottfried, O'Doherty, & Dolan, 2002).

3. *Different conditioning phenomena may involve different brain locations.* This point has been made in a variety of studies with different species. For example, if the hippocampus is removed from a rabbit, the animal will fail to exhibit the blocking effect (Solomon, 1977), but removal of the hippocampus does not prevent the development of conditioned inhibition. In mice, damage to an area near the hippocampus called the entorhinal cortex interferes with the CS pre-exposure effect (Lewis & Gould, 2007). Another brain area, the amygdala, seems important for associations involving both contextual stimuli and typical CSs (Phillips & LeDoux, 1992; Wilson, Brooks, & Bouton, 1995).

4. *Different CRs involve different brain locations.* For example, the cerebellum seems to be important in eyeblink conditioning, whereas other brain areas seem to be involved in heart-rate conditioning. One study compared a group of people with damage to the cerebellum to a group of people without such brain damage. The subjects without brain damage quickly learned a conditioned eyeblink response, whereas the subjects with damage to the cerebellum did not learn this response. However, the air puff itself did elicit an eyeblink UR in these subjects, which shows that they had not simply lost motor control of this response (Daum et al., 1993). The deficit appears to be a problem in forming the necessary associations for the eyeblink CR to a neutral stimulus. This does not mean, however, that the people with damage to the cerebellum suffered a general inability to associate stimuli, because measurements of their heart rates and SCRs showed that they had indeed learned the association between CS and the air puff. These results indicate that different parts of the brain are involved in the conditioning of different response systems.

5. *Individual neurons have been found whose activity appears to be related to the acquisition of CRs.* For example, McCormick and Thompson (1984) found that the firing rates of certain cells in the cerebellum are correlated with behavioral measures of the eyeblink CR. That is, when a rabbit is presented with a series of conditioning trials with a CS such as a tone, the activity of these cells increases at about the same rate as eyeblink response. When the eyeblink CR decreases during extinction, so does the activity of these cells. Moreover, the cellular activity within a single presentation of the CS parallels the pattern of the eyeblink, with the neuron's activity

---

PRACTICE QUIZ (2)

1. Because taste aversions can be learned with long delays between eating and illness, some psychologists said they violated the _____ principle.
2. Rats more easily associate auditory and visual stimuli with _____, and they more easily associate tastes with _____. These can be called examples of _____ associations.
3. Although the evidence is not very strong, there are some indications that people may be predisposed to develop phobias to such stimuli as _____.
4. Morphine produces decreased sensitivity to pain, and a CS associated with morphine produces _____.
5. Research on the neural pathways involved in classical conditioning in *Aplysia* has found that conditioning is the result of _____ in the amount of transmitter released by sensory neurons.
6. For both rabbits and humans, a brain area important for eyeblink conditioning is the _____.

Answers

1. contiguity 2. shock, illness, prepared 3. spiders or snakes 4. increased sensitivity to pain 5. an increase 6. cerebellum

preceding the eyeblink response by about 30 milliseconds. Along with other evidence, this finding suggests that these cells play an important role in the development of the CR. Such neurons are not unique to the cerebellum, however, because neurons with similar properties have been found in the hippocampus, a brain structure suspected of playing a role in learning and memory (Berger & Weisz, 1987). One study used trace conditioning of a fear response (measured by an increased heart rate) with rabbits. For two different groups of rabbits, a CS was followed by shock after a gap of either 10 or 20 seconds. After conditioning, the rabbits received trials in which the CS was presented without shock. The researchers identified individual neurons in the hippocampus whose activity increased after the CS, and peaked either 10 or 20 seconds later (matching the CS–US interval with which the rabbits were trained). These neurons, therefore, seemed to be involved in the timing of the CR (McEchron, Tseng, & Disterhoft, 2003). The discovery of neurons whose activity is so closely related to overt behavior is an important development. Exactly how neurons in different parts of the brain actually contribute to the conditioning process is still being sorted out.

As we have seen, physiological research on classical conditioning is proceeding on a number of different levels, including research on entire brain structures, on individual neurons, and on chemical mechanisms. Both primitive and more advanced species are being studied. Much is still unknown about the brain mechanisms of classical conditioning, but one point seems certain: Anyone hoping for a simple physiological explanation is going to be disappointed. Classical conditioning, one of the simplest types of learning, appears to involve a very complex system of neural and chemical mechanisms.

Summary

In Kamin's experiment on the blocking effect, rats first received conditioning trials with a light paired with shock, and then trials with both the light and a tone paired with the shock. In the test phase, presenting the tone alone produced no fear response. To account for this and similar results, the Rescorla–Wagner model states that conditioning will occur only if there is a discrepancy between the strength of the US and the strength of the subject's expectation. This model can account for many conditioning phenomena, such as overshadowing, conditioned inhibition, and the overexpectation effect. However, the model has difficulty explaining certain phenomena such as the CS preexposure effect. Attentional theories of classical conditioning maintain that the effectiveness of a CS decreases if the CS is not informative. Comparator theories propose that subjects may *learn* a CS–US association but not *perform* a CR unless the CS is a better predictor of the US than are the contextual stimuli.

Many different types of associations can occur in classical conditioning procedures, including both S-S and S-R associations, associations with contextual stimuli, and associations between two CSs. Animals appear to be biologically prepared to learn certain conditioned associations more easily than others. In taste-aversion learning, animals and people can learn to associate a taste with illness, even if the illness occurs several hours after eating. Rats can quickly learn an association between a taste and illness or an association between audiovisual stimuli and shock, but they are slow to learn the opposite associations. Although biological constraints cannot be ignored, the same general principles seem to apply to taste-aversion learning and other forms of classical conditioning.

When a CS has been paired with a drug US, the CS will often elicit compensatory CRs—physiological responses that are the opposite of those produced by the drug—and these compensatory CRs can show up as drug tolerance. Conditioned opponent theories have attempted to describe these compensatory CRs and to predict when a CR will mimic the UR and when it will be the opposite of the UR.

Research with simple creatures such as *Aplysia* has discovered specific neural and chemical changes that occur during conditioning. Research with vertebrates, including humans, has shown that many brain structures may be involved in the development of a simple CR and that different brain structures seem to be involved for different CRs and different conditioning phenomena.

Review Questions

1. Describe Kamin's experiment on the blocking effect. Why was the result surprising?
2. Under what conditions does the Rescorla–Wagner model predict that there will be excitatory conditioning, inhibitory conditioning, or no conditioning? Give a specific example of each case.
3. What are some of the different associations that can form in a simple case of classical conditioning?
4. What is an occasion setter? How does it differ from a typical CS?
5. Why were evidence for long-delay taste-aversion learning and other examples of biological constraints on classical conditioning seen as threats to the general-principle approach to learning? How has this issue been settled?
6. What are conditioned compensatory responses? What role do they play in drug tolerance and addiction? What are some implications for people who suffer from drug addictions?
7. What are some of the main findings and conclusions that can be drawn from physiological research on classical conditioning?

5

Basic Principles of Operant Conditioning

LEARNING OBJECTIVES

After reading this chapter, you should be able to

■ describe Thorndike's Law of Effect and experiments on animals in the puzzle box

■ discuss how the principle of reinforcement can account for superstitious behaviors

■ describe the procedure of shaping and explain how it can be used in behavior modification

■ explain B. F. Skinner's free-operant procedure, three-term contingency, and the basic principles of operant conditioning

■ define instinctive drift, and explain why some psychologists believed that it posed problems for the principle of reinforcement

■ define autoshaping and discuss different theories about why it occurs

Unlike classically conditioned responses, many everyday behaviors are not elicited by a specific stimulus. Behaviors such as walking, talking, eating, drinking, working, and playing do not occur automatically in response to any particular stimulus. In the presence of a stimulus such as food, a creature might eat or it might not, depending on the time of day, the time since its last meal, the presence of other members of its species, other activities available at the moment, and so on. Because it appears that a creature can choose whether to engage in behaviors of this type, people sometimes call them "voluntary" behaviors and contrast them with the "involuntary" behaviors that are part of unconditioned and conditioned reflexes. Some learning theorists state that whereas classical conditioning is limited to involuntary behaviors, operant conditioning influences our voluntary behaviors. The term *voluntary* is difficult to define in a precise, scientific way; therefore, it may be a mistake to use this term to refer to all of our nonreflexive behaviors. Regardless of what we call nonreflexive behaviors, this chapter should make one thing clear: Just because there is no obvious stimulus preceding a behavior, this does not imply that the behavior is unpredictable. Indeed, the extensive research on operant conditioning might be characterized as an effort to discover general principles that can predict what nonreflexive behaviors a creature will produce and under what conditions.

THE LAW OF EFFECT

Thorndike's Experiments

E. L. Thorndike (1898, 1911) was the first researcher to investigate systematically how an animal's nonreflexive behaviors can be modified as a result of its experience. In Thorndike's experiments, a hungry animal (a cat, a dog, or a chicken) was placed in a small chamber that Thorndike called a **puzzle box**. If the animal performed the appropriate response, the door to the puzzle box would be opened, and the animal could exit and eat some food placed just outside the door. For some subjects, the required response was simple: pulling on a rope, pressing a lever, or stepping on a platform. Figure 5-1 shows one of Thorndike's more difficult puzzle boxes, which required a cat to make three separate responses: pulling a string (which lifted one bolt), stepping on the platform (which lifted the other bolt), and reaching through the bars and turning one of the two latches in front

of the door. The first time a subject was placed in a puzzle box (whether simple or complex), it usually took a long time to escape. A typical subject would move about inside the puzzle box and explore the various parts of the chamber in a seemingly haphazard way; during the course of this activity, it would eventually perform the response that opened the door. Based on his careful observations of this behavior, Thorndike concluded that an animal's first production of the appropriate response occurred purely by accident.

To determine how a subject's behavior would change as a result of its experience, Thorndike would return an individual animal to the same puzzle box many times. His measure of performance was *escape latency:* the amount of time it took the subject to escape on each trial. Figure 5-2 presents a typical result from one of Thorndike's cats, which shows that as trials progressed, the cat's latency to escape gradually declined (from 160 seconds on the 1st trial to just 7 seconds on the 24th trial). Thorndike attributed this gradual improvement over trials to the progressive strengthening of an S-R connection: The stimulus was the inside of the puzzle box, and the response was whatever behavior opened the door. To account for the gradual strengthening of this connection, Thorndike (1898) formulated a principle of learning that he called the **Law of Effect**:

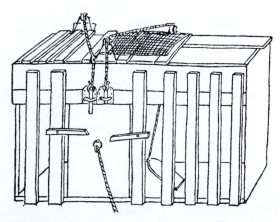

FIGURE 5-1 One of Thorndike's puzzle boxes. A cat could escape from this box by pulling a string, stepping on the platform, and turning one of the two latches on the front of the door. (From Thorndike, 1898)

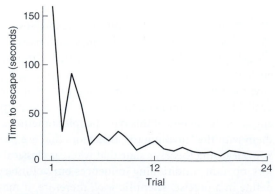

FIGURE 5-2 The number of seconds required by one cat to escape from a simple puzzle box on 24 consecutive trials. (From Thorndike, 1898)

Of several responses made to the same situation, those which are accompanied or closely followed by satisfaction to the animal will, other things being equal, be more firmly connected with the situation, so that, when it recurs, they will be more likely to recur; those which are accompanied or closely followed by discomfort to the animal will, other things being equal, have their connections with that situation weakened, so that, when it recurs, they will be less likely to occur. The greater the satisfaction or discomfort, the greater the strengthening or weakening of the bond. (p. 244)

How can we know what is satisfying or discomforting for an animal subject? Thorndike was careful to define these terms in a way that did not rely on the observer's intuition:

By a satisfying state of affairs is meant one which the animal does nothing to avoid, often doing such things as attain and preserve it. By a discomforting or annoying state of affairs is meant one which the animal commonly avoids and abandons. (p. 245)

The application of the Law of Effect to the puzzle-box experiments is straightforward: Certain behaviors, those that opened the door, were closely followed by a satisfying state of affairs (escape and food), so when the animal was returned to the same situation it was more likely to produce those behaviors than it had been at first. In modern psychology, the phrase "satisfying state of affairs" has been replaced by the term **reinforcer**, but the Law of Effect (or the principle of **positive reinforcement**) remains as one of the most important concepts of learning theory.

Guthrie and Horton: Evidence for a Mechanical Strengthening Process

Two researchers who followed Thorndike, E. R. Guthrie and G. P. Horton (1946), provided more convincing evidence that the learning that took place in the puzzle box involved the strengthening of whatever behavior happened to be followed by escape and food. They placed cats in a puzzle box with a simple solution: A pole in the center of the chamber had only to be tipped in any direction to open the door. A camera outside the chamber photographed the cat at the same instant that the door swung open, thereby providing a permanent record of exactly how the cat had performed the effective response on each trial. The photographs revealed that after a few trials, each cat settled on a particular method of manipulating the pole that was quite consistent from trial to trial. However, different cats developed a variety of methods for moving the pole; for example, one cat would always push the pole with its left forepaw, another would always rub the pole with its nose, and another would lie down next to the pole and roll over into it. Figure 5-3 shows the results from the first 24 trials for one cat. At first the cat's behavior at the moment of reinforcement varied greatly from trial to trial. By the 9th or 10th trial, however, the cat began to develop a stereotyped method of operating the pole—it would walk to the left of the pole and brush against it with its backside. Figure 5-4 shows the behavior of another cat, beginning on trial 52. This cat had developed the behavior of moving the pole by biting it while standing in a particular position.

The findings of Guthrie and Horton can be summarized by stating that after their cats mastered the task, there was relatively little variability from trial to trial for a given cat, but there was considerable variability from one cat to another. These results provide evidence for a particular version of the Law of Effect that Brown and Herrnstein (1975) aptly called the **stop-action principle**. According to this principle, there is a parallel between the action of the camera and the reinforcer in the experiments of Guthrie and Horton. Like the camera, the occurrence of the reinforcer serves to stop the animal's ongoing behavior and strengthen the association between the situation (the puzzle box) and those precise behaviors that were occurring at the moment of reinforcement.

The stop-action principle states that because of this strengthening process, the specific bodily position and the muscle movements

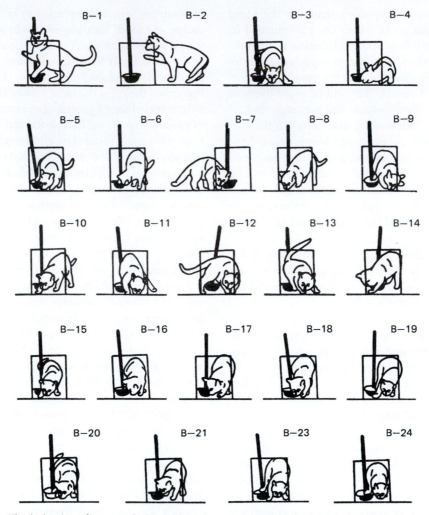

FIGURE 5-3   The behavior of one cat (Subject B) in the puzzle box of Guthrie and Horton. The pictures show the cat's position at the moment of reinforcement on the cat's first 24 trials in the puzzle box, where any movement of the vertical pole caused the door to open. (From Guthrie & Horton, 1946)

occurring at the moment of reinforcement will have a higher probability of occurring on the next trial. If the cat repeats this bodily position and movements on the next trial, this will produce a second reinforcer, thereby further strengthening that S-R association even more. This sort of positive feedback process should eventually produce one S-R connection that is so much stronger than any other that this particular response pattern will occur with high probability, trial after trial. This reasoning provides a simple explanation

of why different cats developed different stereotyped techniques for moving the pole. For each cat, whatever random behavior happened to get reinforced a few times would become dominant over other behaviors.

Superstitious Behaviors

The mechanical nature of the stop-action principle suggests that behaviors may sometimes be strengthened "by accident." Skinner (1948)

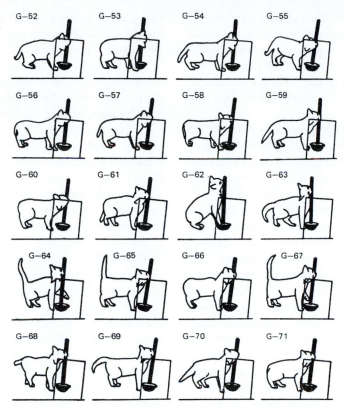

FIGURE 5-4 The behavior of another cat (Subject G) at the moment of reinforcement on trials 52 through 71 in the puzzle box. (From Guthrie & Horton, 1946)

conducted a famous experiment, now often called the **superstition experiment**, that made a strong case for the power of accidental reinforcement. The subjects were pigeons, and each was placed in a separate experimental chamber in which grain was presented every 15 seconds regardless of what the pigeon was doing. After the subject had spent some time in the chamber, Skinner observed the bird's behavior. He found that six of his eight pigeons had developed clearly defined behaviors that they performed repeatedly between food presentations. One bird made a few counterclockwise turns between reinforcers, another made pecking motions at the floor, and a third repeatedly poked its head into one of the upper corners of the chamber. A fourth bird was observed to toss its head in an upward motion, and two others swayed from side to side. These

behaviors occurred repeatedly despite the fact that no behavior was required for reinforcement. Similar results have been found by other researchers who repeated (with some variations) the basic idea of Skinner's experiment (Gleeson, Lattal, & Williams, 1989; Justice & Looney, 1990; Neuringer, 1970).

According to Skinner, these distinctive behaviors developed for the same reasons that the cats of Guthrie and Horton developed distinctive styles of moving the pole: Whatever behavior happened to be occurring when the reinforcer was delivered was strengthened. If the first reinforcer occurred immediately after a pigeon had tossed its head upward, this behavior of head tossing would be more likely to occur in the future. Therefore, there was a good chance that the next reinforcer would also follow a head-tossing motion. The accidental strengthening process is self-perpetuating, because once any one behavior develops a somewhat higher frequency of occurrence than all other behaviors, it has a greater chance of being reinforced, which increases its frequency still further, and so on.

Skinner (1948) proposed that many of the superstitious behaviors people perform are produced by the same mechanism that caused his pigeons to exhibit such peculiar behaviors:

> Rituals for changing one's luck at cards are good examples. A few accidental connections between a ritual and favorable consequences suffice to set up and maintain the behavior in spite of many unreinforced instances. The bowler who has released a ball down the alley but continues to behave as if he were controlling it by twisting and turning his arm and shoulder is another case in point. These behaviors have, of course, no real effect on one's luck or upon a ball half way down an alley, just as in the present case the food would appear as often if the pigeon did nothing—or, more strictly speaking, did something else. (p. 171)

Superstitious behaviors frequently arise when an individual actually has no control over the events taking place, as in card playing or other types of gambling, where winning or losing depends on chance. V. L. Lee (1996) had college students play a computer game in which winning or losing points was out of their control (although they did not know this). She found that the students tended to pick the same computer icons after successfully earning points, but to switch icons after a failure, even though the choice of icons had no effect on success or failure. Matute (1994, 1995) has also observed superstitious behaviors in situations where people have no control over events. In one experiment, college students were exposed to unpleasantly loud tones and were told that they could turn off the tones by typing the correct sequence of keys on a keyboard. In reality, the participants had no control over the

tones, which went on and off no matter what keys they typed. Nevertheless, most of the participants developed superstitious behaviors—they tended to type the same key sequences each time a tone came on. At the end of the experiment, many of the participants said they believed that their typing responses did turn off the tones.

Superstitious behaviors are common among athletes. In a study of college football, track, and gymnastics teams, Bleak and Frederick (1998) found that an average player performed about 10 different superstitious behaviors, such as wearing a lucky charm or item of clothing, eating the same meal before each competition, or taping a part of the body that was not injured. Burger and Lynn (2005) found that superstitious behaviors were widespread among professional baseball players in both the United States and Japan. Some superstitious behaviors occur without the athlete's awareness. Ciborowski (1997) asked college baseball players to describe the behaviors they performed between pitches while batting (e.g., touching parts of the body or clothing, gripping the bat in certain ways, touching the ground or plate with the bat). The players were able to list most of them, but not all. However, when asked how many times they repeated these behaviors, the players' estimates were too low by a factor of four. Amazingly, Ciborowski found that the average player made 82 such movements in one time at bat.

Herrnstein (1966) refined Skinner's analysis of human superstitions. Herrnstein noted that Skinner's analysis is most applicable to idiosyncratic superstitions, like those of a gambler or an athlete. It seems likely that such personalized superstitions arise out of an individual's own experience with reinforcement. On the other hand, superstitions that are widely held across a society (e.g., the belief that it is bad luck to walk under a ladder, or that the number 13 is unlucky) are probably acquired through communication with others, not through individual experience. How these more common superstitions first arose is not known, but Herrnstein suggested that some may be the residue of previous contingencies of reinforcement that are no longer in effect.

As an example, he cited the belief that it is bad luck to light three cigarettes on a single match. This superstition arose in the trenches during World War I. At that time, there was some justification for this belief, because every second that a match remained lit increased the chances of being spotted by the enemy. This danger is not present in everyday life, but the superstition is still passed on from generation to generation. Herrnstein speculated that it may be perpetuated by stories of occasional individuals who violate the rule and meet with an unfortunate fate. Thus, Herrnstein claimed that some superstitions were originally valid beliefs and are now perpetuated by rumor and/or occasional coincidental events. It is easy to imagine how some superstitions (such as the one about walking under a ladder) may have begun, whereas the origins of others are less clear.

In one study on the social transmission of superstitious behaviors, preschool children were taught, either by the words of an adult or by watching another child on a video, that pressing the nose of a mechanical clown might help them earn marbles (Higgins, Morris, & Johnson, 1989). Actually, this behavior had nothing to do with the delivery of marbles, which the clown presented at varying intervals no matter what a child was doing. Nevertheless, the children continued to perform this "superstitious" response, day after day, as long as a marble was delivered now and then.

Skinner's analysis of his superstition experiment is not the only possible interpretation. Staddon and Simmelhag (1971) conducted a careful replication of the superstition experiment, recorded the pigeons' behaviors more thoroughly than Skinner did, and came to different conclusions. In their superstition experiment, Staddon and Simmelhag found that certain behavior patterns tended to occur frequently in many or all of their subjects during the intervals between food deliveries. They found that these behaviors could be grouped in two major categories, which they called **interim behaviors** and **terminal behaviors**. Interim behaviors were defined as those that were frequent in the early part of the interval, when the next reinforcer was still some time

away. Interim behaviors included pecking toward the floor, turning, and moving along the front wall of the chamber. Terminal behaviors were defined as behaviors that seldom occurred early in the interval but increased in frequency as the time of food delivery approached. Two of the most frequent terminal behaviors were orienting toward the food magazine and pecking in the vicinity of the magazine. To recapitulate, interim behaviors are those that occur frequently early in the interval between reinforcers, and terminal behaviors are those that occur frequently toward the end of the interval.

Staddon and Simmelhag proposed that some of the behaviors that Skinner called "superstitious behaviors," such as turning in circles, may actually have been interim behaviors. But interim behaviors are seldom followed by the delivery of food, because they do not often occur at the end of the interval. In other words, Staddon and Simmelhag argued that it is not accidental reinforcement that causes interim behaviors to increase in frequency. Instead, they proposed that interim behaviors are simply behaviors that an animal has an innate predisposition to perform when the likelihood of reinforcement is low. In short, interim behaviors are a reflection of an organism's hereditary endowment, not of the reinforcement process. In addition, certain terminal behaviors, such as pecking, may frequently occur when food is about to be delivered, and their appearance may be unrelated to any accidental reinforcement. Timberlake and Lucas (1985) proposed a similar theory about the possible role of hereditary behavior patterns in Skinner's superstition experiment.

It now seems clear that these alternate accounts of the superstition experiment are at least partly correct. Many studies have shown that the periodic delivery of food or some other reinforcer can give rise to a variety of stereotyped behaviors, which Staddon and Simmelhag called interim and terminal behaviors, and which others have called **adjunctive behaviors**. Thus, not all the behaviors that arise when periodic free reinforcers are delivered are the result of an accidental pairing with reinforcement. Some may simply be innate behaviors that become highly probable when the next reinforcer is some time away and the subject must do something to "pass the time."

Nevertheless, it seems equally clear that Skinner's analysis of superstitious behaviors was also partly correct; that is, sometimes behaviors increase in frequency because of the accidental pairing with reinforcement. In the laboratory, experiments with both adults and children have found that they have a tendency to develop superstitious behaviors when free reinforcers were periodically delivered (Aeschleman, Rosen, & Williams, 2003; Wagner & Morris, 1987). These superstitious behaviors tended to increase just before a reinforcer was delivered, and they were distinctly different for different participants (e.g., one child kissed the nose of the mechanical clown that delivered marbles, another child puckered his mouth, and another child swang his hips). Outside the laboratory, many idiosyncratic superstitions can be easily traced to past reinforcement. The superstitions displayed by many athletes are often the direct result of the success that followed these behaviors in the past, as the athletes themselves will admit.

THE PROCEDURE OF SHAPING, OR SUCCESSIVE APPROXIMATIONS

Even after plenty of practice, both animals and humans show some variability from trial to trial in how they perform an operant response (as can be seen in the performance of the cats in Figures 5-3 and 5-4). This variability in behavior can actually be very helpful for psychological researchers, animal trainers, and behavior therapists. Variability provides the means by which a totally new behavior, never performed by an individual before, can gradually be developed. The procedure that makes use of behavioral variability is known as **shaping**, or the method of successive approximations.

Shaping Lever Pressing in a Rat

Suppose that as part of your laboratory work in a psychology course, you are given a rat in an experimental chamber equipped with a lever the rat can press and a pellet dispenser. You have a remote-control button that, when pressed, delivers one food pellet to the food tray in the chamber. Your task is to train the rat to press the lever at a modest rate. Since you have learned about Thorndike's experiments, you may believe that this task will be very simple: You will simply wait until the rat presses the lever by accident and then deliver a food pellet. Suppose that after a few minutes in the chamber your rat presses the lever, and you immediately press the button to deliver a food pellet. However, the pellet dispenser makes a loud click that startles the rat and causes it to freeze for 10 or 15 seconds. About a minute later, the animal finally discovers the food pellet in the tray and eats it. We have seen that the contiguity between response and reinforcer is an important requirement of the Law of Effect—whatever behavior immediately precedes reinforcement will be strengthened. In this case, the behavior that immediately preceded the rat's discovery of the food pellet was not pressing the lever (as you had intended) but rather approaching the food tray. If it did anything, the reinforcer may have strengthened the rat's tendency to approach or explore the food tray.

The problem is that you need a reinforcer that you can be sure the animal will receive immediately after the correct response is made. A common solution to this problem is to develop the sound of the pellet dispenser into a conditioned reinforcer. A **conditioned reinforcer** is a previously neutral stimulus that has acquired the capacity to strengthen responses because that stimulus has been repeatedly paired with food or some other primary reinforcer. A **primary reinforcer** is a stimulus that naturally strengthens any response it follows. Primary reinforcers include food, water, sexual pleasure, and comfort. If you repeatedly expose your rat to the sound of the pellet dispenser followed by the delivery of a food pellet, the sound of the dispenser should become a conditioned reinforcer. You can be sure that this has been accomplished when the rat will quickly return to the food tray from any part of the chamber as soon as you operate the dispenser.

At this point, your initial plan might work. If you present the sound of the dispenser immediately after the rat presses the lever, the response of lever pressing should be strengthened. However, suppose the lever is 5 inches above the floor of the chamber, and it takes an effortful push from the rat to fully depress the lever. Under these circumstances, you might wait for hours and the rat might never depress the lever. And of course, you cannot reinforce a response that never occurs.

In this situation, the variability inherent in behavior becomes helpful. A good way to start would be to wait until the rat is below the lever and then reinforce any detectable upward head movement. After 5 or 10 reinforcers for such a movement, the rat will probably exhibit an upward head movement soon after consuming the previous food pellet. Once this behavior is well established, the procedure of shaping consists of gradually making your criterion for reinforcement more demanding. For example, the next step might be to wait for an upward head movement of at least half an inch. At first your rat may make a few head movements of less than half an inch (which you do not reinforce), but because of the variability in such behaviors, a movement of the required size will most likely occur. Each reinforcement of such a larger movement will increase the probability of another similar response, and soon the rat will be making these responses regularly. You can then go on to demand upward movements of 1 inch, 1.5 inches, and so on, until the rat is bringing its head close to the lever. The next step might be to require some actual contact with the lever, then contact with one forepaw, then some downward movement of the lever, and so on, until the rat has learned to make a full lever press.

Figure 5-5 provides a graphic illustration of how the procedure of shaping makes use of the variability in the subject's behavior. Suppose that before beginning the shaping process, you simply observed the rat's behavior for 5 minutes, making an estimate every 5 seconds about the height of the rat's head above the floor of the chamber. Figure 5-5 provides an example of what you might find: The y-axis shows the

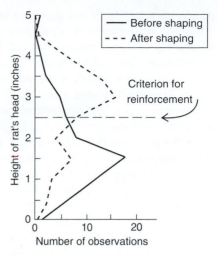

FIGURE 5-5 Hypothetical distributions showing the height of a rat's head as observed at regular intervals before shaping (solid line) and after selective reinforcement of head heights greater than 2.5 inches (dotted line). Rachlin (1970) presents a similar analysis of the shaping process.

height of the rat's head to the nearest half inch, and the x-axis shows the number of times this height occurred in the 5-minute sample. The resulting frequency distribution indicates that the rat usually kept its head about 1.5 inches from the floor, but sometimes its head was lower and sometimes much higher. Given such a distribution, it might make sense to start the shaping process with a requirement that the rat raise its head to a height of at least 2.5 inches before it is reinforced. Figure 5-5 also illustrates how the frequency distribution would probably shift after the shaping process began.

Shaping Behaviors in the Classroom

The procedure of successive approximations can be used to produce totally new behaviors in people as well as in laboratory rats. At many colleges and universities, there are stories about how the students in a large lecture course collaborated to shape the behavior of their professor. In one such story, a professor who usually stood rigidly behind the lectern was reinforced by his students for any movement, and by the end of the hour he was pacing back and forth and gesturing wildly with his arms. In another story, a professor in an introductory psychology course lectured from an elevated stage. The students secretly agreed to reinforce the professor for any movement to the left. The reinforcers they used were listening attentively, nodding their heads in apparent understanding of what he was saying, and taking notes. Whenever the professor moved to the right, however, they stopped delivering these reinforcers—they would stop taking notes, yawn, look bored, and look around the room. This systematic delivery of reinforcers for movement to the left was apparently quite successful, for legend has it that about halfway through the lecture the professor fell off the left side of the stage (which was only about 18 inches high).

Stories of this type suggest that shaping can work even when the subject is unaware of what is going on. If the professors in these stories realized what their students were doing, they probably would have resisted this behavioral control (perhaps on the stubborn belief that it is the behavior of students that should be shaped in the classroom, not the professor's).

Shaping as a Tool in Behavior Modification

Not all examples of shaping are as frivolous as those described in the Shaping Behaviors in the Classroom section. Shaping is frequently used as a method to establish new or better behaviors in a wide range of settings. As one example, Scott, Scott, and Goldwater (1997) used a shaping technique to improve the performance of a university pole vaulter. This 21-year-old had been competing in the sport for 10 years, and he had taken part in international events, but there was one aspect of the skill of pole vaulting that he had difficulty mastering. To obtain the maximum height of a vault, it is important for the athlete to raise his arms and the pole as high overhead as possible when the pole is planted in the ground at the moment of take-off. This vaulter was not extending his arms completely at take-off, and he knew it, but he could not seem to break this bad habit.

Videotapes of the pole vaulter showed that on an average attempt, his arms were extended to a height of 2.25 meters. To train him to reach higher, the researchers set up a photoelectric beam and sensor slightly above this point, at 2.30 meters. On every practice trial, a trainer shouted "Reach!" as he was running down the runway, and if his hands broke the photoelectric beam, there was a beep to signal to that he had extended his arms to the criterion level. Because this beep was associated with a better performance, it can be called a conditioned reinforcer, just as the sound of the pellet dispenser serves as a conditioned reinforcer for a rat learning a new response. Once the pole vaulter achieved a success rate of 90% at one hand height, the criterion was gradually increased (to 2.35 meters, then to 2.40 meters, and so on). The improvement took many months of practice, but eventually the vaulter was extending his arms to just about their maximum possible height. From his perspective, the most important result was that with each increase in the height of the photoelectric beam, the height of the bar that he was able to clear rose to a new personal best. Therefore, this systematic shaping procedure produced the results he was trying to attain.

In another example of shaping, therapists used toys and other desired items as reinforcers to get an 8-year-old boy with mental retardation to use a mask that delivered medication he needed to treat a serious respiratory condition (Hagopian & Thompson, 1999). The boy initially resisted using the mask for any length of time, so the therapists started by giving him a reinforcer when he wore the mask for just 5 seconds. The criterion for reinforcement was gradually increased over a period of several weeks until he was using the mask for the full duration of 40 seconds that he needed.

Shaping can be used with groups as well as with individuals. In a program at a drug treatment clinic, cocaine users were given standard methadone treatment, and a shaping procedure was used to gradually decrease their use of cocaine. Over the course of several weeks, patients received vouchers that could be exchanged for items such as movie tickets if their urine samples showed at least a 25% reduction in cocaine metabolites compared to their previous test. Eventually, they could earn vouchers only if there was no sign of cocaine in their urine samples. The researchers found that this shaping procedure was more effective in reducing cocaine use than requiring complete abstinence from the very start of the program (Preston, Umbricht, Wong, & Epstein, 2001). Similar procedures have been used to help people quit smoking (Stoops et al., 2009).

Because the procedure of shaping can help to improve behaviors even under difficult circumstances, it has become a common component of many behavior modification programs. It has been used to increase school attendance in a teenager with mental retardation (Meyer, Hagopian, & Paclawskyj, 1999) to treat a phobia in a child with autism (Ricciardi, Luiselli, & Camare, 2006) and to eliminate undesirable behaviors of children and adolescents after brain injuries (Slifer & Amari, 2009). These are just a few of the many cases in which shaping has been used to improve the lives of people with a variety of different problems.

Making Shaping More Precise: Percentile Schedules

In some ways, shaping is more of an art than an exact science. Many split-second decisions must be made about which behaviors to reinforce and which not to reinforce, how quickly the criterion for reinforcement should be increased, how large a step in the criterion should be made, what to do when the learner has a setback, and so on. However, in some cases, the procedure of shaping can be made more precise and more effective through the use of what are called **percentile schedules**.

In a percentile schedule, a response is reinforced if it is better than a certain percentage of the last several responses that the learner has made (J. R. Platt, 1973). For example, imagine that a boy is doing poorly in school because he is easily distracted from his work and so does not complete his assignments on time. A behavior therapist might use a percentile schedule to shape more and more rapid completion of his work. Suppose the student is told to work on a series of math problems, and the therapist records how many problems are correctly completed each minute. At the end of every minute, the boy might earn a reinforcer if he completes more problems than he did in 7 of the last 10 minutes. The reinforcers could be points that can later be exchanged for money, snacks, or some other tangible reinforcers. As the boy earns reinforcers, the criterion for future reinforcers should gradually increase, because his performance is always being compared to how well he did in the last 10 minutes. There are several similarities between a percentile schedule and a more informal shaping procedure. In both cases, the criterion for reinforcement begins at a relatively low level that reflects the learner's current behavior. The criterion is set so that the required behavior is well within the learner's current ability level, but only better performances are reinforced. This selective reinforcement of better performances should cause the learner's performance to improve. The difference from the usual shaping procedure, however, is that the rules for reinforcement are very specific, and nothing is left to the discretion of the trainer.

One study used percentile schedules to shape the academic performance of four children with developmental disabilities whose teachers reported that they spent very little class time on their assigned work (Athens, Vollmer, & St. Peter Pipkin, 2007). Under percentile schedules that delivered reinforcers for spending more time on their work, the on-task performance of all four children increased dramatically. Another experiment used percentile schedules as part of a smoking cessation program (Lamb, Morral, Kirby, Iguchi, & Galbicka, 2004). In one group, each smoker gave a breath sample once a day and received a small amount of money if the sample had a lower carbon monoxide level than on at least 4 of the last 9 days. Carbon monoxide levels decreased for most participants, and there were some indications that this procedure was especially helpful for hard-to-treat smokers. The researchers proposed that this might be the case because percentile schedules tailor the treatment goals on an individual basis, so even those who have a difficult time decreasing their smoking can earn reinforcers for small, gradual improvements.

Even a computer can be programmed to deliver reinforcers according to percentile schedules, as long as the computer is capable of recording and evaluating the learner's responses (Galbicka, 1994). Some computer software already used in classrooms does adopt the essence of this approach by keeping track of each student's performance and tailoring the difficulty of the material to each child's rate of improvement. In this way, the slower learners are given additional practice with simpler concepts until they master them, and the faster learners are not held back but are given more difficult material to keep them challenged.

Versatility of the Shaping Process

We have already seen that the applicability of classical conditioning is relatively limited as a theory of learned behaviors: Classical conditioning applies only to those behaviors that are reliably elicited by some stimulus (the unconditioned stimulus [US]). In comparison, the Law of Effect is much more widely applicable, even if we consider only the strict stop-action approach favored by Guthrie and Horton. The stop-action principle applies not only to behaviors that are preceded by a specific stimulus but to any behavior the subject produces. As long as a behavior such as pressing a lever, stepping on a platform, or pulling a chain occurs once in a while, we can patiently wait for the desired behavior to occur, follow it with a reinforcer, and expect the frequency of that behavior to increase. To put it simply, the stop-action principle can be used to increase the frequency of any behavior that is part of the subject's repertoire. However, once the procedure of shaping is added to the Law of Effect, its applicability is extended still further. The procedure of shaping uses the variability inherent in a creature's behavior to develop totally new behaviors, which the

subject has never performed before and probably would never perform in the absence of a shaping program. For instance, a rat can be taught to press a lever that is high above its head or a lever that requires so much effort to operate that the animal must get a running start and throw all of its weight onto the lever. In principle, at least, the applicability of the shaping process is limited only by the capabilities of the subject: If the subject is capable of making the desired behavior, the careful use of the technique of successive approximations should eventually be successful in producing the appearance of the behavior.

THE RESEARCH OF B. F. SKINNER

Whereas Thorndike deserves credit for the first systematic investigations of the principle of reinforcement, it was B. F. Skinner who was

---

PRACTICE QUIZ (1)

1. Thorndike referred to the principle of strengthening a behavior by its consequences as —————; in modern terminology, this is called —————.
2. In photographing cats in the puzzle box, Guthrie and Horton found that the behaviors of an individual cat were ————— from trial to trial, but they were ————— from cat to cat.
3. Superstitious behaviors are more likely to occur when an individual has ————— of the reinforcer.
4. When using food to shape the behavior of a rat, the sound of the food dispenser is a —————, and the food itself is a —————.
5. A shaping procedure in which a behavior is reinforced if it is better than a certain percentage of the last few responses the individual has made is called a —————.

Answers

1. the Law of Effect, reinforcement   2. similar, different
3. little or no control   4. conditioned reinforcer, primary
reinforcer   5. percentile schedule

primarily responsible for the increasing interest in this topic during the middle of the twentieth century. Skinner himself discovered many of the most basic and most important properties of reinforcement. In addition, he trained several generations of students whose ongoing research continues to enrich our knowledge about the ways that reinforcement affects the behavior of people and animals.

Skinner used the terms *operant conditioning* and *instrumental conditioning* to describe the procedure in which a behavior is strengthened through reinforcement. Both of these terms reflect the large degree of control the subject has over the most important stimulus in the environment—the reinforcer. The delivery of the reinforcer is contingent on the subject's behavior; that is, no reinforcer will occur until the subject makes the required response. For example, in Thorndike's puzzle box the reinforcer (escape and food) might occur after 5 seconds or after 500 seconds, depending entirely on when the animal made the appropriate response. The term *operant conditioning* reflects the fact that the subject obtains reinforcement by operating on the environment in this paradigm. The term *instrumental conditioning* is suggestive of the fact that the subject's behavior is instrumental in obtaining the reinforcer.

The Free Operant

In his research on operant conditioning, Skinner modified Thorndike's procedure in a simple but important way. Research with the puzzle box involved a *discrete trial procedure:* A trial began each time a subject was placed in the puzzle box, and the subject could make one and only one response on each trial. The primary dependent variable was response latency. After each trial, the experimenter had to intervene, physically returning the subject to the puzzle box for the next trial. This procedure was time consuming and cumbersome, and only a small number of trials could be conducted each day. Other operant conditioning procedures that were popular in the early part of the century, such as those involving runways or

mazes with a reinforcer at the end, shared these same disadvantages.

Skinner's innovation was to make use of a response that the subject could perform repeatedly without the intervention of the experimenter. In experiments with rats, lever pressing is often the operant response. When the subjects are pigeons, the most frequently measured response is the key peck: One or more circular plastic disks, called response keys, are recessed in one wall of the experimental chamber (Figure 5-6), and the bird's pecks at these keys are recorded. Procedures that make use of lever pressing, key pecking, or similar responses are called **free-operant procedures** to distinguish them from the discrete trial procedures of the puzzle box or maze. The distinguishing characteristics of a free-operant procedure are that (1) the operant response can occur at any time and (2) the operant response can occur repeatedly for as long as the subject remains in the experimental chamber. In addition, responses such as lever pressing and key pecking require so little effort that a subject can make thousands of responses in a single session.

Along with this change in procedures came a change in dependent variables: Instead of using latency as a measure of response strength, Skinner used response rate (usually measured as responses per minute). One major advantage of

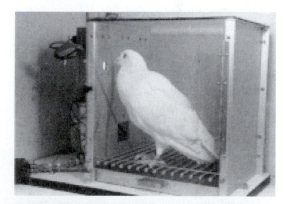

FIGURE 5-6 A pigeon pecking at a lighted key in a typical operant conditioning chamber. Grain is provided as a reinforcer through the square opening beneath the key. (Photo courtesy of James E. Mazur.)

the free-operant procedure, with its large number of responses, is that the experimenter can observe and record the moment-to-moment variations in response rate that occur as a subject learns about the experimental situation or as some external stimulus is changed.

The Three-Term Contingency

In its simplest form, a contingency is a rule that states that some event, B, will occur if and only if another event, A, occurs. Simple classical conditioning provides one example of such a contingency: The US will occur if and only if the CS occurs first. It is sometimes said that in operant conditioning, there is a contingency between response and reinforcer—the reinforcer occurs if and only if the response occurs. Skinner pointed out, however, that there are actually three components in the operant conditioning contingency: (1) the context or situation in which a response occurs (i.e., those stimuli that precede the response); (2) the response itself; and (3) the stimuli that follow the response (i.e., the reinforcer). To be more specific, Skinner noted that the contingency in operant conditioning usually takes the following form: In the presence of a specific stimulus, often called a **discriminative stimulus**, the reinforcer will occur if and only if the operant response occurs. Because of the three components—discriminative stimulus, response, and reinforcer—Skinner called this relationship a **three-term contingency**.

Suppose a pigeon learns to peck a key for food pellets in a chamber that has a bright yellow light just above the key. When the light is on, each response produces a food pellet, but when the light is off, no food pellets are delivered. If the light is periodically turned on and off during the course of the experiment, the pigeon will learn to discriminate between these two conditions and respond only when the light is on. This type of discrimination learning is important in many real-world situations, because a response that is reinforced in one context may not be reinforced in another. For example, a child must learn that the behavior of telling jokes may be reinforced if

it occurs during recess but punished if it occurs during math class. The term **stimulus control** refers to the broad topic of how stimuli that precede a behavior can control the occurrence of that behavior. Chapter 9 will examine this topic in detail.

Basic Principles of Operant Conditioning

Many of the principles of operant conditioning have counterparts in classical conditioning that we have already examined, so a brief discussion of them will suffice here. Thorndike's results (as in Figure 5-2) demonstrate that the **acquisition** of an operant response, like that of a CR, is usually a gradual process. In operant conditioning, the procedure of **extinction** involves no longer following the operant response with a reinforcer, and as in classical conditioning, the response will weaken and eventually disappear. If the subject is returned to the experimental chamber at some later time, **spontaneous recovery** of the operant response will typically be observed, just as it is observed in classical conditioning.

In The Three-Term Contingency section, we saw that **discrimination** learning can occur in operant conditioning as well as in classical conditioning. The opposite of discrimination, **generalization**, is also a common phenomenon in operant conditioning. Let us return to the example of the pigeon that learned to discriminate between the presence and absence of a bright yellow light. Suppose the color of the light changed to green or orange, and no more reinforcers were delivered. Despite this change in color, the pigeon would probably continue to peck at the key for a while, until it learned that no more reinforcers were forthcoming. In other words, the pigeon generalized from the yellow light to a light of another color, even though it had never been reinforced for pecking in the presence of this other color. If we tested a number of different colors, we would probably obtain a typical generalization gradient in which responding was most rapid in the presence of yellow and less and less rapid with colors less and less similar to yellow.

Resurgence

As in classical conditioning, extinction does not permanently eliminate an operant response, as the phenomenon of spontaneous recovery demonstrates. Another interesting phenomenon that makes this same point is called resurgence. **Resurgence** is the reappearance of a previously reinforced response that occurs when a more recently reinforced response is extinguished. For example, R. Epstein (1983) first reinforced key pecking by pigeons, and then this response was extinguished. Next, a different response was reinforced 20 times, and then this response was extinguished. When the new response was no longer reinforced, there was a resurgence of pecking: The pigeons began to peck the key again, at a fairly high rate. Resurgence can occur even when a response has been thoroughly extinguished. In a study by Lieving and Lattal (2003), key pecking was first reinforced and then extinguished for 10 daily sessions. In the last few extinction sessions, the pigeons made few or no key pecks. Then a different response, stepping on a treadle, was reinforced for five sessions, and this was followed by several sessions in which neither response was reinforced. Once treadle pressing was no longer reinforced, all pigeons started to peck the key again, making hundreds of key pecks over the course of several sessions (even though none of these pecks was reinforced).

Resurgence has been observed in other species, including rats (Winterbauer & Bouton, 2010) and humans (Bruzek, Thompson, & Peters, 2009; Doughty, Cash, Finch, Holloway, & Wallington, 2010). It tends to be stronger for behaviors that previously occurred at faster rates (da Silva, Maxwell, & Lattal, 2008). Resurgence of specific response patterns (not just individual responses) can also occur. For instance, Cancado and Lattal (2011) first trained pigeons to peck at a steady pace when a response key was one color and at an accelerating pace when the key was a different color. Then these responses were extinguished and pecking on a different key was reinforced. When pecking on the new key was no longer reinforced, they found a resurgence of both steady and accelerating response patterns on the first key, depending on the color of the key on each trial.

R. Epstein (1996) has suggested that some examples of novel or creative behavior may be the result of resurgence. For example, Epstein and Medalie (1983) trained a pigeon to push a small cardboard box toward different targets. The pigeon was then trained to peck at a metal plate that was at the bottom of one wall of the test chamber, with food as the reinforcer. Later, the metal plate was recessed behind a hole in the wall. The pigeon tried to peck at the metal plate, but it was out of reach. The bird then pushed the cardboard box through the hole in the wall until it touched the metal plate, and then started pecking at the box. This creative solution to the problem of how to operate the metal plate can be at least partly attributed to the resurgence of the previously reinforced behavior of pushing the box when the more recently reinforced behavior was no longer possible.

Conditioned Reinforcement

In operant conditioning, the phenomenon of conditioned reinforcement (also called *secondary reinforcement*) is in many ways analogous to second-order classical conditioning. As discussed in Chapter 3, if some CS (such as a light) is repeatedly paired with a US, that CS can then take the place of the US in classical conditioning with a second CS (say, a tone). If the tone is now repeatedly paired with a light, the tone will start to elicit CRs, which is the same thing that would happen if the tone were paired with the US itself. We might say that the first-order CS, the light, acts as a surrogate for the US in second-order conditioning.

In operant conditioning, the counterpart to the US is the primary reinforcer. The counterpart to the first-order CS is the initially neutral stimulus that becomes a conditioned reinforcer through repeated pairings with the primary reinforcer. The conditioned reinforcer can then act as a surrogate for the primary reinforcer, increasing the strength of any response that it follows.

In an early study on conditioned reinforcement, Skinner (1938) presented rats with repeated pairings of a clicking sound and food. No responses were required during this phase of the experiment. In the second phase of the experiment, food was no longer presented; nevertheless, the rats learned to press a lever when this response produced only the clicking sound. Naturally, since the clicking sound was no longer paired with food, it is not surprising that the lever pressing did not persist for long. This is another way in which first-order CSs and conditioned reinforcers are similar: If a conditioned reinforcer is no longer paired with a primary reinforcer, it eventually loses its capacity to act as a reinforcer, just as a first-order CS loses its ability to condition a second-order CS if it is repeatedly presented without the US.

Skinner used the term **generalized reinforcers** to refer to a special class of conditioned reinforcers—those that are associated with a large number of different primary reinforcers. Perhaps the best example of a generalized reinforcer is money. The potency of this reinforcer in maintaining the behaviors of workers in our society is clear: Few employees would remain on the job if informed that their employer could no longer pay them any salary. Money is a generalized reinforcer (and a powerful one) precisely because it can be exchanged for so many different stimuli that are inherently reinforcing for most people, for example, food, clothing, material possessions, entertainment, and exciting vacations. Although money is a powerful reinforcer, it should be clear that its power, like that of all conditioned reinforcers, depends on its continued association with primary reinforcers. If money could no longer be exchanged for any primary reinforcers, it would be difficult to find individuals willing to work simply to obtain green pieces of paper.

Both laboratory findings and real-world examples of conditioned reinforcers (money, exam grades, praise from a parent, teacher, or boss, etc.) demonstrate the powerful effects that they can have on an individual's behavior. What is still being debated by psychologists, however, is exactly how conditioned reinforcers exert their effects. One basic question is whether conditioned reinforcers affect behavior because they *provide information* (about the future delivery of a primary reinforcer) or because they *add value* to the situation (i.e., they add additional reinforcing value above what the primary reinforcer already provides).

As an example that shows the difference between providing information and adding value, Rachlin (1976) asked readers to imagine two hotels. In hotel A, a dinner bell rings before each meal. This bell should become a conditioned reinforcer because it is paired with the primary reinforcer, food. In hotel B, a dinner bell also rings before each meal, but the bell also rings at other times, when there is no meal. Which hotel will people prefer? If the bell adds value to the situation, hotel B should be preferred, because the bell rings more often. But according to Rachlin, it seems obvious that people would prefer hotel A, where the bell provides accurate information about when meals will be served. An experiment by Schuster (1969) gave pigeons a choice similar to the two hotels. In condition A, pecks at a key occasionally produced a blue light and a buzzer, which were always followed by food. In condition B, there were the same number of pairings of blue light, buzzer, and food, but there were extra presentations of the blue light and buzzer without food. Schuster found that although pigeons pecked more in condition B, when they were given a choice they preferred condition A, where every presentation of the blue light and buzzer were followed by food. This experiment supports the information theory of conditioned reinforcement—the strongest conditioned reinforcers are those that provide the best information about the delivery of primary reinforcers.

Many other studies on conditioned reinforcement have been conducted, and unfortunately they do not offer a simple answer to the question of exactly what conditioned reinforcers do. In some experiments, there seems to be evidence that conditioned reinforcers do add value to the situation (Williams & Dunn, 1991). Taking a somewhat different approach, Fantino (2008) has proposed that the strength of a conditioned reinforcer depends on the *relative improvement* that it signals about the learner's situation. For example, suppose a pigeon is pecking at a response key that only rarely delivers food, but whenever a tone is presented, food is delivered 5 seconds later. The tone should become a strong conditioned reinforcer because it signals a large improvement in the pigeon's situation—a food delivery is now imminent.

Williams (1994) suggested that conditioned reinforcers may play other roles, including marking and bridging. *Marking* is providing immediate feedback for a particular response, as when the sound of the food dispenser immediately after an appropriate response makes it easier for an animal trainer to shape new behaviors. *Bridging* occurs when a conditioned reinforcer fills the time period between a response and the delivery of a primary reinforcer, which may help the learner to associate the response and the reinforcer.

In a review of the many complex and often conflicting laboratory findings about conditioned reinforcers, Shahan (2010) concluded that most of the results are consistent with the idea that conditioned reinforcers act as "signposts" that "serve to guide rather than strengthen behavior" (p. 279). In other words, he argues in favor of the information hypothesis. However, others continue to argue just as strongly for the reinforcing value hypothesis (e.g., McDevitt & Williams, 2010), so this issue is by no means settled.

Response Chains

In Chapter 2, we examined the concept of a reaction chain, which is a sequence of innate behaviors that occur in a fixed order. A similar concept involving learned behaviors is the **response chain**, which is defined as a sequence of behaviors that must occur in a specific order, with the primary reinforcer being delivered only after the final response of the sequence. Some of the clearest examples of response chains are displayed by animals trained to perform complex sequences of behavior for circus acts or other public performances. Imagine a hypothetical performance in which a rat climbs a ladder to a platform, pulls a rope that opens a door to a tunnel, runs through

the tunnel to another small platform, slides down a chute, runs to a lever, presses the lever, and finally receives a pellet of food. Ignoring for the moment how the rat could be trained to do this, we can ask what maintains the behavior once it has been learned.

The first response, climbing the ladder, brings the rat to nothing more than a platform and a rope. These are certainly not primary reinforcers for a rat. Skinner would claim, however, that these stimuli act as conditioned reinforcers for the response of climbing the ladder because they bring the animal closer to primary reinforcement than it was before. Besides serving as conditioned reinforcers, the platform and rope also act as discriminative stimuli for the next response of the chain, pulling the rope. The conditioned reinforcer for this response is the sight of the door opening, for this event brings the subject still closer to primary reinforcement. Like the platform and rope, the open door also serves a second function—it is a discriminative stimulus for the next response, running through the tunnel.

We could go on to analyze the rest of the response chain in a similar fashion, but the general pattern should be clear by now. Each stimulus in the middle of a response chain is assumed to serve two functions: It is a conditioned reinforcer for the previous response and a discriminative stimulus for the next response of the chain. This analysis is depicted graphically in Figure 5-7, where S^D stands for "discriminative stimulus" and S^R stands for "reinforcing stimulus."

How would an animal trainer go about teaching a rat to perform this sequence? One very effective strategy, sometimes called **backward chaining**, is to start with the last response of the chain and work backward. After teaching the rat where to obtain its food reinforcement and establishing the sound of the food dispenser as a conditioned reinforcer, the trainer could start to shape the last response of the chain, pressing the lever. Once this response is well established, the trainer might place the rat on the bottom of the chute. It is very likely that the rat would move from this position to the lever, since the lever will now act as a conditioned reinforcer

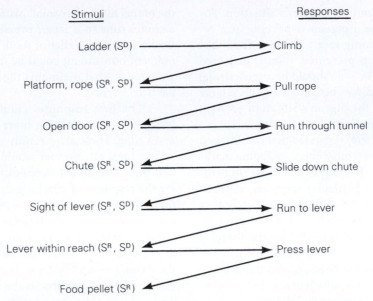

FIGURE 5-7   The alternating sequence of stimuli and responses in the hypothetical response chain described in the text. Each stimulus within the chain serves as a conditioned reinforcer for the previous response and as a discriminative stimulus for the next response.

(having been previously paired with food). By additional shaping, the animal could be trained to slide down the chute to reach the lever, then to travel through the tunnel to reach the chute, and so on. Some shaping with food as a primary reinforcer might be required for some links of the chain (e.g., pulling the rope). Once the response was established, however, the primary reinforcement could be removed and the behavior would be maintained by the conditioned reinforcement provided by the next stimulus of the chain, a stimulus that signaled that the animal was one step closer to the primary reinforcer.

Backward chaining is one effective way to teach a response chain, but it is not the only way. In **forward chaining**, the teacher starts by reinforcing the first response of the chain, then gradually adds the second response, the third response, and so on. For example, in learning to use a laundromat, adolescents with mental retardation were first reinforced just for finding an empty washing machine. Next, they were reinforced for finding an empty machine and putting in the soap, then for finding an empty machine, putting in the

soap, loading the clothes, and so on (McDonnell & McFarland, 1988). Still another training method is the *total task method;* here the individual is taught all of the steps of a response chain at once, using verbal instructions to prompt the correct response at each step. All these methods for teaching response chains (along with other variations) have been used successfully; which is most effective seems to depend on exactly what types of behaviors are being taught (Ash & Holding, 1990; Hur & Osborne, 1993).

Not surprisingly, the behaviors of a response chain will eventually disappear if the primary reinforcement is eliminated. It is also interesting to observe what happens if one of the conditioned reinforcers in the middle of the chain is eliminated. The general rule is that all behaviors that occur before the "broken link" of the chain will be extinguished, whereas those that occur after the broken link will continue to occur. For example, suppose that pulling the rope no longer opens the door to the tunnel. The response of rope pulling will eventually stop occurring, as will the behavior of climbing the ladder that leads to the platform and rope. On the other hand, if the rat is placed beyond the broken link (inside the tunnel or at the top of the chute), the remainder of the chain should continue to occur as long as the final response is followed by the primary reinforcer.

Because they are the farthest from the primary reinforcer, responses near the beginning of a response chain should be the weakest, or the most easily disrupted. Behavior therapists frequently make use of this principle when attempting to break up a response chain that includes some unwanted behaviors (e.g., walking to the drugstore, buying a pack of cigarettes, opening the pack, lighting a cigarette, and smoking it). Efforts to interrupt this chain should be most effective if applied to the earliest links of the chain.

BIOLOGICAL CONSTRAINTS ON OPERANT CONDITIONING

Just as biological factors affect what is learned in classical conditioning, they play an important role in operant conditioning. Two phenomena, instinctive drift and autoshaping, both discovered in the 1960s, raised serious questions about the power of reinforcement to modify and control a creature's behavior. The stories of how these phenomena were discovered and the theoretical debates surrounding them provide valuable lessons about the strengths and limitations of the general principles of learning.

Instinctive Drift

Learning theorists, especially those who specialize in operant conditioning, have generally believed that reinforcement exerts a simple but powerful influence on behavior: Behaviors that are reinforced will increase in frequency, and those that are not will decrease and eventually disappear. When shaping, generalization, chaining, and other basic principles are added to this idea, it should be possible to teach complex and intricate sequences of behavior to both people and animals. Two psychologists who attempted to apply the principles of operant conditioning outside the laboratory were Keller Breland

and Marian Breland. After studying with B. F. Skinner, the Brelands became animal trainers and worked with many different species, teaching complex and frequently amusing patterns of behavior. Their animals were trained for zoos, fairs, television commercials, and other public performances.

The Brelands' business was successful, and over the years they trained several thousand animals. On the surface, at least, it appeared that they had demonstrated that principles from the laboratory were usable in less controlled settings and applicable to creatures ranging from whales to reindeer. Despite the success of their business, however, the Brelands began to notice certain recurrent problems in their use of reinforcement techniques. They referred to these problems as "breakdowns of conditioned operant behavior." In an article entitled "The Misbehavior of Organisms" (Breland & Breland, 1961), they described several of their "failures" in the use of reinforcement. The following is one example:

> Here a pig was conditioned to pick up large wooden coins and deposit them in a large "piggy bank." The coins were placed several feet from the bank and the pig required to carry them to the bank and deposit them, usually four or five coins for one reinforcement. (Of course, we started out with one coin, near the bank.)
>
> Pigs condition very rapidly, they have no trouble taking ratios, they have ravenous appetites (naturally), and in many ways are among the most tractable animals we have worked with. However, this particular problem behavior developed in pig after pig, usually after a period of weeks or months, getting worse every day. At first the pig would eagerly pick up one dollar, carry it to the bank, run back, get another, carry it rapidly and neatly, and so on, until the ratio was complete. Thereafter, over a period of weeks the behavior would become slower and slower. He might run over eagerly for each dollar, but on the way back, instead of carrying the dollar and depositing it simply

and cleanly, he would repeatedly drop it, root it, drop it again, root it along the way, pick it up, toss it up in the air, drop it, root it some more, and so on.

> We thought this behavior might simply be the dilly-dallying of an animal on a low drive. However, the behavior persisted and gained in strength in spite of a severely increased drive—he finally went through the ratios so slowly that he did not get enough to eat in the course of a day. Finally it would take the pig about 10 minutes to transport four coins a distance of about 6 feet. This problem behavior developed repeatedly in successive pigs. (p. 683)

This example differs from the instances of contraprepared associations discussed in Chapter 4. Here, the problem was not that pigs had difficulty learning the required response: At first, a pig would carry the coins to the bank without hesitation. It was only later that new, unreinforced behaviors—dropping and rooting the coins—appeared and increased in frequency. The Brelands noted that the intruding behaviors were those that pigs normally perform as part of their food-gathering repertoires. Because these behaviors appeared to be related to the animal's innate responses, the Brelands called them examples of **instinctive drift**: With extensive experience, the animal's performance drifted away from the reinforced behaviors and toward instinctive behaviors that occur when it is seeking the reinforcer (in this case, food) in a natural environment.

It is interesting to compare the behavior of pigs with that of a raccoon in a similar situation. The task was to pick up coins and place them in a small container. With just one coin, the raccoon learned, with a little difficulty, to pick it up and drop it in the container, after which it received food as a reinforcer. When the raccoon was given two coins simultaneously, however, its behavior deteriorated markedly. Instead of picking up the coins and depositing them quickly (which would provide the most immediate reinforcement), the raccoon would hold onto the coins for several

minutes, frequently rubbing them together, and occasionally dipping them into the container and pulling them out again. Although these behaviors were not reinforced, they became more and more prevalent over time, and the swift sequence of depositing the coins that the Brelands desired was never achieved.

You may recognize a similarity between this raccoon's behaviors and those of the pigs. The raccoon's intruding behaviors resemble those that are part of its food-gathering repertoire. A raccoon may repeatedly dip a piece of food in a stream before eating it, and the rubbing motions are similar to those it might use in removing the shell from a crustacean. Notice, however, that in the present context these behaviors were inappropriate in two respects: (1) The coins were not food, the container was not a stream, and there was no shell to be removed by rubbing the coins together; and (2) the intruding behaviors did not produce food reinforcement—indeed, they actually postponed its delivery.

The Brelands reported that they had found numerous other examples of this sort of instinctive drift, and they claimed that these examples constituted "a clear and utter failure of conditioning theory" (1961, p. 683). The problem was perfectly clear: Animals exhibited behaviors that the trainers did not reinforce in place of behaviors the trainers had reinforced.

Autoshaping

In 1968, P. L. Brown and Jenkins published an article titled "Auto-Shaping of the Pigeon's Key-Peck." They presented their findings as simply a method for training pigeons to peck a key that was easier and less time consuming than manual shaping. Naive pigeons were deprived of food and taught to eat from the grain dispenser. After this, a pigeon was exposed to the following contingencies: At irregular intervals averaging 60 seconds, the response key was illuminated with white light for 8 seconds; then the key was darkened and food was presented. Despite the fact that no response was necessary for the delivery of food, after a number of such trials, all of the pigeons began to peck at the lighted key.

Whereas autoshaping did seem to be an easier way to train the response of key pecking, psychologists soon realized the more important theoretical significance of the Brown and Jenkins result. Key pecking had been used in countless experiments because it was considered to be a "typical" operant response—a response that is controlled by its consequences. Yet here was an experiment in which the key-peck response was not necessary for reinforcement, yet it occurred anyway. Why did the pigeons peck at the key? Several different explanations were proposed.

AUTOSHAPING AS SUPERSTITIOUS BEHAVIOR.
Brown and Jenkins suggested that autoshaping might be an example of a superstitious behavior, as discussed earlier in this chapter. It is possible that approaching, making contact, and pecking the lighted key were accidentally reinforced by the food deliveries that soon followed. However, an experiment by Rachlin (1969) suggested that this hypothesis is not correct. Using a procedure similar to that of Brown and Jenkins, Rachlin photographed pigeons on each trial at the moment reinforcement was delivered. The photographs revealed no tendency for the birds to get progressively closer to the key and finally peck it. On the trial immediately preceding the trial of the first key peck, a pigeon might be far from the key, looking in another direction, at the moment of reinforcement. There was no hint of a gradual shaping process at work.

More evidence against the superstition interpretation came from a study in which the food reinforcer was eliminated from any trial on which the pigeon pecked at the lighted key (Williams & Williams, 1969). The results of this experiment were quite remarkable: Even though no food ever followed a key peck, pigeons still acquired the key-peck response and persisted in pecking at the lighted key on about one third of the trials. This experiment showed quite convincingly that key pecking in an autoshaping procedure is not an instance of superstitious behavior.

AUTOSHAPING AS CLASSICAL CONDITIONING.
A number of researchers have proposed that autoshaping is simply an example of classical conditioning intruding into what the experimenter might view as an operant conditioning situation (Moore, 1973). Pigeons eat grain by pecking at the kernels with jerky head movements. We might say that pecking is the pigeon's unconditioned response to the stimulus of grain. According to the classical conditioning interpretation, this response of pecking is transferred from the grain to the key because the lighted key is repeatedly paired with food. One type of evidence that supports this interpretation comes from experiments in which the researchers either photographed or closely observed the behaviors of their subjects. In an important series of experiments by Jenkins and Moore (1973), illumination of a response key was regularly followed by the presentation of food for some pigeons and by the presentation of water for other pigeons. In both cases the pigeons began to peck at the lighted key. However, by filming the pigeons' responses, Jenkins and Moore were able to demonstrate that the pigeons' movements toward the key differed depending on which reinforcer was used. When the reinforcer was food, a pigeon's response involved an abrupt, forceful pecking motion made with the beak open wide and eyelids almost closed (Figure 5-8, bottom row). These movements are similar to those a pigeon makes when eating. When the reinforcer was water, the response was a slower approach to the key with the beak closed or nearly closed (Figure 5-8, top row). On some trials with water as the reinforcer, swallowing movements and a rhythmic opening and closing of the beak were observed. All of these movements are part of the pigeon's characteristic drinking pattern. Jenkins and Moore proposed that these behaviors were clear examples of Pavlov's concept of stimulus substitution. The lighted key served as a substitute for either food or water, and responses appropriate for either food or water were directed at the key.

Although autoshaping was first observed in pigeons pecking a lighted key (Brown & Jenkins,

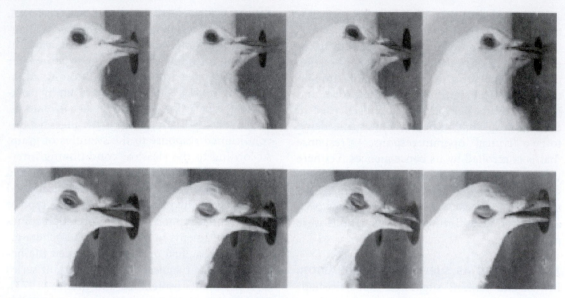

FIGURE 5-8   Photographs of a pigeon's key pecks when the reinforcer was water (top row) and when the reinforcer was grain (bottom row). Notice the different beak and eyelid movements with the two different reinforcers. (From Jenkins & Moore, 1973).

SOURCE: From H.M. Jenkins and B.R. Moore, "The form of the auto-shaped response with food or water reinforcers," *Journal of the Experimental Analysis of Behavior, 20*(2), pages 163–181. Copyright 1973 by the Society for the Experimental Analysis of Behavior, Inc.

1968), this term can refer to any situation in which an animal produces some distinctive behavior in response to a signal that precedes and predicts an upcoming reinforcer. Others have called this phenomenon *sign-tracking,* because the animal watches, follows, and makes contact with a signal for an upcoming reinforcer. In this broader sense, autoshaping (or sign-tracking) has been observed in many species, and many of the examples are consistent with the stimulus substitution theory of classical conditioning. For example, Peterson, Ackil, Frommer, and Hearst (1972) videotaped the behavior of rats to a retractable lever that was inserted into the chamber and illuminated 15 seconds before the delivery of each reinforcer. For some rats, the reinforcer was food; for others, it was electrical stimulation of the brain. Both groups of rats made frequent contact with the lever, but the topographies of their responses were distinctly different. Rats with the food reinforcer were observed to gnaw and lick the lever, whereas those with brain stimulation as a reinforcer would touch the lever lightly with paws or whiskers, or they might sniff

and "explore" the lever. These two different behavior patterns, directed at the lever, resembled the rats' behaviors when food or brain stimulation was actually delivered.

AUTOSHAPING AS THE INTRUSION OF INSTINCTIVE BEHAVIOR PATTERNS.   Whereas the studies just described provide support for the stimulus substitution interpretation of autoshaping, other studies do not. Wasserman (1973) observed the responses of 3-day-old chicks to a key light paired with warmth. In an uncomfortably cool chamber, a heat lamp was turned on briefly at irregular intervals, with each activation of the heat lamp being preceded by the illumination of a green key light. All chicks soon began to peck the key when it was green, but their manner of responding was unusual: A chick would typically move very close to the key, push its beak into the key, and rub its beak from side to side in what Wasserman called a "snuggling" behavior. These snuggling responses resembled behaviors a newborn chick normally makes to obtain warmth from a mother hen: The chick pecks at the feathers on the lower part of the hen's body, then rubs its beak, and pushes its head into the feathers.

On the surface, this study seems to provide another example of stimulus substitution—a warmth-seeking behavior pattern is displayed to a signal for warmth. The problem, however, is that the chicks in the experiment exhibited a very different set of behaviors in response to the heat lamp itself. When the heat lamp was turned on, there was no pecking or snuggling; instead, a chick would extend its wings (which allowed it to absorb more of the heat) and stand motionless. On other trials, a chick might extend its wings, lower its body, and rub its chest against the floor. Thus, although both snuggling and wing extension are warmth-related behaviors for a young chick, there was virtually no similarity between a chick's responses to the key light and its responses to the heat lamp. For this reason, Wasserman concluded that the stimulus substitution account of autoshaping is inadequate and that the physical properties of the signal also determine the form of autoshaped responses.

Other experiments support Wasserman's conclusions. For example, Timberlake and Grant (1975) observed the behaviors of rats when the signal preceding the delivery of a food pellet was the entry of another rat (restrained on a small moving platform) into the experimental chamber. Since a food pellet elicits biting and chewing responses, the stimulus substitution interpretation of autoshaping predicts that a subject should perform these same biting and chewing responses to the restrained rat, because the rat is a signal for food. Not surprisingly, Timberlake and Grant observed no instances of biting or chewing responses directed toward the restrained rat. However, they did observe a high frequency of other behaviors directed toward the restrained rat, including approach, sniffing, and social contact (pawing, grooming, and climbing over the other rat).

In these examples, the behaviors elicited by the signal are different from those elicited by the reinforcer, but they seem to be behaviors involved in obtaining that type of reinforcer in the animal's natural environment. Thus, with rats, which usually feed in groups, the presence of a restrained rat predicting food elicited approach, exploration, and social behaviors—all behaviors that might occur during the course of a food-seeking expedition. With young chicks, a signal preceding the activation of a heat lamp elicited some of these birds' normal warmth-seeking behaviors. In a study with monkeys, Bullock and Myers (2009) presented an image of a gray square that moved along the floor of the chamber, which was followed by delivery of a banana pellet. Video recordings showed that the monkeys made touching, grabbing, licking, and biting responses toward the gray square, behaviors similar to those observed when these monkeys retrieve and consume food.

Timberlake and Grant (1975) suggested the following interpretation:

> As an alternative to stimulus substitution, we offer the hypothesis that autoshaped behavior reflects the conditioning of a system of species-typical behaviors commonly related to the reward. The form of the behavior in the presence of the predictive stimulus will depend on which behaviors in the conditioned system are elicited and supported by the predictive stimulus. (p. 692)

Timberlake (1993, 2001) has called this interpretation of autoshaped behaviors a **behavior-systems analysis** to reflect the idea that different reinforcers evoke different systems or collections of behaviors. An animal may have a system of food-related behaviors, a system of water-related behaviors, a system of warmth-seeking behaviors, a system of mating behaviors, and so on. Exactly which behavior from a given system will be elicited by a signal depends in part on the physical properties of that signal. For instance, in Wasserman's study, the characteristics of the response key (such as a distinctive visual stimulus about head high) evidently lent themselves more readily to snuggling than to wing extension, so that the former was observed rather than the latter.

Notice that the predictions of Timberlake's behavior-systems approach are more ambiguous than those of the stimulus substitution approach. It would be difficult (at least for me) to predict in advance whether a green key light would be more likely to elicit wing extension, snuggling, or some other warmth-related behavior. Nevertheless, the behavior-systems approach does make testable predictions because it states that the behaviors provoked by a signal will depend on the type of reinforcer that usually follows the signal. The theory predicts quite clearly that a signal for warmth should elicit behaviors that are part of the animal's warmth-seeking behavior system, not those that are part of its feeding system or its drinking system. Although these predictions are less specific than those of stimulus substitution theory, they are certainly in closer agreement with the evidence on the form of autoshaped behaviors. Timberlake and his colleagues (Silva & Timberlake, 2000; Timberlake & Lucas, 1989) have shown that the behavior-systems approach can be applied to a variety of learning phenomena (including autoshaping, instinctive drift, preparedness, and backward conditioning).

SUMMARY. Regardless of whether we emphasize the hereditary aspects of autoshaped behaviors or their similarity to classically conditioned CRs, both autoshaped behaviors and instinctive drift seem to pose severe difficulties for operant conditioners. Breland and Breland (1961) summarized the problem nicely: "The examples listed we feel represent clear and utter failure of conditioning theory. . . . The animal simply does not do what it has been conditioned to do" (p. 683).

Reconciling Reinforcement Theory and Biological Constraints

How do those who believe in the general-principle approach to learning, and especially in the principle of reinforcement, respond to these cases where the general principles do not seem to work? First, let us consider the phenomenon of autoshaping.

As we have seen, early discussions of autoshaped behavior suggested that it posed major problems for the general-principle approach because it seemed to defy the rules of operant conditioning. Later analyses suggested that autoshaping is simply an instance of classical

conditioning. Although there may be aspects of autoshaped responses that distinguish them from other types of conditioned responses (Swan & Pearce, 1987; Wasserman, 1973), it is now commonly believed that autoshaping is in fact a good example of classical conditioning. And like taste-aversion learning (see Chapter 4), autoshaping is now widely used as a procedure for studying basic principles of classical conditioning (e.g., Balsam, Drew, & Yang, 2002; Locurto, Terrace, & Gibbon, 1981; Rescorla, 2003). Autoshaping therefore appears to be a type of behavior that is quite consistent with the general-principle approach to learning after all (but with the principles of classical conditioning rather than operant conditioning).

The evidence on instinctive drift in operant conditioning cannot be dealt with so easily. Here, it is not just that reinforced behaviors are slow to be learned. What happens is that totally different, unreinforced behaviors appear and gradually become more persistent. These behaviors are presumably part of the animal's inherited behavioral repertoire. As the Brelands discovered, these behaviors often cannot be eliminated by using standard reinforcement techniques, so it might appear that the principle of reinforcement is simply incorrect—it cannot explain why these behaviors arise and are maintained. Indeed, some researchers have asserted that the concept of reinforcement is inadequate and should be abandoned (Timberlake, 1983).

How might a psychologist who relies heavily on the concept of reinforcement react to this empirical evidence and the theoretical challenges it poses? The reactions of B. F. Skinner are worth examining. First of all, it is important to realize that Skinner has always maintained that an organism's behavior is determined by both learning experiences and heredity. Well before biological constraints on learning became a popular topic, Skinner had written about the hereditary influences on behavior in several places (Heron & Skinner, 1940; Skinner, 1956b, 1966). Later, Skinner (1977) stated that he was neither surprised nor disturbed by phenomena such as instinctive drift or autoshaping. He asserted that these are simply cases where phylogenetic (hereditary) and ontogenetic (learned) influences on behavior are operating simultaneously: "Phylogeny and ontogeny are friendly rivals and neither one always wins" (p. 1009).

In other words, we should not be surprised that hereditary factors can compete with and sometimes overshadow the reinforcement contingencies as determinants of behavior. For example, if reinforcers are delivered at regular, periodic intervals, a variety of unreinforced behaviors appear between reinforcers. As discussed previously, Staddon and Simmelhag (1971) called these interim and terminal behaviors, and collectively they have been called adjunctive behaviors. Adjunctive behaviors can take a variety of forms. If food is delivered at periodic intervals, and if water is available between the food reinforcers, animals may consume substantial amounts of water (Falk, 1961). Other common adjunctive behaviors include aggression (Cohen & Looney, 1973), wheel running (King, 1974), and retreat from the location of food delivery (Cohen & Campagnoni, 1989). Adjunctive behaviors have also been observed with human subjects. In one study, college students played a game of backgammon in which they had to wait for fixed periods of time (and could not watch) as their opponents made their moves. When these waiting periods were long, several behaviors unrelated to playing the game—bodily movement, eating, and drinking—increased in frequency (Allen & Butler, 1990). Although the causes of adjunctive behaviors are still being debated, the main point is that these behaviors appear even though they have nothing to do with earning the reinforcer.

The examples of adjunctive behaviors, autoshaping, and instinctive drift do not mean that the principle of reinforcement is flawed; they simply show that reinforcement is not the sole determinant of a creature's behavior. Critics who use these data to claim that the principle of reinforcement should be abandoned appear to be making a serious logical mistake; that is, they conclude that because a theoretical concept cannot explain everything, it is deficient and should be abandoned. This conclusion does not follow from the premises. It is just as incorrect as the claim of some radical environmentalists (e.g., Kuo, 1921) that all behaviors are learned, none

are innate. This chapter (and each of the next several chapters) provides overwhelming evidence that the delivery of reinforcement contingent upon a response is a powerful means of controlling behavior. No amount of evidence on the hereditary influences on behavior can contradict these findings.

There is a growing consensus in the field of learning that the research on biological constraints does not forecast the end of the general-principle approach, but rather that it has provided the field with a valuable lesson (see, e.g., Domjan, 2008; Green & Holt, 2003; Logue, 1988). This research shows that an animal's hereditary endowment plays an important part in many learning situations, and the influence of heredity cannot be ignored. As we learn more about how these biological factors exert their influence, we will be better able to understand and predict a creature's behavior.

PRACTICE QUIZ (2)

1. Thorndike's research with the puzzle box is an example of a _____ procedure, whereas Skinner's research used a _____ procedure.
2. The three parts of a three-term contingency are the _____, the _____, and the _____.
3. Each stimulus in the middle of a response chain serves as a _____ for the previous response and as a _____ for the next response.
4. The procedure in which pigeons start to peck at a lighted response key when it precedes food deliveries is called _____.
5. The Brelands used the term *instinctive drift* to refer to cases where an animal stopped performing _____ behaviors and started performing _____ behaviors as its training progressed.

Answers

1. discrete trial, free-operant   2. discriminative stimulus, operant response, reinforcer   3. conditioned reinforcer, discriminative stimulus   4. autoshaping   5. reinforced, instinctive

Summary

If a response is followed by a reinforcer, the frequency of that response will increase. Thorndike demonstrated this principle in his experiments with cats in the puzzle box, and he called it the Law of Effect. Using photography, Guthrie and Horton found that whatever motion a cat happened to make at the moment of reinforcement tended to be repeated on later trials. Different cats learned distinctly different styles of making the same response. If a response is strengthened when, by mere coincidence, it is followed by a reinforcer, it is called a superstitious behavior. B. F. Skinner reported seeing superstitious behaviors in a famous experiment with pigeons. Accidental reinforcement may account for the unusual rituals performed by some gamblers and athletes.

The procedure of shaping, or successive approximations, involves reinforcing any small movement that comes closer to the desired response, and then gradually changing the criterion for reinforcement until the desired behavior is reached. Shaping is a common part of many behavior modification procedures.

B. F. Skinner used the term *three-term contingency* to describe the three-part relation between a discriminative stimulus, an operant response, and a reinforcer. Responses can be strengthened by either primary reinforcers or conditioned reinforcers. Contingencies between stimuli and responses can have more than three components, as in a response chain, which consists of an alternating series of stimuli and responses, and only the last response is followed by a primary reinforcer.

While using operant conditioning techniques to train animals, Breland and Breland discovered instinctive drift: The animals would begin to display innate behaviors associated with the reinforcers, even though these behaviors were not reinforced. When Brown and Jenkins repeatedly paired a lighted key with food, pigeons eventually began to peck at the key. They called this phenomenon *autoshaping*. Such examples of biological constraints in operant conditioning do not mean that the principle of reinforcement is incorrect, but they do show that behavior is often controlled by a mixture of learning and hereditary influences.

Review Questions

1. Describe Thorndike's experiments with the puzzle box and how they demonstrated his Law of Effect. What did Guthrie and Horton find when they photographed cats in the puzzle box, and what does this tell us about the principle of reinforcement?

2. Describe Skinner's superstition experiment and his theory about how reinforcement causes superstitious behaviors to develop. What types of superstitions does Skinner's theory explain well, and what types of superstitions need additional explanation?

3. Explain how you could use shaping to teach a dog to jump over a tall hurdle.

4. Give a concrete example of how shaping can be used in a behavior modification program with a human learner.

5. Explain how response chains include all of the following: discriminative stimuli, operant responses, conditioned reinforcers, and a primary reinforcer. Describe at least two different techniques for teaching a response chain.

6. What is autoshaping? Describe three different theories about why autoshaping occurs. Which theory do you think is best, and why?

7. How would you respond to someone who said that examples of biological constraints on learning show that the principle of reinforcement is flawed?

6

Reinforcement Schedules: Experimental Analyses and Applications

LEARNING OBJECTIVES

After reading this chapter, you should be able to

- describe the four simple reinforcement schedules and the types of behavior they produce during reinforcement and extinction

- give examples of reinforcement schedules from everyday life

- explain the difference between contingency-shaped and rule-governed behavior

- describe different theories about why there is a postreinforcement pause on fixed-ratio schedules, and explain which theory is best

- discuss explanations of why responding is faster on variable-ratio schedules than on variable-interval schedules

- give examples of how the principles of operant conditioning have been used in behavior modification with children and adults

A mong B. F. Skinner's many achievements, one of the most noteworthy was his experimental analysis of **reinforcement schedules.** A reinforcement schedule is simply a rule that states under what conditions a reinforcer will be delivered. To this point, we have mainly considered cases in which every occurrence of the operant response is followed by a reinforcer. This schedule is called **continuous reinforcement** (CRF), but it is only one of an infinite number of possible rules for delivering a reinforcer. In the real world, responses are sometimes, but not always, followed by reinforcers. A salesman may make many phone calls in vain for every time he succeeds in selling a magazine subscription. A typist may type dozens of pages, comprised of thousands of individual keystrokes, before finally receiving payment for a completed job. A lion may make several unsuccessful attempts to catch a prey before it finally obtains a meal. Recognizing that most behaviors outside the laboratory receive only intermittent reinforcement, Skinner devoted considerable effort to the investigation of how different schedules of reinforcement have different effects on behavior (Ferster & Skinner, 1957).

PLOTTING MOMENT-TO-MOMENT BEHAVIOR: THE CUMULATIVE RECORDER

Skinner constructed a simple mechanical device, the **cumulative recorder**, which records these responses in a way that allows any observer to see at a glance the moment-to-moment patterns of a subject's behavior. Figure 6-1 shows how the cumulative recorder works. A slowly rotating cylinder pulls a roll of paper beneath a pen at a steady rate, so the *x*-axis of the resultant graph, the cumulative record, represents time. If the subject makes no response, a horizontal line is the result. However, each response causes the pen to move up the page by a small increment (in a direction perpendicular to the movement of the paper), so the *y*-axis represents the cumulative number of responses the subject has made since the start of the session.

As Figure 6-1 shows, a cumulative record tells much more than the overall number of responses. Segments of the record that have a fairly even linear appearance correspond to periods in which the subject was responding at a steady rate—the greater the slope, the faster the response rate. Figure 6-1 also shows how an acceleration or deceleration in response rate would appear in the cumulative record. Finally, small downward deflections in a cumulative record generally indicate those times at which a reinforcer was delivered. With these points in mind, we can now examine how the schedule of reinforcement determines a subject's pattern of responding.

THE FOUR SIMPLE REINFORCEMENT SCHEDULES

Fixed Ratio

The rule for reinforcement in a **fixed-ratio (FR) schedule** is that a reinforcer is delivered after every *n* responses, where *n* is the size of the ratio. For example, in an FR 20 schedule, every 20 responses will be followed by a reinforcer. If an animal begins with an FR 1 schedule (which

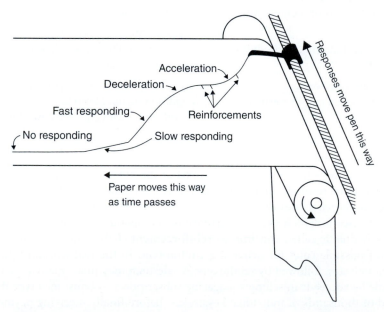

FIGURE 6-1 A simplified drawing of a cumulative recorder and the type of graph it produces.

is the same as CRF) and then the ratio is gradually increased, the animal can be trained to make many responses for each reinforcer. For example, many animals will respond for food reinforcement on FR schedules where 100 or more responses are required for each reinforcer. The behavior of many species (including pigeons, rats, monkeys, and people) on FR schedules has been studied, and in most cases the general characteristics of the behavior are similar. After a subject has performed on an FR schedule for some time and has become acquainted with the requirements of the schedule, a distinctive pattern of responding develops. As Figure 6-2 shows, responding on an FR schedule exhibits a "stop-and-go" pattern: After each reinforcer, there is a pause in responding that is sometimes called a **postreinforcement pause**. Eventually, this pause gives way to an abrupt continuation of responding. Once responding begins, the subject typically responds at a constant, rapid rate (note the steep slopes in the cumulative record) until the next reinforcer is delivered.

Outside the laboratory, perhaps the best example of FR schedules is the "piecework" method used to pay factory workers in some companies. For instance, a worker operating a semiautomatic machine that makes door hinges might be paid $10 for every 100 hinges made. Long ago, I worked in a factory for several summers, and I had the opportunity to observe workers who were paid by the piecework system. Their behavior was quite similar to the FR pattern shown in Figure 6-2. Once a worker started up the machine, he almost always worked steadily and rapidly until the counter on the machine indicated that 100 pieces had been made. At this point, the worker would record the number completed on a work card and then take a break—he might chat with friends, have a soft drink or a cup of coffee, or glance at a newspaper for a few minutes. After this pause, the worker would turn on the machine and produce another 100 hinges. These workers needed very little supervision from their boss. The boss did not have to prod them to work faster or chastise them for taking excessively long breaks.

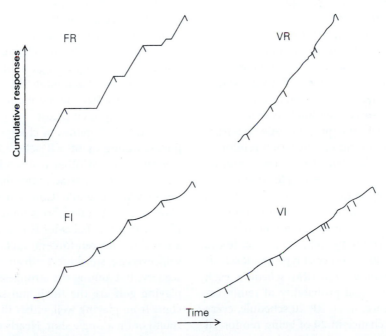

FIGURE 6-2   Idealized cumulative records showing the typical patterns of behavior generated by the four simple reinforcement schedules.

The schedule of reinforcement, which delivered reinforcers in direct proportion to the amount of work done, was all that was needed to maintain the performance of these workers.

With FR schedules, the average size of the postreinforcement pause increases as the size of the ratio increases. For example, with a pigeon pecking a key, the average pause may be only a second or so with an FR 20 schedule, but it may be several minutes long with an FR 200 schedule. In contrast, the subject's rate of responding after the postreinforcement pause remains fairly constant as the size of the ratio increases (Crossman, Bonem, & Phelps, 1987; Powell, 1969). With very large ratios, however, the animal may start to exhibit long pauses at times other than right after reinforcement. The term **ratio strain** is sometimes used to describe the general weakening of responding that is found when large ratios are used.

Variable Ratio

The only difference between an FR schedule and a **variable-ratio (VR) schedule** is that on the latter, the number of required responses is not constant from reinforcer to reinforcer. To be specific, the rule for reinforcement on a VR *n* schedule is that *on average,* a subject will receive one reinforcer for every *n* responses, but the exact number of responses required at any moment may vary widely. When an experiment is controlled by a computer, a VR schedule is sometimes implemented by giving the computer a list of possible ratio sizes from which it selects at random after each reinforcer to determine the number of responses required for the next reinforcer. For example, a list for VR 10 might contain the ratios 1, 2, 3, 4, 5, 6, 10, 19, and 40. In the long run, an average of 10 responses will be required for each reinforcer, but on a given trial, the required number may be as few as 1 or as many as 40. In a special type of VR schedule called a *random ratio (RR) schedule,* each response has an equal probability of reinforcement. For instance, in an RR 20 schedule, every response has 1 chance in 20 of being reinforced regardless of how many responses have occurred since the last reinforcer.

Figure 6-2 shows a typical cumulative record from a VR schedule. The pattern of responding might be described as rapid and fairly steady. The major difference between FR performance and VR performance is that postreinforcement pauses are typically quite brief on VR schedules (Blakely & Schlinger, 1988). They are several times smaller than those found on FR schedules with equal response:reinforcer ratios (Mazur, 1983). Intuitively, the reason for the shorter postreinforcement pauses on VR schedules seems clear: After each reinforcer, there is always the possibility that another reinforcer will be delivered after only a few additional responses.

Many forms of gambling are examples of VR schedules. Games of chance, such as slot machines, roulette wheels, and lotteries, all exhibit the two important characteristics of VR schedules: (1) A person's chances of winning are directly proportional to the number of times the person plays, and (2) the number of responses required for the next reinforcer is uncertain. It is the combination of these two features that makes gambling an "addiction" for some people; that is, gambling behavior is strong and persistent because the very next lottery ticket or the very next coin in a slot machine could turn a loser into a big winner. Ironically, the characteristics of a VR schedule are strong enough to offset the fact that in most forms of gambling, the odds are against the player, so that the more one plays, the more one can be expected to lose.

Although games of chance are among the purest examples of VR schedules outside the laboratory, many other real-world activities, including most sports activities, have the properties of a VR schedule. Consider the behavior of playing golf. As one who is fond of this activity, I know that this behavior is maintained by quite a few different reinforcers, such as companionship, exercise, sunshine, fresh air, and picturesque scenery. But among the strongest reinforcers for playing golf are the thrill and satisfaction that come from playing well, either through an entire round or on a single shot. Nearly every golfer can boast of a few outstanding shots and of occasional days when every iron shot happened to land on the green and every putt seemed to drop. Regardless of what factors cause such occasional excellent performances, what is important from a behavioral perspective is that they are unpredictable. Each time a golfer walks to the first tee, a chance exists that this round will be his or her best. On each shot when the flagstick is within the golfer's range, there is a chance that the ball will end up in the hole or very close to it. This continual possibility of an outstanding round or at least a spectacular shot is probably an important reason why the average golfer keeps returning to the course again and again.

Some other behaviors reinforced on VR schedules include playing practically any competitive sport, fishing, hunting, playing card games or video games, watching the home team play, and going to fraternity parties. The delivery of reinforcers for each of these activities fits the definition of a VR schedule: The occasion of the next reinforcer is unpredictable, but in the long run, the more often the behavior occurs, the more rapidly will reinforcers be received.

Fixed Interval

In all interval schedules, the presentation of a reinforcer depends both on the subject's behavior and on the passage of time. The rule for reinforcement on a **fixed-interval (FI) schedule** is that the first response after a fixed amount of time has elapsed is reinforced. For example, in an FI 60-second schedule, immediately after one reinforcer has been delivered, a clock starts to time the next 60-second interval. Any responses that are made during those 60 seconds have no effect whatsoever. However, at the 60-second mark, a reinforcer is "stored" (i.e., the apparatus is now set to deliver a reinforcer), and the next response will produce the reinforcer.

If the subject had either a perfect sense of time or access to a clock, the most efficient behavior on an FI schedule would be to wait exactly 60 seconds, then make one response to collect the reinforcer. However, because no subject has a perfect sense of time and because a clock is usually not provided for the subject to watch, subjects on

FI schedules typically make many more responses per reinforcer than the one that is required. Figure 6-2 shows the typical pattern of responding found on FI schedules. As on FR schedules, there is a postreinforcement pause, but after this pause, the subject usually starts by responding quite slowly (unlike the abrupt switch to rapid responding on an FR schedule). As the interval progresses, the subject responds more and more rapidly, and just before reinforcement, the response rate is quite rapid. For obvious reasons, the cumulative record pattern from this class of schedule is sometimes called a *fixed-interval scallop*.

The FI schedule does not have many close parallels outside the laboratory, because few real-world reinforcers occur on such a regular temporal cycle. However, one everyday behavior that approximates the typical FI pattern of accelerating responses is waiting for a bus. Imagine that you are walking to a bus stop and that just as you arrive you see a bus leave. Suppose that you are not wearing a watch, but you know that a bus arrives at this stop every 20 minutes; so you sit down on a bench and start to read a book. In this situation, the operant response is looking down the street for the next bus. The reinforcer for this response is simply the sight of the next bus. At first, the response of looking for the bus may not occur at all, and you may read steadily for 5 or 10 minutes before your first glance down the street. Your next glance may occur 1 or 2 minutes later, and now you may look down the street every minute or so. After 15 minutes, you may put away the book and stare down the street almost continuously until the bus arrives.

Other situations in which important events occur at regular intervals can produce similar patterns of accelerating behavior. Mawhinney, Bostow, Laws, Blumenfeld, and Hopkins (1971) measured the study behavior of college students in a psychology course, and they found that the pattern of this behavior varied quite predictably, depending on the schedule of examinations. As mentioned earlier, the conditioned reinforcer of a good grade on an exam can be an important reinforcer for studying. All the readings for the course were available only in a special room in the library, and the materials could not be taken out of this room, so that the students' study behavior could be measured. The amount of time each student spent studying in this room was recorded by observers who watched through a one-way mirror.

During the first 2 weeks of the course, a short quiz (worth 5 points) was scheduled for each class meeting. In the next 3 weeks there were no quizzes, but a longer exam (worth 60 points) was given at the end of the third week. The second half of the term mimicked the first half, with 2 weeks of daily quizzes followed by 3 weeks with a large exam at the end. The weeks with daily quizzes approximated a CRF schedule of reinforcement, for every day of studying might be reinforced with a good grade on the next day's quiz. The exams after 3 weeks were more like an FI schedule, for there was no immediate reinforcer for studying during the early parts of the 3-week period. This arrangement is not exactly like an FI schedule, because on an FI schedule, no response except the last has any effect; in contrast, studying early in the 3-week period presumably had some beneficial effect in terms of the grade on the exam. Despite this difference, Figure 6-3 shows that the patterns of the students' study behavior during the two 3-week periods were similar to typical FI

performance: There was little studying during the early parts of the 3-week period, but the amount of studying steadily increased as the exam approached. In contrast, study behavior was more stable from day to day when the students had daily quizzes. This experiment demonstrates that an instructor's selection of a schedule of quizzes or exams can have a large effect on the study behavior of the students in the course.

Although an accelerating response pattern is a common result when FI schedules are in effect, this scalloping pattern is not always found. For example, some research with both human and animal subjects has found cases in which FI performance looks more like the stop-and-go pattern that is characteristic of FR schedules (Baron & Leinenweber, 1994). In other cases, human subjects exhibit long pauses and very low response rates. The reasons for these different response patterns on FI schedules are still not well understood, but one important factor may be what types of alternative behaviors are available during the intervals between reinforcers. Barnes and Keenan (1993) found the classic scalloped patterns when people could read or watch television during these intervals, but when these activities were not available, they made just a few responses toward the end of the interval.

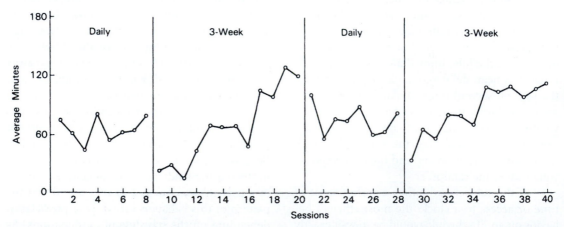

FIGURE 6-3   Results obtained by Mawhinney and colleagues (1971) in their experiment on the study habits of college students. The *y*-axis shows the average number of minutes of study per day when the instructor gave daily quizzes and when a larger exam was given at the end of a 3-week period.

SOURCE: From Mawhinney, et al, "A comparison of students' studying behavior produced by daily, weekly and 3-week testing schedules," *Journal of Applied Behavior Analysis, 4*(4), Winter 1971, Figure 3, page 262. Reprinted by permission.

Variable Interval

Variable-interval (VI) schedules are like FI schedules except that the amount of time that must pass before a reinforcer is stored varies unpredictably from reinforcer to reinforcer. For example, in a VI 60-second schedule, the time between the delivery of one reinforcer and the storage of another might be 6 seconds for one reinforcer, then 300 seconds for the next, 40 seconds for the next, and so on. As on FI schedules, the first response to occur after a reinforcer is stored collects that reinforcer, and the clock does not start again until the reinforcer is collected.

As Figure 6-2 shows, VI schedules typically produce a steady, moderate response rate. This response pattern seems sensible considering the characteristics of the schedule. Because a reinforcer might be stored at any moment, a long pause after reinforcement would not be advantageous. By maintaining a steady response rate, the subject will collect each reinforcer soon after it is stored, thus keeping the VI clock moving most of the time. On the other hand, a very high response rate, such as that observed on a VR schedule, would produce only a minor increase in the rate of reinforcement.

An example of an everyday behavior that is maintained by a VI schedule of reinforcement is checking for mail. The reinforcer in this situation is simply the receipt of mail. Most people receive mail on some days but not on others, and the days when one will find something reinforcing (e.g., letters, as opposed to junk mail or bills) in the mailbox are usually impossible to predict. The delivery of mail approximates a VI schedule because (1) it is unpredictable; (2) if a reinforcer is stored (the mail has been delivered), only one response is required to collect it; and (3) if the reinforcer has not yet been stored, no amount of responding will bring it forth. The resultant behavior is moderate and steady: Most people check the mail every day, but usually only once a day.

Extinction and the Four Simple Schedules

If an individual is performing on one of the four reinforcement schedules and then there is a switch to extinction, how long will the individual continue to respond before quitting? Of course, this depends on the type of schedule and on the size of the ratio or the interval, but some general rules about the **resistance to extinction** of the different simple schedules can be stated. One general finding is that extinction is more rapid after CRF than after a schedule of intermittent reinforcement. This finding is called the **partial reinforcement effect,** an effect that seemed paradoxical to early researchers because it violates Thomas Brown's principle of frequency. Why should a response that is only intermittently followed by a reinforcer be stronger (more resistant to extinction) than a response that has been followed by a reinforcer every time it has occurred? This dilemma has been named **Humphreys's paradox,** after the psychologist who first demonstrated the partial reinforcement extinction effect (Humphreys, 1939).

One explanation of the partial reinforcement effect is called the **discrimination hypothesis** (Mowrer & Jones, 1945). It states that in order for a subject's behavior to change once extinction begins, the subject must be able to discriminate the change in reinforcement contingencies. With CRF, where every response has been reinforced, the change to extinction is easy to discriminate, and so it does not take long for responding to disappear. For example, a vending machine usually dispenses reinforcers (snacks, soft drinks) on a schedule of CRF: Each time the correct change is inserted, a reinforcer is delivered. If the schedule is switched to extinction (the machine breaks down), a person will not continue to put coins in the machine for long.

Compare this situation to a slot machine, which dispenses reinforcers on a VR schedule. If a slot machine broke down in such a way that it appeared to be functioning normally but could never produce a jackpot, a gambler might continue to pour many coins into the machine before giving up. It would take a long time for the gambler to discriminate the change from a VR schedule to extinction.

Although the discrimination hypothesis may be easy to understand, experimental evidence suggests that a slightly different hypothesis, the **generalization decrement hypothesis** (Capaldi, 1966), is better. Generalization decrement is simply a term for the decreased responding one observes in a generalization test when the test stimuli become less and less similar to the training stimulus. For instance, if a pigeon is reinforced for pecking at a yellow key, we should observe a generalization decrement (less rapid responding) if the key is blue in a generalization test. According to the generalization decrement hypothesis, responding during extinction will be weak if the stimuli during extinction are different from those that were present during reinforcement, but strong if these stimuli are similar to those encountered during reinforcement.

According to Capaldi, there is a large generalization decrement when the schedule switches from CRF to extinction, because the subject has never experienced a situation in which its responses were not reinforced. In other words, the animal quickly stops responding because it has never been taught to keep responding when its initial responses are not reinforced. However, suppose an animal has been reinforced on a VR 50 schedule, and now the schedule has been switched to extinction. Here there will be much less generalization decrement, because on many occasions in the past the animal has made a long run of unreinforced responses, and eventually a reinforcer was delivered. For this animal, the stimuli present during extinction (long stretches of unreinforced responses) are quite similar to the stimuli present during the VR schedule. For this reason, the animal will probably continue to respond for a longer period of time.

Other Reinforcement Schedules

Although the four simple reinforcement schedules have been the most thoroughly investigated, they are only four of an infinite number of possible rules for delivering reinforcement. Many other rules for reinforcement have been named and studied. We can take a look at a few of the more common ones.

Under a **differential reinforcement of low rates (DRL) schedule**, a response is reinforced if

and only if a certain amount of time has elapsed since the previous response. For example, under a DRL 10-second schedule, every response that occurs after a pause of at least 10 seconds is reinforced. If a response occurs after 9.5 seconds, this not only fails to produce reinforcement but it resets the 10-second clock to zero, so that now 10 more seconds must elapse before a response can be reinforced. As you might imagine, DRL schedules produce very low rates of responding, but they are not as low as would be optimal. Since subjects cannot estimate the passage of time perfectly, the optimal strategy would be to pause for an average of 12 or 15 seconds, and then respond. In this way, if the subject erred from this average on the short side, the pause might still be longer than 10 seconds and produce a reinforcer. The usual finding, however, is that the average pause is somewhat less than the required duration; as a result, considerably more than half of the subject's responses go unreinforced (Richards, Sabol, & Seiden, 1993). Some subjects seem to use a regular sequence of behaviors to help pace their operant responses. For example, a pigeon on a DRL 5-second schedule might peck at the key, then peck at each of the four corners of the chamber, and then peck at the key again.

The opposite of the DRL contingency is the **differential reinforcement of high rates (DRH) schedule**, in which a certain number of responses must occur within a fixed amount of time. For example, a reinforcer might occur each time the subject makes 10 responses in 3 seconds or less. Since rapid responding is selectively reinforced by this schedule, DRH can be used to produce higher rates of responding than those obtained with any other reinforcement schedule.

Other common reinforcement schedules are those that combine two or more simple schedules in some way. In a **concurrent schedule**, the subject is presented with two or more response alternatives (e.g., several different levers), each associated with its own reinforcement schedule. With more than one reinforcement schedule available simultaneously, psychologists can determine which schedule the subject prefers and how much time is devoted to each alternative. In

chained schedules, the subject must complete the requirement for two or more simple schedules in a fixed sequence, and each schedule is signaled by a different stimulus. For instance, in a chain FI 1-minute FR 10, a pigeon might be presented with a yellow key until the FI requirement is met, then a blue key until 10 more responses are made, and then the reinforcer would be presented. The pigeon's behavior during each link of the chain is usually characteristic of the schedule currently in effect (an accelerating response pattern during the FI component, and a stop-and-go pattern during the FR component). As in the response chains discussed earlier, the strength of responding weakens as a schedule is further and further removed from the primary reinforcer. Thus, an FI schedule will produce less responding if instead of leading to reinforcement it simply leads to an FR schedule.

FACTORS AFFECTING PERFORMANCE ON REINFORCEMENT SCHEDULES

The preceding sections have shown that different reinforcement schedules produce very different rates and patterns of behavior. However, many other factors besides the schedule itself can affect performance on a reinforcement schedule. We will begin with a brief review of some of the most important factors.

It is certainly true that the effectiveness of a reinforcement schedule depends on the nature of the reinforcer that is delivered, and three important features of any reinforcer are its quality, its rate of presentation, and its delay. Neef, Shade, and Miller (1994) investigated the effects of these features on the performance of emotionally disturbed teenagers. The teens were referred to these researchers because they needed practice in math skills and, more generally, in completing school assignments promptly. Computers were programmed to present math problems to each teenager, and the computers reinforced completed problems according to a VI schedule. The *quality* of the reinforcers was varied by using either money (which all subjects preferred) or

points exchangeable for privileges or items in the school store (which were less preferred). *Rate of reinforcement* was varied by using VI schedules of different lengths. *Delay of reinforcement* was manipulated by delivering reinforcers either immediately after the math session was over or not until the next day. Different teens had somewhat different preferences, but in general, they spent more time working on the math problems (1) when the quality of the reinforcer was higher, (2) when the rate of reinforcement was faster, and (3) when the delay was shorter. Neef and colleagues also investigated the factor of *response effort* by varying the difficulty of the math problems, and they found that the students preferred to work on the problems that required less effort.

Another important factor is the *amount of reinforcement*. In the laboratory, animals will usually make more responses on a given reinforcement schedule if the reinforcer is a large amount of food than if it is a small amount of food. In the business world, a salesperson may invest substantial time and effort trying to finalize the sale of a large and expensive item, but will not invest so much effort for a smaller and cheaper item. Finally, the individual's *level of motivation* is an important determinant of how much operant behavior will be seen. A rat that has just eaten a large amount of food will not exhibit much lever pressing; a student who does not care about grades will not do much studying, no matter what the exam schedule may be.

Many of these points may seem obvious, but other factors that can affect performance on reinforcement schedules are not so obvious. Next, we will examine some factors that can easily be overlooked.

Behavioral Momentum

When a heavy object starts moving, it acquires momentum and becomes difficult to stop. Nevin (1992, 1998) has argued that there is an analogy between the momentum of a moving object and the **behavioral momentum** of an ongoing operant behavior. Nevin has found that a behavior's resistance to change (which is a measure of behavioral momentum) depends on the association between the discriminative stimulus and the reinforcer (i.e., on how frequently the behavior has been reinforced in the presence of a certain discriminative stimulus).

An experiment with pigeons (Nevin, 1974) illustrates the concept of behavioral momentum. The pigeons earned food by pecking on a response key that was sometimes green and sometimes red. VI schedules delivered 60 food presentations per hour when the key was green, but only 20 food presentations per hour when the key was red. As expected, the pigeons pecked more rapidly when the key was green. Then, Nevin interrupted the green and red keys with periods during which free food was delivered. In one condition, when the free food deliveries were very rapid, the pigeons' rates of key pecking decreased by about 60% when the key was green, but by over 80% when the key was red. According to Nevin, pecking on the green key had greater momentum because it was associated with a higher rate of reinforcement, so this behavior was less disrupted by the free food deliveries than was pecking on the red key. Studies with humans have also found that behaviors associated with higher rates of reinforcement are harder to disrupt (Dube, Ahearn, Lionello-DeNolf, & McIlvane, 2009; Milo, Mace, & Nevin, 2010).

Nevin and Grace (2000) proposed that the concept of behavioral momentum has a number of implications for attempts to change behavior outside the laboratory. Behavior therapists frequently want to make sure that a newly trained behavior (e.g., working steadily on one's job during work hours) will persist in the presence of potential disruptors (e.g., distractions by friends, reinforcers for competing behaviors). The newly trained behavior will have more momentum and be more likely to persist despite such potential disruptors, if the worker has developed a strong association between the work environment and reinforcement for appropriate work-related behavior.

As another example, the concept of behavioral momentum can help to explain why some undesirable behaviors may relapse when the individual returns to an environment where the behavior occurred in the past (Podlesnik & Shahan, 2010). For instance, a patient who has received treatment for a drug addiction may start taking drugs again when he leaves a treatment center and returns home, because the drugs are strongly associated with a specific discriminative stimulus (the patient's neighborhood and friends). Although the patient may have little problem refraining from drugs in the treatment facility, the association between the patient's neighborhood and drugs has not been broken. Because drug-taking behavior has strong momentum when the individual is in his old neighborhood, it may persist in that environment despite the treatment the patient has received elsewhere. Nevin and Grace (2000) propose that more effective behavior therapies can be devised through a better understanding of how behaviors develop momentum and how the momentum of unwanted behaviors can be disrupted.

Contingency-Shaped versus Rule-Governed Behaviors

As we have seen, each reinforcement schedule tends to produce its own characteristic pattern of behavior (Figure 6-2). B. F. Skinner called these patterns **contingency-shaped behaviors**, because the animal's behavior is gradually shaped into its final form as it gained more and more experience with a particular reinforcement schedule (Ferster & Skinner, 1957). However, some laboratory experiments with human participants have found behavior patterns that were quite different from the typical patterns shown in Figure 6-2. For example, under FI schedules, some humans show the accelerating pattern found with animals, but others respond very quickly throughout the interval, and others make only a few responses near the end of the interval (Leander, Lippman, & Meyer, 1968; Lowe, Harzem, & Bagshaw, 1978). Similar discrepancies between human and animal behaviors have been found with other reinforcement schedules as well (Lowe, 1979). But if these behavior patterns are shaped by the reinforcement contingencies, why should the same reinforcement schedule produce different behavior patterns in humans and nonhumans?

One hypothesis states that the discrepancies between animal and human performance on reinforcement schedules occur because people are capable of both contingency-shaped behavior and **rule-governed behavior**. Skinner (1969) proposed that because people have language, they can be given verbal instructions or rules to follow, and these rules may or may not have anything to do with the prevailing reinforcement contingencies. For example, a mother may tell a child, "Stay out of drafts or you will catch a cold," and the child may follow this rule for a long time, regardless of whether it is truly effective in preventing colds. With respect to laboratory experiments on reinforcement schedules, this theory states that human participants may behave differently from animals because they are following rules about how to respond (e.g., "Press the response button as rapidly as possible," or "Wait for about a minute, and then respond"). They may form these rules on their own, or they may get them from the instructions the experimenter provides before the experiment begins. Once a human participant receives or creates such a rule, the actual reinforcement contingencies may have little or no effect on his or her behavior. For instance, if the experimenter says, "Press the key rapidly to earn the most money," the participant may indeed respond rapidly on an FI schedule even though rapid responding is not necessary on this schedule.

Several types of evidence support the idea that human performance on reinforcement schedules is often rule governed, at least in part. Many studies have shown that the instructions given to participants can have a large effect on their response patterns (e.g., Bentall & Lowe, 1987; Catania, Matthews, & Shimoff, 1982). If participants are given no specific rule to follow, they may form one on their own. Human participants have sometimes been asked, either during an experiment or at the end, to explain why they responded the way they did. Some studies of this type have found a close correspondence between a participant's verbal descriptions and his or her actual response patterns (Wearden, 1988). Other research has shown that infants or young children behave

much more like animals than like older children or adults under simple schedules of reinforcement (Lowe, Beasty, & Bentall, 1983). This may be because the youngest children do not have language at all, and because the language skills of the slightly older youngsters are too meager for them to develop and follow a verbal rule for responding (Pouthas, Droit, Jacquet, & Wearden, 1990).

Not all the evidence supports the hypothesis that the differences between human and nonhuman schedule performance are due to the use of rules by humans. Sometimes when participants are asked to explain what rule they were following, they can give no rule, or the rule they give does not describe their actual behavior pattern (Matthews, Catania, & Shimoff, 1985). Therefore, it seems likely that other variables also contribute to the differences between human and nonhuman performance on reinforcement schedules. For instance, animal subjects are usually deprived of food, and then given a chance to earn a primary reinforcer, food. With humans, the reinforcers in many experiments have been conditioned reinforcers (e.g., points that may later be exchanged for small amounts of money). In addition, animals and humans usually come to the laboratory with very different reinforcement histories, as discussed next.

Reinforcement History

In many laboratory experiments with animals, the subjects have never before been exposed to a reinforcement schedule of any sort. In contrast, adult humans have a long and complex history of exposure to various reinforcement schedules outside the laboratory. Is it possible that the differences between human and nonhuman behavior patterns that are sometimes found with the same reinforcement schedules are a product of these different reinforcement histories? If so, it should be possible to change the response patterns of either animals or humans by giving them prior experience with different reinforcement schedules.

Weiner (1964) had human participants press a response key to earn points in ten 1-hour sessions. Some participants worked on an FR 40 schedule (on which more rapid responding led to more reinforcers). Other participants worked on a DRL 20-second schedule (on which only pauses longer than 20 seconds were reinforced). Then all participants were switched to an FI 10-second schedule. The participants with FR experience responded rapidly on the FI schedule, but those with DRL experience responded very slowly. These large differences persisted even after 20 sessions with the FI schedule.

Similar effects of prior reinforcement history have been found with animals (LeFrancois & Metzger, 1993; Okouchi & Lattal, 2006). In a study by Wanchisen, Tatham, and Mooney (1989), one group of rats received many sessions with only one reinforcement schedule, FI 30 seconds; all of these rats developed the accelerating pattern that is typical for FI schedules. A second group of rats first received 30 sessions with a VR 20 schedule, and then 30 sessions with the FI 30-second schedule. Some of these rats responded rapidly on the FI schedule and some responded very slowly, but none showed an accelerating response pattern. Wanchisen and her colleagues concluded that prior experience with one reinforcement schedule can alter how subjects, both animal and human, later perform on another schedule.

The effects of previous reinforcement history may be especially important in applied settings because people's life experiences are so variable. Two people receiving the same behavioral treatment with the same reinforcement schedule might respond very differently because of their different personal experiences prior to start of treatment. Attempts to reduce unwanted behaviors (such as tantrums or aggression in children) might have different degrees of success with different children because of their prior reinforcement histories. Behavior analysts are currently seeking to obtain a better understanding of reinforcement history effects because of the important influence they may have on treatment programs (St. Peter Pipkin & Vollmer, 2009).

Summary

A large number of variables can affect the type of behavior that is seen with any reinforcement schedule. Factors such as the size and quality of

the reinforcer, the effort involved in the operant response, the individual's level of motivation, and the availability of alternative behaviors can all affect the rate and temporal pattern of an operant response. With human participants, it may be important to know what instructions they were given and what rules about responding they may have formed on their own. With both animals and humans, it may be important to know what reinforcement schedules they have encountered previously, and for how long. Since Skinner's pioneering research, reinforcement schedules have been intensely studied, and there is no doubt that they can exert powerful control over an individual's behavior. It is important to recognize, however, that operant behavior is affected by a multitude of variables, and this makes the task of analyzing the behavior complex and challenging.

PRACTICE QUIZ (1)

1. In a cumulative record, fast responding is indicated by a —————, and no responding is indicated by a —————.
2. Responding on an FR schedule typically shows a(n) ————— pattern, and responding on an FI schedule typically shows a(n) ————— pattern.
3. Responding on ————— schedules is usually rapid and steady, and responding on ————— schedules is usually slower and steady.
4. A behavior has a high ————— if it is not affected much by distractions or environmental changes.
5. ————— behavior is controlled by the schedule of reinforcement; ————— behavior is controlled by instructions subjects are given or form on their own.

Answers

5. contingency-shaped, rule-governed
3. VR, VI   4. behavioral momentum
1. steep line, horizontal line   2. stop-and-go, accelerating

THE EXPERIMENTAL ANALYSIS OF REINFORCEMENT SCHEDULES

Throughout the preceding discussions of reinforcement schedules, the explanations of why particular schedules produce specific response patterns have been casual and intuitive. For example, we noted that it would not "make sense" to have a long postreinforcement pause on a VR schedule, or to respond at a very rapid rate on a VI schedule. This level of discussion can make the basic facts about reinforcement schedules easier to learn and remember. However, such imprecise statements are no substitute for a scientific analysis of exactly which independent variables (which characteristics of the reinforcement schedule) control which dependent variables (which aspects of the subject's behavior). This section presents a few examples that show how a scientific analysis can either improve on intuitive explanations of behavior or distinguish among different explanations, all of which seem intuitively reasonable.

Cause of the FR Postreinforcement Pause

Why do animal subjects pause after reinforcement on FR schedules? Several possible explanations seem intuitively reasonable. Perhaps the postreinforcement pause is the result of fatigue: The subject has made many responses and has collected a reinforcer; now it rests to alleviate its fatigue. A second possibility is satiation: The consumption of the food reinforcer causes a slight decrease in the animal's level of hunger, which results in a brief interruption in responding. A third explanation of the postreinforcement pause emphasizes the fact that on an FR schedule, the subject is farthest from the delivery of the next reinforcer immediately after the occurrence of the previous reinforcer. According to this position, a subject's behavior on an FR schedule is similar to a response chain. We have already seen that the initial responses in the chain, those farthest removed from the primary reinforcer, are the weakest. For convenience, let us call these three explanations of the FR postreinforcement

pause the *fatigue hypothesis*, the *satiation hypothesis*, and the *remaining-responses hypothesis*.

Each of these hypotheses sounds plausible, but how can we determine which is correct? Several types of evidence help to distinguish among them. First, there is the finding that postreinforcement pauses become larger as the size of the FR increases. This finding is consistent with both the fatigue and remaining-responses hypotheses, but it contradicts the satiation hypothesis. Because the subject can collect reinforcers at a faster rate on a small FR schedule, its level of hunger should be lower; so according to the satiation hypothesis, pauses should be longer on shorter FR schedules, not on larger FR schedules.

Data that help to distinguish between the fatigue and remaining-responses hypotheses are provided by studies that combine two or more different FR schedules into what is called a multiple schedule. In a **multiple schedule**, the subject is presented with two or more different schedules, one at a time, and each schedule is signaled by a different discriminative stimulus. For example, Figure 6-4 illustrates a portion of a session involving a multiple FR 10 FR 100 schedule. When the response key is blue, the schedule is FR 100; when it is red, the schedule is FR 10. The key color remains the same until a reinforcer is earned, at which point there is a 50% chance that the key color (and schedule) will switch.

The behavior shown in Figure 6-4, though hypothetical, is representative of the results from several studies that used multiple FR schedules (Crossman, 1968; Mintz, Mourer, & Gofseyeff, 1967). Examine the postreinforcement pauses that occurred at points a, b, c, d, e, and f. Half of these pauses occurred after a ratio of 100 (a, d, f) and half after a ratio of 10 (b, c, e). Notice that there is a long pause at f, as might be expected from the fatigue hypothesis, but contrary to this hypothesis, there are only short pauses after FR 100 at points a and d. The pause after FR 10 is short at point b, but long at points c and e. The data show that we cannot predict the size of the postreinforcement pause by knowing how many responses the subject has produced in the

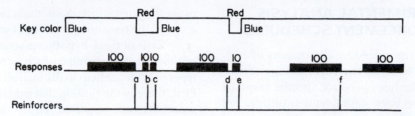

FIGURE 6-4 A hypothetical but typical pattern of response from a multiple schedule where the blue key color signaled that the schedule was FR 100 and the red key color signaled that the schedule was FR 10. The text explains how results like these can be used to distinguish between different theories of the postreinforcement pause.

preceding ratio. This fact forces us to reject the fatigue hypothesis.

On the other hand, it is possible to predict the size of the pause by knowing the size of the *upcoming* ratio. Notice that the pause is short whenever the key color is red (points a, b, and d), which is the discriminative stimulus for FR 10. The pause is long when the key color is blue (points c, e, and f), the discriminative stimulus for FR 100. This pattern is exactly what would be predicted by the remaining-responses hypothesis: The size of the postreinforcement pause is determined by the upcoming FR requirement.

This type of analysis has demonstrated quite clearly that the size of the postreinforcement pause depends heavily on the upcoming ratio requirement, and that the factors of satiation and fatigue play at most a minor role. Derenne and Baron (2002) shed further light on postreinforcement pauses by showing that they are longer if some alternative activity is available. Rats responded for food on FR or VR schedules, and in some conditions a bottle with plain water or saccharin-sweetened water was present in the chamber. The rats' postreinforcement pauses were longer when water was present, mainly because they drank water during this time. Derenne and Baron suggested that when other activities are available, they can compete with responding on a ratio schedule, and the competing activities are most likely to occur when the operant response is weakest (right after reinforcement, when the next reinforcer is furthest away).

Comparisons of VR and VI Response Rates

Experiments with both humans and animals have shown that if a VR schedule and a VI schedule deliver the same number of reinforcers per hour, subjects usually respond faster on the VR schedule (Matthews, Shimoff, Catania, & Sagvolden, 1977). In fact, a study with preschool children, who earned candies by pressing telegraph keys, found faster responding on a VR schedule than on a VI schedule even though the children actually earned candies faster on the VI schedule (Baxter & Schlinger, 1990). In an experiment with pigeons, W. M. Baum (1993) used both VR and VI schedules, with rates of reinforcement ranging from about 20 to several thousand reinforcers per hour. Figure 6-5 shows the results from a typical pigeon. As can be seen, the pigeon consistently responded faster on the VR schedules. Given this consistent finding with both people and animals, the question we will try to answer is: Why is responding faster on VR schedules than on VI schedules when the rates of reinforcement are the same?

One theory about this difference in response rates can be classified as a **molecular theory**, which means that it focuses on small-scale events—the moment-by-moment relationships between responses and reinforcers. The other theory is a **molar theory**, one that deals with large-scale measures of behavior and reinforcement. Of course, the terms *small scale* and *large scale* are relative. To be more specific, molecular

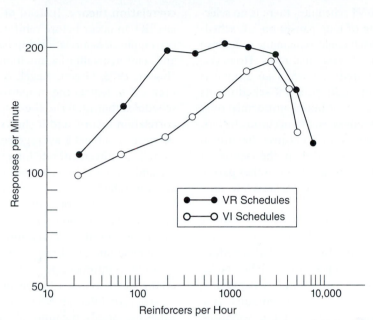

FIGURE 6-5 Response rates of a typical pigeon in Baum's (1993) experiment, showing faster responding on VR schedules than on VI schedules that delivered about the same number of reinforcers per hour.

SOURCE: From Baum, W.M., "Performance on ratio and interval schedules of reinforcement: Data and theory," *Journal of the Experimental Analysis of Behavior*, Vol. 59, 1993, Figure 4, page 251. Copyright 1993 by the Society for the Experimental Analysis of Behavior, Inc.

theories usually discuss events that have time spans of less than 1 minute, whereas molar theories discuss relationships measured over at least several minutes and often over the entire length of an experimental session.

To account for the different response rates on VR and VI schedules, a popular molecular theory is the **interresponse time (IRT) reinforcement theory**. IRT is the time between two consecutive responses. In essence, this theory states that response rates are slower on VI schedules than on VR schedules because long IRTs (long pauses between responses) are more frequently reinforced on VI schedules. This theory was first proposed by Skinner (1938), and later supported by Anger (1956), Shimp (1969), and Platt (1979).

Imagine that a subject has just been switched from CRF to a VI schedule. Some of this subject's IRTs will be short (e.g., less than 1 second will elapse between two responses) and others will be larger (e.g., a pause of 5 or 10 seconds

will separate two responses). On the VI schedule, which of these two responses is more likely to be reinforced—a response after a pause of 0.5 seconds or a response after a pause of 5 seconds? The answer is the latter, because the more time that elapses between two responses, the greater is the probability that the VI clock will time out and store a reinforcer. For example, if the schedule is VI 60 seconds, the probability of reinforcement is roughly 10 times higher for an IRT of 5 seconds than for an IRT of 0.5 seconds. Because longer IRTs are more likely to be followed by a reinforcer, IRT reinforcement theory states that longer IRTs will be selectively strengthened on VI schedules.

Next, let us examine the relationship between IRT size and the probability of reinforcement on a VR schedule. Stated simply, there is no such relationship, because time is irrelevant on a VR schedule: The delivery of reinforcement depends entirely on the number of responses emitted, not on the passage of time.

Therefore, unlike VI schedules, there is no selective strengthening of long pauses on VR schedules, and this in itself could explain the difference between VI and VR response rates. However, Skinner (1938) noted that when an animal is first switched from CRF to a VR schedule, its responses are not distributed uniformly over time. Instead, responses tend to occur in clusters, or "bursts," perhaps simply because the animal makes several responses while in the vicinity of the key or lever, then explores some other part of the chamber, then returns and makes a few more responses, and so on.

Skinner suggested that this tendency to respond in bursts could lead to a selective strengthening of short IRTs on a VR schedule. For simplicity, let us suppose that each burst consists of exactly five responses, each separated by 0.5 seconds, and each pause between bursts is at least 5 seconds long. In each burst of responses, there is only one chance for a long IRT to be reinforced (the first response after the pause), but there are four chances for a 0.5-second IRT to be reinforced (the next four responses). Skinner concluded that short IRTs were selectively strengthened on a VR schedule simply because they were reinforced more frequently.

To provide evidence for their viewpoint, proponents of IRT reinforcement theory have arranged schedules that reinforce different IRTs with different probabilities. For example, Shimp (1968) set up a schedule in which only IRTs between 1.5 and 2.5 seconds or between 3.5 and 4.5 seconds were reinforced. As the theory of selective IRT reinforcement would predict, IRTs of these two sizes increased in frequency. In another experiment, Shimp (1973) mimicked the pattern of IRT reinforcement that occurs in a typical VI schedule: He did not use a VI clock but simply reinforced long IRTs with a high probability and short IRTs with a low probability. The result of this "synthetic VI" schedule was a pattern of responding indistinguishable from that of a normal VI schedule—moderate, steady responding with a mixture of long and short IRTs.

A molar theory of the VI–VR difference might be called the **response–reinforcer**

correlation theory. Instead of focusing on the last IRT to occur before reinforcement, this theory emphasizes a relationship between responses and reinforcement of a much more global nature (Baum, 1973; Green, Kagel, & Battalio, 1987). Figure 6-6 depicts the properties of VI and VR schedules that underlie the response–reinforcer correlation theory, and it shows the relationship between a subject's average response rate and overall reinforcement rate for a typical VR schedule and a typical VI schedule. On VR 60, as on all ratio schedules, there is a linear relationship between response rate and reinforcement rate. For instance, a response rate of 60 responses per minute will produce 60 reinforcers per hour, and a response rate of 90 responses per minute produces 90 reinforcers per hour. The relationship on the VI 60-second schedule (as on all VI schedules) is very different. No matter how rapidly the subject responds, it cannot obtain more than the scheduled 60 reinforcers per hour. The reason that reinforcement rate drops with very low response rates is that the VI clock will sometimes be stopped (having stored a reinforcer), and it will not start again until the subject makes a response and collects a reinforcer. But as long as the subject

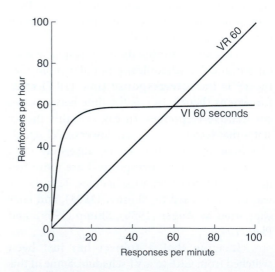

FIGURE 6-6   The relationship between a subject's rate of response and the rate of reinforcement on a VR 60 schedule and a VI 60-second schedule.

responds at a modest rate, it will obtain close to 60 reinforcers per hour.

The relationships depicted in Figure 6-6 apply only in the long run. Because of the variable nature of VI and VR schedules, in the short run the actual rate of reinforcement will often be much higher or much lower. According to the response–reinforcer correlation theory, however, animals can ignore these short-term fluctuations and learn about the long-term relationships between response rate and reinforcement rate. Let us consider how this could cause the response rate difference between VI and VR. Suppose that after extensive experience on VR 60, a pigeon's response rate stabilizes at about 60 responses per minute (where the two functions cross in Figure 6-6), producing about 60 reinforcers per hour. Now suppose the schedule is switched to VI 60 seconds, under which this same response rate would also produce 60 reinforcers per hour. However, the pigeon's response rate is not completely steady, and by occasionally responding at rates above and below 60 responses per hour, the pigeon learns that variations in response rate have little effect on reinforcement rate on the VI schedule. The pigeon's behavior may gradually drop to, say, 20 responses per hour without a substantial decrease in the rate of reinforcement. Speaking loosely, we could say that on VI 60 seconds, the pigeon has learned that the extra 40 responses per hour are "not worth it," for they would produce only a negligible increase in reinforcement rate.

Probably the best way to decide between the molar and molecular theories is to use a schedule in which the molar contingencies favor rapid responding and the molecular contingencies favor slow responding (or vice versa). This is not possible with normal VR or VI schedules, but experiments with pigeons (Vaughan, 1987) and rats (Cole, 1999) used some complex schedules that had these properties. For instance, one schedule used by Vaughan had the molar features of a VR schedule (with more reinforcers for faster response rates) but the molecular features of a VI schedule (with reinforcement more likely after a long IRT). As predicted by IRT reinforcement theory, the pigeons responded slowly on this

schedule (and thereby lost reinforcers in the long run). Conversely, the pigeons responded rapidly on a schedule in which the molecular contingencies favored rapid responding (short IRTs) but the molar contingencies favored slow responding (so once again the pigeons lost reinforcers in the long run). With rats, Tanno and Sakagami (2008) used a variety of complex schedules to compare the effects of molar and molecular variables. They found that the long-term correlation between response rates and reinforcement had very little effect on the rats' responding. However, they responded rapidly on schedules where short IRTs were selectively reinforced, and slowly on schedules where long IRTs were selectively reinforced. All of these results clearly favor the molecular approach, for they indicate that the animals were sensitive to the short-term consequences of their behavior, but not to the long-term consequences.

APPLICATIONS OF OPERANT CONDITIONING

Within the field of behavior modification, operant conditioning principles have been applied to so many different behaviors that they are too numerous to list, let alone describe, in a few pages. Operant conditioning principles have been used to help people who wish to improve themselves by losing weight, smoking or drinking less, or exercising more. They have been applied to a wide range of children's problems, including classroom disruption, poor academic performance, fighting, tantrums, extreme passivity, and hyperactivity. They have been used in attempts to improve the daily functioning of adults and children who have more serious behavior problems and must be institutionalized. These principles have also been applied to problems that affect society as a whole, such as litter and pollution, the waste of energy and resources, workplace accidents, delinquency, shoplifting, and other crimes. Because of the number and diversity of these applications, this section can do no more than describe a few representative examples. For those who wish to know more, there are many books devoted to the systematic use of operant conditioning principles in real-world settings (Martin & Pear, 2010; Miltenberger, 2011; Wheeler & Richey, 2009).

Teaching Language to Children with Autism

Autism is a severe disorder that affects roughly 1 in every 100 children, usually appearing when a child is a few years old. One major symptom of autism is extreme social withdrawal. The child shows little of the normal interest in watching and interacting with other people. Children with autism do not acquire normal language use: They either remain silent or exhibit echolalia, which is the immediate repetition of any words they hear. These children frequently spend hours engaging in simple repetitive behaviors such as rocking back and forth or spinning a metal pan on the floor. Despite considerable research, the causes of autism remain a mystery, but one certainty is that typical psychiatric and institutional care produces little, if any, improvement in these children (Kanner, Rodriguez, & Ashenden, 1972).

During the 1960s, Ivar Lovaas developed an extensive program based on operant conditioning principles designed to teach children with severe autism to speak, to interact with other people, and in general to behave more normally (Lovaas, 1967, 1977). Lovaas's methods make use of many of the operant conditioning principles we have already discussed, plus some new ones. At first, a therapist uses a spoonful of ice cream or some other tasty food as a primary reinforcer, and starts by reinforcing the child simply for sitting quietly and looking at the experimenter. Next, using the procedure of shaping, the therapist rewards the child for making any audible sounds, and then for making sounds that more and more closely mimic the word spoken by the therapist. For instance, if the child's name is Billy, the therapist may say the word "Billy" as a discriminative stimulus, after which any verbal response that approximates this word will be reinforced. So as not to rely entirely on food as a reinforcer (which would lose its effectiveness rapidly because of satiation), the therapist begins to develop other stimuli into conditioned reinforcers. Before presenting the food, the therapist might say "Good!" or give the child a hug—two stimuli that can eventually be used as reinforcers by themselves.

Early in this type of training, the therapist might use her hand to aid the child in his mouth and lip movements. This type of physical guidance is one example of a **prompt**. A prompt is any stimulus that makes a desired response more likely. In this example, the therapist's prompt of moving the child's lips and cheeks into the proper shape makes the production of the appropriate response more likely. Whenever a prompt is used, it is usually withdrawn gradually, in a procedure known as **fading**. The therapist may do less and less of the work of moving the child's lips and cheeks into the proper position, then perhaps just touch the child's cheek lightly, then not at all. This type of training demands large amounts of time and patience on the part of the therapist, especially in the beginning when progress is slowest. It may take several days of training, conducted for several hours each day, before the child masters his first word. However, the pace of a child's progress quickens as additional words are introduced, and after a few weeks the child may master several new words each day.

At this stage of training, the child is only imitating words he hears. The next step is to teach him the meanings of these words. Training begins with concrete nouns such as *nose, shoe,* and *leg.* The child is taught to identify the correct object in response to the word as a stimulus (e.g., by rewarding an appropriate response to the instruction, "Point to your nose") and to produce the appropriate word when presented with the object (Therapist: "What is this?" Billy: "Shoe."). As in the imitative phase, the child's progress accelerates as the labeling phase proceeds, and soon the child is learning the meanings of several new words each day. Later in training, similar painstaking techniques are used to teach the child the meanings of verbs and adjectives, of prepositions such as *in* and *on,* and of abstract concepts such as *first, last, more, less, same,* and *different.* This program can produce dramatic improvements in the behavior of children who typically show negligible improvement from any other type of therapy. Over the course of several months, Lovaas typically found that a child who was initially aloof and completely silent became friendly and affectionate and learned to use language to answer questions, to make requests, or to tell stories.

How successful is this behavioral treatment in the long run? Lovaas (1987) compared children who had received extensive behavioral treatment for autism (40 hours a week for 2 or more years) with children who had received minimal treatment (10 hours a week or less). At age 6 or 7, all children were given some standard IQ tests, and their performance in school was evaluated. The differences between groups were dramatic: Nearly half of the children from the treatment group had normal IQs and academic performance, as compared to only 2% of the children from the control group. A follow-up 6 years later, when the children were about 13 years old, found that the children in the treatment group continued to maintain their advantage over those in the control group. Some of the children in the treatment group performed about as well as average children of the same age on tests of intelligence and adaptive behavior (McEachin, Smith, & Lovaas, 1993). These results are encouraging, for they suggest that if extensive behavioral treatment is given to young children with autism, it can essentially eliminate the autistic symptoms in at least some of them.

Behavior therapy is the only method of treating autism that has been shown to reduce or eliminate some of the main symptoms of this disorder (Mulick & Butter, 2002). To be most effective, the treatment should begin at an early age, and it should be intensive, that is, the child should receive many hours of treatment per week, for a period of several years. Although this treatment is expensive, Jacobson, Mulick, and Green (1998) used a cost–benefit analysis to show that giving children with autism early intensive behavioral treatment actually yields substantial savings to society in the long run, because it reduces the need for special education and government support throughout the individual's life. In addition, there is, of course, the improved quality of life that occurs for the child and the child's family.

Token Reinforcement

In behavioral psychology, a **token** is defined as "an object or symbol that is exchanged for goods or services" (Hackenberg, 2009, p. 257). Research with various species of animals suggests that tokens can act as conditioned reinforcers—that is, their delivery can strengthen operant responses. In early research, Wolfe (1936) taught chimpanzees to insert poker chips into a vending machine to receive small amounts of food or water. The poker chips could then be used as reinforcers to establish and maintain new behaviors, such as lifting a weighted lever arm. Studies with rats using marbles as tokens (Malagodi, 1967) and with pigeons using illuminated lights as tokens (Bullock & Hackenberg, 2006) have found that they produce response patterns that are very similar to those obtained with primary reinforcers such as food. For instance, Malagodi's rats exhibited stop-and-go responding when marbles were delivered on an FR schedule, and slower, steady responding when they were delivered on a VI schedule.

In human applications, tokens may be physical objects such as poker chips or gold stars on a bulletin board, or they may simply be points added in a record book. Token systems have been used in classrooms, psychiatric institutions, prisons, and homes for juvenile delinquents (Kazdin, 1977). What all token systems have in common is that each individual can earn tokens by performing any of a number of different desired behaviors and can later exchange these tokens for a variety of "backup" or primary reinforcers.

Schaefer and Martin (1966) used a token system in an attempt to improve the functioning of 40 adult female patients with chronic schizophrenia in a large state hospital. They noted that these patients appeared "apathetic" and seemed to lack "interest and motivation." For instance, a patient might stare at a wall all day or continually pace around the ward. Schaefer and Martin sought to determine whether the contingent delivery of tokens for more varied and normal behaviors would improve the functioning of these patients. The patients were randomly divided into two groups. Patients in the control group received a supply of tokens regardless of their behavior. Patients in the experimental group received tokens for specific behaviors from three broad categories: personal hygiene, social interaction, and adequate work performance. Some examples of reinforced behaviors in the first category were thoroughness of showering, brushing teeth, combing hair, use of cosmetics, and maintenance of an attractive appearance. Among the reinforced social behaviors were everyday greetings (e.g., "Good morning"), speaking in group-therapy sessions, and playing cards with other patients. Work assignments included such activities as emptying wastepaper baskets, wiping tables, and vacuuming. Notice that all of the reinforced behaviors would generally be considered normal and desirable not only within the hospital but also in the outside world. The tokens were used to purchase both necessities and luxuries, including food, cigarettes, access to television, and recreational activities. The token program remained in effect for 3 months, and during this time the variety and frequency of "adaptive" behaviors increased in the experimental group, whereas there was no visible change in the control group.

Other studies on token systems in psychiatric institutions have also found that such procedures can produce impressive improvements in the personal, social, and work-related behaviors of patients. However, the use of token systems in psychiatric hospitals and other institutions has declined over the years, for several reasons (Glynn, 1990). First, token systems require a long time to produce lasting changes in behavior, whereas the average duration of hospitalization has decreased greatly over the years. Second, token systems are difficult to implement, and they require the cooperation and hard work of a well-trained staff. Third, there has been an increasing emphasis on pharmacological treatments for psychiatric patients. There have also been some court rulings that restrict what can legally be done with token systems. For these reasons, it seems unlikely that token systems will be used extensively in psychiatric institutions in the near future.

Although their use with psychiatric patients has declined, token systems are now very commonly used in classrooms. Tokens may be delivered for good academic performance or for good behavior. In one example, the classroom behavior of special education students was improved by giving them tokens for such behaviors as paying attention, using appropriate language, cooperating with others, and following instructions (Cavalier, Ferretti, & Hodges, 1997). Teachers can set up a system in which tokens are exchanged for snacks, small prizes, or access to special activities.

For more than two decades, a token system of behavior management was used in a student housing cooperative at the University of Kansas. This residence hall for 30 students achieved lower rents and high student satisfaction by giving the students responsibility for many of the tasks needed to keep the house functioning. The students were in charge of advertising vacancies, collecting rents, purchasing food and preparing meals, cleaning, making routine repairs, and many other tasks. To make certain that these chores got done, detailed job descriptions were created for every work assignment, supervisors checked to see that the tasks were completed correctly and recorded the performance of each worker, and the students earned rent reductions by doing their assigned tasks. At the same time, monetary fines were imposed if a student failed to perform a large percentage of his assigned tasks.

To determine whether this behavior-management system was indeed responsible for the smooth functioning of the residence, the token system was suspended for a period of 4 weeks, and students received their maximum rent reductions whether or not they completed their tasks (Johnson, Welsh, Miller, & Altus, 1991). Figure 6-7 shows the results of this experiment. For 5 weeks in which the behavior-management system was in effect, the students completed about 85% of their assigned tasks. During the 4 weeks in which the system was suspended, the number of completed tasks steadily declined to under 60%. Performance quickly improved when the system

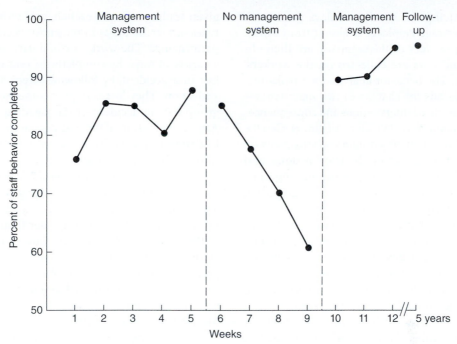

FIGURE 6-7   The percentage of tasks in a student housing cooperative that were completed when a behavior-management system was in effect, when the system was suspended, and when it was reinstated.

SOURCE: From Johnson et. al., "Participatory management: Managing staff performance in a university housing cooperative," *Journal of Applied Behavior Analysis, 24*(1), Spring 1991, Figure 1, page 124. Reprinted by permission.

was reinstated, and a follow-up 5 years later showed a continued high level of task completion. One especially encouraging feature of this project is that the students took an active role in designing the behavior-management system, and the system continued to function successfully with only minimal supervision by a behavior analyst.

Using a combination of token reinforcement and modern technology, Dallery, Glenn, and Raiff (2007) offered vouchers to smokers for reducing their levels of carbon monoxide (which measures how much they had been smoking). The entire project was conducted over the Internet. Twice a day, participants used a webcam to record themselves taking a breath test for carbon monoxide. Over a 4-week period, they earned vouchers for greater and greater decreases in carbon monoxide levels, and the vouchers could be used to buy items from merchants on the Internet. The individual results were variable, but many participants showed dramatic reductions in smoking as the treatment progressed.

Organizational Behavior Management

An area of applied behavior analysis known as **organizational behavior management** is devoted to using the principles of behavioral psychology to improve human performance in the workplace (Johnson, Redmon, & Mawhinney, 2001). Researchers in this field have addressed such matters as worker productivity, supervisor effectiveness, accident prevention, quality improvement, and customer satisfaction. The idea of organizational behavior management is to apply a scientific approach to workplace behavior.

When behavior analysts serve as consultants for a business organization, the process usually involves several different steps. The organization's leaders must decide on the goals they wish to achieve and describe them in concrete terms (e.g., reducing the number of days per month that the average employee is absent from work). Current practices of the company are then observed, and data are collected on the workers' behaviors. The behavior analysts then make recommendations for changes of two main types—antecedent-based interventions and consequence-based interventions (Wilder, Austin, & Casella, 2009). Antecedent-based interventions focus on events that occur before the work is done, and they focus on such matters as providing appropriate worker training, clarifying tasks, and setting goals. Consequence-based interventions focus on the events that occur after the work is done, and they can include the use of praise, monetary rewards, and feedback. As in all applied behavior analysis, data are collected to evaluate whether the changes are having their desired effects, and further adjustments are made as needed.

An early study by Wallin and Johnson (1976) illustrates the potential benefits of this approach. In a small electronics company where worker tardiness and absenteeism had become a problem, workers were allowed to participate in a monthly lottery if their attendance record had been perfect for the past month. The names of all workers who had perfect attendance records were placed in a basket and a random drawing determined the winner of a $10 prize. Since the lottery was an example of a VR schedule, we might predict that it should produce steady behavior, assuming that the size of the reinforcer was sufficient. Apparently it was, for in the first 11 months of the lottery system, employee absenteeism was 30% lower than in the previous 11 months. This simple program saved the company thousands of dollars in sick-leave expenditures. But monetary reinforcers are not always necessary. G. A. Werner (1992) found that simply recognizing employees with good attendance by awarding them certificates and displaying these certificates publicly could produce a substantial decrease in absenteeism.

Reinforcement procedures have also been used to decrease workplace accidents. For instance, Fox, Hopkins, and Anger (1987) described how workers in two open-pit mines were given trading stamps (exchangeable for various types of merchandise) in return for accident-free performance. The workers could earn stamps in a variety of ways: by completing a year without a lost-time accident, by following safety standards, and so on. They lost stamps if someone in their group had an accident or damaged equipment. After the adoption of the trading-stamp program, lost-time accidents decreased by more than two thirds in both mines and continued at this lower level over a period of several years. The program was also cost effective for the mining companies: The monetary savings from reduced accident rates were at least 15 times greater than the cost of the trading-stamp program. Quite a few other studies have found that such reinforcement programs can both reduce workplace accidents and save companies substantial amounts of money (McAfee & Winn, 1989; Sulzer-Azaroff, Loafman, Merante, & Hlavacek, 1990).

Many applications of behavior analysis in the workplace involve not just one specific change but a treatment package consisting of several components. For instance, in a hospital's operating room, behavior analysts used a combination of goal setting, task clarification, and feedback to increase the use of safe methods of passing sharp surgical instruments from one person to another. Baseline measurements showed that surgeons and staff frequently used unsafe techniques that increased the risk of a cut or puncture wound. In a meeting with operating room personnel, a "challenging but realistic" goal for improvement was agreed upon. Task clarification was accomplished by having staff model safe and unsafe techniques so that everyone understood the proper techniques. For feedback, the operating room procedures were observed and recorded, and each week the percentage of safe transfers was reported to the staff. Under this program, the use of safe techniques increased by a factor of two (Cunningham & Austin, 2007).

Organizational behavior management has been used for many different types of companies, both large and small, in many different sectors of the economy, including human services, manufacturing, transportation, and education.

Some researchers have compared different ways of delivering feedback to workers about their job performance (Alvero, Bucklin, & Austin, 2001). Others have studied different ways of giving workers monetary incentives for their work (Bucklin & Dickinson, 2001). Of course, no two companies are exactly alike, but by comparing the results from many different cases, researchers can start to draw general conclusions about what methods of behavior change are the most effective.

Behavior Therapy for Marital Problems

Some therapists have used behavioral principles to aid couples who seek help for marital problems. Jacobson and Dallas (1981) recognized that in unhappy married couples, each spouse tends to resort to threats, punishment, and retaliation in an attempt to get what he or she wants from the other. For this reason, the initial phases of therapy are designed to promote more positive interactions between partners. To encourage a reciprocal exchange of reinforcers between spouses, a contingency contract is often used. A **contingency contract** is a written agreement that lists the duties (behaviors) required of each party and the privileges (reinforcers) that will result if the duties are performed (Stuart, 1971). In most cases, both spouses play active roles in creating the contract and indicate their agreement with the terms of the contract by signing it.

A contingency contract can help to encourage the exchange of reinforcers and to let each partner know what behaviors the other desires. For instance, the husband may agree to do the dishes in the evening if and only if the wife took the children to school that morning. Conversely, the wife agrees to take the children to school the next morning if and only if the husband did the dishes the night before. Jacobson and Dallas (1981) claim that the use of a written contract has several advantages: "it constitutes a public commitment to change; it decreases the likelihood of forgetting; and it prevents each spouse from retrospectively distorting the terms of the agreement" (p. 390). This part of behavioral marital therapy is called *behavior*

exchange because each spouse makes an effort to perform specific behaviors that will please the other.

Behavior exchange is just one part of behavioral marital therapy. Another important component is training in communication and problem-solving skills. N. S. Jacobson (1977) observed that unhappy couples often have difficulty communicating, and they find it difficult to solve even the simplest of problems that may arise. As part of their therapy, a couple first reads a book about problem solving in marriage; then they try to solve a very minor problem as the therapist watches. For instance, the wife may complain that she does not like always having to remind the husband to take out the garbage. The couple then tries to find a solution to this small problem that satisfies both spouses. Whenever one spouse responds in an inappropriate way, the therapist interrupts, points out the flaw, and suggests a better alternative. After a little trial and error, the couple usually finds a solution to this minor problem. Over time, they gradually work up to bigger problems, and they are typically given "homework assignments" in which they engage in problem solving on a regular basis between meetings with the therapist (Coop Gordon, Dixon, Willett, & Hughes, 2009).

Behavior therapy (or *cognitive-behavior therapy,* as it is often called because of its emphasis on problem solving and communication) seems to offer a promising approach to the treatment of marital discord: One review of 17 separate studies concluded that a couple's chances of successfully resolving their marital difficulties more than doubled if the couple received this type of therapy (Halweg & Markman, 1988). Although these techniques do not work for everyone, they can help many unhappy couples improve the quality of their marriages. As with most types of behavior modification, behavioral therapy for couples is not a fixed and unchanging system; it continues to evolve as therapists experiment with new techniques and measure their effectiveness.

Conclusions

The successful application of the principles of reinforcement to a wide array of behavior problems provides one of the strongest pieces of evidence that the research of the operant conditioning laboratory is relevant to real-world behavior. One common criticism of behavior modification is that these principles are nothing new—that people have always used reward and punishment to try to control the behavior of others. Kazdin (1980) argued that this criticism is unfair for several reasons. First, many people are apparently unaware of how their own actions affect the behavior of others; as a result, they inadvertently reinforce the very behaviors they would like to eliminate. The parent who eventually gives in to a child's demands after the child whines or has a tantrum is reinforcing whining and tantrums on a VI schedule. The psychiatric nurse who listens sympathetically when a patient complains of imaginary illnesses or tells unbelievable stories is reinforcing this unusual verbal behavior with attention. These and countless other examples show that many people have little understanding of the basic principles of reinforcement.

Kazdin also noted that whereas the rules for reinforcement are applied systematically and consistently in a behavior-modification program, they seldom are when the average person uses reinforcers. A parent may begin with a rule that a child can earn an allowance by drying the dishes each night. However, the parent may sometimes excuse the child and give the allowance anyway if the child complains of being tired (and complaining is thereby reinforced). On another day, when the parent is in a bad mood, the same complaint of being tired might result in the child being spanked.

One final argument against the statement that the principles of operant conditioning are "commonsense" ideas is that knowing something about the principles of reinforcement is not the same as knowing everything. Behavior therapists certainly do not know everything about how reinforcement works, but they do know much more than the average person. Consider how many of the principles of operant conditioning you understood (at least at a commonsense level) before you started this chapter compared to those you know now. You may have had some idea of how primary and conditioned reinforcers can alter

behavior, but unless you have had experience training animals, you were probably unfamiliar with the principles of shaping, backward chaining, prompting, fading, and discrimination learning. You would probably find it difficult to predict the different behavior patterns produced by the four simple reinforcement schedules, either during acquisition or subsequent extinction. (If you do not believe this, try describing the four simple schedules to a friend with no training in psychology to see whether he or she can predict the different behaviors these schedules generate.) The subtleties and complexities of operant behavior are not obvious, and it has taken careful experiments to uncover them. With further research in this area, psychologists should continue to develop a more complete understanding of how "voluntary" behaviors are affected by their consequences.

PRACTICE QUIZ (2)

1. Research results favor the _____ theory of FR postreinforcement pauses over the _____ and _____ theories.
2. IRT reinforcement theory states that longer IRTs are more likely to be reinforced on _____ schedules, but bursts of responding are more likely to be reinforced on _____ schedules.
3. _____ theories deal with long-term relationships between behavior and reinforcement, whereas _____ theories deal with moment-to-moment relationships between behavior and reinforcement.
4. Physically guiding the movements of a learner is an example of a _____; gradually removing this physical guidance is called _____.
5. In behavioral marital therapy, a written agreement between spouses is called a _____.

Answers

1. remaining-responses, fatigue, satiation 2. VI, VR 3. molar, molecular 4. prompt, fading 5. contingency contract

Summary

An FR schedule delivers a reinforcer after a fixed number of responses, and it typically produces a postreinforcement pause followed by rapid responding. A VR schedule delivers a reinforcer after a variable number of responses, and it typically leads to rapid, steady responding. On an FI schedule, the requirement for reinforcement is one response after a fixed amount of time. Subjects often exhibit a postreinforcement pause and then an accelerating response pattern. VI schedules are similar except that the time requirement is variable, and they typically produce moderate, steady responding.

Performance on a reinforcement schedule can be affected by the quality and amount of reinforcement, response effort, and the individual's level of motivation and past experience. People may also respond according to rules they have been taught or have learned on their own. When reinforcement is discontinued, extinction is usually rapid after CRF, slower after FI or FR, and slowest after VI or VR.

Experimental analysis has shown that the postreinforcement pause on FR schedules occurs primarily because each reinforcer is a signal that many responses must be completed before the next reinforcer. Regarding the question of why VR schedules produce faster responding than VI schedules, IRT reinforcement theory states that long pauses are often reinforced on VI schedules, whereas bursts of rapid responses are more likely to be reinforced on VR schedules. A different theory states that subjects learn that more rapid responding yields more reinforcers on VR schedules, but not on VI schedules.

Reinforcement schedules are frequently used in behavior therapy. Children with autism have been taught to speak by using positive reinforcement, shaping, prompting, and fading. Token systems and other reinforcement techniques have been used in some psychiatric hospitals, schools, and businesses. In behavior therapy for couples, contingency contracts help partners increase the exchange of positive reinforcers.

Review Questions

1. For each of the four basic reinforcement schedules, describe the rule for reinforcement, the typical response pattern, and the rate of extinction.

2. From your own experience, describe a situation that resembles one of the four simple reinforcement schedules. How is the reinforcement schedule in your example similar to the laboratory example? Are there any important differences between the two? Is the behavior pattern in real life similar to behavior in the laboratory?

3. What are some factors that can affect performance on a reinforcement schedule? Illustrate using concrete examples.

4. What is the difference between the molecular and molar theories of behavior? Describe a molecular theory and a molar theory of why responding is usually faster on VR schedules than on VI schedules.

5. Give a few examples of how the principles of operant conditioning have been used in behavior therapy. In describing the methods, identify as many different terms and principles of operant conditioning as you can.

CHAPTER

7

Avoidance and Punishment

LEARNING OBJECTIVES

After reading this chapter, you should be able to

- identify different procedures for increasing or decreasing behavior

- describe three theories of avoidance and explain their strengths and weaknesses

- discuss the phenomenon of learned helplessness as it occurs in animals and in people

- describe factors that determine whether punishment will be effective

- explain the disadvantages of using punishment as a method of controlling behavior

- describe different types of behavior decelerators and how they are used in behavior therapy

Chapters 5 and 6 were devoted to the topic of positive reinforcement, a procedure in which a response is followed by a particular stimulus (a reinforcer) and the response is strengthened as a result. However, positive reinforcement is only one of four possible relationships between a behavior and its consequences. Figure 7-1 presents these four possibilities in the form of a two-by-two matrix. First, after a behavior occurs, a stimulus can be presented, or a stimulus can be removed or omitted. In each of these cases, the result could be either an increase or a decrease in the behavior, depending on the nature of the stimulus that is either presented or removed. We have already thoroughly examined the procedure in cell 1 of the matrix (positive reinforcement). This chapter will focus on the other three cells.

We can begin with some definitions. With **negative reinforcement** (cell 3), a behavior increases in frequency if some stimulus is removed after the behavior occurs. For example, suppose a person with a headache takes some ibuprofen, and the headache promptly goes away. In this case, the individual **escapes** from the pain of the headache by performing some behavior. As a result, this behavior should be strengthened in the future: The next time the person has a headache, he is likely to take ibuprofen again. The term *negative reinforcement* also includes instances of **avoidance** in which a response prevents an unpleasant stimulus from occurring in the first place. For example, paying your income tax avoids the unpleasant consequences of

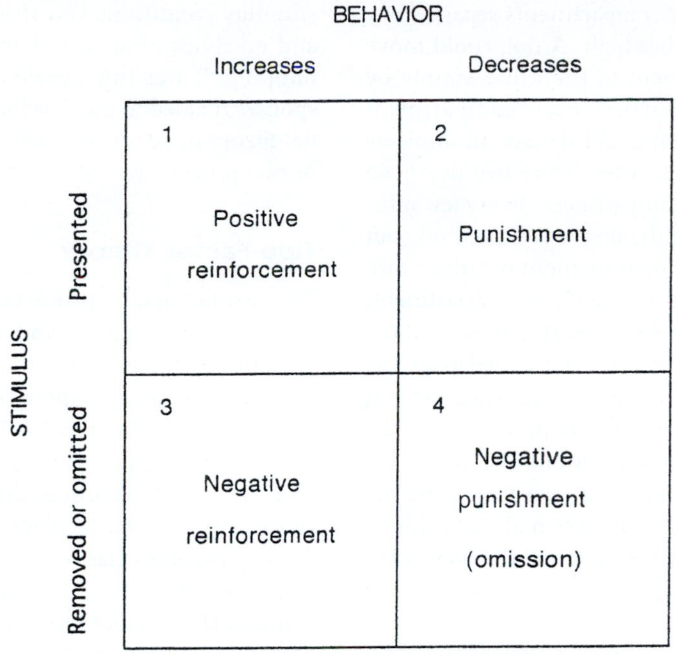

BEHAVIOR

Increases   Decreases

FIGURE 7-1 A two-by-two matrix depicting two types of reinforcement and two types of punishment.

failing to do so. Both positive and negative reinforcement strengthen or increase the likelihood of the behavior involved. The term *positive* indicates that a stimulus is presented if a behavior occurs; the term *negative* indicates that a stimulus is subtracted (removed or avoided entirely) if a behavior occurs.

Cells 2 and 4 are similar to cells 1 and 3, respectively, except that the opposite type of stimulus is used. Cell 2 represents the procedure of **punishment** in which a behavior is followed by an unpleasant stimulus. To emphasize the fact that a stimulus is presented, we might call this procedure *positive punishment,* but this term is seldom used. Cell 4 represents **negative punishment** in which a pleasant stimulus is removed or omitted if a behavior occurs. The term **omission** is often used instead of negative punishment. If a parent refuses to give a child her usual weekly allowance after some bad behavior (such as staying out too late), this is an example of negative punishment.

The first part of this chapter surveys a number of experiments on negative reinforcement, and it discusses some of the theoretical issues about avoidance that psychologists have debated over the years. Next, we will look at the two types of punishment procedures. Although punishment is, in theory, the opposite of reinforcement, some psychologists have concluded that punishment is not an effective form of behavioral control. We will consider the evidence and attempt to draw some conclusions. Finally, we will examine some of the ways that punishment has been used in behavior modification.

AVOIDANCE

A Representative Experiment

Solomon and Wynne (1953) conducted an experiment that illustrates many of the properties of negative reinforcement. Their subjects were dogs and their apparatus was a **shuttle box**—a chamber with two rectangular compartments separated by a barrier several inches high. A dog could move from one compartment to the other simply by jumping over the barrier. Each compartment had a metal floor that could deliver an unpleasant stimulus, a shock. There were two overhead lights, one for each compartment. Every few minutes, the light above the dog was turned off (but the light in the other compartment remained on). If the dog remained in the dark compartment, after 10 seconds the floor was electrified and the dog received a shock until it hopped over the barrier to the other compartment. Thus the dog could *escape* from the shock by jumping over the barrier. However, the dog could also *avoid* the shock completely by jumping over the barrier before the 10 seconds of darkness had elapsed. The next trial was the same, except that the dog had to jump back into the first compartment to escape or avoid the shock.

For the first few trials a typical dog's responses were escape responses—the dog did not jump over the barrier until the shock had started. After a few trials, a dog would start making avoidance responses—it would jump over the barrier soon after the light went out, and if it jumped in less than 10 seconds it did not receive the shock.

After a few dozen trials, a typical dog would almost always jump over the barrier just 2 or 3 seconds after the light went out. Many dogs never again received a shock after their first successful avoidance response. From then on, they always jumped in less than 10 seconds after the light went out. Results such as these had led earlier theorists (Mowrer, 1947; Schoenfeld, 1950) to ponder a question that is sometimes called the **avoidance paradox**: How can the *nonoccurrence* of an event (shock) serve as a reinforcer for the avoidance response? Reinforcement theorists had no problem explaining *escape* responses, because the response produced an obvious change in an important stimulus (e.g., shock changed to no shock when the escape response was made). The problem for reinforcement theorists was with *avoidance* responses, because here there was no such change in the stimulus. Some theorists felt it did not make sense to say that no change in the

stimulus conditions (no shock before the jump and no shock after) could act as a reinforcer for jumping. It was this puzzle about avoidance responses that led to the development of an influential theory of avoidance called **two-factor theory**, or two-process theory.

Two-Factor Theory

The two factors, or processes, of this theory are classical conditioning and operant conditioning, and according to the theory, both are necessary for avoidance responses to occur (Eelen & Vervliet, 2006; Mowrer, 1947). These two factors can be illustrated in the experiment of Solomon and Wynne. One unconditioned response to shock is fear, and fear plays a critical role in the theory. Through classical conditioning, this fear response is transferred from the unconditioned stimulus (US) (shock) to some conditioned stimulus (CS) (a stimulus that precedes the shock). In the Solomon and Wynne experiment, the CS was the 10 seconds of darkness that preceded each shock. After a few trials, a dog would presumably respond to the darkness with fear. This conditioning of a fear response to an initially neutral stimulus is the first process of the theory.

The second factor, based on operant conditioning, is escape from a fear-provoking CS. In the Solomon and Wynne experiment, a dog could escape from a dark compartment to an illuminated compartment by jumping over the barrier. It is important to understand that in two-factor theory, what we have been calling "avoidance responses" is redefined as escape responses. The theory says that the reinforcer for jumping is not the avoidance of the shock, but rather the escape from a fear-eliciting CS. This theoretical maneuver is two-factor theory's solution to the avoidance paradox. We no longer have to wonder how no change in a stimulus (shock) can reinforce a behavior. Removing the fear-evoking CS (darkness) is an observable change in the stimulus environment that could certainly act as a negative reinforcer. In summary, according to two-factor theory, ending the signal for shock in avoidance behavior has the same status as ending the shock in escape behavior—both are actual stimulus changes that can serve as reinforcers (i.e., negative reinforcers, because they are removed when a response is made).

Evidence Supporting Two-Factor Theory

Because the role of the fear-eliciting CS is so crucial to two-factor theory, many experiments have investigated how CSs can influence avoidance behavior. One class of experiments has involved creating a fear-eliciting CS in one context and observing its effects when it is presented during a different situation, where an animal is already making avoidance responses. For example, Rescorla and LoLordo (1965) first trained dogs in a shuttle box where jumping into the other compartment postponed a shock. Then the dogs received conditioning trials in which a tone was paired with shock. Finally, the dogs were returned to the avoidance task, and occasionally the tone was presented (but no longer followed by shock). Whenever the tone came on, the dogs dramatically increased their rates of jumping over the barrier. This result shows that a stimulus that is specifically trained as a CS for fear can amplify ongoing avoidance behavior.

Other experiments supporting two-factor theory have shown that the signal for shock in a typical avoidance situation does indeed develop aversive properties, and that animals can learn a new response that terminates the signal. N. E. Miller (1948) attempted to turn a white compartment into an aversive stimulus by shocking rats while they were in that chamber. From this point on, no further shocks were presented, but Miller found that a rat would learn a new response, turning a wheel, when this response opened a door and allowed the rat to escape from the white chamber. In the next phase, wheel turning was no longer an effective response; instead, a rat could escape from the white chamber by pressing a lever. Eventually, Miller's rats learned this second novel response.

These studies provided support for two-factor theory by showing that a CS for shock can accelerate ongoing avoidance behavior, and its removal can be used as a reinforcer to teach an animal totally new responses. However, not all the evidence on two-factor theory has been favorable; the Problems with Two-Factor Theory section discusses some results that pose problems for the theory.

Problems with Two-Factor Theory

AVOIDANCE WITHOUT OBSERVABLE SIGNS OF FEAR.
One problem with two-factor theory concerns the relationship between fear and avoidance responses. If the theory is correct, we should be able to observe an increase in fear when the signal for shock is presented and a decrease in fear once the avoidance response is made. However, it has long been recognized that observable signs of fear disappear as subjects become more experienced in avoidance tasks (e.g., Starr & Mineka, 1977). For example, Solomon and Wynne (1953) noted that early in their experiment a dog would exhibit various signs of fear (whining, urination, shaking) when the light was turned off. However, once the animal became proficient in making the avoidance response, such overt signs of emotion disappeared. But according to two-factor theory, fear should be greatest when avoidance responses are the strongest, since fear is supposedly what motivates the avoidance response.

To deal with this problem, other versions of two-factor theory have downplayed the role of fear in avoidance learning. For example, Dinsmoor (2001) has maintained that it is not necessary to assume that the CS in avoidance learning produces fear (as measured by heart rate or other physical signs). We only need to assume that the CS has become aversive (meaning that it has become a stimulus the animal will try to remove). Studies such as those described in the previous section clearly show that a CS paired with shock can develop this property of aversion.

EXTINCTION OF AVOIDANCE BEHAVIOR.
As noted earlier, many of the dogs in the Solomon and Wynne experiment quickly became proficient at the avoidance task, so after a few trials they never again received a shock. From the perspective of two-factor theory, each trial without the shock is avoided is an extinction trial: The CS (darkness) is presented, but the US (shock) is

not. According to the principles of classical con-ditioning, the CR of fear (or aversion, if we use Dinsmoor's approach) should gradually weaken on such extinction trials until it is no longer elic-ited by the CS. But if the darkness no longer elicits fear or aversion, the avoidance response should not occur either. Therefore, two-factor theory pre-dicts that avoidance responding should gradually deteriorate after a series of trials without shock. However, once avoidance responses fail to occur, the dog will again receive darkness–shock pairings, and the aversion should be reconditioned. Then, as soon as avoidance responses again start to occur, the aversion to darkness should once again start to extinguish. In short, two-factor theory seems to predict that avoidance responses should repeatedly appear and disappear in a cyclical pattern.

Unfortunately for two-factor theory, such cycles in avoidance responding have almost never been observed. Indeed, one of the most notewor-thy features of avoidance behavior is its extreme resistance to extinction. In the experiments of Solomon and Wynne, many dogs responded for several hundred trials without receiving a shock (Solomon, Kamin, & Wynne, 1953; Solomon & Wynne, 1954). In addition, their response laten-cies continued to decrease during these trials even though no shock was received. This suggests that the strength of the avoidance response was increas-ing, not decreasing, during these shock-free trials.

These findings were troublesome for two-factor theory, and many psychologists viewed the slow extinction of avoidance behavior as a major problem for the theory. To try to deal with these problems, two other important theories of avoid-ance were developed, one-factor theory and cog-nitive theory.

One-Factor Theory

To put it simply, **one-factor theory** states that the classical conditioning component of two-factor theory is not necessary. There is no need to assume that escape from a fear-eliciting CS is the reinforcer for an avoidance response, because, contrary to the assumptions of two-factor theory, avoidance of a shock can in itself serve as a reinforcer. An experi-ment by Murray Sidman illustrates this point.

Sidman (1953) developed an avoidance procedure that is now called either the **Sidman avoidance task** or simply **free-operant avoid-ance.** In this procedure, there is no signal preced-ing shock, but if the subject makes no responses, the shocks occur at perfectly regular intervals. For instance, in one condition of Sidman's experi-ment, a rat would receive a shock every 5 seconds throughout the session if it made no avoidance response (Figure 7-2a). However, if the rat made an avoidance response (pressing a lever), the next shock did not occur until 30 seconds after the

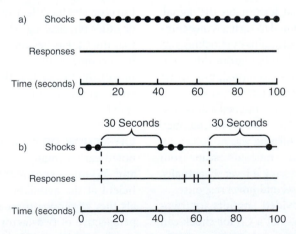

FIGURE 7-2   The procedure in one condition of Sidman's (1953) avoidance task. (a) If the subject makes no responses, a shock is delivered every 5 seconds. (b) Each response postpones the next shock for 30 seconds.

response. Each response postponed the next shock for 30 seconds (Figure 7-2b). By responding regularly (say, once every 20 to 25 seconds), a rat could avoid all the shocks. In practice, Sidman's rats did not avoid all the shocks, but they did respond frequently enough to avoid many of them.

On the surface, these results seem to pose a problem for two-factor theory because there is no signal before a shock. If there is no CS to elicit fear or aversion, why should an avoidance response occur? Actually, two-factor theorists had a simple answer to this question, as Sidman himself realized. The answer is that although Sidman provided no external stimulus, the passage of time could serve as a stimulus because the shocks occurred at regular intervals. That is, once a rat was familiar with the procedure, its fear might increase as more and more time elapsed without a response. The rat could associate fear with the stimulus "a long time since the last response," and it could remove this stimulus (and the associated fear) by making a response.

To make a stronger case for one-factor theory, we need an experiment in which neither an external stimulus nor the passage of time could serve as a reliable signal that a shock was approaching. An experiment by Herrnstein and Hineline (1966) met these requirements. The basic idea of the procedure was that by pressing a lever, a rat could switch from a schedule that delivered shocks at a rapid rate to one that delivered shocks at a slower rate. For example, in one condition there was a 30% chance of shock if the rat had not recently pressed the lever, but only a 10% chance if the rat had recently pressed the lever. Obviously, to reduce the number of shocks, the animal should remain on the 10% schedule as much as possible. However, the key feature of this procedure was that pressing the lever did not ensure any amount of shock-free time. Sometimes, just by chance, a rat would press the lever and get a shock from the 10% schedule almost immediately. This is because lever pressing in this procedure only produced a lower rate of shocks on average; it did not guarantee any fixed shock-free time.

Herrnstein and Hineline (1966) found that 17 of their 18 rats eventually acquired the avoidance response. They concluded (1) that animals can learn an avoidance response when neither an external CS nor the passage of time is a reliable signal for shock, and (2) that to master this task, animals must be sensitive to the average shock frequencies when they respond and when they do not respond. Herrnstein (1969) reasoned that if the rats were sensitive to these two shock frequencies in the procedure, then it is a needless complication to assume that fear or aversion to a CS controls the avoidance responses in the typical avoidance experiment: Why not simply assume that a reduction in shock frequency is the reinforcer for the avoidance response? For this reason, one-factor theory of avoidance is sometimes called the *shock-frequency reduction theory* (Hineline, 2001).

SLOW EXTINCTION AS A FAILURE OF DISCRIMINATION. One-factor theory, which relies solely on the principles of operant conditioning, has a simple explanation for the slow extinction of avoidance responses. We have seen that once an avoidance response is acquired, the animal may avoid every scheduled shock by making the appropriate response. Now suppose that at some point the experimenter turns off the shock generator. From the animal's perspective, the subsequent trials will appear no different from the previous trials: The stimulus comes on, the subject responds, the stimulus goes off, no shock occurs. Since the animal can discriminate no change in the conditions, there is no change in behavior either, according to this reasoning.

Cognitive Theory

Seligman and Johnston (1973) developed a **cognitive theory of avoidance** that they suggested was superior to both two-factor and one-factor theories. They proposed that an animal's behavior can only change in an avoidance task if there is a discrepancy between expectancy and observation. On the first trial of a signaled avoidance experiment, an animal can have no expectations about shock or how to avoid it. Consequently, the animal makes no avoidance response on the first trial. However, as the trials proceed, the animal gradually develops the expectations that (1) no shock will occur if it makes a certain response, and (2) shock will occur if it does not make the response. Because the animal prefers the first option over the second option, it makes the response.

Once these two expectations have been formed, Seligman and Johnston assumed that the animal's behavior will not change until one or both of the expectations are violated. This can explain the slow extinction of avoidance behavior. As long as the animal responds on each extinction trial, all it can observe is that a response is followed by no shock. This observation is consistent with the animal's expectation, so there is no change in its behavior. Presumably, extinction will only begin to occur if the animal eventually fails to make a response on some trial (perhaps by mistake, or because it is distracted, or for some such reason). Only on a trial without an avoidance response can the animal observe an outcome (no response leads to no shock) that is inconsistent with its expectations.

A more recent cognitive theory proposed by Lovibond (2006) maintains that individuals can learn more detailed expectations that include information about the three parts of the three-term contingency (discriminative stimulus, operant response, and consequence). For instance, an individual might learn that in the presence of one warning signal, a specific response will avoid one type of aversive event, but if another warning signal occurs, a different avoidance response is required to avoid a different aversive event. Research with college students by Declercq, De Houwer, and Baeyens (2008) has found that they can and do develop these more elaborate three-part expectations in avoidance tasks.

THE PROCEDURE OF RESPONSE BLOCKING (FLOODING). The slow extinction of avoidance responses is not inevitable: Extinction can be speeded up by using a procedure called **response blocking**, or **flooding**. As its name suggests, response blocking involves presenting the signal that precedes shock but preventing the subject from making the avoidance response. For example,

Page and Hall (1953) conducted an avoidance experiment in which rats learned to avoid a shock by running from one compartment to another. After the response was learned, one group of rats received normal extinction trials. A second group had the extinction trials preceded by five trials in which a rat was retained in the first compartment for 15 seconds, with the door to the second compartment closed. Thus these rats were prevented from making the avoidance response, but unlike in the acquisition phase, they received no shocks in the first compartment. Page and Hall found that extinction proceeded much more rapidly in the response-blocking group. The other term for this procedure, *flooding,* connotes the fact that subjects are "flooded" with exposure to the stimulus that used to precede shock. (In the Page and Hall experiment, this stimulus was simply the inside of the first compartment.) There is considerable evidence that response blocking is an effective way to speed the extinction of avoidance responses (Baum, 1966, 1976).

Cognitive theory offers a simple explanation of why response blocking works. The subject is forced to observe a set of events—no response followed by no shock—that does not match the animal's expectation that no response will be followed by shock. A new expectation, that no shock will follow no response, is gradually formed; as a result, avoidance responses gradually disappear.

Can the other theories of avoidance account for the effects of response blocking? An obvious explanation based on two-factor theory is that the forced exposure to the CS produces extinction of the conditioned fear or aversion. An explanation based on one-factor theory might proceed as follows: Normal avoidance extinction is slow because there is nothing to signal the change from acquisition to extinction conditions. However, the procedure of response blocking introduces a drastic stimulus change: There is now a closed door that prevents the animal from entering the other compartment. This change in stimuli gives the subject a cue that things are now different from the preceding acquisition phase. It is not surprising that subsequent extinction proceeds more quickly.

Biological Constraints in Avoidance Learning

As if the theoretical analysis of avoidance was not confusing enough, the picture is further complicated by evidence that biological constraints can also play an important role in avoidance learning, just as they can in classical conditioning and with the use of positive reinforcement. Robert Bolles (1970) proposed that animals exhibit a type of preparedness in avoidance learning. In this case, the preparedness does not involve a stimulus–stimulus association, but rather a propensity to perform certain behaviors in a potentially dangerous situation. Bolles was highly critical of traditional theories of avoidance learning, especially two-factor theory. He suggested that a two-factor account of avoidance learning in the wild might go as follows: A small animal in the forest is attacked by a predator and is hurt but manages to escape. Later, when the animal is again in this part of the forest, it encounters a CS—a sight, sound, or smell that preceded the previous attack. This CS produces the response of fear, and the animal runs away to escape from the CS, and it is reinforced by a feeling of relief. According to the two-factor account, then, avoidance behavior occurs because animals learn about signals for danger (CSs) and then avoid those signals. Bolles (1970) claimed, however, that this account is

> utter nonsense. . . . Thus, no real-life predator is going to present cues just before it attacks. No owl hoots or whistles 5 seconds before pouncing on a mouse. And no owl terminates its hoots or whistles just as the mouse gets away so as to reinforce the avoidance response. Nor will the owl give the mouse enough trials for the necessary learning to occur. What keeps our little friends alive in the forest has nothing to do with avoidance learning as we ordinarily conceive of it or investigate it in the laboratory. . . . What keeps animals alive in the wild is that they have very effective innate defensive reactions which occur when they encounter any kind of new or sudden stimulus. (pp. 32–33)

Bolles called these innate behavior patterns **species-specific defense reactions (SSDRs)**. As the name implies, SSDRs may be different for different animals, but Bolles suggested that they usually fall into one of three categories: freezing, fleeing, and fighting (adopting an aggressive posture and/or behaviors). Bolles proposed that in laboratory studies of avoidance, an avoidance response will be quickly learned if it is identical with or at least similar to one of the subject's SSDRs. If the required avoidance response is not similar to an SSDR, the response will be learned slowly or not at all. To support this hypothesis, Bolles noted that rats can learn to avoid a shock by jumping or running out of a compartment in one or only a few trials. The rapid acquisition presumably reflects the fact that for rats, fleeing is a highly probable response to danger. However, it is very difficult to train a rat to avoid shock by pressing a lever, presumably because this response is unlike any of the creature's typical responses to danger.

The important point here is that the difficulty in learning new responses such as lever pressing depends on the nature of the reinforcer. When the reinforcer is avoidance of shock, lever pressing is a difficult response for rats to acquire, and some rats never learn it. Yet when the reinforcer is food or water, lever pressing is a relatively easy response for rats to learn. As another example, we have seen that it is quite easy to shape a pigeon to peck a key when food is the reinforcer. In comparison, it is very difficult to train a pigeon to peck a key to avoid a shock. The problem is apparently that a pigeon's most usual response to an intense aversive stimulus is to fly away, a response that has almost nothing in common with standing in place and pecking. Because of examples like this, Fanselow (1997) has argued that the basic principle of negative reinforcement (which states that any response that helps to avoid an aversive event will be strengthened) is not especially useful when SSDRs take over: Even a simple response such as pressing a lever or pecking a key may be difficult for the animal to learn.

A few studies have shown that it is possible to train animals to make an arbitrary operant response in an avoidance situation by somehow making the desired response more compatible with the SSDRs of that species. For example, in response to mild shock, a pigeon may exhibit SSDRs from the "fighting" category, including flapping its wings. Beginning with this response of wing flapping, Rachlin (1969) trained pigeons to operate a "key" that protruded into the chamber in order to avoid the shock. With rats, Modaresi (1990) found that lever pressing was much easier to train as an avoidance response if the lever was higher on the wall, and especially if lever presses not only avoided the shocks but produced a "safe area" (a platform) on which the rats could stand. Through a careful series of experiments, Modaresi showed that these two features coincided with the rats' natural tendencies to stretch upward and to seek a safe area when facing a potentially painful stimulus. Both of these studies are consistent with Bolles's claim that the ease of learning an avoidance response depends on the similarity between that response and one of the animal's SSDRs.

Conclusions About the Theories of Avoidance

First, let us consider once again the difference between one-factor theory and cognitive theory. In the final analysis, the differences between these two theories are to a large extent semantic: Wherever cognitive theory speaks of a violation of expectations or a change in expectations, one-factor theory can point to changes in discriminative stimuli. Those who like to speculate about an animal's expectations will probably favor cognitive theory; strict behaviorists, who avoid such speculation about internal events, will prefer the terminology of one-factor theory.

Over the years, two-factor theory has been a popular theory of avoidance behavior, but it has several problems. Avoidance learning can occur when there is no external signal for shock (Herrnstein & Hineline, 1966). In addition, two-factor theory has difficulty explaining the slowness of extinction in avoidance tasks. Both one-factor theory and cognitive theory avoid these problems by assuming that a fear-eliciting

CS is not an indispensable requirement for avoidance behavior. However, we have seen evidence that fear does play a role in some avoidance situations, and this evidence favors two-factor theory. For this and other reasons, some learning theorists still favor two-factor theory over the other two theories (Levis, 1989; Zhuikov, Couvillon, & Bitterman, 1994).

The debate between one-factor theorists and two-factor theorists is, in part, a debate between those who favor a molar approach to behavior analysis and those who favor a molecular approach. As explained in Chapter 6, molar theories assume that behavior is controlled by long-term relationships between behavior and its consequences, whereas molecular theories assume that moment-to-moment consequences are important. One-factor theorists favor the molar approach, because they maintain that animals are sensitive to long-term consequences, such as an overall reduction in shock frequency that occurs when an avoidance response is made (Baum, 2001; Hineline, 2001). Two-factor theorists favor the molecular approach because they assume that the immediate consequences control avoidance responses. For example, Dinsmoor (2001) has suggested that bodily feedback from the act of making an avoidance response can serve as an immediate reinforcer because, even in procedures such as those of Herrnstein and Hineline (1966), responding leads to a relative degree of safety.

After several decades of research and debate, the question of which theory of avoidance is best has not been settled to everyone's satisfaction. This may be a sign that each theory is partially correct. Perhaps fear does play an important role in some avoidance situations, but it is not a necessary role; avoidance responding may sometimes occur in the absence of fear, as the one-factor and cognitive theories propose.

Flooding as Behavior Therapy

Regardless of which theory best accounts for the effects of response blocking or flooding, this procedure has been adopted by some behavior therapists as a treatment for phobias. The major difference between flooding and systematic de-sensitization (Chapter 3) is that the hierarchy of fearful events or stimuli is eliminated. Instead of beginning with a stimulus that elicits only a small amount of fear, a therapist using a flood-ing procedure starts immediately with a highly feared stimulus and forces the patient to remain in the presence of this stimulus until the patient's external signs of fear subside. For example, an in-dividual with a snake phobia might be required to remain in a small room where the therapist is handling a live snake. Of course, it is the thera-pist's duty to describe the details of the flooding procedure to the patient in advance, to point out that the fear the patient will experience may be quite unpleasant, and to obtain the patient's con-sent before proceeding.

Morganstern (1973) reviewed a number of studies that compared the effectiveness of flood-ing and systematic desensitization, and he con-cluded that these procedures are about equally effective. Since systematic desensitization (which never allows the patient to experience a high level of fear) is a more pleasant form of therapy, Morganstern argued that there is little justifica-tion for using flooding in therapy. This viewpoint seems reasonable, but flooding can sometimes succeed in eliminating a phobia when system-atic desensitization has failed. As one example, an 11-year-old boy with a fear of loud noises was exposed to the noise of many bursting balloons in a small room (with the boy's full consent and that of his parents). He was encouraged by the thera-pist to break balloons himself, and within two ses-sions his fear of the noises had disappeared (Yule, Sacks, & Hersov, 1974). Although flooding was successful in this case, Yule and colleagues sug-gest that it should be used with caution. They suggest that long-duration sessions are essential: The therapist should first observe the onset of fear, and then continue with the procedure until a definite reduction in fear is seen. If the session is terminated too soon, the patient's phobia might actually increase. Indeed, there are a few reports of cases where patients' fears worsened after short-duration therapy sessions of this type (Staub, 1968). Despite these drawbacks, flooding

can be an effective form of treatment for pho-bias when used carefully (Zoellner, Abramowitz, Moore, & Slagle, 2009).

Other behavioral treatments also rely on prolonged stimulus exposure to eliminate fears or other undesirable responses. For example, patients with post-traumatic stress disorder (an anxiety disorder that results from a traumatic ex-perience such as a rape or a wartime experience) can be given *prolonged exposure therapy* in which they receive long-duration exposure to stimuli (either real or in their imaginations) that elicit their anxiety reactions (Hembree, Rauch, & Foa, 2003). Patients with obsessive-compulsive disor-ders (which involve repeatedly and excessively engaging in rituals such as hand-washing, check-ing to make sure doors are locked, etc.) can be treated by exposing them to the stimuli that trig-ger these reactions while preventing them from performing the ritualistic behaviors (Abramowitz & Foa, 2000). Research on these stimulus expo-sure therapies has shown that they can be effec-tive in reducing patients' fears or compulsive behaviors.

LEARNED HELPLESSNESS

Aversive stimuli can do more than produce fear and avoidance responses. Abundant research with both animals and people has shown that repeated exposure to aversive events that are un-predictable and out of the individual's control can have long-term debilitating effects. Seligman and his colleagues (Maier & Seligman, 1976; Peterson, Maier, & Seligman, 1993) have proposed that in such circumstances, both animals and people may develop the expectation that their behavior has little effect on their environment, and this expectation may generalize to a wide range of situations. Seligman calls this general expectation **learned helplessness**.

Consider the following experiment. A dog is first placed in a harness where it receives a se-ries inescapable shocks. On the next day, the dog is placed in a shuttle box where it receives escape/avoidance trials similar to those administered by Solomon and Wynne (1953): A 10-second period of darkness is followed by shock unless the dog jumps into the other compartment. But whereas the dogs in Solomon and Wynne's study learned the task within a few trials, about two thirds of the animals in Seligman's procedure never learned either to escape or avoid the shock. (In Seligman's procedure, the shock ended after 60 seconds if a dog did not respond.) For a few trials, a dog might run around a bit, but eventually the dog would simply lie down and whine when the shock came on, making no attempt to escape. Seligman concluded that in the initial training with inescapable shock, the dog developed an expectation that its behavior has no effect on the aversive consequences it experiences, and this expectation of helplessness carried over to the shuttle box.

Parallel experiments have been conducted with humans. For instance, in one study (Hiroto & Seligman, 1975) college students were first presented with a series of loud noises that they could not avoid. They were then asked to solve a series of anagrams. These students had much greater difficulty solving the problems than students who were not exposed to the unavoidable noises. A typical control participant solved all the anagrams, and got faster and faster as the trials proceeded. A typical participant in the noise group would fail on most of the problems, apparently giving up on a problem before the allotted time had expired. Seligman's explanation is the same for both the animal and human cases: Early experience with uncontrollable aversive events produces a sense of helplessness that carries over into other situations, leading to learning and performance deficits.

The appearance of learned helplessness after exposure to inescapable aversive events has been found in many different species, from rats (Enkel, Spanagel, Vollmayr, & Schneider, 2010) to cockroaches (Brown, Hughes, & Jones, 1988). In fact, research on rats by Grau and his colleagues has shown learned helplessness can be observed at the level of the spinal cord, without any influence of the brain (Crown, Ferguson, Joynes, & Grau, 2002; Grau et al., 2006). These findings suggest that learned helplessness is a very basic phenomenon of associative learning, one that can

be found in a wide range of species and even in the more primitive regions of the nervous system.

Many psychologists believe that learned helplessness can contribute to the severe and prolonged periods of depression that some people experience (e.g., Vedeniapin, Cheng, & George, 2010). As one example, Seligman (1975) described the case of a middle-aged woman whose children had gone off to college and whose husband was often away on business trips. These unpleasant events were out of the woman's control—nothing she did could bring her family back. Apparently as a result of these experiences, the woman developed a case of profound depression. She often stayed in bed most of the day, for just getting dressed seemed like a great chore. As with Seligman's dogs, the simplest of tasks became difficult for this woman. Since Seligman's initial work, hundreds of studies have been published on learned helplessness in humans, and this research has branched in many directions. Psychologists have applied the concept of learned helplessness to the problems of patients suffering from long-term illnesses (Chaney et al., 1999), to women who have been the victims of domestic violence (Walker, 2009), to the ability of the elderly to cope with their problems (Flannery, 2002), to the work efficiency and satisfaction of industrial employees (Sahoo & Tripathy, 1990), and to many other situations where people might feel that they have little control over important events in their lives.

The theory of learned helplessness has even been applied to the performance of professional football teams. What happens after a team loses a game by a lopsided score? We might expect that in the next game the team will rebound and perform better than expected, perhaps because the players work harder in preparation or because the coaching staff makes adjustments. The theory of learned helplessness makes the opposite prediction, however. A bad loss one week should lead to feelings of helplessness, and the team's performance in the next game should also be below average. Reisel and Kopelman (1995) tested these opposing predictions using 3 years' worth of data from all teams in the National Football League, and the results supported the theory of learned helplessness. They found that (1) if a team was badly beaten in one game, the team tended to perform worse than expected in the next game, and (2) this was especially true if the team faced a difficult opponent in the next game. (According to the theory, learned helplessness should indeed be most pronounced when the upcoming task appears insurmountable.)

Some researchers have used Seligman's procedures to establish learned helplessness in animals and then examine possible connections between brain chemistry and depression. Animals that are given certain pharmacological agents show less learned helplessness than control animals (Besson, Privat, Eschalier, & Fialip, 1999; Joynes & Grau, 2004). This research may provide a better understanding of depression in humans, and it may lead to better treatments for this disorder.

The work of Seligman and his colleagues has also suggested possible remedies for helplessness that do not involve drugs. One form of treatment has already been alluded to: If helpless dogs are guided across the barrier for enough trials, they will eventually start making the response on their own. In more general terms, Seligman suggests that the best treatment is to place the subject in a situation where it cannot fail, so that gradually an expectation that one's behavior has some control over the consequences that follow will develop. More interesting are studies showing that learned helplessness can be prevented in the first place by what Seligman calls *immunization.* For example, a rat might first be exposed to a situation where some response (such as turning a wheel) provides escape from shock. Thus the rat's first exposure to shock occurs in a context where it can control the shock. Then, in a second situation, inescapable shocks are presented. Finally, the rat is tested in a third situation where a new response (say, switching compartments in a shuttle box) provides escape from shock. Studies have shown that this initial experience with escapable shock blocks the onset of learned helplessness (Williams & Lierle, 1986).

As one possible implication of this finding, Seligman (1975) suggests that feelings of helplessness in a classroom environment may be prevented by making sure that a child's earliest classroom experiences are ones where the child succeeds (ones where the child demonstrates a mastery over the task at hand). McKean (1994) has made similar suggestions for helping college students who exhibit signs of helplessness in academic settings. Such students tend to view course work as uncontrollable, aversive, and inescapable. They assume that they are going to do poorly and give up easily whenever they experience difficulty with course assignments or other setbacks. To assist such students, McKean suggests that professors should make their courses as predictable and controllable as possible (e.g., by clearly listing all course requirements on the syllabus, by explaining the skills students will need to succeed in the course, and by suggesting how to develop these skills). Initial course assignments should be ones that students are likely to complete successfully, so they gain confidence that they have the ability to master the requirements of the course.

In his more recent work, Seligman (2006) has proposed that another method for combating learned helplessness and depression is to train people in **learned optimism**. The training involves a type of cognitive therapy in which people practice thinking about potentially bad situations in more positive ways. For instance, a middle-aged woman taking a college course might be disappointed with her exam grade, and think, "I am too old for this. I bet everyone else did better than I did. It was a mistake for me to return to college now." Seligman proposes that this type of helpless thinking can be changed if a person learns to recognize and dispute such negative thoughts. For instance, the woman could think, "A grade of B- is not that bad. I am working full time and did not have as much time to prepare as I would like. Now that I know what to expect, I will do better on the next exam." Seligman argues that by regularly practicing the technique of disputing one's thoughts of helplessness and dejection, a person can learn to avoid them.

PRACTICE QUIZ (1)

1. Two types of negative reinforcement are _____ and _____.
2. According to the two-factor theory of avoidance, a _____ develops to an initially neutral stimulus that precedes an aversive event.
3. Extinguishing an avoidance response by physically preventing the individual from making the response is called _____.
4. _____ are behaviors such as fleeing, freezing, or fighting that animals tend to make in dangerous situations.
5. According to Seligman, teaching people to think about potentially bad situations in more positive ways can lead to _____.

Answers

1. escape, avoidance   2. fear response   3. response blocking or flooding   4. SSDRs   5. learned optimism

Some writers have questioned the effectiveness of Seligman's techniques to teach optimism (e.g., Kelley, 2004), but results from a number of studies suggest that they can be beneficial (Gilboy, 2005; Seligman, Schulman, & Tryon, 2007). Perhaps it should not be too surprising that just as learned helplessness can occur as a result of experience with uncontrollable aversive events, there may be other learning experiences that can result in learned optimism.

PUNISHMENT

Figure 7-1 suggests that punishment has the opposite effect on behavior as positive reinforcement: Reinforcement produces an increase in behavior, and punishment produces a decrease in behavior. Whether punishment is indeed the opposite of reinforcement is an empirical question, however, and such illustrious psychologists as Thorndike and Skinner have concluded that it is not. Based on their own research, each concluded that the effects of punishment are not exactly opposite to those of reinforcement. However, their experiments are not very convincing.

For example, Skinner (1938) placed two groups of rats on variable-interval (VI) schedules of lever pressing for three sessions; then each animal had two sessions of extinction. For one group, nothing unusual happened during extinction; responding gradually decreased over the two sessions. For the second group, however, each lever press during the first 10 minutes of extinction was punished: Whenever a rat pressed the lever, the lever "slapped" upward against the rat's paws. This mild punishment was enough to reduce the number of responses during these 10 minutes to a level well below that of the first group. However, when the punishment was removed, response rates increased, and by the end of the second session, the punished animals had made just about as many responses as the unpunished animals. From these results, Skinner concluded that the effects of punishment are not permanent and that punishment produces only a "temporary suppression" of responding.

The problem with Skinner's conclusion is that although the effects of punishment were temporary in his experiment, so was the punishment itself. We know that the effects of positive reinforcement are also "temporary" in the sense that operant responses will extinguish after the reinforcer is removed. Since Skinner's early experiment, many studies have addressed the question of whether punishment is the opposite of reinforcement in its effects on behavior. The section Is Punishment the Opposite of Reinforcement? describes a few of these studies.

Is Punishment the Opposite of Reinforcement?

We can attempt to answer this question by examining the two words used by Skinner: *temporary* and *suppression*. If, unlike in Skinner's experiment, the punishment contingency is permanent, is the decrease in behavior still temporary? Sometimes it can be: Some studies have shown that subjects may habituate to a relatively mild punisher. In an experiment by Azrin (1960), pigeons were responding steadily for food on a VI schedule, and then punishment was introduced—each response produced a mild shock. Response rates decreased immediately, but over the course of several sessions, they returned to their preshock levels. Despite such results, there is no doubt that suitably intense punishment can produce a long-term decrease or disappearance of the punished behavior. When Azrin used more intense shocks, there was little or no recovery in responding over the course of the experiment.

Although Skinner did not define the term *suppression,* later writers took it to mean a general decrease in behavior that is not limited to the particular behavior that is being punished. Does the use of punishment lead to a general reduction in all behavior, or does only the punished behavior decrease? An experiment by Schuster and Rachlin (1968) investigated this question. Pigeons could sometimes peck at the left key in a Skinner box, and at other times they could peck at the right key. Both keys offered identical VI schedules of food reinforcement, but then different schedules of shock were introduced on the two keys. When the left key was lit (signaling that the VI schedule was available on this key), some of the pigeon's key pecks were followed by shock. However, when the right key was lit, shocks were presented regardless of whether the pigeon pecked at the key. Under these conditions, responding on the left key decreased markedly, but there was little change in response rate on the right key.

Studies like this have firmly established the fact that punishment does more than simply cause a general decrease in activity. When a particular behavior is punished, that behavior will exhibit a large decrease in frequency while other, unpunished behaviors usually show no substantial change in frequency. To summarize, contrary to the predictions of Thorndike and Skinner, research results suggest that the effects of punishment are directly opposite to those of reinforcement: Reinforcement produces an increase in whatever specific behavior is followed by the hedonically positive stimulus, and punishment produces a decrease in the specific behavior that is followed by the aversive stimulus. In both cases, we can expect these changes in behavior to persist

as long as the reinforcement or punishment contingency remains in effect.

Factors Influencing the Effectiveness of Punishment

We now know a good deal more about punishment besides the fact that its effects can be permanent and that the response-punisher contingency is important. Researchers have examined a number of variables that determine what effects a punishment contingency will have. Several decades ago, Azrin and Holz (1966) reviewed some of these variables, and to their credit, all of their major points appear as valid now as when their findings were published. Several of their points are described in this section.

MANNER OF INTRODUCTION. If one's goal is to obtain a large, permanent decrease in some behavior, then Azrin and Holz (1966) recommended that the punisher be immediately introduced at its full intensity. We have already seen that subjects can habituate to a mild punisher, and several studies have shown that this habituation seems to generalize to higher intensities of punishment. The end result is that a given intensity of punishment may produce a complete cessation of behavior if introduced suddenly, but it may have little or no effect on behavior if it is gradually approached through a series of successive approximations. Azrin, Holz, and Hake (1963) reported that a shock of 80 volts following each response was sufficient to produce a complete suppression of pigeons' key-peck responses if the 80-volt intensity was used from the outset. However, if the punishment began at lower intensities and then slowly increased, the pigeons would continue to respond even when the intensity was raised to as much as 130 volts. Since the goal when using punishment is to eliminate an undesirable behavior, not to shape a tolerance of the aversive stimulus, the punisher should be at its maximum intensity the first time it is presented.

IMMEDIACY OF PUNISHMENT. Just as the most effective reinforcer is one that is delivered immediately after the operant response, a punisher that immediately follows a response is most effective in decreasing the frequency of the response. Baron, Kaufman, and Fazzini (1969) studied the behavior of rats that were responding on a Sidman avoidance task. Some of the rats' avoidance responses were punished with shock, but in different conditions the delay between a response and the punishment was varied between 0 and 60 seconds. There was an orderly relationship between punishment delay and response rate: The more immediate the punishment, the greater the decrease in responding.

The importance of delivering punishment immediately may explain why many common forms of punishment are ineffective. For example, the mother who tries to decrease a child's misbehavior with the warning, "Just wait until your father gets home," is describing a very long delay between a behavior and its punishment. It would not be surprising if this contingency had little effect on the child's behavior. The same principle applies in the classroom where a scolding from the teacher is most effective if the teacher scolds a child immediately after the child has misbehaved, not after some time has passed (Abramowitz & O'Leary, 1990). It has also been suggested that one reason some people engage in crimes even though they are likely to get caught eventually is that they receive the rewards immediately but the punishment is delayed. A large-scale study of adolescents in the United States concluded that those who were involved in crimes such as burglary or car theft tended to be less sensitive to delayed consequences than those who never engaged in these criminal activities (Nagin & Pogarsky, 2004).

SCHEDULE OF PUNISHMENT. Like positive reinforcers, punishers need not be delivered after every occurrence of a behavior. Azrin and Holz concluded, however, that the most effective way to eliminate a behavior is to punish every response rather than to use some intermittent schedule of punishment. In one experiment, rats pressed levers to earn food, but some lever presses were punished with a brief shock. The shocks were delivered on fixed-ratio (FR) schedules ranging from FR 1 (every response followed by shock) to FR 1,000 (every thousandth response followed by shock). As you might expect, the smaller FR punishment schedules produced the greater decreases in responding (Azrin, Holz, & Hake, 1963). The same general rule applies to human behavior: Using an intermittent schedule of punishment may sometimes be enough to eliminate an unwanted behavior, but the most powerful way to reduce behavior is to punish every occurrence (Cipani, Brendlinger, McDowell, & Usher, 1991; Hare, 2006).

The schedule of punishment can affect the patterning of responses over time as well as the overall response rate. When Azrin (1956) superimposed a fixed-interval (FI) 60-second schedule of punishment on a VI 3-minute schedule of food reinforcement, he found that pigeons' response rates declined toward zero as the end of each 60-second interval approached. In other words, the effect of the FI schedule of punishment (a decelerating pattern of responding) was the opposite of that typically found with FI schedules of reinforcement (an accelerating pattern of responding). In a similar fashion, Hendry and Van-Toller (1964) punished rats' lever presses on an FR 20 schedule and found that response rates decreased as the 20th response was approached. Response rates increased suddenly after each shock was delivered. This pattern is also the opposite of that produced by FR reinforcement schedules, in which there is a pause after each reinforcer is delivered. In other research, Galbicka and his colleagues showed that certain lengths of interresponse times (IRTs) could be decreased through punishment: When long IRTs were punished, monkeys produced fewer long IRTs and more short IRTs (Galbicka & Branch, 1981; Galbicka & Platt, 1984). This result parallels the studies showing that certain durations of IRTs can be increased through selective reinforcement (Chapter 6).

These and other studies on schedules of punishment bolster the argument that punishment is the opposite of reinforcement in its effects on behavior: Where a particular reinforcement schedule produces an accelerating response pattern, the same schedule of punishment produces a decelerating pattern. Where reinforcement produces a pause-then-respond pattern, punishment produces a respond-then-pause pattern. Where reinforcement increases IRTs of certain sizes, punishment decreases them.

MOTIVATION TO RESPOND. Azrin and Holz noted that the effectiveness of a punishment procedure is inversely related to the intensity of the subject's motivation to respond. Azrin, Holz, and Hake (1963) demonstrated this point quite clearly by observing the effects of punishment on pigeons' food-reinforced responses when the birds were maintained at different levels of food deprivation. Punishment had little effect on response rates when the pigeons were very hungry, but when these animals were only slightly food deprived, the same intensity of punishment produced a complete cessation of responding. This finding is not surprising, but it does emphasize a strategy for increasing the effectiveness of a punishment procedure without increasing the amount of punishment: Attempt to discover what reinforcer is maintaining the behavior, and decrease the value of that reinforcer. Thus, if a mother believes that her young child engages in destructive behaviors as a way of getting the mother's attention, she can (1) punish the undesired behaviors and simultaneously (2) give the child more attention before the youngster resorts to the undesirable behaviors. A related strategy, as discussed next, is to deliver the same reinforcer for a different, more desirable response.

REINFORCEMENT OF ALTERNATIVE BEHAVIORS. Based on their research with animals, Azrin and Holz concluded that punishment is much more effective when the individual is provided with an alternative way to obtain the reinforcer. For instance, it is much easier to use punishment to stop a pigeon from pecking at a response key that delivers food if another key is available that also produces food (without punishment). For this reason, when behavior therapists decide that it is necessary to use punishment to eliminate some unwanted behavior

(e.g., fighting among children), they almost always pair this punishment with reinforcement for an alternative behavior that is incompatible with the unwanted behavior (e.g., cooperative play).

One study with four children who engaged in frequent self-injurious behaviors (hitting themselves, head banging) demonstrated that sometimes the mere availability of an alternative source of reinforcement can increase the effectiveness of a punishment procedure (Thompson, Iwata, Conners, & Roscoe, 1999). Before treatment began, a suitable reinforcer was found for each child, such as a toy, a game, or a string of beads. During treatment, every instance of a self-injurious behavior was followed by mild punishment (such as brief physical restraint, or a reprimand—"Don't do that!"). On some days, the alternative reinforcer preferred by each child was available, whereas on other days the alternative reinforcer was not available. Figure 7-3 shows that for each child, the punishment was more

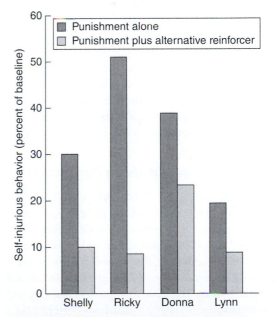

FIGURE 7-3 Frequency of self-injurious behavior (plotted as a percentage of the frequency before treatment began) is shown for four children under conditions with punishment alone and with punishment plus the availability of an alternative reinforcer. (Based on Thompson et al., 1999)

effective in reducing self-injurious behavior when the alternative reinforcer was available.

PUNISHMENT AS A DISCRIMINATIVE STIMULUS. Besides having aversive properties, a punisher can also sometimes function as a discriminative stimulus; that is, a signal predicting the availability of other stimuli, either pleasant or unpleasant. Imagine an experiment in which a pigeon's responses go unpunished during some portions of the session but are followed by shock during other parts of the session. Each time the shock begins, the pigeon's response rate increases! This behavior seems paradoxical until we learn that the pigeon can obtain food only during those periods when its responses are punished; an extinction schedule is in effect during the periods when responses are not shocked (Holz & Azrin, 1961). In other words, the shocks following responses served as discriminative stimuli for the availability of food reinforcement, for they were the only stimuli that differentiated between the periods of reinforcement and extinction. Azrin and Holz suggested that similar explanations may account for some instances of self-injurious behaviors that appear equally paradoxical at first glance. Because self-injurious behaviors often bring to the individual the reinforcers of sympathy and attention, the aversive aspects of this type of behavior (pain) may serve as discriminative stimuli that reinforcement is imminent.

Disadvantages of Using Punishment

Although Azrin and Holz (1966) concluded that punishment can be a method of behavior change that is at least as effective as reinforcement, they warned that it can produce a number of undesirable side effects. First, they noted that punishment can elicit several emotional effects, such as fear and anger, that are generally disruptive of learning and performance. A study on guard dogs that had been trained through the use of a shock collar found that these dogs exhibited signs of fear and stress whenever their owner was present, even when they were not in the training situation (Schilder & van der Borg, 2004). Balaban, Rhodes, and Neuringer

(1990) found that college students performing a memory task worked more slowly and made more mistakes when each mistake was punished by a shock than when each mistake was simply signaled by a tone. Therefore, if the teacher's goal is to reduce mistakes and increase correct responses, the strategy of punishing mistakes can backfire.

Second, punishment can sometimes lead to a general suppression of all behaviors, not only the behavior being punished. Imagine that a child in a classroom raised his hand, asked a question, and the teacher replied, "Well, that's a very stupid question." The teacher's remark might be intended to try to reduce the number of stupid questions that children ask, but the likely result would be a decrease in all questions, good or bad, both from that child and from everyone else in the class.

A third disadvantage is that in real-world situations the use of punishment demands the continual monitoring of the individual's behavior. In contrast, use of reinforcement does not necessarily demand such monitoring, because it is in the individual's interest to point out instances of a behavior that is followed by a reinforcer. If a child receives a reinforcer for cleaning up her room, she will probably make sure her parents see the room after it is cleaned. On the other hand, if the child is punished for a messy room, she is unlikely to call her parents to see the messy room so that she can be punished.

Along the same lines, a practical problem with the use of punishment is that individuals may try to circumvent the rules or escape from the situation entirely. Azrin and Holz (1966) described the behavior of a clever rat that was scheduled to receive shocks for some of its lever presses while working for food reinforcement. The rat learned to avoid the shocks by lying on its back while pressing the lever, thereby using its fur as insulation from the shocks delivered via the metal floor of the chamber. We might expect people to be even more ingenious in their tricks to circumvent a punishment contingency. If punishment is a teacher's primary method of behavioral control, a child may try to hide evidence of misbehavior. In addition, the child may attempt to escape from the situation by feigning sickness or by playing hooky.

Another problem with using punishment is that it can lead to aggression against either the punisher or whoever happens to be around. The constant risk of bodily harm faced by prison guards (and by prisoners) attests to this fact. Aggression as a response to aversive stimulation is not unique to humans. Ulrich and Azrin (1962) reported a study in which two rats were placed in an experimental chamber. The animals behaved peaceably until they began to receive shocks, at which point they began to fight. Similar results have been obtained with pigeons, mice, hamsters, cats, and monkeys.

A final problem with using punishment (one not mentioned by Azrin and Holz) is that in institutional settings, the people who must actually implement a behavior modification program may be reluctant to use punishment. Various studies have examined the attitudes of personnel who work with institutionalized patients, such as individuals with a developmental handicap. The staff in such institutions preferred other techniques for changing behavior, such as instruction, modeling, and reinforcement, over punishment (Davis & Russell, 1990). Perhaps these individuals have learned, through their daily work experiences, about some of the disadvantages of punishment described in the preceding paragraphs.

Given the numerous disadvantages of punishment, Azrin and Holz suggested that it should be used reluctantly and with great care. A final argument against using punishment is an ethical one. If an individual's behavior can be changed in the desired way with either reinforcement or punishment, why should the more unpleasant procedure of punishment be used? Unfortunately, there are cases in which reinforcement is ineffective, and in these cases punishment is sometimes used as a last resort. Some people strongly believe that aversive techniques should never be used as a means of controlling another person's behavior. Perhaps they are right, but Azrin and Holz pointed out that punishment will always be a part of our environment. It might be possible to legislate punishment out of existence in institutions such as prisons, schools, and psychiatric hospitals. It would be much more difficult, however, to eliminate punishment in everyday interpersonal interactions (between parent and child, between spouses, etc.). Finally, the physical environment is full of potential punishers that are impossible to eliminate. Just think of the possible punishing consequences that might follow the wrong behavior while one is driving a car, walking through a forest, swimming, skiing, cooking, or performing almost any behavior. As Vollmer (2002, p. 469) put it, "Punishment happens." Since punishment cannot be eliminated from our environment, it is important for behavioral psychologists to continue to study this phenomenon in order to increase our understanding of how it influences behavior.

In a review of the use of punishment in treating behavior disorders, Lerman and Vorndran (2002) concluded that many questions about the effective use of punishment have never been adequately studied. There is not much research on the long-term effects of punishment, on how punishing a behavior in one situation may produce generalization to other situations, or on how to minimize the disadvantages of punishment in applied settings. Additional research should help to find better ways to use punishment and avoid its undesirable side effects. For example, we have seen that punishment can be quite ineffective if it is delayed, but sometimes it is not possible for a teacher or caregiver to punish a bad behavior immediately. However, there may be ways to "bridge the gap" between an unwanted behavior and punishment and still maintain the punisher's effectiveness. Working with children who were developmentally disabled, Rolider and Van Houten (1985) found that delayed punishment could be effective if they used a tape recorder to replay the sounds of a child's disruptive behavior from earlier in the day, and then deliver the punisher (physical restraint or scolding). This is just one example of a creative solution to one of the problems of using punishment, and others will surely be discovered as research in this area continues.

Negative Punishment

Cell 4 in Figure 7-1 represents the procedure of negative punishment, or omission, in which some stimulus is removed if a response occurs, resulting in a decrease in responding. The possibility of losing a reinforcer can have strong effects on behavior. In one study, college students played a game in which they could win or lose money by clicking on moving targets on a computer screen. Whenever money could be lost by choosing a particular target, the students showed a strong tendency to avoid that target. Based on a quantitative analysis of the students' choices, the researchers estimated that the punishing effect of losing money was about three times as powerful as the reinforcing effect of winning the same amount of money (Rasmussen & Newland, 2008). In another study, college students earned money by pressing buttons on a response panel. The researchers found that, just as with positive punishment, the contingency between responding and money loss was critical. The students' response rates did not change much if the payoffs were simply delivered at a slower rate, but their response rates decreased substantially if a response occasionally led to the loss of some of the money they had already earned (Pietras, Brandt, & Searcy, 2010).

As with positive punishment, omission procedures are most effective if the omission occurs immediately after the undesired behavior, every time the behavior occurs. In one case, therapists used time-outs to discourage an adult with mental retardation from putting his hands in his mouth (which caused his hands to become red and swollen). Time-outs reduced hand-mouthing action to near-zero levels if they occurred on a schedule of continuous punishment, but the time-outs had much less effect if they were delivered on FI schedules (Lerman, Iwata, Shore, & DeLeon, 1997). Thus, with both positive and negative punishment, immediacy and consistency are important. Because negative punishment is a means of reducing behavior without using an aversive stimulus, it has become a popular tool in behavior modification, as discussed in the Behavior Decelerators in Behavior Therapy section.

BEHAVIOR DECELERATORS IN BEHAVIOR THERAPY

The term **behavior decelerator** is sometimes used to refer to any technique that can lead to a slowing, reduction, or elimination of unwanted behaviors. Punishment and omission are two of the most obvious methods for reducing undesired behaviors, but they are by no means the only ones. Behavior therapists have cataloged a variety of other useful behavior-deceleration techniques, and we will examine some of the most common ones.

Positive Punishment

Wherever possible, behavior therapists avoid using punishment because the comfort and happiness of the patient is one of their major concerns. However, if a behavior is dangerous or otherwise undesirable, and if other techniques are impractical or unsuccessful, the use of punishment may be deemed preferable to doing nothing at all. This section describes some representative situations in which behaviors have been reduced or eliminated with punishment. As will be seen, the aversive stimuli used are often quite mild.

PUNISHMENT OF "VOLUNTARY" BEHAVIORS. One nonphysical form of punishment that is frequently used by parents and teachers is scolding and reprimanding a child for bad behavior. This tactic can certainly influence a child's behavior, but not always in the way the adult wants. The problem is that a reprimand is a form of attention, and we have already seen that attention can be a powerful reinforcer. Furthermore, a child who is scolded or reprimanded frequently also receives attention from siblings or classmates, and this attention from peers may serve as further reinforcement for the undesired behavior. O'Leary, Kaufman, Kass, and Drabman (1970) found that the manner in which a reprimand is given is a major factor determining its effectiveness. Most teachers use loud or public reprimands that are heard not only by the child involved but by all others in the classroom. However, when second-grade teachers were instructed to use "soft" or private reprimands wherever possible (i.e., to walk up to the child and speak quietly, so that no other children could hear), they observed a 50% decrease in disruptive behavior.

Stronger forms of punishment are sometimes necessary when a child's behavior is a more serious problem than a mere classroom disturbance. For example, some children with autism or developmental disabilities engage in self-injurious behaviors such as repeatedly slapping themselves in the face, biting deep into their skin, or banging their heads against any solid object. Because of the risk of severe injury, these children are sometimes kept in physical restraints around the clock, except when a therapist is in the immediate vicinity. Prochaska, Smith, Marzilli, Colby, and Donovan (1974) described the treatment of one 9-year-old girl named Sharon. She would hit her nose and chin with her fist at a rate of about 200 blows per hour if she was not restrained. Behavior therapists first tried to decrease her head banging with negative punishment and with positive reinforcement for other behaviors, but with Sharon, these procedures were ineffective. They then began to use a shock to her leg as a punisher for head banging, and her behavior was continuously monitored at school and at home. Under these conditions, Sharon's head banging dropped to zero within a week. The disappearance of head banging generalized to times when the shock generator was removed, and eventually the punishment procedures were terminated with no return of the behavior. There were also improvements in other behaviors: Sharon's crying spells (previously frequent) ceased, so she could now go with her parents to public places such as shopping malls and restaurants.

The use of shock as a punisher with children is a controversial matter, but to be fair, the aversive features of this procedure must be weighed against the negative consequences of failing to implement the punishment procedure. In Sharon's case, the pain of several dozen half-second shocks seems small when compared to the alternative: a life of self-injury, physical restraint, and inability to play with peers or go out in public.

One promising development in the treatment of self-injurious behaviors is the finding that sometimes punishers much milder than electric shock can be effective. For example, Fehr and Beckwith (1989) found that head hitting by a 10-year-old boy with a handicap could be reduced by spraying a water mist in the child's face. This treatment was especially effective when used in combination with reinforcement for other, better behavior. Water mist has also been successfully used to reduce aggression and other unwanted behaviors (Matson & Duncan, 1997).

PUNISHMENT OF "INVOLUNTARY" BEHAVIORS. You may be surprised to learn that so-called involuntary or reflexive behaviors, which seem to occur automatically in response to some stimulus, can be reduced through punishment. Heller and Strang (1973) described the use of a mild punisher to reduce the frequency of bruxism in a 24-year-old man. Bruxism is the gnashing and grinding of one's teeth while asleep, a problem found in about 5% of college students. This behavior sometimes results in serious tooth damage. To measure the rate of bruxism automatically, Heller and Strang used a voice-operated relay that was activated by the sound of the teeth grinding. The client wore an earplug while he slept, and each instance of bruxism recorded by the voice-operated relay was followed immediately by a 3-second burst of noise in the client's ear. As soon as this punishment contingency was introduced, the rate of bruxism decreased from a baseline rate of about 100 occurrences per hour to about 30 per hour. The remaining instances of bruxism were often too soft to trigger the equipment and therefore went unpunished. It is interesting to note that although the client was asleep when the bruxism occurred, the character of this behavior changed in a way that partially circumvented the punishment contingency (it became quieter). Presumably, the rate of bruxism would have decreased further if more sensitive recording equipment had been used.

Aversive stimuli have also been used to eliminate other types of involuntary behaviors, such as chronic coughing or sneezing, that are not due to any obvious medical problem (Creer, Chai, & Hoffman, 1977; Kushner, 1968). Punishment techniques have been used to treat involuntary muscle spasms (Sachs & Mayhall, 1971), frequent vomiting (Cunningham & Linscheid, 1976), gagging (Glasscock, Friman, O'Brien, & Christopherson, 1986), and hallucinations (Bucher & Fabricatore, 1970). Of course, we should not expect a punishment contingency to eliminate a symptom caused by some physical disorder (e.g., coughing due to a respiratory illness). However, if physicians have determined that no medical problem is responsible for a persistent behavioral symptom, punishment may be an effective (albeit unpleasant) treatment.

Negative Punishment: Response Cost and Time-Out

It is easy to incorporate a negative punishment contingency in any token system: Whereas tokens can be earned by performing desirable behaviors, some tokens are lost if the individual performs an undesirable behavior. The loss of tokens, money, or other conditioned reinforcers following the occurrence of undesirable behaviors is called **response cost.** Token systems that include a response-cost arrangement have been used with children, prison inmates, and patients in mental institutions. E. L. Phillips (1968) described how response cost was used as part of a token system for boys, in their early teens or younger, who had committed minor violations of the law and were sent by authorities to live together in a home supervised by two "house parents." Each boy was on a token system under which he could earn points through such behaviors as doing homework, getting good grades, keeping his room clean, and doing household chores. The points could be used to purchase snacks or an allowance, or for privileges such as watching television, staying up late, or going into town. Behaviors that lost points were arguing or fighting, disobeying the house parents, displaying poor manners, or being late. The response-cost contingency produced substantial improvements in the boys' behaviors. As might be expected, the loss of points affected only those behaviors that were included under the rules. For instance, when fines were established for being late from school, the boys became prompt in returning home from school, but not in returning from errands.

Probably the most common form of negative punishment is the **time-out**, in which one or more desirable stimuli are temporarily removed if the individual performs some unwanted behavior. In one case study, time-out was combined with reinforcement for alternative behaviors to eliminate the hoarding behavior of a patient in a psychiatric hospital (Lane, Wesolowski, & Burke, 1989). This case study illustrates what researchers call an **ABAB design**. Each "A" phase is a baseline phase in which the patient's behavior is recorded, but no treatment is given. Each "B" phase is a treatment phase. Stan was an adult with a brain injury, and he frequently hoarded such items as cigarette butts, pieces of dust and paper, food, and small stones by hiding them in his pockets, socks, or underwear. In the initial 5-day baseline phase, the researchers observed an average of about 10 hoarding episodes per day. This was followed by a treatment phase (days 6 through 15) in which Stan was rewarded for two alternative behaviors—collecting baseball cards and picking up trash and throwing it away properly. During this phase, any episodes of hoarding were punished with a time-out period in which Stan was taken to a quiet area for 10 seconds. The number of hoarding episodes decreased during this treatment phase. In the second baseline phase, the treatment was discontinued; during these 4 days, Stan's hoarding behavior increased. Finally, in the second treatment phase, the time-outs and reinforcement for alternative behaviors resumed, and Stan's hoarding gradually declined and eventually stopped completely. In a follow-up 1 year later, no hoarding was observed. This ABAB design demonstrated the effectiveness of the treatment procedures, because Stan's hoarding occurred frequently in the two baseline phases and decreased dramatically in the two treatment phases.

Time-outs are often used with children, as when a parent tells a child to go to his or her room for misbehaving. In classroom situations, time-outs in which a child is sent to an isolated room can reduce aggressive or disruptive behaviors. Time-outs can also be effective if teachers simply remove a child from some ongoing activity. For example, because fourth-grade children in one elementary school were constantly unruly and disruptive during gym class, their teachers set up a time-out contingency. Any child who behaved in a disruptive way was immediately told to stop playing and to go sit on the side of the room, where he or she had to remain until all the sand had flowed through a large hourglass (which took about 3 minutes). Children who repeatedly misbehaved also lost free play time and other desirable activities (a response-cost contingency). This omission procedure was very effective, and disruptive behavior during gym class soon dropped by 95% (White & Bailey, 1990).

In a few cases, time-out procedures used in schools have been challenged in court: Parents claim that schools do not have the right to exclude their children from academic activities, even if the children are being disruptive. Yell (1994) reviewed these cases and reported that in every instance the courts ruled that time-out can be used in classrooms, provided it is used appropriately. Nevertheless, Yell recommends that educators be aware of state and local policies about the use of time-out, and he suggests a number of guidelines that should be followed when using this procedure. Although these procedures may be criticized by some, both time-out and response cost have become increasingly popular with teachers and behavior therapists, because they are effective ways to reduce unwanted behaviors without presenting any aversive stimulus.

Other Techniques for Behavior Deceleration

OVERCORRECTION. In some cases, if an individual performs an undesired behavior, the parent, therapist, or teacher requires several repetitions of an alternate, more desirable behavior. This technique is called **overcorrection**, and it often involves two elements: restitution (making up for the wrongdoing) and positive practice (practicing a better behavior). The corrective behavior is usually designed to require more time and effort than the original bad behavior. For example, Adams and Kelley (1992) taught parents how to use an overcorrection procedure to reduce aggression against siblings. After an instance of physical or verbal aggression against a sibling, restitution might consist of an apology, and the positive practice might involve sharing a toy, touching the sibling gently, or saying something nice. This positive practice was repeated several times. If the child did not practice these behaviors appropriately, the practice trials started over from

the beginning. This procedure produced a significant reduction in aggression between siblings.

Overcorrection has frequently been used with individuals who have mental disabilities to reduce aggression and other undesirable behaviors. For example, Sisson, Hersen, and Van Hasselt (1993) used overcorrection as part of a treatment package to teach adolescents with profound retardation to package items and sort them by zip code. Maladaptive behaviors included stereotyped motions such as flapping hands, rocking back and forth, and twirling and flipping the items. After each occurrence of such a behavior, the therapist guided the patient through three repetitions of the correct sequence of behaviors.

Overcorrection meets the technical definition of a punishment procedure, because a sequence of events (the correction procedure) is contingent on the occurrence of an undesired behavior, and the behavior decreases as a result. A difference from other punishment techniques, however, is that during the corrective exercises, the learner is given repeated practice performing a more desirable behavior. This may be the most beneficial component of the overcorrection procedure, because providing the learner with a more desirable alternative behavior is an important ingredient in many behavior reduction treatments.

EXTINCTION. If an undesired behavior occurs because it is followed by some positive reinforcer, and if it is possible to remove that reinforcer, the behavior should eventually disappear through simple extinction. One of the most common reinforcers to maintain unwanted behaviors is attention. In the home, the classroom, or the psychiatric hospital, disruptive or maladaptive behavior may occur because of the attention it attracts from parents, peers, teachers, or hospital staff. These behaviors will sometimes disappear if they are ignored by those who previously provided their attention. For example, a woman had a skin rash that did not go away because she continually scratched herself in the infected areas. The therapist suspected that this scratching behavior was maintained by the attention the woman received concerning her rash from her family and fiancé (who applied skin cream to the rash for her). The therapist asked her family and fiancé to avoid all discussion of the rash and not to help her treat it. The scratching behavior soon extinguished and the rash disappeared (Walton, 1960).

Ducharme and Van Houten (1994) noted that using extinction as a behavior decelerator is not free of problems. Extinction is sometimes slow, especially if the unwanted behavior has been intermittently reinforced in the past. In addition, the unwanted behaviors sometimes increase rather than decrease at the beginning of the extinction process. (Parents who decide to ignore tantrums in an effort to extinguish them may initially witness one of the worst tantrums they have ever seen.) As with any extinguished behavior, episodes of spontaneous recovery may occur. Nevertheless, when used properly, extinction can be a very useful method of eliminating unwanted behaviors. One of the most effective ways to use extinction is to combine it with the reinforcement of other, more desirable behaviors.

ESCAPE EXTINCTION.   This procedure can be used when an undesired behavior is maintained by escape from some situation the individual does not like. For instance, some children with developmental disabilities exhibit food refusal: They will not eat, nor will they swallow food put in their mouths. Of course, the longer this behavior continues, the greater the risks to the child's health. Why this behavior occurs is not clear, but researchers have observed that food refusal often leads to escape from the situation—the caregiver does not force the child to eat, and the attempt to feed the child eventually ends. In escape extinction, the caregiver does not allow the child to escape from the situation until the child eats. This may involve keeping a spoonful of food in the child's mouth until the child swallows the food. Although some might question such a forceful technique, keep in mind how serious a problem refusing to eat can be. Studies have found that this method is very effective in reducing food refusal behaviors (Piazza, Patel, Gulotta, Sevin, & Layer, 2003; Tarbox, Schiff, & Najdowski, 2010).

As another example, therapists at one institution found that a few children with developmental disabilities would engage in self-injurious behavior (head banging, hand biting, etc.) whenever they were instructed to work on educational tasks, and by doing so they escaped from their lessons. The therapists therefore began an extinction procedure in which the child's tutor would ignore the self-injurious behavior, tell the child to continue with the lesson, and manually guide the child through the task if necessary. In this way, the reinforcer (escape from the lesson) was eliminated and episodes of self-injurious behavior decreased dramatically (Pace, Iwata, Cowdery, Andree, & McIntyre, 1993).

RESPONSE BLOCKING.   For behaviors that are too dangerous or destructive to wait for extinction to occur, an alternative is response blocking, which is physically restraining the individual to prevent the inappropriate behavior. Most parents of young children probably use response blocking quite often to prevent their youngsters from doing something that would be harmful to themselves or to others. Behavior therapists have used response blocking to reduce or eliminate such behaviors as self-injury, aggression, and destruction of property by children or adults with mental retardation (Fisher, Lindauer, Alterson, & Thompson, 1998; Smith, Russo, & Le, 1999).

Response blocking can have both short-term and long-term benefits. First, by preventing the unwanted behavior, immediate damage or injury can be avoided. Second, as the individual learns that the behavior will be blocked, attempts to initiate this behavior usually decline. For example, to prevent a girl with mental retardation from poking her fingers in her eyes, Lalli, Livezey, and Kates (1996) had the girl wear safety goggles. Unlike cases of response blocking in which the therapist manually restrains the patient, this use of goggles had the advantage of blocking the unwanted behaviors even when the girl was alone. After she stopped trying to poke at her eyes, the goggles were gradually replaced with her normal eyeglasses, and her eye-poking behavior did not reappear.

DIFFERENTIAL REINFORCEMENT OF ALTERNATIVE BEHAVIOR.   A classic study by Ayllon and Haughton (1964) offers a good illustration of how extinction of inappropriate behaviors can be combined with reinforcement of more appropriate behaviors—a procedure known as **differential reinforcement of alternative behavior (DRA)**. Ayllon and Haughton worked with patients in a psychiatric hospital who engaged in psychotic or delusional speech. They found that this inappropriate speech was often reinforced by the psychiatric nurses through their attention, sympathy, and conversation. Ayllon and Haughton conducted a two-part study. In the first part, the nurses were explicitly instructed to reinforce psychotic speech with attention and tangible items (gum, candy, etc.). Psychotic speech increased steadily during this part of the study. In the second phase, the nurses were told to ignore psychotic speech, but to reinforce normal speech (e.g., conversations about the weather, ward activities, or other everyday topics). This study demonstrated both the power of attention as a reinforcer and how attention can be withheld from inappropriate behaviors and delivered for more desirable alternative behaviors.

This chapter has already mentioned several other cases in which reinforcement of alternative behaviors has been successfully combined with other behavior-deceleration techniques. In modern behavior therapy, DRA is a common part of treatment packages for behavior reduction. Petscher, Rey, and Bailey (2009) reviewed over 100 studies in which DRA was used with successful results. It has been used effectively for such problems as food refusal, aggression, disruptive classroom behavior (LeGray, Dufrene, Sterling-Turner, Olmi, & Bellone, 2010) and self-injurious behavior (Shimoyama & Sonoyama, 2010). The logic is that most behavior-reduction techniques teach a person *what not to do,* but they do not teach the patient *what to do.* DRA remedies this deficiency, and it provides more acceptable behaviors to fill the "behavioral vacuum" that is created when one behavior is reduced.

STIMULUS SATIATION. If it is not feasible to remove the reinforcer that is maintaining an undesired behavior, it is sometimes possible to present so much of the reinforcer that it loses its effectiveness due to **stimulus satiation**. Ayllon (1963) described a female psychiatric patient who hoarded towels in her room. Despite the nurses' efforts to remove them, she usually had more than 20 towels

in the room. A program of stimulus satiation was begun in which the nurses brought her many towels each day. At first, the woman seemed to enjoy touching, folding, and stacking them, but soon she started to complain that she had enough and that the towels were in her way. Once the number of towels in her room reached about 600, she started removing them on her own. The nurses then stopped bringing her towels, and afterward, no further instances of hoarding were observed.

One unusual example of stimulus satiation involved no physical objects at all. A psychiatric patient who complained of hearing voices was given ample time to listen to these voices. For 85 half-hour sessions, the patient was instructed to sit in a quiet place and record when the voices were heard, what they said, and how demanding the tone of voice was. By the end of these sessions, the rate of these hallucinations was close to zero (Glaister, 1985). This version of stimulus satiation has also been used to treat obsessive thoughts.

PRACTICE QUIZ (2)

1. In Skinner's experiment, the effects of punishment were ——————, but so was the punishment itself.
2. To minimize the chance that the learner will habituate to a punishing stimulus, it should be introduced ——————.
3. In terms of timing, the most effective punisher is one that is delivered ——————.
4. In practice, it is always best to couple punishment of an undesired behavior with reinforcement of ——————.
5. In an ABAB design, each "A" represents a —————— period, and each "B" represents a —————— period.
6. If an undesired behavior is being maintained by the attention it receives, it can usually be decreased by using ——————.

Answers

1. temporary 2. at full intensity 3. immediately
4. an alternative behavior, or a more desirable behavior
5. baseline, treatment 6. extinction

Summary

In negative reinforcement, an aversive stimulus is removed or eliminated if a response occurs. Two variations of negative reinforcement are escape and avoidance. The two-factor theory of avoidance states that avoidance involves (1) learning to fear a previously neutral stimulus and (2) responding to escape from this stimulus. A number of studies have supported the two-factor theory, but some findings pose problems for the theory: Well-practiced subjects continue to make avoidance responses while showing no measurable signs of fear, and extinction of avoidance responses is very slow.

The one-factor theory of avoidance states that removing a fear-provoking CS is not necessary for avoidance responding, and that avoidance of the aversive event is in itself the reinforcer. Studies supporting one-factor theory have shown that animals can learn avoidance responses when there is no CS to signal an upcoming shock. The cognitive theory of avoidance states that subjects learn to expect that (1) if they respond, no aversive event will occur and (2) if they do not respond, an aversive event will occur. To teach a subject that the second expectation is no longer correct, response blocking (or flooding) can be used.

Seligman showed that if animals are presented with aversive stimuli that they cannot avoid, they may develop learned helplessness. He suggested that unavoidable aversive events can lead to helplessness and depression in people, and this theory has been applied to many aspects of human behavior.

In punishment, an aversive stimulus is presented if a response occurs, and the response is weakened. Many factors influence the effectiveness of punishment, including its intensity, immediacy, and schedule of presentation, and the availability of alternative behaviors. There are disadvantages to using punishment: It requires continual monitoring of the subject, and it can lead to undesirable side effects, such as aggression, a decrease in other behaviors, or attempts to escape from the situation.

Behavior therapists usually do not use punishment unless there is no feasible alternative; nevertheless, punishment can be an effective way of reducing a variety of unwanted behaviors (e.g., aggression, classroom misbehavior, and involuntary behaviors such as bruxism and chronic coughing). Other methods for reducing unwanted behaviors include response cost, time-out, overcorrection, extinction, escape extinction, response blocking, reinforcement of alternative behavior, and stimulus satiation.

Review Questions

1. What factors comprise the two-factor theory of avoidance? What types of evidence support two-factor theory? What are the main pieces of evidence that pose problems for the theory?

2. What is the one-factor theory, and how does this theory account for (a) the acquisition of avoidance responses and (b) the slowness of extinction of avoidance responses? How does the cognitive theory of avoidance account for these effects?

3. Considering the research on how learned helplessness develops, explain what types of experiences could lead to learned helplessness in (a) a freshman in college, (b) a baseball pitcher traded to a new team, or (c) an elderly resident in a nursing home.

4. Name several factors that determine the effectiveness of a punishment procedure. Give a concrete example to illustrate each factor. What are some potential disadvantages of using punishment?

5. Imagine a toddler who has developed the habit of disrupting any games his older brothers and sisters are playing. Describe at least two different techniques of behavior deceleration that a parent might use in this situation.

6. Describe some examples of how punishment has been successfully used in behavior therapy, and discuss some details that probably helped ensure the success of the procedures.

8

Theories and Research on Operant Conditioning

LEARNING OBJECTIVES

After reading this chapter, you should be able to

- discuss whether performing a response and receiving a reinforcer are essential in the learning and in the performance of a new behavior

- describe studies on how reinforcement can be used to control visceral responses, and explain how these techniques have been used in biofeedback

- list five different theories about how we can predict what will serve as a reinforcer, and

- discuss the strengths and weaknesses of the different theories

- explain how a functional analysis of reinforcers can be used to determine the causes of unusual or puzzling behaviors

- give examples of how the field of behavioral economics has been applied to animal and human behaviors

The theoretical issues examined in this chapter are very broad, and they deal with matters of importance to the entire field of learning. The topics concern such basic issues as what ingredients, if any, are essential for learning to take place, and under what conditions a supposed reinforcer will strengthen the behavior it follows. Most of the issues we will examine have been pondered by learning theorists for many years. Some are fairly well-resolved, but others are the subject of continuing research.

The topics of this chapter can be divided into four general categories. First, we will consider whether both the performance of a response and the reinforcement of that response are necessary for learning to take place. Second, we will examine attempts to use reinforcement to control "visceral" responses—responses of the body's glands and organs that usually occur without our awareness. Third, we will trace the history of attempts to develop a method for predicting which stimuli will be effective reinforcers for a given individual and which will not. A successful method for predicting the effectiveness of a reinforcer would have obvious practical utility, and we will see that it would be equally important from a scientific standpoint. Finally, we will survey recent efforts to analyze the effects of reinforcers using concepts from economics.

THE ROLE OF THE RESPONSE

Operant conditioning might be described as "learning by doing": An animal performs some response and experiences the consequences, and the future likelihood of that response is changed. For Thorndike, the performance of the response was a necessary part of the learning process. After all, if a response does not occur, how can it be strengthened by reinforcement? Convinced that a pairing of response and reinforcer is essential for learning, Thorndike (1946) proposed the following experiment:

> Put the rat, in a little wire car, in the entrance chamber of a maze, run it through the correct path of a simple maze and into the food compartment. Release it there and let it eat the morsel provided. Repeat 10 to 100 times according to the difficulty of the maze under ordinary conditions. . . . Then put it in the entrance chamber free to go wherever it is inclined and observe what it does. Compare the behavior of such rats with that of rats run in the customary manner. (p. 278)

Thorndike predicted that a rat that was pulled passively through a maze would perform like a naive subject in the later test, since the animal had no opportunity to perform a response. On this and several other issues, Thorndike's position was challenged by Edward C. Tolman (1932, 1951, 1959), who might be characterized as an early cognitive psychologist (although he worked decades before the emergence of the field of cognitive psychology). According to Tolman, operant conditioning involves not the simple

strengthening of a response but the formation of an expectation. In a maze, for example, a rat develops an expectation that a reinforcer will be available in the goal box. In addition, Tolman proposed that the rat acquires a **cognitive map** of the maze—a general understanding of the spatial layout of the maze. Tolman proposed that both of these types of learning could be acquired by passive observation as well as by active responding, so that animals should be able to learn something in the type of experiment Thorndike described.

One study fashioned according to Thorndike's specifications was conducted by McNamara, Long, and Wike (1956), who used two groups of rats in an elevated T-maze. Rats in the control group ran through the maze in the usual fashion, and a correct turn at the choice point brought the animal to some food. If the rat went to the wrong arm of the maze, it was confined there for 1 minute. Control rats received 16 trials in the maze, and by the end of training, they made the correct turn on 95% of the trials. Rats in the experimental group received 16 trials in which they were transported through the maze in a wire basket. Each experimental rat was paired with a control subject; that is, it was transported to the correct or incorrect arm of the maze in exactly the same sequence of turns that its counterpart in the control group happened to choose (therefore receiving the same number of reinforcers as its counterpart). This training was followed by a series of extinction trials in which all rats ran through the maze, but no food was available. During these extinction tests, the experimental animals performed just as well as the control group even though they had never been reinforced for running through the maze.

Similar findings of learning without the opportunity to practice the operant response have been obtained in other studies (Dodwell & Bessant, 1960; Keith & McVety, 1988). Dodwell and Bessant found that rats benefited substantially from riding in a cart through a water maze with eight choice points. This shows that animals can learn not only a single response but also a complex chain of responses, without practice. These studies make it clear that, contrary to Thorndike's prediction, active responding is not essential for the acquisition of an operant response.

THE ROLE OF THE REINFORCER

Is Reinforcement Necessary for Operant Conditioning?

From a literal point of view, the answer to this question is obviously yes, since by definition operant conditioning consists of presenting a reinforcer after the occurrence of a specific response. But we have seen that, loosely speaking, operant conditioning can be called a procedure for the learning of new "voluntary," or nonreflexive, behaviors. A better way to phrase this question might be "Is reinforcement necessary for the learning of all new voluntary behaviors?" Prominent early behaviorists such as Hull (1943), Mowrer (1947), and Thorndike believed

that it was, but on this issue as well, Tolman took the opposite position. A famous experiment by Tolman and Honzik (1930), called the **latent learning** experiment, provided evidence on this issue.

In the Tolman and Honzik experiment, rats received 17 trials in a maze with 14 choice points, one trial per day. The rats were divided into three groups. Group 1 was never fed in the maze; when they reached the goal box, they were simply removed from the maze. Rats in Group 2 received a food reinforcer in the goal box on every trial. In Group 3, the conditions were switched on day 11: For the first 10 trials there was no food in the goal box, but on trials 11 through 17 food was available.

On each trial, Tolman and Honzik recorded the number of errors (wrong turns) a rat made; Figure 8-1 shows the averages from each group. Rats in Group 2 (consistently reinforced) displayed a typical learning curve, with

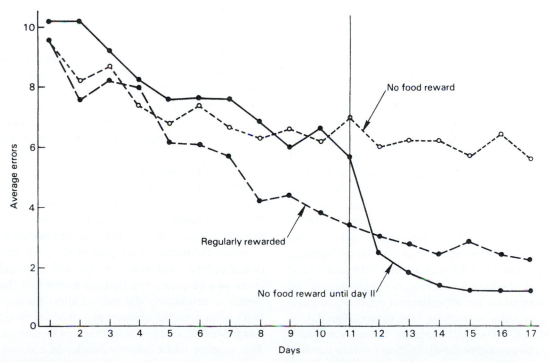

FIGURE 8-1 Mean number of errors on each trial for the three groups in the Tolman and Honzik (1930) experiment on latent learning. Copyright 1930 by the University of California Press.

the number of errors decreasing to about three per trial by the end of the experiment. Rats in Group 1 (never reinforced) showed much poorer performance. Their error rate dropped slightly but leveled off at about seven errors per trial. The results from Group 3 are the most interesting. On the first 11 trials, their results resembled those of Group 1. This makes sense since both groups received no food on trials 1 to 10, and on trial 11 the rats in Group 3 had no way of knowing that food was available until they reached the goal box. On trial 12, however (i.e., after only one trial with food), the performance of Group 3 improved dramatically, and their average number of errors was actually slightly lower than that of Group 2 for the remainder of the experiment. In other words, as soon as rats in Group 3 learned that food was available in the goal box, their performance became equal to that of rats that had been consistently reinforced since the beginning of the experiment.

Since Group 2 required some 12 trials to drop to an error rate of three per trial, it would be implausible to propose that Group 3 learned an equivalent amount on a single trial (trial 11). Instead, Tolman and Honzik asserted that although the rats in Group 3 received no food on trials 1 to 10, they nevertheless learned just as much about the maze as rats in Group 2. However, because they initially received no food in the maze, Group 3 rats were not motivated to display what they had learned. Only after food was available did the rats in Group 3 translate their learning into performance. Tolman and Honzik concluded that reinforcement is not necessary for the *learning* of a new response, but it is necessary for the *performance* of that response. Several dozen experiments on latent learning were conducted between the 1920s and 1950s, most of which found evidence that learning can occur when the experimenter provides no obvious reinforcer such as food (MacCorquodale & Meehl, 1954). All learning theorists are now acutely aware of the distinction between learning and performance, largely because of Tolman's influential work.

Expectations About the Reinforcer

Although latent learning can occur without a reinforcer, the strengthening power of a reinforcer is shown most clearly when a reinforcer is presented after the required response is made. In such situations, exactly what is the function of the reinforcer? Some theorists, such as Thorndike (1946) and Hull (1943), suggested that the reinforcer is merely a sort of catalyst; that is, it strengthens an S-R association between the discriminative stimulus and the operant response, but the reinforcer itself is not included in that association. Opposing this view is the idea that a reinforcer not only stimulates associative learning but also becomes a part of the associative network (Mackintosh & Dickinson, 1979; Tolman, 1932). If so, the associative learning in operant conditioning would involve three distinct elements: the discriminative stimulus, the operant response, and the reinforcer. According to this view, we might say that the animal "develops an expectation" that a particular reinforcer will follow a particular response.

An early experiment by Tinklepaugh (1928) tested these competing ideas. A monkey was first trained on a discrimination task in which a slice of banana was placed beneath one of two containers. After waiting a few seconds, the monkey could choose one of the containers, earning the slice of banana if it chose correctly. The monkey almost always succeeded on this easy task. Then, on a test trial, the experimenter secretly replaced the slice of banana with a piece of lettuce (a less potent reinforcer for the monkey). If the monkey had learned only an S-R association (between the correct container and the reaching response), then the switch to lettuce should go unnoticed. If, however, the monkey had developed an expectation about the usual reinforcer, the lettuce should come as a surprise. Tinklepaugh found that the switch in reinforcers did indeed affect the animal's behavior: The monkey appeared surprised and frustrated, and it refused to accept the lettuce. The monkey had evidently developed a strong expectation about what type of reinforcer was forthcoming.

Colwill and Rescorla (1985) obtained similar findings with rats under more controlled conditions. Two different responses produced two different reinforcers: Pressing a lever earned food pellets and pulling a chain earned a few drops of sugar water. The rats learned to make both responses. Later, each rat was given either free food pellets or free sugar water (with the lever and chain unavailable), and then each animal was made ill with a poison. This procedure was designed to devalue one of the two reinforcers by associating that food with illness. In the test phase, each rat was again presented with the lever and the chain, but this time no food was available. The question of interest was whether a rat would respond more on the lever or the chain in the extinction test. Colwill and Rescorla found that rats poisoned after eating food pellets made few lever presses but many chain pulls, and the opposite was true for those rats poisoned after drinking sugar water. They concluded that the rats associated lever pressing with food pellets and chain pulling with sugar water, and the animals avoided whichever response was associated with the food paired with illness.

Other studies have provided a more complete picture of the different associations formed during operant conditioning (see Balleine, 2009; Colwill, 1996). In one series of experiments, Colwill and Rescorla (1986, 1988) found that pairwise associations are formed among all three components of Skinner's three-term contingency (the discriminative stimulus, the operant response, and the reinforcer). For instance, they found that rats learned to associate two different discriminative stimuli with two different reinforcers (a light with food pellets and a noise with sugar water, or vice versa). Similarly, animals can learn to associate a particular response with a particular discriminative stimulus. These findings parallel those that demonstrate the existence of associations among the three main components of classical conditioning situations—the CS, the US, and the response (see Chapter 4).

These experiments demonstrate conclusively that reinforcers are more than catalysts that strengthen S-R associations. In operant conditioning, animals learn something more complex than merely "In the presence of stimulus A, make response B." They evidently learn the three-term contingency "In the presence of stimulus A, response B is followed by reinforcer C." Furthermore, if more than one stimulus, response, and reinforcer are used, animals can keep track of several three-term contingencies at once. Not surprisingly, similar associations have been demonstrated in operant conditioning with human participants (Gámez & Rosas, 2005, 2007). Thus in operant conditioning, just as in classical conditioning, subjects appear to develop a richer and more diverse array of associations than was once supposed.

Can Reinforcement Control Visceral Responses?

In a theoretical debate that began before theories of avoidance learning were developed (Chapter 7), two-factor theorists were those who believed that classical conditioning and operant conditioning are two distinctly different types of learning. Konorski and Miller (1937), who favored two-factor theory, proposed that although operant responses are clearly controlled by their consequences, classically conditioned responses are not. They hypothesized that reinforcement can control the behavior of the skeletal muscles (those involved in movement of the limbs) but not visceral responses (the behavior of the glands, organs, and the smooth muscles of the stomach and intestines). On the other hand, one-factor theorists believed that reinforcement and punishment are universal principles of learning that can be used to control all types of behavior, including the responses of an individual's glands, organs, and smooth muscles.

For many years it was impossible to perform a meaningful experiment about this matter because scientists had no way to separate skeletal and visceral responses. Suppose a misguided one-factor theorist offered to deliver a reinforcer, a $20 bill, if you increased your heart rate by at least 10 beats per minute. You could easily accomplish this by running up a flight of stairs or by doing a few push-ups. This demonstration of the control of heart rate through reinforcement would not convince any two-factor theorist, who would simply point out that what the reinforcer increased was the activity of the skeletal muscles, and the increase in heart rate was an automatic, unlearned response to the body's increase in activity. That is, the increase in heart rate was not a direct result of the reinforcement; rather, it was a by-product of skeletal activity. To perform a convincing study, it would be necessary to eliminate any possible influence of the body's skeletal muscles.

During the 1960s, N. E. Miller and his colleagues devised a procedure that met this requirement. Their subjects were rats that were temporarily paralyzed by an injection of a drug called curare. Curare blocks movement of the skeletal muscles, including those necessary for breathing, so an artificial respirator was needed to keep the rats alive. The normal activity of the glands and organs is not affected by curare, so it might be possible to observe the direct control of visceral responses by reinforcement. But what could serve as an effective reinforcer for a paralyzed rat? To solve this problem, Miller made use of a finding by Olds and Milner (1954) that a mild, pulsating electrical current delivered via an electrode to certain structures in the brain acts as a powerful reinforcer. Rats will press a lever at high rates for many hours, ceasing only at the point of exhaustion, if this type of **electrical stimulation of the brain** (ESB) is made contingent on this response.

Figure 8-2 shows the experimental procedure used by Miller and his colleagues in many of their experiments. A curarized rat is artificially respirated, has an electrode implanted in its brain for the delivery of ESB, and is connected to recording equipment to monitor heart rate (or other visceral responses). In an early set of experiments, Miller and DiCara (1967) attempted to increase or decrease the heart rates of different rats, using ESB as reinforcement. After measuring a rat's baseline heart rate (which averaged about 400 beats per minute), the experimenters began a shaping procedure. If the goal was an increase in heart rate, reinforcement would be provided for some small (e.g., 2%) increase. The criterion for reinforcement was then gradually raised. With other rats, Miller and DiCara used a similar procedure to try to shape decreases in heart rate. They obtained substantial changes in heart rate in both directions: By the end of a session, the average heart rate was over 500 beats per minute for subjects reinforced for a rapid heart rate, and about 330 beats per minute for subjects reinforced for a slow heart rate.

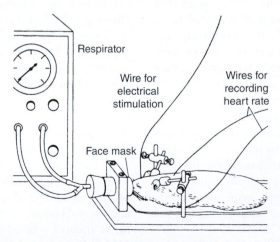

FIGURE 8-2 The experimental arrangement used by Miller and DiCara in their experiments on the operant control of heart rate.

SOURCE: Reprinted by permission of Donald G. Garber, executor of the Estate of Bunji Tagawa.

Miller's research group also found that reinforcement could control many visceral responses besides heart rate (see DiCara, 1970, for a review). They found that curarized rats could either dilate or constrict the blood vessels of the skin, increase or decrease the activity of the intestines, and increase or decrease the rate of urine production by the kidneys. The specificity of these responses made it difficult to argue that they were caused by some general property of the drug, of the artificial respiration procedure, and so forth. Unfortunately, later studies by both Miller and others found it difficult to replicate the early results that showed control of heart rate by ESB reinforcement. Sometimes such control was demonstrated, but often it was not, and there was no obvious pattern in the successes and failures (Miller & Dworkin, 1974). If we must try to draw some conclusions from these conflicting data, it seems that reinforcement can exert direct control over some visceral responses when the activity of the skeletal muscles has been eliminated, but this control is not as easy to obtain as the early studies seemed to suggest.

From a practical standpoint, however, it can be important to know whether reinforcement can be used to control certain internal bodily processes *under any circumstances,* not just in the extreme case where the animal is temporarily paralyzed with curare. Some interesting studies by Gruber and Taub (1998) showed that reinforcement could be used to teach monkeys (1) to control muscle tension in their limbs, or (2) to increase or decrease the temperature of their hands. In the case of temperature control, a column of lights served as stimuli indicating the monkey's hand temperature, and a sip of a preferred beverage was used as a reinforcer to shape either temperature increases or decreases. Over a series of training sessions, the monkeys were able to learn first to increase and then to decrease the temperature of their hands. This experiment does more than simply demonstrate the power of reinforcement; the ability to control hand temperature or other bodily processes can help treat many different medical problems, as explained in the Biofeedback section.

Biofeedback

Some psychologists have speculated that one reason we have so little control over many of our bodily functions is that feedback from our organs and glands is weak or nonexistent. The term **biofeedback** refers to any procedure designed to supply the individual with amplified feedback about some bodily process. The reasoning is that improved feedback may be accompanied by the possibility of better control.

The general design of many biofeedback experiments can be illustrated by examining one study on the control of muscle tension in the forehead. Excessive tension in the forehead muscles is the cause of muscle-contraction headaches, which some people experience at a high frequency. Budzynski, Stoyva, Adler, and Mullaney (1973) attempted to train a group of individuals who suffered from chronic muscle-contraction headaches to relax these muscles. These people experienced some headache pain almost every day before the start of treatment. During therapy sessions, each patient received electromyogram (EMG) biofeedback: Electrodes attached to the patient's forehead monitored muscle tension, and the level of tension was translated into a continuous train of clicks the patient could hear. The patient was instructed to slow down the rate of clicking, thereby decreasing the tension in these muscles. Patients learned to accomplish this task almost immediately, and their average muscle tension levels were about 50% lower in the first biofeedback session than in the preceding baseline sessions. After biofeedback training, patients could produce low-forehead tension without the biofeedback equipment, and this ability was retained in a 3-month follow-up. Patients were instructed to practice this muscle relaxation at home, twice a day for about 20 minutes. This combination of biofeedback training and home practice led to a marked reduction in headache activity in about 75% of the patients, and these improvements were maintained in a 3-month follow-up. On average, patients reported a decrease of about 80% in the frequency and severity of their headaches, and many were able to decrease or eliminate medication they had been taking. A review of over 100 studies on biofeedback treatments for headaches concluded that they can be quite effective for tension and migraine headaches both in the short term and in follow-ups of a year or more (Nestoriuc, Martin, Rief, & Andrasik, 2008).

Using EMG biofeedback in the opposite way—to increase muscle tension—can also have therapeutic benefits. Johnson and Garton (1973) used biofeedback to treat 10 patients with hemiplegia (paralysis on one side of the body), who could walk only with the aid of a leg brace. All of them had suffered from this problem for at least a year, and they had failed to improve with traditional muscular-rehabilitation training. With electrodes connected to the paralyzed muscles of the leg, a patient received auditory feedback on the level of muscle tension (which was initially very low, of course). Any increase in muscle tension would produce a louder sound, and a patient's task was to increase the loudness of the signal. All patients rapidly learned how to do this. They received daily biofeedback sessions, first in the hospital and later at home with a portable EMG feedback device. All patients showed some improvement in muscle functioning, and five improved to the point where they could walk without the leg brace. This study and others have demonstrated quite convincingly that EMG biofeedback can be a useful supplement to traditional rehabilitation therapy for certain muscular disorders, producing improvements that would not be obtained without the biofeedback.

Feedback from an EMG device is only one of many types of biofeedback; some other examples include feedback on heart rate, cardiac irregularities, blood pressure, skin temperature, electrical activity of the brain, stomach acidity, and intestinal activity. Biofeedback has been tried as a treatment for many different problems with varying degrees of success (Schwartz & Andrasik, 2003). For instance, training patients to increase the temperature of their hands has been found to be an effective treatment for migraine headaches in both children and adults (Nestoriuc & Martin, 2007; Scharff, Marcus, & Masek, 2002). In one study, a combination of skin temperature

biofeedback and training in other skills (including progressive relaxation techniques) produced substantial improvement in patients suffering from irritable bowel syndrome, a disorder with symptoms that include frequent intestinal pain, gas, and diarrhea (Schwartz, Taylor, Scharff, & Blanchard, 1990). In treating patients who complained of shortness of breath and other breathing difficulties during panic attacks, therapists found that these symptoms could be reduced by providing respiratory biofeedback, including feedback on the depth and regularity of their breathing (Meuret, Wilhelm, & Roth, 2004).

A type of biofeedback called **neurofeedback** (also known as electroencephalogram, EEG, biofeedback) has been used to treat children diagnosed with attention-deficit hyperactivity disorder (ADHD). In one study (Linden, Habib, & Radojevic, 1996), children with this diagnosis were given 40 sessions of neurofeedback in which each child received feedback on the electrical activity of his or her brain. The purpose of the training was to increase a particular brain wave pattern called beta waves, which are thought to be associated with an attentive and alert mental state. A child received feedback whenever beta waves were present in the EEG recording. After their training sessions were completed, these children obtained higher scores on an IQ test and exhibited greater attentiveness. Several other studies have found beneficial effects of neurofeedback as a treatment for ADHD, sometimes as part of a larger treatment package (Little, Lubar, & Cannon, 2010). Neurofeedback is also being tested as a treatment for a variety of other medical problems, such as epilepsy and chronic pain (Carmagnani & Carmagnani, 1999).

Other researchers have examined whether neurofeedback can be used to enhance the cognitive performance of normal adults. Zoefel, Huster, and Herrmann (2011) gave college students five sessions of neurofeedback training to increase alpha waves—brain waves that have a distinct cyclical pattern occurring at a frequency of about 10 cycles per second. By the fifth session, their EEGs showed a clear increase in alpha waves. As a measure of cognitive functioning, the students were given a mental rotation test (in which they had to decide which of two objects presented in different orientations in a visual display were identical). Their performance on this task was better than before the neurofeedback training, and better than that of a control group that did not receive the training. These are preliminary findings, and further research is needed to determine if there are any long-term benefits to this type of training. However, one clear conclusion from this line of research is that neurofeedback can be used to modify a variety of different types of brain wave patterns.

Not all attempts to treat medical problems with biofeedback have been successful. For instance, some attempts to use biofeedback as a treatment for high blood pressure have not obtained good results, whereas others have found substantial decreases in blood pressure levels in most patients (Nakao, Nomura, Shimosawa, Fujita, & Kuboki, 2000). Weaver and McGrady

(1995) suggested that it may be possible to use various measures to identify which patients will respond to biofeedback for high blood pressure and which will not. If so, biofeedback treatment could be targeted at those individuals who are most likely to benefit from the treatment.

Research on biofeedback has grown substantially over the years, and biofeedback techniques have been applied to an increasingly diverse array of medical disorders. The effectiveness of biofeedback must be judged on a problem-by-problem basis. For some medical problems, biofeedback may be ineffective. For other problems, it may be only as effective as other, less expensive treatments. For still others, it may produce health improvements that are superior to those of any other known treatment.

HOW CAN WE PREDICT WHAT WILL BE A REINFORCER?

The past several chapters should leave no doubt that the principle of reinforcement is one of the most central concepts in the behavioral approach to learning. This concept has also been the subject of considerable debate and controversy between behavioral psychologists on one hand and critics of the behavioral approach on the other. Critics have frequently argued that the definition of reinforcement is circular, and therefore that the concept is not scientifically valid (Chomsky, 1959, 1972b; Postman, 1947). This is a serious criticism, so let us examine what they mean by the term *circular*.

Consider this brief definition of a reinforcer: a stimulus that increases the future probability of a behavior which it follows. Suppose a behavioral psychologist presents a stimulus, a small quantity of beer, to a rat each time the rat presses a lever, and the probability of lever pressing increases. By the foregoing definition, the psychologist would conclude that beer is a reinforcer for the rat. This conclusion, however, provides no explanation; it is nothing more than a restatement of the facts. If asked "Why did the rat's lever pressing increase?" the behaviorist would answer "Because it was reinforced by the presentation of beer." If asked

---

PRACTICE QUIZ (1)

1. Tolman claimed that rats could still learn a maze if they were carried through it because they developed a _____.
2. Experiments on latent learning have shown that reinforcement is necessary for the _____ on an operant response, but not for the _____ of the response.
3. In experiments on the control of heart rate by reinforcement, _____ was used as a reinforcer for rats that were temporarily paralyzed with curare.
4. In using EMG biofeedback for tension headaches, patients listen to clicks that indicate _____, and they are told to try to reduce the rate of the clicks.
5. The technique of reinforcing particular types of brain waves is called _____.

Answers

1. cognitive map 2. performance, learning 3. ESB
4. tension in their forehead muscles 5. neurofeedback

"How do you know beer is a reinforcer?" the reply would be "Because it caused an increase in lever pressing." The circularity in this sort of reasoning should be clear: A stimulus is called a reinforcer because it increases some behavior, and it is said to increase the behavior because it is a reinforcer. As stated, this simple definition of a reinforcer makes no specific predictions whatsoever. If there were no increase in lever pressing in the beer experiment, this would pose no problem for the behavioral psychologist, who would simply conclude, "Beer is not a reinforcer for the rat."

If there were nothing more to the concept of a reinforcer than this, then critics would be correct in saying that the term is circular and not predictive. Because of the seriousness of this criticism, behavioral psychologists have made several attempts to escape from this circularity by developing independent criteria for determining which stimuli will be reinforcers and which will not. The problem boils down to finding some rule that will tell us in advance whether a stimulus will act as a reinforcer. If we can find such a rule, one that makes new, testable predictions, then the circularity of the term *reinforcer* will be broken. Several attempts to develop this sort of rule are described next.

Need Reduction

In his earlier writings, Clark Hull (1943) proposed that all primary reinforcers are stimuli that reduce some biological need, and that all stimuli that reduce a biological need will act as reinforcers. The simplicity of this **need-reduction theory** is appealing, and it is certainly true that many primary reinforcers serve important biological functions. We know that food, water, warmth, and avoidance of pain are all primary reinforcers, and each also plays an important role in the continued survival of an organism. Unfortunately, it does not take much thought to come up with exceptions to this rule. For example, sexual stimulation is a powerful reinforcer, but despite what you may hear some people claim, no one will die if deprived of sex indefinitely. Another example of

a reinforcer that serves no biological function is saccharin (or any other artificial sweetener). Saccharin has no nutritional value, but because of its sweet taste it is a reinforcer for both humans and nonhumans. People purchase saccharin and add it to their coffee or tea, and rats choose to drink water flavored with saccharin over plain water.

Besides reinforcers that satisfy no biological needs, there are also examples of biological necessities for which there is no corresponding reinforcer. One such example is vitamin B_1 (thiamine). Although intake of thiamine is essential for maintaining good health, animals such as rats apparently cannot detect the presence or absence of thiamine in their food by smell or taste. As a result, rats suffering from a thiamine deficiency will not immediately select a food that contains thiamine. If they have the opportunity to sample various diets over a period of days, however, they will eventually settle on the diet that improves their health (Rodgers & Rozin, 1966). This result shows that it is better health, not the presence of thiamine in the rat's food, that is actually the reinforcer for selecting certain foods.

It makes sense that most biological necessities will function as reinforcers, because a creature could not survive if it were not strongly motivated to obtain these reinforcers. As a predictor of reinforcing capacity, however, the need-reduction hypothesis is inadequate because there are many exceptions to this principle—reinforcers that satisfy no biological needs, and biological needs that are not translated into reinforcers.

Drive Reduction

Recognizing the problem with the need-reduction hypothesis, Hull and his student N. E. Miller (1948, 1951) became advocates of the **drive-reduction theory** of reinforcement. This theory states that strong stimulation of any sort is aversive to an organism, and any reduction in this stimulation acts as a reinforcer for the immediately preceding behavior. The term *drive reduction* was chosen because many of the strong stimuli an animal experiences are frequently called drives (the hunger drive, the sex drive, etc.). In addition, the theory asserts that other strong stimuli, which are not normally called drives (e.g., loud noise, intense heat, and fear), will also provide reinforcement when their intensity is reduced. A reduction in stimulation of any sort should serve as a reinforcer.

There are at least two major problems with the drive-reduction theory. First, if we measure the intensity of stimulation using an objective, physical scale of measurement, not all reductions in stimulation act as reinforcers. For example, reducing the room temperature from 100°F to 75°F (which is the reduction of a stimulus, heat) would probably serve as a reinforcer for most animals, but reducing the room temperature from 25°F to 0°F (an equally large reduction in heat) would not. Common sense tells us that 100°F is "too hot" and 0°F is "too cold," but that is beside the point; one reduction in heat serves as a reinforcer and the other does not.

Second, there are many examples of reinforcers that either produce no decrease in stimulation or actually produce an increase in stimulation. Sheffield, Wulff, and Backer (1951) found that male rats would repeatedly run down an alley when the reinforcer was a female rat in heat. This reinforcer produced no decrease in the male's sex drive because the rats were always separated before ejaculation occurred, yet the male rat's high speed of running continued trial after trial. Similarly, we know that sexual foreplay is reinforcing for human beings even when it does not culminate in intercourse. People will engage in a variety of behaviors for the opportunity to engage in sexual activities that do not include orgasm and the resultant reduction in sex drive. The popularity of pornographic magazines and films provides further evidence on this point.

Reinforcers that consist of an actual increase in stimulation are common for creatures of a wide range of species and ages. Human infants, kittens, and other young animals spend long periods of time playing with toys and other objects that produce ever-changing visual, auditory, and tactile stimulation. The opportunity to run in a running wheel can serve as a reinforcer for rats (Belke & Pierce, 2009). Photographs presented as a slide show can serve as reinforcers for monkeys, and motion pictures are even stronger reinforcers (Blatter & Schultz, 2006). Butler (1953) found that monkeys would learn a complex response when the reinforcer was simply the opening of a window that let them see outside the experimental chamber. A great variety of stimuli and activities that increase sensory stimulation can serve as reinforcers for adult humans: music, engaging in sports and exercise, mountain climbing, skydiving, horror films, and the like. There seems to be no way to reconcile these facts with the drive-reduction hypothesis.

Trans-situationality

The failures of both need-reduction and drive-reduction theories suggest that there is no simple way to classify reinforcers and nonreinforcers on the basis of their biological or stimulus properties. The problem is compounded by the existence of individual differences; for example, horror films may be reinforcers for some people but not for others. Because of these difficulties, theorists such as Paul Meehl (1950) turned to a more modest theoretical position, but one that still offered the possibility of making new predictions and thereby avoiding the circularity of the term *reinforcer*. Meehl invoked the concept of **trans-situationality**, which simply means that a stimulus that is determined to be a reinforcer in one situation will also be a reinforcer in other situations. Suppose that at the outset we do not know whether water sweetened with saccharin will be a reinforcer for a mouse. By performing a simple experiment, we might find that the mouse will learn to run in an activity wheel if every several revolutions of the wheel are reinforced with a few seconds of access to the saccharin solution. After we have determined that saccharin is a reinforcer in this one experiment, the principle of trans-situationality implies that we should be able to make new predictions. For instance, we should be able to use saccharin as a reinforcer for lever pressing, climbing a ladder, learning the correct sequence of turns in a maze, and so on.

In reality, the principle of trans-situationality works quite well in many cases. Reinforcers such as food, water, and escape from pain can be used to strengthen a multitude of different behaviors. The problem is that there are some cases in which a reinforcer in one situation does not act as a reinforcer in another situation. The first person to document clear exceptions to the principle of trans-situationality was David Premack, whose influential experiments and writings changed the way many psychologists think about reinforcement.

Premack's Principle

The procedure of reinforcement is often described as a contingency between a behavior (the operant response) and a stimulus (the reinforcer). An implication of this description is that the two elements of a reinforcement contingency are members of two distinct classes of events: reinforceable behaviors on one hand and reinforcing stimuli on the other. One of Premack's major contributions was to demonstrate that there is no clear boundary between these two classes of events, and in fact it may be counterproductive to talk about two separate classes at all. Premack followed the lead of earlier writers such as Sheffield (1948) in pointing out that nearly all reinforcers involve both a stimulus (such as food) and a behavior (such as eating), and it may be the latter that actually strengthens the operant response. Is it water or the act of drinking that is a reinforcer for a thirsty animal? Is a toy a reinforcer for a child or is it the behavior of playing with the toy? Is a window with a view a reinforcer for a monkey or is it the behavior of looking? Premack proposed that it is more accurate to characterize the reinforcement procedure as a contingency between one behavior and another than as a contingency between a behavior and a stimulus. For example, he would state that in many operant conditioning experiments with rats, the contingency is between the behavior of lever pressing and the

behavior of eating—eating can occur if and only if a lever press occurs.

At least for the moment, let us accept Premack's view and see how it relates to the principle of trans-situationality. If the principle is correct, then there must be some subset of all behaviors that we might call *reinforcing behaviors* (e.g., eating, drinking, playing) and another subset of behaviors that are *reinforceable behaviors* (e.g., lever pressing, running in a wheel, pecking a key). According to the principle of trans-situationality, any behavior selected from the first subset should serve as a reinforcer for any behavior in the second subset. However, Premack's experiments have shown a number of ways in which trans-situationality can be violated.

To replace the principle of trans-situationality, Premack (1959, 1965) proposed an alternative theory, now called **Premack's principle**, which provides a straightforward method for determining whether one behavior will act as a reinforcer for another. The key is to measure the durations of the behaviors in a baseline situation, where all behaviors can occur at any time without restriction. Premack's principle states that *more probable behaviors will reinforce less probable behaviors*. The phrase *more probable behavior* means the behavior that the subject performed for a larger fraction of the time in the baseline session. Premack suggested that instead of postulating two categories of behaviors—reinforceable behaviors and reinforcing behaviors—we should rank behaviors on a scale of probability that ranges from behaviors of high probability to those of zero probability. Behaviors higher on the probability scale will reinforce behaviors lower on the probability scale.

A study Premack (1963) conducted with Cebus monkeys highlights the advantages of Premack's principle and the weaknesses of the trans-situationality principle. These monkeys are inquisitive animals that will explore and manipulate any objects placed in their environment. Premack allowed the monkeys to play with different mechanical objects. His findings can be illustrated by examining the results from one monkey, Chicko. Figure 8-3 shows that in baseline conditions, operating a lever had the highest probability, operating a plunger had the lowest, and opening a small door had an intermediate probability.

Later, in contingency sessions, different pairs of items were presented. One item served as the "operant response" and the other as the potential "reinforcer"—the reinforcer was locked and could not be operated until an operant response occurred. In six different phases, every possible combination of operant response and reinforcer was tested, and Figure 8-3 shows the results. The lever served as a reinforcer for both door opening and plunger pulling. Door opening reinforced plunger pulling but it did not reinforce lever pressing. Plunger pulling did not reinforce either of the other behaviors. You should see that each of these six results is in agreement with the principle that more probable behaviors will reinforce less probable behaviors.

Notice that door opening, the behavior of intermediate probability, violated the principle of trans-situationality. When it was contingent on plunger pulling, door opening was a reinforcer. When it led to the availability of lever pressing, it played the role of a reinforceable response. Which was door opening, then, a reinforcer or a reinforceable response? Premack's answer is that it can be either, depending on the behavior's relative position on the scale of probabilities. A behavior will act as a reinforcer for behaviors that are lower on the probability scale, and it will be a reinforceable response for behaviors higher on the probability scale. For this reason, Premack's principle is sometimes called a principle of **reinforcement relativity**: There are no absolute categories of reinforcers and reinforceable responses, and which role a behavior plays depends on its relative location on the probability scale.

PREMACK'S PRINCIPLE AND PUNISHMENT. Premack (1971a) proposed a principle of punishment that is complementary to his reinforcement principle: *Less probable behaviors will punish more probable behaviors.* Since a subject may

L = Lever Pressing
D = Door Opening
P = Plunger Pulling

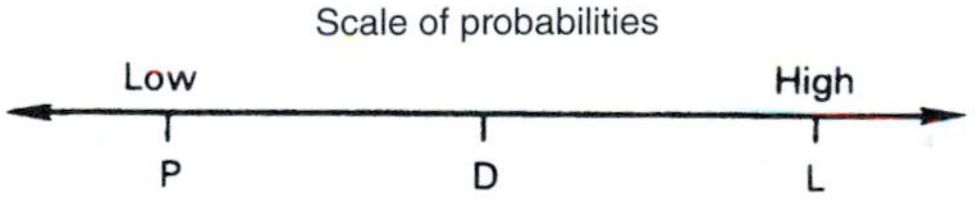

Scale of probabilities

Low   High

     P   D   L

Contingency Conditions	Result	Conclusion
1. D → L	D Increases	L Reinforces D
2. P → L	P Increases	L Reinforces P
3. L → D	L Does Not Increase	D Does Not Reinforce L
4. P → D	P Increases	D Reinforces P
5. L → P	L Does Not Increase	P Does Not Reinforce L
6. D → P	D Does Not Increase	P Does Not Reinforce D

FIGURE 8-3 The procedure used in Premack's (1963) experiment, and the results from one monkey, Chicko. The notation D→L means that Chicko was required to open the door before being allowed to operate the lever.

not perform a low-probability behavior if given a choice, it is necessary to require that the low-probability behavior be performed to demonstrate that this principle is correct. One way to accomplish this is to use a **reciprocal contingency**, which ensures that two behaviors occur in a fixed proportion. For example, in an experiment I conducted many years ago (Mazur, 1975), rats were required to engage in 15 seconds of wheel running for every 5 seconds of drinking, but the rats could choose to complete many such cycles of running and drinking or none at all.

The results from one typical rat will show how this experiment simultaneously verified Premack's reinforcement and punishment rules. In baseline sessions, this rat spent about 17% of the session drinking and about 10% of the session running, as shown in Figure 8-4. But when the rat was required to spend 15 seconds running for every 5 seconds of drinking, the percentage of time spent running increased compared to baseline, whereas drinking time decreased compared to baseline. In other words, the higher probability behavior, drinking, reinforced running, and at the same time, the running requirement punished

drinking. All the other rats in this experiment showed similar results: In the reciprocal contingency, drinking time decreased and running time increased, just as Premack's principles of reinforcement and punishment predicted. Other studies have also found support for Premack's rules (Amari, Grace, & Fisher, 1995; Hanley, Iwata, Roscoe, Thompson, & Lindberg, 2003).

THE USE OF PREMACK'S PRINCIPLE IN BEHAVIOR MODIFICATION. Although we have focused on the theoretical implications of Premack's principle, this theory has had a large impact on the applied field of behavior modification, in several ways. First, it has stressed that behaviors themselves can serve as reinforcers, thereby encouraging behavior therapists to use such reinforcers in their work. Therapists now frequently instruct clients to use "Premackian reinforcers," such as reading, playing cards, phoning a friend, or watching television, as reinforcers for desired behaviors such as exercising, studying, or avoiding smoking. Premackian reinforcers have also been widely adopted in institutional settings. Imagine the difficulties the staff of a

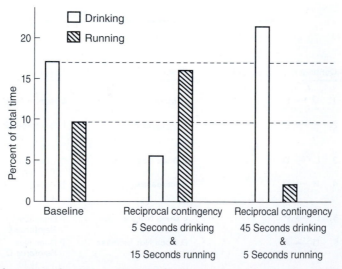

FIGURE 8-4 The performance of one rat in Mazur's (1975) experiment. In the first reciprocal contingency, running time increased and drinking time decreased compared to their baseline levels. In the second reciprocal contingency, running time decreased and drinking time increased compared to their baseline levels.

psychiatric hospital would face in setting up a token system if they relied only on tangible reinforcers such as food, beverages, cigarettes, and money. The costs of reinforcing patients with such items would be prohibitive, and problems of satiation would be commonplace. However, by making certain activities contingent on good behavior, therapists gain access to a wide variety of inexpensive reinforcers.

Premack's principle was used by the parents of a 7-year-old boy who refused to eat all but a few very specific foods and who would become aggressive if they tried to feed him anything else. His parents were concerned about his health on such a restricted diet, so behavior therapists devised the following plan. At mealtimes, the parents would tell the boy that if he ate a small amount of a new food, he could then eat one of his favorite foods. If he refused to eat the new food, he would not be allowed to eat his favorite food (but he was given a less preferred food so he would not go hungry). As a result of this simple strategy, the boy gradually began to eat a wider variety of foods, and he was calmer when presented with new foods (Brown, Spencer, & Swift, 2002).

Homme, deBaca, Devine, Steinhorst, and Rickert (1963) used Premack's principle to control the behavior of a class of nursery-school children. Among the most probable behaviors of these children were running around the room, screaming, pushing chairs about, and so on. The teacher's instructions and commands initially had little impact on the children's behaviors. A program was then established in which these high-probability behaviors were made contingent on low-probability behaviors, such as sitting quietly and listening to the teacher. After a few minutes of such a low-probability behavior, the teacher would ring a bell and give the instructions "run and scream," at which point the children could perform these high-probability behaviors for a few minutes. Then the bell would ring again and the teacher would give instructions for another behavior, which might be one of high or low probability. (One of their favorite high-probability behaviors was pushing the teacher

around in a desk chair with casters.) After a few days, the children's obedience of the teacher's instructions was nearly perfect.

A similar procedure was used by Azrin, Vinas, and Ehle (2007) with two 13-year-old boys diagnosed with ADHD. They were so active and disruptive in the classroom that it was a problem for the whole class. The researchers observed that when they were allowed in the school's recreation room, the boys spent most of their time engaged in vigorous physical activity with the play equipment. This high-probability behavior was therefore used as a reinforcer for sitting quietly and attentively during class. After several minutes of appropriate behavior, the teacher would say, "You can now play because you have been so calm and attentive," and the boys were allowed to play in the recreation room for a few minutes. Under this arrangement, the boys' behaviors during class improved dramatically.

These examples illustrate just a few of the many ways that Premack's principle has been used in applied settings. Although the next section shows that the principle has limitations, it has proven to be a successful rule of thumb for deciding which events will be reinforcers and which will not.

Response Deprivation Theory

Research has shown that Premack's principle will reliably predict reinforcement and punishment effects (1) if a schedule requires more of the low-probability behavior than of the high-probability behavior, or (2) if a schedule requires equal amounts of the two behaviors. However, if a schedule requires much more of the high-probability behavior than the low-probability behavior, Premack's principle may be violated. My experiment with rats in a reciprocal contingency between running and drinking (Mazur, 1975) illustrates how this can happen.

Recall that one rat spent about 17% of the time drinking and 10% running in baseline sessions (Figure 8-4). This animal's ratio of drinking time to running time was therefore about 1.7 to 1. In one of the reciprocal contingencies, 45 seconds of drinking were required for every 5 seconds of running. This is a 9:1 ratio of drinking to running, which is higher than the ratio exhibited in the unrestricted, baseline conditions. Figure 8-4 shows that in this reciprocal contingency, running time decreased to about 2% of the session time, while drinking time actually increased to 21%. Thus, contrary to Premack's principle, in this case a low-probability behavior actually reinforced a high-probability behavior.

To handle results of this type, Timberlake and Allison (1974; Allison, 1993) proposed the **response deprivation theory** of reinforcement, which is actually a refinement of Premack's principle. The essence of this theory is that whenever a contingency restricts an individual's access to some behavior compared to baseline (when there are no restrictions on any behavior), the restricted behavior will serve as a reinforcer, regardless of whether it is a high-probability or a low-probability behavior. To understand how this theory works, imagine that a man typically spends 30 minutes a day working out with his home exercise equipment, and he spends 60 minutes a day studying for a difficult graduate course. He decides that he should be spending more time on this course, but he has trouble making himself study any longer. To use response deprivation theory, the man makes an agreement with his wife (who will act to enforce the rule) that for every 20 minutes he spends studying, he earns 5 minutes of exercise time (see Figure 8-5). Notice that if the man continued to study just 60 minutes a day, he would earn only 15 minutes of exercise time, so this would deprive him of the 30 minutes of exercise that he used to have. Therefore, according to response deprivation theory, this contingency produces a relative deprivation of exercise. Because of this, the theory predicts that the man

will strike some compromise between studying and exercising—for example, he might increase his studying to 100 minutes a day, which would earn him 25 minutes of exercise time (which is closer to his baseline level of 30 minutes). Upon observing this increase in studying compared to baseline, we would say that exercising (the lower-probability behavior) has served as a reinforcer for studying.

In summary, response deprivation theory states that unless a schedule happens to require exactly the same ratio of two behaviors that an individual chooses in baseline conditions, one of the behaviors becomes a relatively precious commodity because of its restricted availability. Regardless of whether it is the high- or low-probability behavior, the more restricted behavior will act as a reinforcer for the less restricted behavior.

Although it may be a bit more difficult to understand than Premack's principle, response deprivation theory is the most reliable predictor of reinforcer effectiveness of all the theories we have examined. The theory allows us to predict whether an activity will serve as a reinforcer by observing the probability of that behavior (and of the behavior to be reinforced) in a baseline situation. This theory has been tested both in laboratory experiments with animals and in applied settings with people, and it has proven to be an accurate way to predict when a contingency will produce an increase in a desired behavior and when it will not (Klatt & Morris, 2001; Timberlake & Farmer-Dougan, 1991). For example, Konarski (1987) set up different contingencies between two behaviors in a population of adults with mental retardation, and this allowed him to make a direct comparison of the predictions of Premack's principle and response deprivation theory. The predictions of Premack's principle succeeded in

Baseline:	60 minutes studying, 30 minutes exercising
Contingency:	Every 20 minutes studying earns 5 minutes exercising
Results:	100 minutes studying, 25 minutes exercising
Conclusion:	Exercising has served as a reinforcer for studying

FIGURE 8-5 A hypothetical example of response deprivation theory. Because the contingency deprives the man of his usual amount of exercise time, exercising should serve as a reinforcer for studying.

some cases and failed in others, but the predictions of response deprivation theory proved to be correct almost 100% of the time. Because response deprivation theory allows us to predict, in advance, what will serve as a reinforcer, the definition of a reinforcer is no longer circular.

The Functional Analysis of Behaviors and Reinforcers

Response deprivation theory offers a good way to predict when an activity will serve as an effective reinforcer. However, a different problem that often challenges behavior therapists is to determine what reinforcer is maintaining some undesired behavior. Those who work with children or adults who have autism or mental retardation often see bizarre or inappropriate behaviors that seem to occur for no obvious reason. Examples include the destruction of toys or other objects, aggression against peers or caregivers, screaming, self-injurious behaviors (SIBs), and chewing on inedible objects. One useful first step toward eliminating these behaviors is to conduct a **functional analysis**, which is a method that allows the therapist to determine what reinforcer is maintaining the unwanted behavior.

These maladaptive behaviors may occur for many possible reasons. An aggressive act may allow a child to seize a desired toy (a positive reinforcer). Destroying objects may lead to attention from the caregiver (another positive reinforcer). Screaming or disruptive behavior may produce an interruption in an unwanted lesson or activity (a negative reinforcer). In addition, some behaviors (e.g., chewing on inedible objects, repetitive motions, or SIBs) may produce what is called **automatic reinforcement**; that is, sensory stimulation from the behavior may serve as its own reinforcer (Fisher, Adelinis, Thompson, Worsdell, & Zarcone, 1998).

How can the cause of a particular maladaptive behavior be determined? Using the method of functional analysis, the patient's environment is systematically changed in ways that allow the therapist either to support or to rule out possible explanations of the inappropriate behavior. For example, Watson, Ray, Turner, and Logan (1999) used functional analysis to evaluate the SIB of a 10-year-old boy who was mentally disabled. In his classroom, the boy would frequently bang his head on the table, slap his face, and scratch at his face with his fingernails. On different days, the boy's teacher reacted to episodes of SIB in different ways. On some days, the teacher immediately said "Don't do that" after each instance of SIB, to see if the behavior was being reinforced by the teacher's attention. On other days, the boy was given a toy or other item after each instance of SIB, to see if tangible reinforcers might be strengthening this behavior. To assess the possibility that the SIB might be producing automatic reinforcement, the boy was sometimes placed in a room by himself, where he could receive no attention or tangible reinforcers if he engaged in SIB. Finally, on some days, whatever task the boy was working on was terminated after an instance of SIB, to determine whether the behavior might be reinforced by escape from unpleasant tasks.

Figure 8-6 shows the results from these tests. Look at these results, and try to decide what was causing the SIB. Compared to the normal classroom situation (labeled "Baseline"), the rate of SIB was much lower in the situations testing the effects of attention, tangible reinforcers, and automatic reinforcement, but it was higher when it allowed the boy to escape from the ongoing task. The researchers therefore concluded that the SIB was actually escape behavior. As a treatment, they instructed the boy's teacher to allow him to end a nonpreferred task and switch to a more preferred task if he completed it without any instance of SIB. After this approach was adopted, the boy's SIB virtually disappeared.

Functional analysis must be done on a case-by-case basis, because the same behaviors may occur for different reasons for different people. In one survey of more than 100 individuals who engaged in SIB, functional analysis found that for about a third of them, the behavior was being maintained by attention from the caregiver. For these individuals, the SIB was greatly reduced by having the caregiver ignore instances of SIB but give the patients attention when they were engaged in other behaviors (Fischer, Iwata, & Worsdell, 1997). In another example of functional

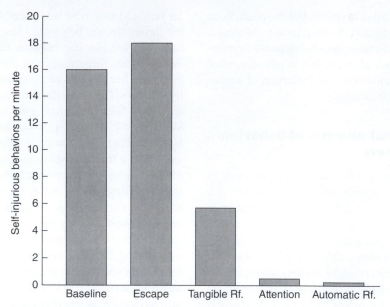

FIGURE 8-6   An example of functional analysis. The rates of SIB exhibited by a boy with a mental disability are shown for five different experimental conditions. (From Watson et al., 1999)

analysis, researchers found that finger sucking by two children was being maintained not by attention or by escape from unpleasant tasks but by automatic reinforcement (the sensory stimulation of the fingers). When bandages or rubber gloves were put on the children's fingers, their finger sucking decreased (Ellingson et al., 2000). Functional analysis can also be used for adults with psychological disorders who display unusual or disturbing behaviors (Rehfeldt & Chambers, 2003; Wilder, White, & Yu, 2003).

The power of functional analysis is that the therapist need not simply watch helplessly and wonder why a maladaptive behavior is occurring. By the appropriate manipulation of the environment, possible sources of reinforcement can be evaluated, and based on this information, an appropriate treatment plan can be tailored to the needs of each individual.

BEHAVIORAL ECONOMICS

This chapter has described several different theories about reinforcement. To achieve a better understanding of this concept, some psychologists

have turned to theories from the field of economics. Microeconomics, which is concerned with the behavior of individual consumers, and the study of operant conditioning, which is concerned with the behavior of individual organisms, have several common features. Both disciplines examine how the individual works to obtain relatively scarce and precious commodities (consumer goods in economics, reinforcers in operant conditioning). In both cases the resources of the individual (money in economics, time or behavior in operant conditioning) are limited. Both disciplines attempt to predict how individuals will allocate their limited resources to obtain scarce commodities.

Because of these common interests, some psychologists and economists have begun to share theoretical ideas and research techniques. The field of **behavioral economics** is a product of these cooperative efforts (Bradshaw, 2010; Diamond & Vartiainen, 2007). This section describes a few of the ways in which economic concepts have been applied to human and animal behaviors, both inside and outside the laboratory.

Optimization: Theory and Research

OPTIMIZATION AS A BASIC ASSUMPTION IN MICROECONOMICS. A basic question for microeconomists is how individual consumers will distribute their incomes among all the possible ways it can be spent, saved, or invested. Suppose a woman brings home $800 a week after taxes. How much of this will she spend on food, on rent, on household items, on clothing, on entertainment, on charitable contributions, and so on? **Optimization theory** provides a succinct and reasonable answer: She will distribute her income in whatever way maximizes her "subjective value" (or loosely speaking, in whatever way gives her the most satisfaction). Although this principle is easy to state, putting it into practice can be extremely difficult. How can we know whether buying a new pair of shoes or giving that same amount of money to a worthy charity will give the woman greater satisfaction? For that matter, how does the woman know? Despite these difficulties, optimization theory maintains that people can and do make such judgments and then distribute their income accordingly.

A simple example may help to illustrate the assumptions of optimization theory. Suppose that you are an avid reader of both autobiographies and science fiction, and that as a birthday present you receive a gift certificate good for any 10 paperbacks at a local bookstore. How many autobiographies will you buy, and how many books of science fiction? Optimization theory cannot give us a definite answer, but it does provide some guidelines. A common assumption is that as a consumer obtains more and more items of a given type, the value of each additional item of that same type decreases. For example, the value of one new science fiction novel may be relatively high, but a second science fiction novel will be a bit less valued, and the tenth new science fiction novel may have fairly little value. This assumption is based on the concept of satiation.

Similarly, your first new autobiography should be the most valued, the second a bit less valued, and so on. These assumptions are illustrated graphically in the two left panels of Figure 8-7. The y-axis shows the (hypothetical) cumulative value of different numbers of science fiction novels (left panel) and autobiographies (center panel). The steps depict the additional value provided by one more paperback of each type. The consistently higher curve for science fiction novels means that for this illustration, we will assume that you enjoy science fiction novels somewhat more than autobiographies. From these two graphs, the total value of any possible combination of science fiction novels and autobiographies can be calculated. The results are plotted in the right panel of Figure 8-7.

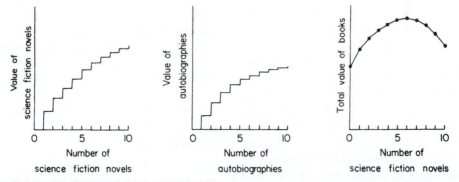

FIGURE 8-7 An illustration of the predictions of optimization theory for a case where a person must choose any combination of science fiction novels and autobiographies, for a total of 10 books. The left panel shows that the subjective value of a set of science fiction novels increases with each additional novel, but the increment in value is progressively smaller. The center panel shows a similar pattern for autobiographies. The right panel shows that a person with precisely these preferences for the two types of books would maximize subjective value by choosing six science fiction novels and four autobiographies.

Even before looking at this graph, you can probably guess that the optimal package will consist of some mixture of the two types of books, since the first autobiography has more value than the 10th science fiction novel, and the first science fiction novel has more value than the 10th autobiography. For the specific functions drawn in the two left panels, it turns out that the combination of six science fiction novels and four autobiographies leads to the highest total value. Optimization theory therefore predicts that this combination would be chosen by a person who had this particular set of preferences for the two types of books.

The decisions of anyone who earns an income are obviously much more complex than in this simple example, but optimization theory suggests that the decision-making process is essentially the same; that is, the consumer searches for the maximum subjective value. Although a good deal of economic theory is based on this principle, uncertainty about the exact shape of any individual's value functions makes the principle of optimization difficult to test. The next section shows that the principle has also been applied to animal behavior where researchers have been able to gather concrete evidence to support it.

OPTIMIZATION AND BEHAVIORAL ECOLOGY. Behavioral ecologists study the behaviors of animals in their natural habitats or in semi-naturalistic settings, and they attempt to determine how the behavior patterns of different species are shaped by environmental factors and the pressures of survival. It is easy to see why the concept of optimization is appealing to behavioral ecologists, with their interest in the relationship between evolution and behavior: Animals whose behaviors are more nearly optimal should increase their chances of surviving and of breeding offspring that will have similar behavioral tendencies. Behavioral ecologists have documented many cases where an animal's behaviors are close to optimal; these cases involve such varied pursuits as foraging for food, searching for a mate, and choosing group size (Krebs & Davies, 1978).

Here is one example of how the principle of optimization can be applied to animal behavior.

When searching for its prey, any predator must make decisions. If a large prey is encountered, it should of course be captured. On the other hand, if a small prey is encountered, the predator's decision is trickier. If a long time is required to chase, capture, and eat the small prey, it may not be worthwhile to go after it, because during this time the predator will miss the opportunity to capture any larger prey that might come along. A general rule is that if the density of large prey is low (so that encounters with large prey are rare), the predator should go after any prey, large or small. If the density of large prey is high, however, the predator should ignore all small prey, because in chasing them it would lose valuable time during which a large prey might come along.

Werner and Hall (1974) tested these predictions by placing 10 bluegill sunfish in a large aquarium with three sizes of prey (smaller fish). When prey density was low (20 of each type), the sunfish ate all three types of prey as often as they were encountered. When prey density was high (350 of each type), the sunfish ate only the largest prey. When prey density was intermediate (200 of each type), the sunfish ate only the two largest prey types. By measuring the time the sunfish required to capture and eat prey of each type, Werner and Hall were able to calculate that the behaviors of the sunfish were exactly what optimization theory predicted for all three situations.

This example shows how scientists have applied optimization theory to the behaviors of animals in naturalistic settings. Operant conditioning experiments have also provided some support for the theory (Silberberg, Bauman, & Hursh, 1993). In the psychological laboratory, optimization theory can be put to a more rigorous test, and its predictions can be compared to those of alternative theories. Some of this research will be described in Chapter 13.

Elasticity and Inelasticity of Demand

In operant research, many studies have been done to see how behavior changes as the requirements of a reinforcement schedule become more severe, such as when a ratio requirement is increased from fixed ratio (FR) 10 to FR 100. This question is similar to the economic question of how the *demand* for a commodity changes as its price increases. Economists use the term **elastic demand** if the amount of a commodity purchased decreases markedly when its price increases. Demand is typically elastic when close substitutes for the product are readily available. For example, the demand for a specific brand of cola would probably drop dramatically if its price increased by 50%, because people would switch to other brands, which taste about the same. Conversely, the term **inelastic demand** means changes in price of a product have relatively little effect on the amount purchased. This is generally the case for products with no close substitutes. In modern society, the demand for gasoline is fairly inelastic because many people have no alternative to driving their cars to work, school, shopping centers, and so on.

One way behavioral economists can measure demand with people is simply by using a questionnaire format. In one study, college students were asked to estimate how much alcohol they would consume during an evening at a bar, depending on the prices of the drinks (which ranged from free drinks to $9 per drink). Figure 8-8 shows that the students' answers conformed to a typical **demand curve**—they estimated that they would drink a lot if the drinks were free or inexpensive, but their estimated consumption decreased steadily as the prices of the drinks increased (Murphy, MacKillop, Skidmore, & Pederson, 2009).

Demand curves can be obtained from animals by measuring how much they respond for a particular type of reinforcer while increasing the "price" by requiring more and more responses per reinforcer. For example, Madden, Smethells, Ewan, and Hursh (2007) had rats press a lever for food pellets on schedules that ranged from FR 1 to FR 200 or higher. The food pellets were formulated to satisfy all the rats' dietary needs. The data are shown as triangles in Figure 8-9. As the size of the FR schedule increased, the rats' demand for food decreased, but only slightly. In another phase of this experiment, the researchers used the

same procedure to obtain demand curves when the reinforcer was fat (a liquid consisting of corn oil mixed in water, which provided calories but was not a complete diet). As shown by the open circles in Figure 8-9, the demand for fat was more elastic than for food pellets—as the size of the FR schedules increased, the rats' consumption of fat decreased much more sharply.

Besides providing examples of two reinforcers with different elasticities of demand, this experiment shows that deciding which of two reinforcers is "stronger" is a complex question with no simple answer. Notice that with very small FR schedules, the rats earned more fat reinforcers than food pellets, but with larger FR schedules they earned more food pellets than fat reinforcers. Which, then, is the more effective reinforcer? One possible answer to this question is to determine which reinforcer has the higher *peak output* (the reinforcement schedule at which the individual makes the most total responses, which can be calculated by multiplying the number of reinforcers earned times the size of the ratio schedule). In Figure 8-9, these points are marked

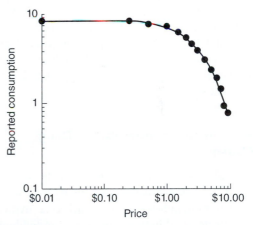

FIGURE 8-8 A demand curve obtained by asking college students about how much alcohol they would consume in an evening at different prices per drink.

SOURCE: From Murphy, J.G., MacKillop, J., Skidmore, J.R., Pederson, A.A., "Reliability and validity of a demand curve measure of alcohol reinforcement," *Experimental and Clinical Psychopharmacology, 17*(6), December 2009, 396–404, ©American Psychological Association. Reprinted with permission.

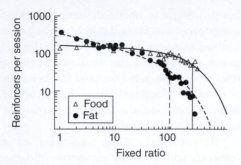

FIGURE 8-9 Demand curves for food pellets and for fat, obtained by having rats work for these two reinforcers on different FR schedules. (From Madden et al., 2007).

by the vertical lines, and they show that food pellets had a higher peak output than fat. However, other researchers have proposed other ways to compare the strengths of two different reinforcers, such as by measuring which is preferred in a choice situation, which can sustain the highest response ratio before an animal stops responding, and other measures (Herrnstein, 1961; Hursh & Silberberg, 2008). Unfortunately, these different measures of reinforcer strength do not always give the same answer (Bickel, Marsch, & Carroll, 2000; Shahan, Bickel, Madden, & Badger, 1999). Psychologists and behavioral economists are still debating this matter, but for now at least, a seemingly simple question "Which of two reinforcers is stronger?" does not appear to have a simple answer.

Behavioral Economics and Drug Abuse

Animal experiments can often provide valuable information about matters that are of great importance to human behavior. One such area involves the effects of addictive drugs on an individual's behavior. Many laboratory experiments have examined how animals respond when given the opportunity to work to obtain drugs such as alcohol, heroin, or cocaine. One general finding is that these drugs can serve as powerful reinforcers for animals ranging from rats to monkeys. In addition, it is possible to use economic concepts to analyze the effects of a drug more precisely.

For example, some studies have used animal subjects to measure the elasticity of different drugs. Animals may be allowed to work for drugs on FR schedules of different sizes to determine how the "price" of the drug affects consumption. Surprisingly, studies with animals have found that some drugs considered to be highly addictive have relatively elastic demand. For instance, one experiment with rats found that demand for cocaine was much more elastic than demand for food (Christensen, Silberberg, Hursh, Huntsberry, & Riley, 2008).

Research with animals has also found that other factors besides price can affect demand for a drug, such as the availability of substitutes and competition from other reinforcers. For instance, in one study, baboons had to choose between food and intravenous injections of heroin. When both were plentiful (a choice was available every 2 minutes), the baboons chose the two alternatives about equally often, and as a result they consumed a good deal of heroin. But when the two reinforcers were less plentiful (a choice was available only every 12 minutes), the baboons chose food most of the time, and their consumption of heroin decreased dramatically (Elsmore, Fletcher, Conrad, & Sodetz, 1980). Studies like these show that even addictive drugs conform to standard economic principles of supply and demand, and that drug consumption will decrease if the cost gets high enough. Furthermore, it does not always take a manipulation as extreme as decreasing the availability of food to reduce drug consumption. Carroll (1993) showed that rhesus monkeys' demand for the drug PCP could be substantially reduced simply by giving them access to saccharin as an alternative reinforcer, and similar results have been obtained with other addictive drugs.

Research using the behavioral economic approach to drug addiction has also been conducted with human participants, involving such drugs as nicotine, caffeine, alcohol, and heroin. As with the animal studies, this research has shown that economic principles can be applied to drugs just as well as to other commodities. For instance, as the price of a drug increases, or as substitute reinforcers become more available, drug consumption declines (Bickel, DeGrandpre, & Higgins, 1995). This research can help to analyze the effectiveness of different treatments for drug addictions. Consider the strategy of treating heroin addicts by giving them methadone as a substitute. In economic terms, methadone is an imperfect substitute for heroin because it delivers some but not all of the reinforcing properties of heroin. More specifically, methadone prevents the withdrawal symptoms associated with heroin abstinence, but it does not provide the euphoria, or "high," that heroin does. In addition, for a drug user, the clinical setting in which methadone is administered may not be as reinforcing as the social environment in which heroin is typically used (Hursh, 1991). For these reasons, it would be a mistake to expect the availability of methadone treatment to eliminate heroin use, even if the treatment were freely and easily available to all those who currently use heroin.

Vuchinich (1999) has argued that to reduce drug abuse in our society, a multifaceted approach is best. First, the cost of using drugs should be increased through stricter drug enforcement policies that reduce the supply. Second, the community must make sure that reinforcers are available for other, non-drug activities. For young people who may be tempted to experiment with drugs, sports and recreational programs that require participants to avoid drugs may be effective. For recovering addicts, the alternative reinforcers can be provided by supportive family and friends, and a job that demands a drug-free employee. Third, Vuchinich emphasizes that the reinforcers for non-drug activities should be ones that can be delivered promptly, because delayed reinforcers are notoriously ineffective.

Other Applications

Behavioral economic principles have been applied to other behavior problems, including smoking, overeating, and compulsive gambling (Bickel & Vuchinich, 2000; Cherukupalli, 2010). One important theme of the behavioral economic approach is that although it can sometimes be difficult to change such behaviors, it is not impossible. Behavioral economists and psychologists

argue that these problem behaviors should not be viewed as incurable diseases, but rather as economic behaviors that follow the same principles as do other behaviors (Heyman, 2009). Whether one uses the terminology of economics (supply, demand, elasticity) or of learning theory (reinforcement, punishment, stimulus control), these behaviors can be changed by appropriate modifications in the individual's environment.

As the field of behavioral economics has grown, researchers have used behavioral principles to analyze an increasing variety of topics, such as how much time supermarket shoppers take to make decisions on high-priced versus low-priced items (Oliveira-Castro, 2003), when customers do and do not use a maximization strategy when choosing between different brands of products (Foxall & Schrezenmaier, 2003), and what factors affect how Internet shoppers choose between similar items that are offered at different prices (Suri, Long, & Monroe, 2003). It seems likely that in future years, many other economic questions will be analyzed using behavioral principles.

PRACTICE QUIZ (2)

1. The fact that such things as sex and artificial sweeteners are reinforcers is a problem for _____ theory.
2. The fact that visual stimulation, exercise, and horror films can be reinforcers is a problem for _____ theory.
3. According to Premack's principle, _____ behaviors will reinforce _____ behaviors.
4. The procedure of using a series of test conditions to determine what is maintaining a person's maladaptive behavior is called _____.
5. If the demand for a product decreases sharply when its price increases, demand for the product is called _____.

Answers

1. need-reduction 2. drive-reduction 3. more probable, less probable 4. functional analysis 5. elastic

Summary

Thorndike predicted that an individual must actively respond for learning to occur, but experiments in which animals were passively transported through mazes showed that they learned without active responding. In the latent learning experiment of Tolman and Honzik, rats showed immediate improvement in their performance once food was presented at the end of a maze. Tolman and Honzik concluded that the rats had learned the maze without reinforcement, but that reinforcement was necessary before they would perform the correct responses.

Studies have shown that animals develop expectations about what reinforcer will be delivered and may appear surprised if the reinforcer is changed. Other research has shown that animals develop specific associations among all three components of the three-term contingency—the discriminative stimulus, the operant response, and the reinforcer.

Studies with animals found that reinforcement can control visceral responses such as heart rate and stomach activity, but some of these findings have been difficult to replicate. Nevertheless, research with human patients has found many useful medical applications of biofeedback, in which a person is given continuous feedback about some bodily process and attempts to control it. Biofeedback has been used successfully for headaches, some types of muscular paralysis, stomach and intestinal disorders, and a variety of other ailments.

How can we predict what will be a reinforcer? Hull's need-reduction and drive-reduction theories have obvious shortcomings. The principle of trans-situationality states that a reinforcer in one situation will be a reinforcer in other situations. Premack's principle states that more probable behaviors will reinforce less probable behaviors. But the best general rule for predicting what will be a reinforcer seems to be response deprivation theory, which states that whenever a contingency is arranged between two behaviors, the more restricted behavior should act as a reinforcer for the less restricted behavior.

The field of behavioral economics combines the techniques of operant research and the principles of economics. Optimization theory, which states that individuals will distribute their money, time, or responses in a way that optimizes subjective value, has been applied to many cases of animal behavior in natural settings. Other research has tested economic principles about supply and demand, elasticity, and substitutability among reinforcers using animal subjects in controlled environments.

Review Questions

1. How were the three different groups of rats treated in Tolman and Honzik's classic experiment on latent learning? How did each of the three groups perform, and what did Tolman and Honzik conclude?

2. Describe two experiments, using different procedures, that showed that animals develop expectations about the reinforcer in operant conditioning.

3. Describe one biofeedback procedure used to treat a medical problem. What type of feedback is given, how do subjects respond, and how effective is the treatment in the long run?

4. What are need-reduction theory, drive-reduction theory, and the principle of trans-situationality? What are their weaknesses? How do Premack's principle and response deprivation theory predict what will serve as a reinforcer?

5. What are some reasons why children with psychological problems may exhibit bizarre behaviors? How can a functional analysis determine the cause of such behaviors?

6. How can economic concepts such as price, elasticity, and substitutability be applied to drug abuse? How do addictive drugs compare to other reinforcers?

Stimulus Control and Concept Learning

LEARNING OBJECTIVES

After reading this chapter, you should be able to

- discuss the debate over whether generalization gradients are innate or learned, and evaluate the evidence for each position

- discuss the debate over whether stimulus control is absolute or relational, and evaluate the evidence for each position

- define behavioral contrast and discuss different theories of why it occurs

- define errorless discrimination learning and give examples of its use in behavior modification

- explain what is known about the structure of natural concepts, and describe the research on natural concept learning by animals

- describe some of the ways that stimulus control techniques are used in behavior modification

The relationship between stimuli and the behaviors that follow them is the topic of this chapter, a topic frequently called **stimulus control**. As we have seen throughout this book, predicting what response will occur in the presence of a given stimulus is a challenging task, even when the same stimulus is presented again and again in a controlled laboratory environment. But in the real world, all creatures are repeatedly confronted with stimuli and events they have never experienced before, and their survival may depend on an adaptive response. The topic of stimulus control also encompasses research on how creatures respond to such novel stimuli. In previous chapters we used the term *generalization* to describe an individual's tendency to respond to novel stimuli in much the same way that it has previously responded to similar, familiar stimuli. Now we will examine the process of generalization more closely.

In its overall organization, this chapter progresses from simple to increasingly complex relations among stimuli. We will begin with analyses of generalization among stimuli that differ only in their location on a single physical continuum, such as size or wavelength of light. Next, we will examine a more abstract sort of generalization in which the stimuli presented in two tasks are completely different and it is only the structures of the tasks that are similar. For instance, if an animal first masters a task in which one color signals reinforcement and another color signals extinction, will this experience help it learn a subsequent discrimination task involving not colors but two different shapes? Finally, we will consider the topic of concept learning, which involves the classification of different objects into a single category (e.g., "trees"), even though their visual appearances may sometimes have little in common.

GENERALIZATION GRADIENTS

Measuring Generalization Gradients

Suppose that we have trained a pigeon to peck at a yellow key by reinforcing pecks with food on a variable-interval (VI) schedule, and the bird now pecks at the key at a fairly steady rate. Now we wish to determine how much generalization there will be to other key colors, such as blue, green, orange, and red. How can we collect this information? One way is to use *probe trials,* in which the other colors are briefly presented to measure the pigeon's responding but no reinforcer is given. The probe trials are occasionally inserted among reinforced trials with the training stimulus. For instance, 90% of the trials might involve the yellow key light and the VI schedule, but 10% of the trials would include the other key colors and an extinction schedule. The advantage of embedding probe trials among reinforced trials with the training stimulus is that the procedure can continue indefinitely without the threat of extinction until sufficient data are collected. The main disadvantage of this procedure is that the pigeon may begin to form a discrimination between the yellow key and all other key colors, so that there will be progressively less generalization as the training proceeds.

Another method for obtaining generalization gradients is to start with the same type of training phase, in which the pigeon learns to respond steadily to the yellow key light, and then follow it with a series of extinction trials with both the yellow light and other colors. In this method, the trick is to obtain enough trials with each stimulus before responding extinguishes. Often this can be accomplished by keeping the durations of the extinction trials short.

With human subjects, other techniques for measuring generalization are available. For example, Droit-Volet (2002) first asked young children to listen to several presentations of a 4-second tone. The children were then given test trials with tones of different durations; they were told to respond by saying "yes" if it was the same 4-second tone and "no" if it was a different-duration tone. Droit-Volet obtained a fairly symmetrical generalization gradient, with the most "yes" responses to the 4-second tone and fewer "yes" responses to shorter or longer tones.

What Causes Generalization Gradients?

Why should reinforcement of a behavior in the presence of one stimulus cause this behavior to occur to similar stimuli that have never been used in training? Pavlov's (1927) answer was that generalization is an automatic by-product of the conditioning process. His basic idea was that the effects of conditioning somehow spread across to nearby neurons in the cerebral cortex. Although the details of Pavlov's theory are not accurate, his more general view that generalization is an inherent property of the nervous system seems quite sensible. Some more recent theories also try to explain the shapes of generalization gradients using reasonable assumptions about the wiring of the nervous system (e.g., Gluck, 1991).

A very different hypothesis was proposed by Lashley and Wade (1946). They theorized that some explicit discrimination training along the dimension in question (such as wavelength of light or frequency of tone) is necessary before the typical peaked generalization gradient is obtained. For instance, if the dimension of interest is color, they would claim that the learner must receive experience in which reinforcers are delivered when a particular color is present but not when the color is absent. Without such discrimination training, Lashley and Wade proposed that the generalization gradient would be flat; that is, the individual would respond just as strongly to all colors—there would be no discrimination among them. In short, whereas Pavlov proposed that generalization gradients are innate, Lashley and Wade proposed that they depend on learning experiences.

HOW EXPERIENCE AFFECTS THE SHAPE OF GENERALIZATION GRADIENTS. A nice set of experiments by Jenkins and Harrison (1960, 1962) provided support for the position of Lashley and Wade by showing that an animal's experience can have a major effect on the shape of its generalization gradient. Three groups of pigeons responded on a VI schedule for food reinforcement in the presence of a 1,000-Hz tone. The pigeons in the first group received **nondifferential training**, in which every trial was the same—the key light was lit, the 1,000-Hz tone was on, and the VI schedule was in effect. Once they were responding steadily, they received a series of extinction trials with different tone frequencies, and some trials had no tone at all. The results are presented in the top panel of Figure 9-1. As Lashley and Wade predicted, the pigeons in this group produced generalization gradients that were basically flat: Response rates were roughly the same at all tone frequencies!

Why did tone frequency have no effect on the pigeons' response rates? Jenkins and Harrison noted that for this group of pigeons, many stimuli were equally good predictors of the reinforcer: the tone, the illuminated key light, and the many other sights, sounds, and smells of the experimental chamber. If one of these stimuli (such as the key light) happened to be particularly salient, it might overshadow the other stimuli, just as one CS may overshadow another in classical conditioning. Perhaps the illuminated key light did indeed overshadow the tone, and as a result the tone exerted no control over responding—the pigeons pecked just as rapidly when the frequency of the tone was changed or when there was no tone at all.

Pigeons in the second group received **presence–absence training**, which included two types of trials: (1) trials with the 1,000-Hz tone and the VI schedule for food, exactly as in the first group, and (2) trials without the tone, during which the key light was lit as usual but no food was ever delivered. The 1,000-Hz tone would be called an S^+ (a discriminative stimulus for reinforcement) and the absence of the tone would be called an S^- (a discriminative stimulus for the absence of reinforcement). When these pigeons were later tested with other tone frequencies, they produced typical generalization gradients with sharp peaks at 1,000 Hz, as shown in the center panel in Figure 9-1. Notice that in this condition, the tone was the only stimulus reliably correlated with reinforcement (because the key light and the other sights and smells of the chamber were present both on reinforced trials and on extinction trials). Because it was the best signal for the availability of reinforcement, the tone came to exert control over the pigeons' responding, as witnessed by the sharp declines in response rate that occurred when the tone's frequency was changed.

A third group tested by Jenkins and Harrison (1962) received discrimination training in which the 1,000-Hz tone was the S^+ and a 950-Hz tone was an S^-. In other words, food was available on trials with the 1,000-Hz tone, but not on trials with the 950-Hz tone. This type of training is called **intradimensional training** because S^+ and S^- came from the same stimulus dimension (tone frequency). When tested with different tones in extinction, these pigeons produced much narrower generalization gradients, as shown in the bottom panel of Figure 9-1. These results provided further evidence that an animal's experience can have major effects on the shape of its generalization gradients. To account for this result, Jenkins and Harrison (1962) pointed out that a tone had many separate features—frequency, loudness, location, and so on. For the pigeons that received intradimensional training, the only reliable predictor of reinforcement was the tone's frequency, so the other features of this tone, such as loudness and location, should lose their control over responding. The sharper gradients from the

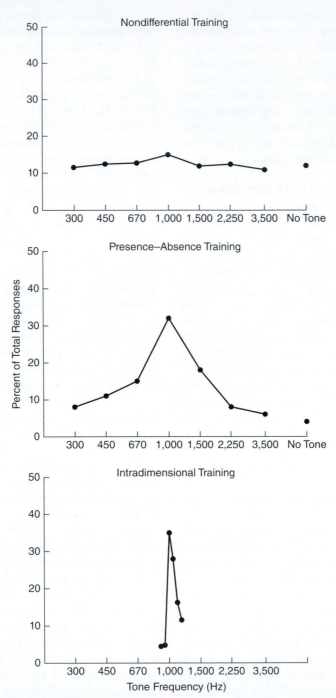

FIGURE 9-1 Generalization gradients for tone frequency in the experiments of Jenkins and Harrison (1960, 1962) after nondifferential training (top panel) and presence–absence training with a 1,000-Hz tone (center panel) and intradimensional training with a 1,000-Hz tone as S+ and a 950-Hz tone as S− (bottom panel). From H.M. Jenkins and R.H. Harrison, "Generalization gradients of inhibition following auditory discrimination learning," *Journal of the Experimental Analysis of Behavior, 5*(4), pages 435–441. Copyright 1962 by the Society for the Experimental Analysis of Behavior, Inc. Reprinted with permission.

pigeons that received intradimensional training are consistent with this analysis.

In summary, these results support Lashley and Wade's hypothesis that generalization gradients are dependent on an individual's experience. The story is not so simple, however. Other studies have shown that peaked generalization gradients can sometimes be obtained with nondifferential training. For example, Guttman and Kalish (1956) found peaked gradients with different key colors after pigeons received nondifferential training with a yellow key light. Results like these seem to support Pavlov's theory that no special training is necessary for generalization gradients to appear. In defense of their theory, Lashley and Wade suggested that although animals might receive only nondifferential training within an experiment, they may have learned from their everyday experiences prior to the experiment that different stimuli along the dimension in question can signal different consequences. Thus, the pigeons in the Guttman and Kalish experiment might have learned from their everyday experiences that color is frequently an informative characteristic of a stimulus; as a result, they were predisposed to "pay attention" to the color of the key in the experimental chamber.

HOW SENSORY DEPRIVATION AFFECTS THE SHAPE OF GENERALIZATION GRADIENTS. Once the possibility of pre-experiment learning is entertained, the Lashley and Wade theory becomes quite difficult to test: It becomes necessary to prevent the possibility of discrimination learning along the dimension in question from the moment an animal is born. Rudolph, Honig, and Gerry (1969) conducted such an ambitious experiment by raising chickens and quail in an environment that was illuminated with a monochromatic green light of 530 nanometers. (One nanometer, abbreviated nm, equals one billionth of a meter.) Because this special light emitted only a single wavelength, all objects appeared green regardless of their actual color in white light. (To envision what this visual experience is like, imagine watching a black-and-white movie while wearing green-tinted glasses: Everything on the screen would appear as a mixture of green and black.)

The birds were also trained to peck a green key for food. When tested with other key colors, the birds displayed typical generalization gradients, with peaks at 530 nm. Other experiments of this type found similar results (Malott, 1968; Tracy, 1970). These results clearly contradict the theory of Lashley and Wade, because they found normal generalization gradients with birds that had absolutely no prior experience with different colors.

To summarize, the research on the relationship between experience and generalization has shown that Pavlov's theory and Lashley and Wade's theory are both partially right and partially wrong. The experiments of Jenkins and Harrison found flat generalization gradients for the pigeons that had no discrimination training, and the type of training the pigeons received had major effects on the shapes of their gradients. In contrast, the experiments on sensory deprivation showed that peaked generalization gradients can sometimes be observed even when animals have no prior experience with a particular stimulus dimension. The results suggest a compromise position: In some cases, discrimination learning may be necessary before stimulus control is obtained; in other cases, no experience may be necessary. The evidence that, for birds, such experience is necessary for tones but not for colors is consistent with the idea that vision is a dominant sensory modality for these creatures. Perhaps we might say that birds are "prepared" to associate the color of a stimulus with the consequences that follow, but are "unprepared" to associate the pitch of a tone with subsequent events.

Now that we have seen that discrimination training can affect the shape of a generalization gradient, we will turn to a different but related topic. The next section examines the question of exactly what an animal learns when it receives intradimensional discrimination training, when one stimulus serves as S$^+$ and another as S$^-$.

IS STIMULUS CONTROL ABSOLUTE OR RELATIONAL?

Imagine a simple experiment on discrimination learning in which a chicken is presented with two discriminative stimuli, a medium gray card and a dark gray card. Approaching the medium gray card is reinforced, but approaching the dark gray card is not. This training is called a **simultaneous discrimination procedure** because the two stimuli are presented together and the chicken must choose between them. With enough training, the chicken will learn to choose the medium gray card. But exactly what has the animal learned? According to the **absolute theory of stimulus control**, the animal has simply learned about the two stimuli separately: It has learned that choosing the medium gray color produces food and choosing the dark gray color produces no food.

On the other hand, according to the **relational theory of stimulus control**, the animal has learned something about the *relationship* between the two stimuli: It has learned that the *lighter* gray is associated with food. The absolute position assumes that the animal responds to each stimulus without reference to the other; the relational position assumes that the animal responds to the relationship between the two. C. Lloyd Morgan (1894), an early writer on animal behavior, favored the absolute position because he believed that nonhumans are simply not capable of understanding relationships such as *lighter, darker, larger,* or *redder.* These relationships are abstract concepts that are not part of any single stimulus, and he felt that animals do not have the capacity to form such abstractions. An early advocate of the relational position was the German psychologist Wolfgang Kohler (1939). Now, many decades later, the question of whether animals can learn about relationships continues to be of interest to modern psychologists (Wright & Lickteig, 2010). Let us look at the evidence on both sides of this debate and attempt to come to some resolution.

Transposition and Peak Shift

In support of the relational position, Kohler (1939) presented evidence for a phenomenon called **transposition**. After training several chickens on the simultaneous discrimination task just described, Kohler gave the chickens several trials on which the two stimuli were (1) the medium gray card that had previously served as the S⁺ and (2)

a card with a lighter gray. Which stimulus would the chickens choose? If the absolute theory is correct, the chickens should choose the medium gray, because choosing that particular shade of gray had been reinforced in the past. However, if the chickens had learned to respond to the relation between the two training stimuli (choosing the lighter gray), they should choose the novel, light gray card. Across several extinction trials, all of the chickens showed a preference for the light gray card over the previously reinforced medium gray card. The term *transposition* is meant to convey the idea that the animal has transferred the relational rule ("Choose the lighter gray") to a new pair of stimuli (one of which happens to be the previous S⁺).

Kohler also found evidence for transposition with chimpanzees, and similar results have been obtained with several other species, including penguins (Manabe, Murata, Kawashima, Asahina, & Okutsu, 2009), rats (Lawrence & DeRivera, 1954), and human children (Alberts & Ehrenfreund, 1951). These results constitute one of the main pieces of evidence for the relational theory.

In research on generalization gradients, Hanson (1959) discovered a phenomenon called **peak shift** that is in some ways similar to transposition. Notice that whereas transposition is found in simultaneous discrimination tasks, generalization gradients are usually obtained by using a **successive discrimination procedure**—the stimuli are presented one at a time. In Hanson's experiment, pigeons in a control group received several sessions of training in which pecking at a 550-nm key light occasionally produced food, and they had no training with any other key color. In an experimental group, pigeons received intradimensional training with the 550-nm key light as S⁺ and a 555-nm key light as S⁻. After this training, Hanson measured the birds' responses to a range of different key colors during extinction so as to obtain generalization gradients.

The control group produced a typical generalization gradient with a peak at 550 nm, as expected. In contrast, the group that received intradimensional training produced a peak around 530 to 540 nm rather than at the previously reinforced wavelength. In fact, there was very little responding to the S⁺ (the 550-nm key light) in the generalization test. The term *peak shift* thus refers to a shift in the generalization gradient in a direction away from the S⁻.

Peak shift has also been observed with many other stimuli besides colors, such as stimulus duration (Spetch & Cheng, 1998) and the number of objects in an array (Honig & Stewart, 1993). It has been found with many species, including humans (Derenne, 2010; Okouchi, 2003).

The absolute position would seem to predict a peak at 550 nm for both groups, since this was the stimulus that had previously signaled the availability of reinforcement. The peak shift seems to favor the relational position, for the following reason. Lights of both 550 and 555 nm are greenish yellow, but the shorter wavelength is a bit greener. The pigeons that received intradimensional training might have learned that the *greener* of the two stimuli was a signal for reinforcement. This would explain why they responded more to the 530- and 540-nm stimuli, which are greener still. However, the relational position cannot explain why responding was much lower with wavelengths between 500 and 520 nm, which are the purest greens.

Spence's Theory of Excitatory and Inhibitory Gradients

A clever version of the absolute theory developed by Kenneth Spence (1937) can account quite nicely for both transposition and peak shift. The essence of the absolute position is that the subject learns only about the two stimuli individually and learns nothing about the relation between the two. Beginning with this assumption, Spence proposed that in intradimensional training, an excitatory generalization gradient develops around the S⁺ and an inhibitory gradient develops around the S⁻. Let us see how this process might apply to Hanson's experiment. Figure 9-2a depicts an excitatory generalization gradient around 550 nm and an inhibitory gradient centered around 555 nm. The term *associative strength* refers to the ability of each stimulus to elicit a response. Spence proposed that the net associative strength of any

stimulus can be determined by subtracting its inhibitory strength from its excitatory strength. For each wavelength, the result of this subtraction is shown in Figure 9-2b.

Notice that the S⁺, at 550 nm, has the highest excitatory strength, but it also has a good deal of inhibitory strength because of its proximity to the S⁻. On the other hand, a stimulus in the vicinity of 530 to 540 nm has considerable excitatory strength but relatively little inhibitory strength (because it is farther away from the S⁻). The result is that stimuli around 530 to 540 nm actually have a higher net associative strength than the S⁺ of 550 nm. If we assume (as Spence did) that the strength of responding in the presence of any stimulus depends on its associative strength, then Figure 9-2b predicts the type of peak shift that Hanson actually obtained.

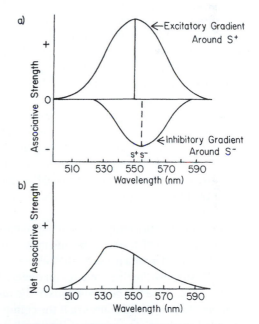

FIGURE 9-2 An analysis of peak shift based on Spence's (1937) theory. (a) Intradimensional training is assumed to produce an excitatory gradient around S⁺ (550 nm) and an inhibitory gradient around S⁻ (555 nm). (b) The net associative strength of each wavelength equals the difference between its excitatory strength and inhibitory strength. Because of the inhibitory gradient around S⁻, the peak of this gradient is shifted from S⁺ in a direction away from S⁻.

Recall that the relational theory cannot explain why responding was so low with stimuli of 500 to 520 nm. Spence's theory has no problem explaining these results. As Figure 9-2 shows, we need only assume that these wavelengths are so far from both S+ and S− that they acquired little excitatory or inhibitory strength. In short, Spence's theory can explain both the peak shift and the decreased responding with stimuli farther away from S+. It does a very good job of accounting for the results from successive discrimination experiments.

The Intermediate-Size Problem

Whereas Spence's theory does a good job of accounting for the results from experiments on transposition and peak shift, it does not predict the results on a test called the **intermediate-size problem**. Gonzalez, Gentry, and Bitterman (1954) conducted an experiment on the intermediate-size problem with chimpanzees. Their stimuli were nine squares of different sizes. Their smallest square (called Square 1) had an area of 9 square inches, and their largest square (Square 9) had an area of about 27 square inches. During training, the chimpanzees were always presented with Squares 1, 5, and 9, and they were reinforced if they chose the intermediate square, Square 5. (Of course, the left-to-right locations of the squares varied randomly from trial to trial so that a subject could not use position as a discriminative stimulus.)

On test trials, the chimpanzees were presented with different sets of three squares, and they were reinforced no matter which square they chose. As an example, suppose the three squares on one trial were Squares 4, 7, and 9. The predictions of the relational position are straightforward: If the chimps had learned to choose the square of intermediate size, they should choose Square 7. Figure 9-3 helps to explain the predictions of Spence's theory. The initial training should have produced an excitatory gradient around Square 5 and inhibitory gradients around Squares 1 and 9. Because Square 5 is flanked on each side by an inhibitory gradient, there is no peak shift in this case; instead, the inhibitory

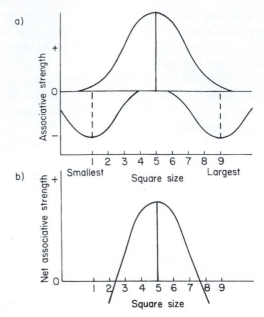

FIGURE 9-3 An application of Spence's (1937) theory to the intermediate-size problem. (a) In initial training, an excitatory gradient develops around S+ (Square 5) and inhibitory gradients develop around the two S−s (Squares 1 and 9). (b) Because of the two symmetrical inhibitory gradients, there is no peak shift in the gradient of net associative strength. There is only a sharpening in the generalization gradient.

gradients simply sharpen the gradient of net associative strength around Square 5. Thus, a chimpanzee should choose whichever stimulus is closer to Square 5 (Square 4 in the earlier example). The actual results favored the relational theory over Spence's theory: The chimps usually chose the square of intermediate size on test trials regardless of which three squares were presented. In short, the chimps behaved as though they were responding to the relationships among the stimuli, not their absolute sizes.

Other Data, and Some Conclusions

Lazareva and her colleagues have conducted a careful series of experiments designed to re-examine the debate over absolute versus relational stimulus control (Lazareva, Miner, Wasserman, & Young, 2008; Lazareva, Wasserman, & Young, 2005). Their subjects were pigeons, who were

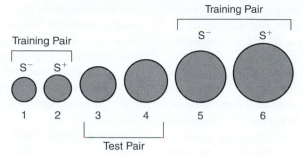

FIGURE 9-4   Examples of the types of stimuli and tests used by Lazareva and colleagues to compare the absolute and relational theories of stimulus control. After discrimination training with Circle 1 versus Circle 2, and training with Circle 5 versus Circle 6, pigeons were tested with a new pair of stimuli—Circle 3 versus Circle 4.

trained in simultaneous discriminations involving circles of different sizes. Figure 9-4 gives one example of the type of procedure they used. On some trials, the pigeons were trained with Circle 1 as S^- and Circle 2 as S^+. On other trials, they were trained with Circle 5 as S^- and Circle 6 as S^+. Therefore, in both cases, a choice of the larger circle was reinforced. Then the pigeons were given a choice between two new stimuli, Circles 3 and 4. Notice that Circle 3 is similar in size to Circle 2 (an S^+) and Circle 4 is similar to Circle 5 (an S^-). Therefore, Spence's theory predicts that through the process of generalization, the pigeons should choose Circle 3 over Circle 4. However, if the pigeons learned the relational rule of always picking the larger circle, they should choose Circle 4. The pigeons did show a preference for Circle 4 over Circle 3, which supported the prediction of the relational theory.

Lazareva and her colleagues concluded that although there may be some situations where animals respond to the absolute properties of stimuli as Spence theorized, most of the evidence now favors the relational approach to stimulus control. They also found that relational responding was stronger when their animals were trained with more examples (e.g., four different pairs of circles, with the larger circle serving as S^+ in every pair). It makes sense that giving animals more examples, all of them consistent with the same relational rule, should help them learn the rule better. In summary, they concluded that there is "strong

support for the idea that animals are indeed capable of relational responding" (Lazareva et al., 2005, p. 43).

BEHAVIORAL CONTRAST

Phenomena such as peak shift and transposition show that it is often impossible to predict how one stimulus will affect an individual's behavior unless we also take into account other stimuli— either those that are currently present or those the individual has encountered in the past. The phenomenon of **behavioral contrast** (Reynolds, 1961) offers another example that shows that stimuli cannot be judged in isolation.

An experiment by Gutman (1977) provides a good example of behavioral contrast. Like many experiments on behavioral contrast, Gutman's study used a type of successive discrimination procedure known as a **multiple schedule**. As discussed in Chapter 6, in a multiple schedule, two or more reinforcement schedules are presented one at a time, in an alternating pattern, and each schedule is associated with a different discriminative stimulus. The different reinforcement schedules that comprise a multiple schedule are called the *components* of the multiple schedule. In Phase 1 of Gutman's experiment, rats were exposed to a two-component multiple schedule in which the component schedules were identical: One VI 30-second schedule was signaled by a noise, and a separate VI 30-second schedule was signaled by a light. The light and noise were alternately presented every 3 minutes throughout a session. Not surprisingly, response rates to the noise and light were about the same in this first condition, as shown in Figure 9-5. In Phase 2, the schedule operating during the noise was switched from VI 30 seconds to extinction. Figure 9-5 shows that, as expected, responding became slower and slower during the noise. What was more surprising, however, was that response rates increased dramatically in the presence of the light, even though the reinforcement schedule for the light was not changed. This phenomenon, in which responding to one stimulus changes as a result of a change in the reinforcement conditions for another stimulus, is called behavioral contrast.

To be more specific, Gutman's study provided an example of **positive contrast**, because it involved an increase in responding during the unchanged light component. The opposite effect has also been observed. For example, suppose the noise schedule was switched and three times as many reinforcers

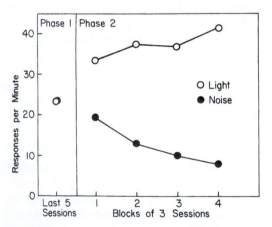

FIGURE 9-5   Results from Gutman's (1977) experiment on behavioral contrasts in rats. When both the light and the noise signaled VI 30-second schedules (Phase 1), response rates were about the same for both stimuli. When the noise signaled a period extinction (Phase 2), response rates declined toward zero when the noise was present but increased substantially above those of Phase 1 when the light was present. From A. Gutman, "Positive contract, negative induction, and inhibitory stimulus control in the rat," *Journal of the Experimental Analysis of Behavior, 27*(2), pages 219–233. Copyright 1977 by the Society for the Experimental Analysis of Behavior, Inc. Reprinted with permission.

were delivered in the presence of the noise. The likely result would be an increase in responding during the noise and a decrease in responding during the light. This decrease in responding during the unchanged light component would be called **negative contrast**.

Behavioral contrast has been observed with many different types of reinforcers and with many different species, from bumble bees to humans (Tarbox & Hayes, 2005; Waldron, Wiegmann, & Wiegmann, 2005). There are plenty of different theories about why it occurs. According to the *behavioral reallocation hypothesis,* faster responding in the unchanged component (positive contrast) is possible because of the slower responding that occurs in the component that is changed to extinction. The slower responding in the extinction component might allow the subject to recover from fatigue, so the "well-rested" animal can respond faster in the unchanged component. In addition, during the extinction component, the animal may be able to spend more time performing various activities that would normally compete for its time in the unchanged component (e.g., grooming, exploring the chamber). That is, the animal may pack more of these extraneous behaviors into the extinction component, so it has more time to perform the operant response in the unchanged component (Dougan, McSweeney, & Farmer-Dougan, 1986).

Another theory of behavioral contrast is the *reinforcer habituation/satiation hypothesis* (McSweeney & Weatherly, 1998). The basic idea behind this theory is the well-established finding that the more frequently a reinforcer is presented over a short period of time, the less effective it becomes, because of habituation, satiation, or both. Comparing Phases 1 and 2 in Gutman's (1977) experiment as an example, it should be clear that more reinforcers were presented in Phase 1 (when VI schedules delivered food during both the light and noise components) than in Phase 2 (when no VI schedule operated during the noise component). Therefore, there was probably less habituation and satiation to the food in Phase 2, which could explain why there was faster responding in the light component than in Phase 1.

A third theory of behavioral contrast focuses on the decrease in reinforcement in the changed component (Herrnstein, 1970). According to this account, an animal's rate of response in one component of a multiple schedule depends not only on the reinforcement available during that component but also on the rate of reinforcement in the adjacent components. To speak loosely, it is as though the animal judges the value of one component by comparing it to its neighbors. In the first phase of Gutman's experiment, the schedule during the light component was "nothing special," since the same schedule was available during the noise component. The light therefore produced only a moderate rate of response. On the other hand, during the second phase of the experiment, the light component was quite attractive compared to the extinction schedule of the noise component, so the light produced a high response rate.

In a thorough review of the many experiments and theories about behavioral contrast, B. A. Williams (2002) concluded that there are several different causes of behavioral contrast and that no single theory can account for all of the data. The effects of habituation and satiation probably contribute to the effect, as suggested by McSweeney and Weatherly (1998). In addition, there is evidence to support the sort of comparison process proposed by Herrnstein (1970) in which the value of a reinforcer is affected by what reinforcers are available in the neighboring components. However, Williams (2002) presented evidence that behavioral contrast is to a large extent based on anticipation of the upcoming component, rather than a reaction to the preceding component. For example, if a multiple schedule includes three components—A, B, and C—that are repeatedly presented in this order, responding in component B is affected by the schedule in component C, but not by the schedule in component A. Behavioral contrast is a complex phenomenon, and it is probably the product of a few different factors.

Although its causes are not completely understood, behavioral contrast demonstrates once again that it can be dangerous to study reinforcement schedules as though they were isolated entities. An individual's behavior on one reinforcement schedule may be greatly influenced by events occurring before and after the schedule is in effect.

> ## PRACTICE QUIZ (1)
>
> 1. Lashley and Wade proposed that generalization gradients were the result of experience, and without discrimination training, animals would show _____ generalization gradients.
> 2. In _____ training, one stimulus serves as a S⁺ and another stimulus on the same dimension serves as S⁻.
> 3. In the phenomenon of peak shift, the peak of the generalization shifts from the S⁺ in the direction _____ the S⁻.
> 4. Results from the intermediate-size problem favor the _____ theory of stimulus control.
> 5. Suppose an animal first receives reinforcers for responding in the presence of either blue or yellow stimuli, but then the schedule for the yellow stimulus switches to extinction. We would expect responding in the presence of the blue stimulus to _____, which is called _____ behavioral contrast.
>
> *Answers*
>
> 4. relational 5. increase, positive
> 1. flat 2. intradimensional 3. away from

"ERRORLESS" DISCRIMINATION LEARNING

Suppose that as a laboratory exercise for a course on learning, your assignment is to teach a pigeon a strong discrimination between red and green key colors. The red key will signal a VI 1-minute schedule, and you would like moderate, steady responding to this key color. The green key will signal extinction, so you would like no responding during the green key. You could begin by using food to shape pecking at the red key. At first, you would reinforce every response, and then gradually shift to longer and longer VI schedules (e.g., VI 15 seconds, then VI 30 seconds, and finally VI 1 minute). After several sessions with a VI 1-minute schedule on the red key, the pigeon would probably respond steadily throughout the session, and you could then introduce the green key color and its extinction schedule. From now on, sessions might alternate between 3-minute red components and 3-minute green components. At first, we would expect the pigeon to respond when the key was green because of generalization, but eventually responses to green should decrease to a low level.

This might sound like a sensible plan for developing a good red/green discrimination, but Terrace (1966) listed several reasons why it is not ideal. One major problem is that this method of discrimination training takes a long time, and along the way the animal makes many "errors" (unreinforced responses on the green key). Because the training must continue for several sessions before a good discrimination is achieved, there are likely to be many setbacks owing to the spontaneous recovery of responding to the green key at the start of each session. Perhaps because of the numerous errors, it appears that this type of discrimination training is aversive for the animal. For one thing, the pigeon may exhibit aggressive behavior, such as wing flapping. If another pigeon is present in an adjacent compartment, the pigeon may engage in an aggressive display and eventually attack the other animal. Such attacks typically occur soon after the transition from S⁺ to S⁻. A final problem with this procedure is that even after months of training, the animal's performance is usually not perfect—there are occasional bursts of responding to the S⁻.

Terrace (1963) showed that there is a better method of discrimination training, which he called **errorless discrimination learning** because the learner typically makes few or no responses to the S⁻. The errorless discrimination procedure differs from the traditional procedure in two main ways. First, rather than waiting for strong, steady responding to the S⁺, the experimenter introduces the S⁻ early in the training procedure. Terrace first presented the S⁻ within 30 seconds of the pigeon's first peck at the red key. Second, a fading procedure is used to make it unlikely that the learner will respond to the S⁻. Notice that in the procedure described earlier, the green key would remain on for 3 minutes the

first time it was presented. This would give the pigeon plenty of time to respond to the green key (and each response to green would be an "error" since these responses never produced food). However, in Terrace's procedure, the S⁻ was presented for only 5 seconds at a time at first, which gave the pigeon little chance to respond in its presence. In addition, Terrace knew that pigeons usually do not peck at a dark key, so at first, the S⁻ was not an illuminated green key but a dark key. Using a fading procedure, Terrace gradually progressed from a dark key to a dimly lit green key, and over trials the intensity of the green light was increased. In summary, in Terrace's procedure the S⁻ was introduced early in training, it was presented very briefly at first, and it was initially a stimulus that was unlikely to elicit responding.

Terrace's errorless discrimination procedure is an effective way to decrease the number of responses to the S⁻ and improving the learner's long-term discrimination performance. In one experiment, pigeons trained with a conventional discrimination procedure made an average of more than 3,000 responses to the S⁻ during 28 sessions, whereas pigeons trained with the errorless procedure averaged only about 25 responses to the S⁻. Because errorless discrimination learning can produce very good stimulus control in a minimum amount of time, variations of Terrace's techniques have been used in educational settings. B. F. Skinner (1958) maintained that classroom curricula should be designed so that the student almost never makes a mistake. His reasoning is that if we do not want children to avoid learning experiences, and if making an incorrect response (and thereby failing to receive reinforcement) is aversive, then we should try to eliminate these aversive episodes as much as possible.

In one example of an educational application of errorless discrimination learning, Duffy and Wishart (1987) used a fading procedure to teach children with Down syndrome to identify basic shapes such as ovals and rectangles. Some of the children were taught using a conventional trial-and-error method, using cards with three shapes, such

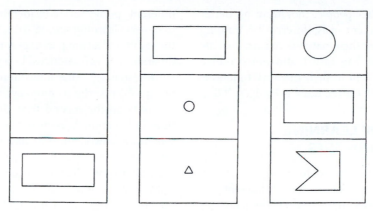

FIGURE 9-6   Examples of the types of cards used by Duffy and Wishart (1987) to teach children with Down syndrome the names of shapes. Errorless learning started with only the correct shape (left), then small incorrect shapes were added (center), and the incorrect shapes gradually became larger until they were the same size as the correct shape (right).

as the right-hand card in Figure 9-6. A child would be asked to "point to the rectangle" and would be praised if he or she made a correct response. If the child made an error (which happened frequently in the conventional procedure), the teacher would say, "No, that is not right. Try again the next time." The errorless learning procedure was exactly the same, except that at first the cards had only the correct shape and two blank spaces, as on the left-hand card in Figure 9-6. Not surprisingly, the children had little problem pointing to the correct shape. Then, very small incorrect shapes were added, as on the center card in Figure 9-6; over trials, the sizes of the incorrect shapes were gradually increased until they were the same size as the correct shape. Duffy and Wishart found that with the errorless procedure, the children made very few mistakes during training, and their performance remained slightly better at the end of training. They also reported that the children's attitudes toward the learning situation seemed to be better with the errorless procedure, perhaps because they did not suffer many failures.

Because of these advantages, errorless learning procedures, along with other techniques that gradually increase the difficulty of the discriminations, have frequently been incorporated in teaching procedures for children with mental handicaps (Mueller & Palkovic, 2007). However, there may be some drawbacks to using errorless discrimination

procedures with these children. After errorless training, the children may have difficulty learning discrimination reversals, in which the roles of S^+ and S^- are reversed (McIlvane, Kledaras, Iennaco, McDonald, & Stoddard, 1995). They may also have difficulty generalizing and maintaining their discrimination skills in new situations (Jones & Eayrs, 1992). Educators must therefore carefully consider the advantages and disadvantages when deciding whether to use errorless discrimination training or alternative techniques.

Adult learners can also benefit from errorless discrimination training. It has been used to teach job-related skills to patients with schizophrenia (Kern, Liberman, Kopelowicz, Mintz, & Green, 2002). It has been widely used to reteach adults information they have lost as a result of Alzheimer's disease or other brain disorders (Haslam, Moss, & Hodder, 2010; Robinson, Druks, Hodges, & Garrard, 2009). In one study, 12 patients in the early stages of Alzheimer's disease were given errorless training to help them relearn names of people they had forgotten. As a result of this training, the patients were significantly better at remembering the names of these people when they saw their faces, and the improvement in the memories persisted 6 months later. The improvement, however, was specific to those names and faces they had studied; when trying to remember the names of other people, they were no better than before. In other words, the errorless training techniques helped these patients relearn specific information they had lost; it did not produce overall improvement in their memory functioning (Clare, Wilson, Carter, Roth, & Hodges, 2002).

TRANSFER OF LEARNING AND LEARNING SETS

If animals are given many discrimination tasks, one after another, each of which has a different pair of stimuli as S⁺ and S⁻, they can get faster and faster at solving each new problem. Harry Harlow (1949) was the first to demonstrate this phenomenon. In a famous experiment, Harlow presented two monkeys with more than 300 different discrimination problems. Two different stimulus objects were presented on a trial. The choice of one stimulus led to food, and the choice of the other did not. The same objects were used as S⁺ and S⁻ for six trials, which constituted one discrimination problem. Then another two objects served as S⁺ and S⁻ for the second discrimination problem (another six trials), then another two objects for the third problem, and so on. On the first few discrimination problems, the monkeys' performance improved gradually over trials, reaching a level of only about 75% correct by the sixth and final trial. However, on later problems, the monkeys learned each new discrimination more and more quickly. After about 250 discrimination problems, they were able to master each new discrimination by the second trial (i.e., after only one trial of learning). They needed only one trial to determine which stimulus object was the S⁺, and starting with trial 2, they chose this object nearly 100% of the time. This performance suggests that the monkeys had learned a "strategy" that they could apply to each new problem: If your choice is reinforced on the first trial, choose this same object on the next five trials; if not, choose the other object on the remaining trials.

This improvement in the rate of learning across a series of discrimination problems has been given several different names: It has been called a **learning set**, *learning to learn*, and *transfer from problem to problem.* Some evidence suggests that

different species vary considerably in their ability to develop learning sets. Warren (1965) compared the results of learning-set experiments with several different species (conducted by a number of different researchers). After a few hundred discrimination problems, rhesus monkeys chose the correct stimulus on the second trial almost 90% of the time. Other animals, such as cats, develop learning sets more slowly, and rats and squirrels showed only modest transfer from problem to problem, even after more than a thousand discrimination tasks. Warren noted that there is a clear tendency for animals higher on the phylogenetic scale to develop stronger learning sets. It seems that one noteworthy characteristic of higher species is the ability to acquire more abstract information from a learning situation. That is, besides learning which specific stimuli are S⁺ and S⁻ in each discrimination problem, the higher species may be better at recognizing the similarities between problems and at developing a behavioral strategy that improves performance on subsequent problems.

Such cross-species comparisons must be viewed with caution, however, because the success or failure of one species may depend on exactly how the experiment was conducted. Although early studies suggested that rats show little transfer even after extended training, more recent studies with rats found substantial transfer after only a few dozen problems when odors or spatial locations were used instead of visual stimuli (Fagan, Eichenbaum, & Cohen, 1985; Zeldin & Olton, 1986). These results show that with stimuli of the right modality, rats can develop substantial learning sets after all.

Harlow's (1949) procedure of repeated discrimination problems provides just one example of a learning set. Another situation in which a learning set can develop is the *discrimination reversal procedure.* In this procedure, a subject first acquires one discrimination, and then the roles of S⁺ and S⁻ are periodically switched. For example, Harlow studied the behavior of eight monkeys in an experiment where S⁺ and S⁻ were switched every 7, 9, or 11 trials. Early in the experiment, the monkeys performed incorrectly for several trials after each reversal (which is not surprising since they had previously been reinforced for choosing the now-incorrect stimulus). However, after many reversals, they needed only one trial to correct their behavior; that is, after one unreinforced choice, they would switch to the other stimulus. In short, they had learned how to perform this task with a minimum number of errors.

Difficulty in switching choices in a discrimination reversal task can be an indicator of brain damage or psychological disorders. Rats with damage to the prefrontal cortex are slower to shift choices when S^+ and S^- are abruptly switched than control rats (Tait & Brown, 2007). Human adults with schizophrenia can also have difficulty shifting from S^+ to S^- when the reinforcement contingencies are switched (Turnbull, Evans, Kemish, Park, & Bowman, 2006). It is interesting to note that this sort of higher level discrimination learning can be disrupted in these cases even though simpler discrimination learning may be unaffected.

CONCEPT LEARNING

Many of the discrimination tasks we have examined in this chapter might seem quite artificial for three reasons: (1) The stimuli involved were simple, idealized images that an animal would be unlikely to encounter in the natural environment (e.g., a perfect square, uniformly red, on a plain white background); (2) only a small number of stimuli were used (the simplest of discrimination tasks involves only two stimuli, S^+ and S^-); and (3) from an objective point of view, the distinction between positive and negative instances was well defined and unambiguous. For instance, the S^+ might be a red square and the S^- a green square, and the animal would not be presented with any other shapes, nor with any squares that were a mixture of red and green.

In research on the topic of *concept learning,* or *categorization,* all three of these restrictions are removed. This research is designed to mimic more closely the types of discrimination an animal must learn in the natural environment. For example, when an animal learns to discriminate between predators and nonpredators or between edible plants and poisonous plants, (1) the stimuli

will generally not be simple, idealized forms, (2) there may be countless examples from each category of stimuli, and (3) the distinction between positive and negative instances of a category may not always be easy to make. Research on concept learning has explored how both animals and people learn to make such complex discriminations.

The Structure of Natural Categories

Eleanor Rosch (1973, 1975, 1977) conducted a series of experiments on how people respond to different members of "natural" categories— categories of objects found in the real world, such as birds, vegetables, or vehicles. Two of her most important conclusions were that the boundaries of these categories are not distinct, and that people tend to judge some members of a category as "good" or "typical" examples of the category and others as "bad" or "atypical" examples. Rosch used the terms **central instances** and **peripheral instances** to refer to typical and atypical examples, respectively. In one experiment, Rosch (1973) simply asked people to estimate the typicality of different examples of various categories. A 7-point rating scale was used, with 1 signifying a very typical instance and 7 a very atypical example.

Rosch reported that her participants found this an easy task, and different instances received very different rankings. For example, in the category of birds, *robin* received a mean ranking of 1.1, *chicken* a mean ranking of 3.8, and *bat* a mean ranking of 5.8. Thus, robins were judged to be typical birds and chickens much less typical; bats were treated as very marginal examples of birds. The example of bats illustrates how the boundaries of a natural category may be indistinct. Bats are not really birds at all, but many people probably do not know this, and they may consider bats as (atypical) members of the bird category. Conversely, whereas an olive is a fruit, many people do not classify it as such, and in Rosch's study it received a mean rating of 6.2.

Rosch described three important characteristics of natural categories. First, people tend to agree about which examples are central and which are peripheral. A second characteristic, related to the first, is that when people are asked to list the members of various categories, they list central instances more frequently. For instance, when Battig and Montague (1969) asked people to make lists of birds, *robin* was listed by 377 subjects, *chicken* by 40 subjects, and *bat* by only 3 subjects. A third characteristic is that in reaction-time tests, people take longer to decide that peripheral examples are members of the category.

It is interesting to speculate about how children learn to identify members and nonmembers of various natural categories. Language might play an important role: A parent may point to a robin and say "That is a bird." Later, the parent may tell the child that it is a robin, and that robins are one type of bird. Yet language alone cannot explain why natural categories have the structure they do (with central instances, peripheral instances, and ambiguous boundaries). Consider the fact that a child may be repeatedly taught "A robin is a bird" and "A chicken is a bird," yet the child will still judge the latter to be an atypical bird, and will be a bit slower to agree that a chicken is a bird. How can we explain this behavior?

Cognitive psychologists have proposed many different theories of human concept learning, including exemplar theories, prototype theories, and feature theories (with many variations of each). According to **exemplar theories** (e.g., Jäkel, Schölkopf, & Wichmann, 2008), a category such as *bird* consists of the memory of many individual examples of birds the person has seen. If a newly encountered instance is similar to the examples in memory, it will be judged to be a member of the bird category. According to **prototype theories** (e.g., Hampton, 2006), through experience with many birds, a person develops a prototype—an idea of what an ideal or typical bird is like. If a new instance is very similar to the prototype, it will be considered a central instance of a bird. If it is only moderately similar to the prototype, it will be considered a peripheral instance. If it is very unlike the prototype, it will not be considered a member of the bird category. According to **feature theories**, a person judges whether a given instance is a member of a category by checking for specific features (e.g., Spalding & Ross, 2000).

Members of the bird category might include the following features, among others: It has wings, feathers, a beak, and two legs, it sings, it flies, it perches in trees. A robin has all of these features, so it is judged to be a typical bird; a chicken does not, so it is judged to be less typical. There has been extensive debate about which theory of concept learning is best.

Regardless of how people manage to classify natural objects, the task is a complex one. Consider the natural concept of *tree*. For many people, the ideal tree might be something like a full-grown maple tree, with a sturdy brown trunk and a full canopy of large green leaves. Yet people can correctly identify objects as trees even when they have none of the characteristics of this ideal tree (e.g., a small sapling with no leaves, half buried in snow). Recognizing the impressive concept-formation abilities that people possess, some psychologists wondered whether any other animals have the ability to learn natural concepts.

Animal Studies on Natural Concept Learning

Quite a few experiments have examined natural concept learning by animals. Herrnstein and his colleagues conducted the first experiments on natural concept learning by animals, by having pigeons view slides of everyday objects or scenes (Herrnstein & Loveland, 1964; Herrnstein, Loveland, & Cable, 1976). In one experiment, Herrnstein (1979) chose to study the natural concept of *tree*: If a slide contained one tree, several trees, or any portion of a tree (e.g., a branch, a part of the trunk), it was a positive instance, and pecking at the response key was reinforced on a VI schedule. If the slide contained no tree or a portion of a tree, it was a negative instance—pecking produced no food, and the slide remained on the screen until 2 seconds elapsed without a peck.

In each session, a pigeon saw 80 different slides, half positive instances and half negative. In most sessions, the same 80 slides were presented, but in several generalization tests, some completely new slides were used. The first thing

Herrnstein found was that the pigeons quickly learned to discriminate between positive and negative instances. After only a few sessions, the pigeons were responding significantly faster to the positive slides than to negative slides. You might think that the pigeons did not learn anything about the general category of tree, but simply learned about the 80 slides individually. However, the generalization tests showed that the pigeons' accurate discrimination was not limited to the 80 slides used in training. When presented with slides they had never seen before, the pigeons responded about as rapidly to the positive slides and about as slowly to the negative slides as they did to old positive and negative slides, respectively. In other words, they were able to classify new slides as trees or non-trees about as well as the old slides.

Similar concept-formation experiments with pigeons have used many other categories besides trees. Among the concepts that pigeons have successfully learned are *people* (Herrnstein & Loveland, 1964), *water* (Herrnstein, Loveland, & Cable, 1976), *fish* (Herrnstein & de Villiers, 1980), and *artificial objects* (Lubow, 1974). They have also been trained to distinguish among the different letters of the alphabet (Blough, 1982). The ability to learn natural concepts has also been found in many other species, including monkeys (Schrier & Brady, 1987), orangutans (Marsh & MacDonald, 2008), dogs (Range, Aust, Steurer, & Huber, 2008), and mynahs (Turney, 1982).

One question that arises from this research is whether animals recognize that the two-dimensional slides or pictures that they view are actually images of three-dimensional objects. This is a difficult question to answer, but some research suggests that they can. Delius (1992) presented pigeons with actual three-dimensional objects that were either spherical (marbles, peas, ball bearings, etc.) or nonspherical (dice, buttons, nuts, flowers, etc.), and each choice of a spherical object was reinforced with food. The pigeons quickly learned to choose the spherical objects. They were then tested with photographs or black-and-white drawings of spherical and nonspherical objects,

and they chose the pictures of spherical objects with a high level of accuracy. In a related study, Honig and Stewart (1988) found that pigeons responded to photographs taken at two distinctive locations in ways that suggested they had formed concepts of the actual physical locations represented in the photographs. These studies show that, at least under certain conditions, animals can learn the correspondence between pictures and three-dimensional objects.

In a clever experiment by Watanabe, Sakamoto, and Wakita (1995), pigeons were taught to discriminate between the paintings of two artists, the impressionist Monet and the abstract painter Picasso. After they learned this discrimination with one set of paintings for each artist, they were able to correctly categorize new paintings by Monet and Picasso that they had not seen before. Furthermore, without further training, they were also able to distinguish between the works of other impressionist painters (Renoir and Cezanne) and other abstract painters (Matisse and Braque). The experimenters also tested the birds with some familiar paintings, but presented upside down or reversed left to right. With the abstract paintings of Picasso, this had little effect on the birds' accuracy. However, with Monet's paintings, which depict more realistic three-dimensional objects to the human eye, the birds made more errors with the upside-down or reversed images. This finding provides a bit more evidence that pigeons can respond to two-dimensional images as representations of three-dimensional objects.

Perhaps the most basic question about animal concept learning is the same one that is asked about human concept learning: How do they do it? The three classes of theories developed for human concept learning (prototype theories, exemplar theories, and feature theories) have also been applied to animal concept learning, and as in with human concept learning, there is no agreement about which type of theory is best (Huber & Aust, 2006). Nevertheless, a good deal has been discovered about animal concept learning, and there are some interesting similarities to human concept learning. A number of studies have shown that, like people, animals differentiate between central and peripheral instances of a category. For example, they respond more slowly to instances that contain only a few features of the positive category than instances that contain more positive features (Jitsumori, 2006). In some cases, they may display a stronger response to a prototypical example they have never seen before than to less central examples that they have seen before (Pearce, 1989).

Like humans, animals do not categorize complex visual stimuli simply on the basis of which individual features are present, but on how the features are arranged into a whole. Kirkpatrick-Steger, Wasserman, and Biederman (1996) taught pigeons to discriminate between line drawings of four objects: a watering can, an iron, a desk lamp, and a sailboat. They then tested the birds with line drawings in which the pieces of these objects were scrambled in various ways, to see if the pigeons could still discriminate the objects. The pigeons' correct and incorrect responses showed some interesting patterns. For example, one bird performed well with scrambled drawings of the watering can as long as the handle was above the base, but poorly if the handle was below the base. With drawings of the sailboat, this bird performed well when the two sails were properly aligned, side by side, but poorly if they were misaligned. Other birds showed similar sensitivity to the spatial arrangement of the objects' parts. These results indicate that the pigeons were not just responding to individual features in isolation; rather, relationships among the features were also important in their ability to recognize the objects.

Another characteristic of concept learning that is shared by people and animals is flexibility—animals can learn to classify stimuli according to a variety of different criteria, depending on what the task demands (Lazareva & Wasserman, 2010). They can classify instances as positive or negative either on the basis of the overall characteristics of the image or on the basis of small details. For instance, pigeons in one experiment had to categorize computer-modified pictures of human faces as male or female. The pigeons

could successfully use small textural details (the smoothness of the face) or large-scale features (the overall shape of the face), whichever was relevant for the particular set of slides with which they were trained (Troje, Huber, Loidolt, Aust, & Fieder, 1999).

As another example of flexibility, animals can also learn concepts that vary in their level of generality. Vonk and MacDonald (2004) tested orangutans' abilities to learn three classification tasks. The first, and most concrete, task was to distinguish between orangutans and other primates. The second task, which involved more general categories, was to distinguish between primates and other animals. The third task, involving the broadest and most general categories, was to distinguish between animals and non-animals. Notice that in the most concrete task, the positive instances (pictures of different orangutans) would have many perceptual similarities, whereas in the most general task, the positive instances (pictures of different animals) were perceptually much more varied. Nevertheless, the orangutans were able to learn all three tasks quite well. Others animals, including pigeons and monkeys, have also been able to learn more general concepts similar to those used with the orangutans, with varying degrees of success (Roberts & Mazmanian, 1988).

One area where the abilities of animals have been questioned is in learning concepts that involve abstract relationships. A simple example is learning to classify two instances as *same* or *different*. It might seem that deciding whether two examples are the same or not would be an easy decision, but it has proven to be surprisingly difficult to demonstrate this ability in animals. There has been considerable debate about whether learning abstract concepts is a uniquely human ability. There are, however, some studies with primates (J. Smith, Redford, Haas, Coutinho, & Couchman, 2008) and even with pigeons (Schmidtke, Katz, & Wright, 2010) that seem to demonstrate success at same/different discriminations. Whether animals can learn even more challenging abstract relations, such as analogies, will be examined in Chapter 10.

Developing Stimulus Equivalence

We have seen that both people and animals have a fairly easy time learning natural categories, such as trees, water, or even artists' styles. But what would happen if subjects were asked to learn a "category" of arbitrarily chosen objects—stimuli that have nothing in common except that the experimenter chose to put them all in a single group? Can subjects learn to treat an arbitrary group of objects as a category, and exactly what will they learn about the relationships among individual stimuli? The answer seems to depend on both who the subjects are and how they are taught.

If the subjects are human, a phenomenon known as **stimulus equivalence** can develop. Stimulus equivalence refers to a situation in which subjects learn to respond to all stimuli in a category as if they are interchangeable, even though they have been taught only a few relations between stimuli, not all possible relations. This is a fairly abstract statement, so let us take a concrete example. Suppose a young child is trained with six different geometrical shapes as stimuli. The shapes are not similar in an obvious way, but we will call them A, B, C, D, E, and F. On every trial, one shape is presented as a stimulus, and the child must choose between two other shapes by touching one or the other. On some trials, shape A is the stimulus, and the correct response is shape B, with shape D, E, or F as the incorrect alternative (see Figure 9-7). On other trials, B is the stimulus, and the correct response is C (again with D, E, or F as the incorrect alternative). The child is also taught to pick E if D is the stimulus, and to pick F if E is the stimulus. This training has therefore involved only four relations: A→B, B→C, D→E, and E→F. After this training, the child is tested with new choices that were never presented before. If C is the stimulus and the possible choices are B and D, the child will choose B. If A is the stimulus and the possible choices are C and F, the child will choose C. Do you see the pattern that is emerging?

Sample		Correct Choice	Incorrect Choices
A	→	B	D, E, or F
B	→	C	D, E, or F
D	→	E	A, B, or C
E	→	F	A, B, or C

FIGURE 9-7   Each letter represents a geometrical shape in an experiment on stimulus equivalence training. On each trial, a child is presented with one geometrical shape as a sample and two choices, one "correct" and one "wrong." In this example, the children are trained with four relations: A→B, B→C, D→E, and E→F. If they are then tested with new combinations, their choices will likely show that they have formed two equivalence sets, as illustrated by the two circles at the bottom.

Using a training procedure similar to this one and then testing with new combinations of stimuli and responses, Sidman and Tailby (1982) found that the children in their experiment had formed two equivalence sets, with A, B, and C in one set and D, E, and F in the other (as illustrated in the bottom of Figure 9-7), and they treated all members of one set as interchangeable. (Actually, Sidman and Tailby used more than six stimuli and two equivalence sets, but this simplified description gives the general idea of their experiment.) The important point is that these equivalence sets emerged even though the children were trained with only a few of the possible stimulus–response combinations.

This exercise with arbitrary shapes may sound like a strange intellectual game for children, and you may wonder why psychologists are interested in the development of stimulus equivalence. One reason is the belief that the ability to learn equivalence sets is similar to the ability to learn language. After all, written and spoken words are arbitrary stimuli that refer to objects or events in the world. For example, a child in elementary school must learn that the spoken word "six," the written word "six," the number "6," and the Roman numeral "VI" all refer to the same quantity. These different symbols constitute an equivalence set: They can be used interchangeably by a person who understands spoken and written English.

All language involves learning an arbitrary connection between some object or event in the world and a sound—the spoken word for that object or event. Some psychologists have therefore suggested that the ability to learn equivalence sets is closely related to the ability to learn language, and animals that do not use language should not exhibit stimulus equivalence. Indeed, some studies with nonhumans found no evidence for the development of stimulus equivalence, even after extended training (Dugdale & Lowe, 2000; Sidman et al., 1982).

Vaughan (1988) tried to show that pigeons could form equivalence sets if they were given suitable training. He presented 80 slides of trees to the pigeons, and he randomly assigned 40 slides to the positive category (in which pecking led to food) and another 40 to the negative category (in which pecking did not lead to food). Within a few sessions, the pigeons learned to peck at the positive slides and not to peck at the negative slides. This showed that the pigeons could learn the correct response for 80 individual slides, but it does not tell us whether they had learned to associate the 40 slides of each category. Vaughan then repeatedly reversed the positive and negative roles of all 80 slides every few days (with all positive slides becoming negative and vice versa). After a while, the pigeons demonstrated that they had learned to partition the 80 slides into two categories, which we might call equivalence sets. On any given day, if the first several slides of one category were positive, the birds would peck when other slides from that category were presented. Conversely, if the first several slides of one category were negative, the birds would not respond to other slides from that category. Vaughan concluded that the birds had learned two equivalence sets of 40 slides each.

Researchers using other experimental techniques have found additional evidence for stimulus equivalence in pigeons (Jitsumori, Siemann, Lehr, & Delius, 2002; Urcuioli, 2006; 2008) and in a variety of other species, from rats (Nakagawa, 1999) to sea lions (Kastak & Schusterman, 2002). It now appears that those who proposed that only humans can learn equivalence sets underestimated what other species could do. If they are given appropriate training, animals show an impressive ability to group unrelated stimuli into categories and to treat the members of a category as if they were interchangeable.

STIMULUS CONTROL IN BEHAVIOR MODIFICATION

Almost every instance of behavior modification involves stimulus control in one way or another. For instance, treatments of phobias are designed to eliminate a response (a fear reaction) that is under the control of a certain class of stimuli (the phobic objects or situations). What is special about the following examples, however, is that one of the main features of the behavioral treatment is the development of appropriate stimulus control.

Stimulus Equivalence Training

Procedures that were first used to teach stimulus equivalence in laboratory experiments, as described in the preceding section, are now being used in a variety of therapeutic settings. In some cases, stimulus equivalence training can assist children who are having difficulty learning to read. For example, one group of children was given practice in matching written words to spoken words and in writing printed words by copying them. After this practice, the children were able to read the written words (which they could not do before), even though the practice did not involve reading the written words out loud. Evidently, this training helped the children learn equivalences between (1) hearing a spoken word, (2) seeing the written word, and (3) reading the word out loud. Besides learning to read the words they had practiced, the children were also able to read other words that used the same syllables in different combinations (Melchiori, de Sousa, & de Rose, 2000). Similar procedures have been used to teach children with visual disabilities the braille alphabet by training equivalence relations among printed letters, braille letters, and spoken letters (Toussaint & Tiger, 2010). Stimulus equivalence training can also be used for more advanced academic skills. In one study, equivalence-based training was given to college students in introductory psychology in an attempt to teach them a difficult topic (the concept of a statistical interaction). On a post-test, students who were given the training obtained an average score of 92%, compared to 57% in a control group that did not receive the training (Fields, Travis, Roy, Yadlovker, De Aguiar-Rocha, & Sturmey, 2009). If stimulus equivalence training continues to produce encouraging results such as these, it will surely be used in more clinical and academic settings in the future.

Study Habits and Health Habits

Many different reasons explain why some students do poorly in school. One frequent problem among students who do poorly is that no matter where they are, studying is a low-probability behavior. Such a student may intend to study regularly but may actually succeed in doing productive work only rarely. The problem is simply that there are no stimuli that reliably occasion study behavior. A student may go to her room after dinner, planning to study, but may turn on the television or stereo instead. She may go to the library with her reading assignments but may find herself socializing with friends or taking a nap instead of reading.

Recognizing that poor study habits are frequently the result of ineffective stimulus control, L. Fox (1962) devised the following program for a group of college students who were having difficulty. The students were assigned a specific hour of the day, and they were instructed to spend at least a part of this hour, every day, studying their most difficult course. Furthermore, this studying was to be done in the same place every day (usually in a small room of a library or a classroom building). The student was told to take only materials related to the course into that room, and not to use that room on other occasions.

A student was not necessarily expected to spend the entire hour in that room: If the student began to daydream or became bored or restless, he was to read one more page and then leave immediately. The purpose of this procedure was to establish a particular time and place as a strong stimulus for studying a particular subject by repeatedly pairing this time and place with nothing but study behavior. Fox's reasoning was that other stimuli did not lead to study behavior because they were associated with competing activities (watching television, talking with friends), so it was best to select a new setting where it would be difficult for competing activities to occur.

At first, the students found it difficult to study for long in this new setting, and they would leave the room well before the hour was over. Gradually, however, their study periods grew longer, and eventually they could spend the entire hour in productive study. At this point, the therapist chose the student's second most difficult course, and the stimulus control procedure was repeated. Before long, each student was studying each of his courses for 1 hour a day at a specific time and place. If the student needed to spend more time on any course, he could do this whenever he wished, but not in the special room.

All of Fox's students exhibited substantial improvement in their grades. It is not certain how much of this improvement was due to better stimulus control, because the students were also given training in other techniques, including the SQ3R method (survey, question, read, recite, and review). However, setting a time and place for studying is at least an important first step. Other evidence suggests that combining stimulus control techniques with other behavioral methods such as self-reinforcement can lead to improved academic performance (Richards, 1981).

Stimulus control techniques have also been used to promote healthier lifestyles and combat obesity. Some of the techniques are designed to reduce overeating. For instance, because people often eat excessively while watching television, a simple but helpful strategy is never to allow yourself to eat snacks in front of the television (Gore, Foster, DeiLillo, Kirk, & West, 2003). Other techniques are aimed at increasing physical activity and reducing sedentary behaviors such as watching television and using computers. One group of researchers worked with obese children and their parents to try to reduce sedentary behaviors. The methods included having the children keep logs to record the amount of time they engaged in sedentary behaviors, posting signs around the house encouraging more physical activity, and limiting the number of hours the television was on (a technique known as **narrowing**, because the opportunities to engage in an undesirable activity are restricted). These methods proved effective—the children's levels of daily physical activity increased, and they lost weight (Epstein, Paluch, Kilanowski, & Raynor, 2004).

Insomnia

Most people have experienced occasional insomnia, but persistent, severe insomnia can be a serious problem. A person who lies in bed awake most of the night is unlikely to function well the next day. Although some cases of chronic insomnia are due to medical problems, many are the result of inappropriate stimulus control. That is, the stimulus of one's bed does not reliably produce the behavior of sleeping. The role of stimulus control becomes apparent if we compare the behavior of insomniacs with those of people without sleeping problems. A normal person exhibits one sort of stimulus control: She is able to sleep well in her own bed, but she may have some difficulty falling asleep in a different place, such as on a couch or in a hotel room. An insomniac may exhibit exactly the opposite pattern: He may have difficulty falling asleep in his own bed, but he may fall asleep on a couch, in front of the television, or in a different bed. This pattern shows that insomnia is often not a general inability to fall asleep, but a failure to fall asleep in the presence of a particular stimulus, one's own bed.

The reason a person's own bed may fail to serve as a stimulus for sleeping is fairly clear: The bed may become associated with many activities that are incompatible with sleeping, including reading, watching television, eating, and thinking about the day's events or one's problems. To make one's bed a more effective stimulus for sleeping, some behavior therapists recommend that the client never do anything but sleep there. Bootzin (1972) described the case of a man who would lie in bed for several hours each night worrying about everyday problems before falling asleep with the television on. The man was instructed to go to bed each night when he felt sleepy, but not to watch television or do anything else in bed. If he could not get to sleep after a few minutes, he was to get out of bed and go into another room. He could then do whatever he liked, and he was not to go back to bed until he felt sleepy. Each time he went to bed, the same instructions were to be followed: Get up and leave the room if you do not fall asleep within a few minutes. At first, the client had to get up many times each night before falling asleep, but after a few weeks he would usually fall asleep within a few minutes the first time he got in bed.

The techniques first devised by Bootzin have been used with many insomniac patients with good results (Taylor & Roane, 2010). The procedure is effective for at least two reasons. First, since the clients are instructed to remain out of bed when they cannot sleep, their need for sleep increases early in the program, when they spend a good portion of the night out of bed. Thus, when they go to bed, their chances of falling asleep are greater. Second, since the bed is used only for sleeping, its associations with other behaviors gradually decrease and at the same time its association with sleep increases. This type of behavioral intervention can now be delivered more precisely with the assistance of modern computer technology. Riley, Mihm, Behar, and Morin (2010) gave adults with insomnia small hand-held computers that recorded their sleeping and waking patterns. The computers provided the patients with customized instructions and prompts about when to go to bed, when to get out of bed if they were still awake, and so on. This technology is still being tested and refined, but preliminary results suggest that it can improve the sleep quality of people with chronic insomnia.

The usefulness of these procedures for training stimulus control may hinge on the reduction of incompatible behaviors. The student in a quiet room of the library will have little to do but study. In addition, those few behaviors other than studying that can occur (such as daydreaming) are prevented because the student is instructed to leave the room immediately if he or she stops studying. Similarly, the therapy for insomnia involves preventing the client from engaging in any behavior other than sleeping in one's bed. In a sense, then, these stimulus control techniques are the opposite of the procedure of reinforcing incompatible behaviors so as to eliminate an undesirable behavior. In the former, incompatible behaviors are prevented, and in the latter, they are reinforced.

PRACTICE QUIZ (2)
1. In _____, the S⁻ is introduced early in training, and it is presented in a way that makes it unlikely that the learner will respond to it.
2. A robin would be called a _____ example of a bird, whereas an ostrich would be called a _____ example.
3. To provide convincing evidence that an animal has learned a natural concept such as *fish*, it is essential to include _____ as test stimuli.
4. Treating all the examples in a category as being interchangeable, even the examples that were placed in the category at random, is called _____.
5. In some cases, a person may have difficulty studying in a particular location because that location is associated with _____.

Answers

5. many behaviors other than studying
3. examples never seen before 4. stimulus equivalence
1. errorless discrimination learning 2. central, peripheral

Summary

Pavlov proposed that generalization is an automatic by-product of the conditioning process, whereas Lashley and Wade proposed that experience is necessary for typical gradients to occur. Each theory seems to be correct in some cases and wrong in others. Some experiments found that discrimination training was necessary before typical generalization gradients appeared. However, experiments on sensory deprivation supported Pavlov's position by finding generalization gradients for color with birds that were raised in an environment with only one color.

Another question is whether stimulus control is absolute or relational. Spence's theory of absolute stimulus control can account for peak shifts in generalization gradients by assuming that an excitatory gradient develops around the S⁺ and an inhibitory gradient develops around the S⁻. However, this theory cannot explain results from the intermediate-size problem, which favor the position that animals can respond to relationships between stimuli. Other evidence also suggests that animals are capable of learning relational rules.

Terrace developed an "errorless" discrimination training procedure, in which the S⁻ is introduced very early in training, but under conditions in which the subject is not likely to respond to this stimulus. Errorless discrimination training has been successfully used in behavior-modification programs with children who have mental handicaps and with other populations.

Concept formation occurs when individuals learn to treat one class of stimuli as positive and another class as negative. Studies with pigeons and other animals show that they can learn such categories as tree, water, and people. Humans can also learn equivalence sets, in which random stimuli are arbitrarily assigned to different categories. Some psychologists have proposed that only humans can learn such arbitrary categories, but others claim to have evidence that animals can also learn them.

Stimulus control techniques are used in behavior modification when a desired response seldom occurs in the presence of the appropriate stimulus. For students who do poorly, a special location can be trained as a strong discriminate stimulus for study behavior. If a person's insomnia is due to poor stimulus control, the person's bed can be trained as a strong discriminative stimulus for sleeping.

Review Questions

1. What was Pavlov's theory about the cause of generalization gradients? What is another theory about them? What do experiments on discrimination training and on sensory deprivation tell us about this issue?

2. Describe the difference between the absolute and relational theories of stimulus control. What do studies on transposition, peak shift, and the intermediate-size problem indicate about these theories?

3. Give examples of positive and negative behavioral contrast. What are some plausible explanations of why they occur?

4. What is errorless discrimination learning? Describe how this technique could be used to teach young children the names of different types of flowers.

5. Describe some findings about natural categories in humans and some findings about natural category learning by pigeons. What do these studies demonstrate about concept formation by animals?

6. Give one or two examples of how stimulus control techniques have been used in behavior-modification programs. Describe some specific procedures that the client must practice in order for the treatment to work.

10

Comparative Cognition

LEARNING OBJECTIVES

After reading this chapter, you should be able to

- describe how short-term memory and rehearsal have been studied with animals

- describe how long-term memory has been studied with animals

- explain what is known about animals' abilities to measure time, to count, and to learn serial patterns

- discuss different attempts to teach language to animals and evaluate their success

- describe research on animals' abilities in the areas of object permanence, analogies, and metacognition

I n recent years there has been increasing interest in applying concepts from cognitive psychology (which previously focused almost exclusively on people) to animals. Through this interest a new field has emerged, and it has been called **animal cognition or comparative cognition**. A major purpose of this field is to compare the cognitive processes of different species, including humans. By making such comparisons, researchers hope to find commonalities in the ways different species receive, process, store, and use information about their world. Of course, when psychologists compare species as different as humans, chimps, rodents, and birds, differences in learning abilities are likely to emerge as well, and these differences can be just as informative as the similarities. The comparative approach can give us a better perspective on those abilities that we have in common with other species, and it can also help us understand what makes the human species unique.

This chapter will survey some of the major topics of traditional cognitive psychology, including memory, problem solving, reasoning, and language. We will try to determine how animals' abilities in each of these domains compare to those of people.

MEMORY AND REHEARSAL

A prevalent view about human memory is that it is important to distinguish between **long-term memory**, which can retain information for months or years, and **short-term memory**, which can only hold information for a matter of seconds. The facts in your long-term memory include such items as your birthday, the names of your friends, the fact that $4 + 5 = 9$, the meaning of the word *rectangle,* and thousands of other pieces of information. On the other hand, an example of an item in short-term memory is a phone number you have just looked up for the first time. If someone distracts you for a few seconds after you have looked up the number, you will probably forget the number and have to look it up again. Researchers who study animal memory have also found it important to distinguish between long-term and short-term memory, so it will be convenient for us to examine these two types of memory separately in the following sections. We will also examine animal research on rehearsal, a process that is important for both types of memory.

Short-Term Memory, or Working Memory

Besides being short-lived, short-term memory is also said to have a very limited capacity compared to the large capacity of long-term memory. Although your short-term memory is large enough to hold a seven-digit phone number long enough to dial it, you would probably have great difficulty remembering two new phone numbers at once. (If you do not believe this, look up two phone numbers at random and try to recall them 10 seconds later.) According to cognitive psychologists, because of the brevity and limited capacity of short-term memory, information must be transferred to long-term memory if it is to have any permanence.

In both human and animal research, the term **working memory** is now frequently used instead of short-term memory (Baddeley, 2010). This change in terminology reflects the view that the information in working memory is used to guide whatever tasks the individual is currently performing. For example, suppose you are working on a series of simple addition problems, without the aid of a calculator. At any given moment, your working memory would contain several different pieces of information: that you are adding the hundreds column, that the total so far is 26, that the next number to be added is 8, and so on. Notice that the information must continually be updated: Your answers would be incorrect if you remembered the previous total rather than the present one, or if you failed to add the hundreds column because you confused it with the hundreds column of the previous problem. In many tasks like this, people need to remember important details about their current task and to ignore similar details from already completed tasks. In a similar way, a butterfly searching for nectar may need to remember which patches of flowers it has already visited today, and it must not confuse today's visits with yesterday's.

Research with animals has examined different properties of working memory, such as its duration, its capacity, and factors that affect accuracy of performance. The following sections describe two techniques that are frequently used to study working memory in animals.

DELAYED MATCHING TO SAMPLE. As an introduction to this procedure, Figure 10-1a diagrams the simpler task of **matching to sample** as it has been used in experiments with pigeons. A suitable experimental chamber is one with three response keys mounted in one wall. Before each trial, the center key is lit with one of two colors (e.g., red or green). This color is called the *sample stimulus.* Typically, the pigeon must peck at this key to light the two side keys: The left key will then become green and the right key red, or vice versa. These two colors are called the *comparison stimuli.* The pigeon's task is to peck at the side key that has the same color as the center key. A correct response produces a food reinforcer; an incorrect response produces no food. Matching to sample is an easy task for pigeons and other animals, and at asymptote they make the correct choice on nearly 100% of the trials (Blough, 1959).

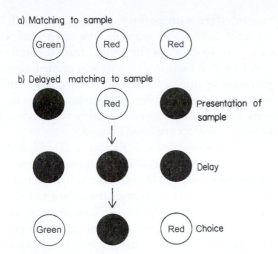

a) Matching to sample

b) Delayed matching to sample

Presentation of sample

Delay

Choice

FIGURE 10-1 (a) The procedure of simple matching to sample. The right key matches the center key, so a peck at the right key is the correct response. (b) DMTS. A peck at the right key is again the correct response, but now the pigeon must remember the sample color through the delay interval.

Figure 10-1b diagrams the slightly more complex procedure of **delayed matching to sample (DMTS)**. In this case, the sample is presented for a certain period of time, then there is a delay during which the keys are dark, and finally the two side keys are lit. Once again, the correct response is a peck at the comparison stimulus that matches the sample, but because the sample is no longer present, the pigeon must remember its color through the delay if it is to perform better than chance. Since one of the two keys is correct, chance performance is 50%. If the animal is correct more than 50% of the time, this means it has remembered something about the sample through the delay interval.

By using delays of different durations in the DMTS procedure, we can measure how long information about the sample is retained in working memory. The answer is different for different species. For example, the filled circles in Figure 10-2a show the accuracy of pigeons in an experiment by Grant (1975), in which the delay was varied from 0 to 10 seconds. The average percentage of correct choices decreased steadily with longer delays, and with the 10-second delay, the pigeons made the correct choice about 66% of the time. The results

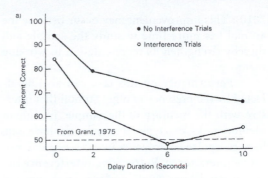

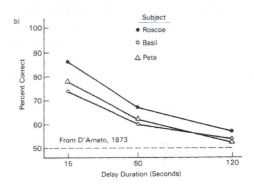

FIGURE 10-2 (a) Performance of pigeons in a delayed matching-to-sample task, where the delay between sample and choice stimuli was varied. (From Grant, 1975). Copyright 1975 by the American Psychological Association. Adapted by permission. (b) Performance of three capuchin monkeys in a delayed matching-to-sample task. Note that the scale on the *x*-axis is different in the two panels. From Grant, D.S., "Proactive interference in pigeon short-term memory," *Journal of Experimental Psychology: Animal Behavior and Processes, 1*(3), July, 1975, 207–220, © American Psychological Association. Adapted with permission.

from a similar study with three capuchin monkeys (D'Amato, 1973) are shown in Figure 10-2b. These monkeys were able to perform well with much longer delays, maintaining about a 66% success rate with delays of 60 seconds.

It is important to realize that functions like these do not depict a fixed or immutable time course of working memory for these species, because many factors can significantly alter the rate at which performance deteriorates as a function of delay. For example, the performance of pigeons on DMTS improves if the sample is presented for a longer duration (Kangas, Vaidya, & Branch,

2010). This improvement may occur because the animal has more time to study the sample and thereby strengthen its representation in working memory.

Performance on this task can also be affected by the presence of other stimuli that interfere with the memory of the sample. In human memory tasks, two types of interference have long been recognized: retroactive interference and proactive interference. **Retroactive interference** occurs when the presentation of some new material interferes with the memory of something that was learned earlier (i.e., the interfering material works backward in time—retroactively—to disrupt previously learned material). For example, suppose that in a list-learning task like the one used by Ebbinghaus (Chapter 1), a person memorizes List A, then List B, and then is tested on List A. The memorization of List B will impair the subject's memory of List A and lead to poorer performance than if the person never had to learn List B. **Proactive interference** occurs when previously learned material impairs the learning of new material. (In this case, the interfering material works forward in time—proactively—to disrupt subsequent learning.) For example, it might be easy to memorize one list, List D, in isolation, but this list may be much harder to learn if it is preceded by the memorization of Lists A, B, and C.

Both types of interference have been found with animals in DMTS. Retroactive interference can be demonstrated by presenting various sorts of stimuli during the delay interval. Not surprisingly, when the sample and comparison stimuli are different colors, matching performance is impaired if colored lights are presented during the delay interval (Jarvik, Goldfarb, & Carley, 1969). In fact, any sort of surprising or unexpected stimulus presented during the delay interval is likely to impair performance on the matching task.

To demonstrate the existence of proactive interference in DMTS, studies have shown that stimuli presented *before* the sample can impair performance (White, Parkinson, Brown, & Wixted, 2004). Proactive interference can occur if a series of trials are presented in rapid succession, because the memory of the preceding trials can interfere with performance on later trials (Wright, 2006). For example, the open circles in Figure 10-2a show the results from a condition in which each DMTS trial was immediately preceded by one or more interference trials, on which the opposite color was correct. As can be seen, performance was considerably worse when these interference trials were added.

A procedure that is similar to DMTS, but a bit more complex, is the **conditional discrimination task**. In a conditional discrimination task, the sample and comparison stimuli are not the same. For example, the sample stimuli might be red and green, and the comparison stimuli might be a horizontal black line and a vertical black line, each on a white background. The correct response rules might be these: If red, choose horizontal, and if green, choose vertical. In analyzing performance on this task, psychologists have tried to determine whether animals use retrospective or prospective coding to retain information in working memory. **Retrospective coding** involves "looking backward" and remembering what has already happened (e.g., "The sample was red"). **Prospective coding** involves "looking forward" and remembering what response should be made next (e.g., "Peck the key with the horizontal line").

An experiment by Roitblat (1980) found evidence that pigeons use a prospective strategy on a conditional discrimination task. (He was able to determine this by examining the pigeon's error rates when different sample stimuli were easy to confuse versus when different comparison stimuli were easy to confuse.) To put it simply, the pigeons appeared to be remembering which response to make, not which sample stimulus they had seen. However, Urcuioli and Zentall (1986) found evidence for retrospective coding when the sample stimuli were easy to discriminate and the comparison stimuli were not. A study with monkeys found that they also used both prospective and retrospective coding in a discrimination task and that these two types of coding were accompanied by activation of different parts of the cerebral cortex (Rainer, Rao, & Miller, 1999).

Variations of the DMTS task have also been used with humans. For instance, a participant may be presented with one or more sample stimuli (such as nonsense syllables or unfamiliar shapes). After a delay, a comparison stimulus is presented and the person must decide if it was one of the sample stimuli. Using the DMTS task along with brain recording techniques such as functional magnetic resonance imaging, researchers can identify which parts of the brain are involved in working memory (e.g., Kim, Matthews, & Park, 2010), and this research can help to understand various brain disorders. For instance, individuals with schizophrenia perform worse than normal adults on the DMTS task, and they also show different patterns of brain activity when they perform this task (Koychev, El-Deredy, Haenschel, & Deakin, 2010).

THE RADIAL-ARM MAZE. The DMTS task is quite different from anything an animal is likely to encounter in its natural environment. A somewhat more realistic task that involves working memory is provided by the **radial-arm maze**: It simulates a situation in which an animal explores a territory in search of food. Figure 10-3 shows the floor plan of a typical eight-arm maze for rats used. The entire maze is a platform that rests a few feet above the floor; the maze has no walls, so the rat can see any objects that may be in the

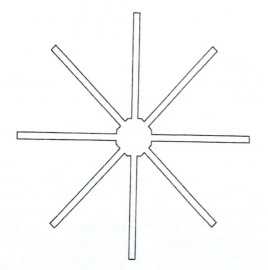

FIGURE 10-3 The floor plan of an eight-arm maze for rats.

room (windows, doors, desks, etc.). At the end of each arm is a cup in which a bit of food can be stored. In a typical experiment, some food is deposited at the end of each arm. The rat is placed in the center area to start a trial and is given time to explore the maze and collect whatever food it can find. Once the rat collects the food in one arm, it will find no more food in that arm if it returns later during the same trial. The most efficient strategy for obtaining food is therefore to visit each arm once and only once.

A good way for a rat to perform this task would be simply to start at one arm and then go around the maze in a clockwise (or counterclockwise) pattern. The rat could visit all the arms and make no errors, and this strategy would place few demands on working memory. However, there is good evidence that rats do not follow this type of strategy. Instead, they seem to select successive arms in a haphazard manner (Olton, 1978). Other studies have shown that rats do not use the smell of food to guide them and that they do not use scent markings to avoid repeat visits. What they do use to orient their travels within the maze are visual landmarks in the room surrounding the maze. The landmarks help the animals identify individual arms and keep track of which ones they have already visited (Babb & Crystal, 2003; Mazmanian & Roberts, 1983).

Perhaps the most remarkable feature of an average rat's performance on this task is its accuracy. The first visit to any arm is considered a correct response and any repeat visit is an error, because there will be no food. If a trial is ended after the rat visits eight arms (including any repeat visits), it will usually make seven or eight correct responses (Olton, 1978). This performance means that the rat is very skillful at avoiding the arms that it has already visited on the current trial. With larger, 17-arm mazes, rats still average about 15 correct responses out of 17 visits (Olton, Collison, & Werz, 1977), and similar performance has been obtained from gerbils (Wilkie & Slobin, 1983). Of course, the spatial working memory of rats does have limits: One study found a gradual decline in performance as the size of a maze was increased from 8 to 48 arms (Cole & Chappell-Stephenson, 2003).

It is commonly said that human working memory can retain only about seven unrelated items at once (e.g., seven words or seven random digits). With this number as a point of comparison, the nearly flawless performance of rats in a 17-arm maze is especially impressive. Equally impressive are the time intervals over which rats can remember which arms they have visited. Beatty and Shavalia (1980) allowed rats to visit four arms of an eight-arm maze, after which they were removed from the maze. If they were returned to the maze as much as 4 hours later, the rats were almost perfect in their selection of the four arms they had not previously visited. This finding shows why working memory is probably a more appropriate term than short-term memory. In research with people, short-term memory has generally referred to information that is lost in a matter of seconds, but a rat's memory for its travels in the radial-arm maze can last 100 times longer.

Do rats use retrospective or prospective coding in the radial-arm maze? Cook, Brown, and Riley (1985) found evidence for both types of coding, using a 12-arm maze for rats. Each 12-visit trial was interrupted for 15 minutes after 2, 4, 6, 8, or 10 visits. The rats' pattern of errors suggested that the rats used primarily retrospective coding during the first six visits or so and then switched to primarily prospective coding. Notice how this switch in coding strategies can serve to lessen the demands on working memory. For example, after two visits, a rat could use either retrospective coding to remember these 2 arms or prospective coding to list the 10 yet-to-be-visited arms. Obviously, the retrospective strategy is easier. But later in the trial, when faced with the choice of remembering, say, 9 visited arms or 3 to-be-visited arms, the prospective strategy of remembering the to-be-visited arms is easier. It therefore seems that rats (and other animals) have the capacity to use both retrospective and prospective coding, and they may tend to use whichever makes a task easier to perform (Zentall, 2010). However, there may be differences among species in the types of coding they can use. DiGian and Zentall (2007) had pigeons perform a task that was analogous to

a radial-arm maze, and they found evidence for only prospective coding, not retrospective coding.

SUMMARY. Research with DMTS and the radial-arm maze has substantially increased our understanding of animal working memory, which turns out to have many of the same properties as human working memory. Depending on the species and the task at hand, information in working memory may last only a few seconds or as long as several hours. Because the amount of information that can be stored in working memory is quite small, this information is very susceptible to disruption by either proactive or retroactive interference. Many studies have investigated exactly what type of information is stored in working memory, and these studies have provided evidence for both retrospective coding (remembering what has just happened) and prospective coding (remembering what remains to be done). Which type of coding dominates in a particular situation often seems to depend on which is easier to use in that situation.

Rehearsal

The concept of **rehearsal** is easy to understand when thinking about human learning. We can rehearse a speech by reading it aloud or by reading it silently. It seems natural to think of rehearsal as overt or silent speech in which we repeatedly recite whatever we wish to remember. Theories of human memory state that rehearsal has several different functions: It can keep information active in short-term memory (which is called **maintenance rehearsal**), it can promote the transfer of this information into long-term memory (sometimes called **associative rehearsal**), and it can help to plan future actions.

Because we tend to equate rehearsal with speech, it may surprise you to learn that psychologists have found good evidence for rehearsal in animals. Since animals do not use language, what does it mean to say that they can engage in rehearsal? With animals, rehearsal is more difficult to define, but it refers to an active processing of stimuli or events after they have occurred. Rehearsal cannot be observed directly; its existence can only be inferred from an animal's behavior on tasks that make use of short- or long-term memory. The available data suggest that rehearsal seems to serve the same functions for animals as it does for people.

MAINTENANCE REHEARSAL. We have already seen that information is retained in working memory for a short period of time and then is lost. Some researchers have attempted to show that animals can control how long information is retained in working memory. Their purpose is to demonstrate that working memory involves more than a passive memory trace that decays over time; rather, by using rehearsal, an animal can actively maintain information in working memory (Grant, 1981). This process of rehearsal can be thought of as a sort of covert behavior that an animal can learn to use or not use as the situation demands.

Evidence for maintenance rehearsal in animals comes from a technique called **directed forgetting**. When this technique is used with human participants, items such as pictures or words are presented, and after each item the person is instructed either to remember it or to forget it. The typical finding is that people recall more of the items they were instructed to remember, presumably because they rehearsed them (e.g., Quinlan, Taylor, & Fawcett, 2010). To examine directed forgetting with animals, a conditional discrimination task can be used (Roper & Zentall, 1993). On each trial, after the sample stimulus is presented, either a "remember cue" or a "forget cue" is presented during the delay that follows the sample stimulus. The remember cue tells the animal that it is important to remember the sample because a test is coming up (i.e., the comparison stimuli will soon follow). The forget cue tells the animal that it is safe to forget the sample because there will be no test on this trial. Therefore, the animal is "directed" either to remember or to forget the sample. If an animal can choose whether to engage in rehearsal, it should eventually learn to follow the directions and rehearse the sample when it sees the remember cue but not when it sees the forget cue. Once an animal is well trained on this task, occasional

probe trials are included—the forget cue is presented, but then (in what should be a surprise to the animal) the comparison stimuli are presented, and a correct choice is reinforced. The idea is that if the animals had learned not to bother rehearsing on trials with the forget cue, they should perform poorly on these occasional surprise quizzes. In one study with pigeons, this is exactly what was found: On probe trials that followed the forget cues, the pigeons averaged about 70% correct choices, compared to about 90% on trials with the remember cue (Maki & Hegvik, 1980).

Evidence for directed forgetting has been obtained with other species, including monkeys and rats (Miller & Armus, 1999; Roberts, Mazmanian, & Kraemer, 1984). In another experiment with pigeons, Milmine, Watanabe, and Colombo (2008) recorded the activity of individual neurons in the prefrontal cortex (a part of the brain associated with working memory), and they found significantly greater activity during the delay intervals after remember cues than after forget cues. Taken together, these studies on directed forgetting make a strong case that, like people, nonhuman animals can choose whether to rehearse information they have recently received.

ASSOCIATIVE REHEARSAL. Research on human memory has shown that rehearsal increases the strength of long-term memory. If people are given a list of items to remember and then given a distraction-free period (in which they presumably recite or rehearse the material in some way), their ability to recall the list items at a later time will be improved. In a clever series of experiments, Wagner, Rudy, and Whitlow (1973) demonstrated that rehearsal also contributes to the strength of long-term learning in classical conditioning with rabbits. They demonstrated that the acquisition of a conditioned response (CR) proceeds more slowly if some *posttrial episode* (*PTE*) that "distracts" the animal occurs shortly after each conditioning trial. They also showed that surprising PTEs are more distracting (interfere more with learning) than expected PTEs. Expected PTEs were sequences of stimuli that the rabbits had seen many times, whereas surprising PTEs were arrangements of stimuli that the animals had not seen before. During classical conditioning, the rabbits received a series of trials on which a conditioned stimulus (CS) was paired with an unconditioned stimulus (US) (a mild shock in the vicinity of the eye, which produced an eyeblink). For all rabbits, a PTE occurred 10 seconds after each conditioning trial. However, for half of the rabbits, the PTE was an expected sequence of stimuli, and for the other half, it was a surprising sequence of stimuli. The eyeblink conditioning to the CS developed much more slowly in the rabbits that received surprising PTEs.

The researchers reasoned that in order for a long-term CS–US association to develop, an animal needs a distraction-free period after each conditioning trial during which rehearsal takes place. The surprising PTEs distracted the rabbits and interrupted their rehearsal of the events that had just occurred, so the rate of conditioning was slowed. The expected PTEs caused less disruption of rehearsal because the rabbits had seen these PTEs before, so they had more time to rehearse, and they learned faster.

If this reasoning is correct, then the sooner a surprising PTE occurs after the conditioning trial, the greater should be the disruption of conditioning. To test this prediction, Wagner, Rudy, and Whitlow varied the time between the trial and the surprising PTE from 3 to 300 seconds for different groups of subjects. Figure 10-4 shows the median percentages of CRs to the new CS over the first 10 conditioning trials. As can be seen, the PTEs had their greatest disruptive effects when they closely followed each conditioning trial, and thereby kept rehearsal to a minimum.

REHEARSAL IN PLANNING BEHAVIORS. In their everyday activities, people will often engage in mental rehearsal to plan behaviors before actually performing them. Before you raise your hand to make a comment in a class discussion, you may think through the points that you are going to make. Before pushing your shopping cart down the aisles of a supermarket, you may think about the items you need and plan your route through the store. There is some evidence from behavioral and neurophysiological studies that nonhuman animals also engage in this type of mental rehearsal to plan behaviors before performing them.

In one study, monkeys were trained to watch a visual display in which the colors and

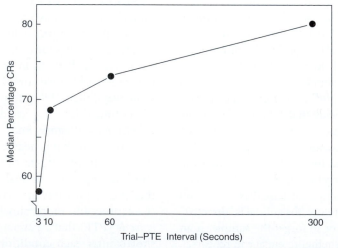

FIGURE 10-4 The four data points show the percentage of conditioned eyeblink responses in four different groups of rabbits in the Wagner et al. (1973) experiment. For each group, the x-axis shows the amount of time that elapsed between each conditioning trial and a surprising PTE. From Wagner, A.R., Rudy, J.W., Whitlow, J.W., "Rehearsal in animal conditioning" *Journal of Experimental Psychology, 97*(3) March 1973, 407–426, © American Psychological Association. Reprinted with permission.

movements of the objects indicated the direction in which they should move a pendulum with their hands (Cisek & Kalaska, 2004). If a monkey moved the pendulum in the correct direction, it received a sip of juice as a reinforcer. Once a monkey learned the task well, (1) its eyes moved toward the correct location on the display before the objects moved (which shows that it had learned to anticipate which way objects of different colors moved), and (2) individual neurons in the premotor cortex started to fire before the monkey moved the pendulum (with different neurons firing for different directions of movement). These results are not very surprising, because the premotor cortex is known to be involved in the control of bodily movements. More interesting, however, were the results from conditions in which a monkey watched the display and received juice, but its hand was not on the pendulum and no hand movement was required. Even though the monkeys did not move their hands in these conditions, (1) their eye movements again anticipated the movements of the targets on the screen, and (2) the same individual neurons in the premotor cortex fired as when they were actually performing the movements. The researchers suggested that the neural firings reflected mental rehearsal—the monkeys were anticipating the correct movements, even when they did not actually perform them. Other research has also found neural activity in the premotor cortex of monkeys that seems to be related to the mental rehearsal of previously learned behaviors (Dushanova & Donoghue, 2010).

Long-Term Memory, Retrieval, and Forgetting

Besides their different durations, probably the biggest distinction between short- and long-term memory is their different storage capacities. In contrast to the very limited size of short-term memory, the storage capacity of long-term memory is very large. It is probably safe to say that no one has yet found a way to measure and quantify this capacity for either animals or people, but some studies have demonstrated impressive feats of learning and remembering.

Vaughan and Greene (1983, 1984) trained pigeons to classify slides of everyday scenes as either "positive" (because responses to these slides were reinforced with food) or "negative" (because responses to these slides were never reinforced). Each slide was randomly assigned to the positive or negative category, so the first time a pigeon saw a slide there was no way to know if it was positive or negative, and on later presentations the bird could respond correctly only if it remembered that specific slide. Vaughan and Greene started with 40 positive slides and 40 negative slides. After about 10 daily sessions, the pigeons were discriminating between positive and negative slides with better than 90% accuracy. This procedure was repeated with three more sets of 80 news slides, which were learned in just a few sessions each. Finally, the birds were tested with all 320 slides, and their accuracy was still above 90%. Even when tested after a 2-year delay, the pigeons responded with over 70% accuracy, significantly better than the chance level of 50%. Taking this method even further, Cook, Levison, Gillett, and Blaisdell (2005) trained pigeons with over 1,600 slides, and they found accuracy levels above 75%. Equally impressive memory for pictures has been found with humans (Shepard, 1967).

Studies with other species of birds have demonstrated similar feats of memory, often involving memory for caches—sites where the birds have stored food. For example, a bird known as Clark's nutcracker gathers more than 20,000 pine seeds each fall and stores them in the ground in several thousand different locations. To survive the winter, the bird must recover a large portion of these seeds. Field observations and laboratory experiments have shown that nutcrackers do not use random searching or olfactory cues in recovering their caches. Although they may use certain characteristics of cache sites to aid their searches (e.g., the appearance of the soil above a cache), the birds' memories of specific visual landmarks and spatial cues are much more important (Kelly, Kamil, & Cheng, 2010; Vander Wall, 1982).

Research with scrub jays has shown that birds' long-term memory for caches is not limited to remembering the locations where food is stored. In one set of experiments, the jays were given both perishable and nonperishable food items to store in different cache sites, and they were allowed to search for the food items either 4 hours later (when the perishable items were still fresh) or 4 days later (when the perishable items were no longer edible). The jays would search at the sites of the perishable items after a 4-hour delay, but after a 4-day delay they would only go to the sites of the nonperishable foods. These experiments showed that the birds remembered not only where food was stored, but what type of food was stored at each location, whether it was perishable or not, and how long ago it was stored (Clayton, Yu, & Dickinson, 2001).

Other studies with animals have investigated the time course of forgetting from long-term memory, just as Ebbinghaus tested his recall of nonsense syllables after different intervals to construct a forgetting curve (see Chapter 1). The general shape of forgetting curves for animals is similar to the pattern in Figure 1-4: Forgetting is rapid at first, with a substantial loss during the first 24 hours, but subsequent forgetting proceeds at a much slower rate (Gleitman, 1971).

What causes the forgetting of information in long-term memory? For humans, a prevalent view is that interference from other stimuli and events, to which we are constantly exposed in daily life, is a major cause of forgetting (Wixted, 2004), and this view has substantial empirical support. Both proactive and retroactive interference have been observed in studies of animal long-term memory (Amundson & Miller, 2008; Engelmann, 2009). As an example of proactive interference, suppose that a pigeon receives several days of training on a discrimination task in which S⁻ is a pure green and S⁺ is a slightly blue-green. Then the roles of S⁻ and S⁺ are reversed for one session, and the bird learns to respond to the blue-green stimulus. If the bird is then tested on the following day,

the early training with green as the S⁻ is likely to interfere with the bird's memory of the more recent training, and it may respond more to green and less to blue-green. This is an instance of proactive interference because the memory of prior training impairs the memory of subsequent training.

If an individual forgets something that was learned long ago, is this because the memory has been lost forever, or is the problem one of retrieval failure (the memory is still there but it is difficult to find)? In research on human memory, there is evidence that many instances of forgetting are really cases of retrieval failure. Although you may not be able to recall some information on your first attempt (e.g., the Democratic elected president of the United States in 1980), you may succeed if you are given a hint (e.g., peanuts).

One phenomenon that supports the concept of retrieval failure is the **context-shift effect**: if you learn some new information in one context (such as a particular room), your recall of the information will be better if you are tested in the same context than in a new context (a different room). The context-shift effect has been found with both humans and animals (Millin & Riccio, 2004; Smith & Vela, 2001), and it shows how specific cues can help one remember things that would otherwise be forgotten.

Based on the idea that forgetting is often a problem of retrieval failure, many experiments with animals have shown that "forgotten" memories can be recovered if the animal is given an appropriate clue or reminder (Spear, 1971). For example, Gordon, Smith, and Katz (1979) trained rats on an avoidance task in which a subject had to go from a white room to a black room to avoid a shock. Three days after training, rats in one group were given a reminder of their previous avoidance learning: They were simply confined in the white compartment for 15 seconds, with no shock. Rats in a control group were not returned to the test chamber. Twenty-four hours later, both groups were tested in extinction to see how quickly they would move into the black chamber. The rats that had received the reminder treatment entered the black room significantly faster, presumably because the reminder served to revive their memories of their earlier avoidance training. The general conclusion from this line of research is that any stimulus that is present during a learning experience (including the room or chamber in which the learning takes place) can later serve as a reminder and make it more likely that the experience will be remembered.

The topic of memory is a very large one, and this survey has only highlighted some of the main theories and findings. There are, of course, differences between human and nonhuman memory, but we have seen that many characteristics of short- and long-term memory are similar in people and other animals. Both short- and long-term memory are important for many of the other cognitive tasks we will now consider. Whether an animal is solving a problem, learning an abstract concept, or counting stimuli, it must rely on long-term memory for background information about the current task, and on short-term memory for information about what has already happened and what is likely to happen next.

PRACTICE QUIZ (1)

1. DMTS is a procedure used to study _____ memory.
2. When the presentation of new material interferes with the memory of something learned earlier, this is called _____.
3. _____ rehearsal serves to keep information in short-term memory.
4. If a surprising event occurs soon after a classical conditioning trial, this will result in _____ conditioning than would have occurred without the surprising event.
5. If an animal seems to have forgotten some new learning, it is sometimes possible for the animal to recover the learning if given a _____.

Answers

1. short-term or working 2. retroactive interference
3. maintenance 4. less 5. reminder, or clue

TIME, NUMBER, AND SERIAL PATTERNS

Can animals sense the passage of time and estimate the duration of an event? Can they count objects, and if so, how many and how accurately? Can they detect orderly sequences of events in their environment? These questions are interesting because they all deal with abstract properties of stimuli. A 30-second television commercial may have nothing in common with a 30-second traffic light, yet a person can easily understand the abstract feature (duration) that makes these two events similar. In the same way, even young children can recognize what four blocks, four cookies, and four crayons have in common, even though the physical properties of these objects are very different. Determining whether animals can also recognize and respond to such abstract dimensions as time and number is not an easy task, but substantial progress has been made in recent years.

Experiments on an "Internal Clock"

Try to imagine what would happen in the following experiment. A rat is first trained on an FI 40-second schedule. A light is turned on to signal the start of each 40-second interval, and after the reinforcer, the light is turned off during an intertrial interval, and then the next trial begins. Training on this schedule continues until the animal's response rate in each interval consistently shows the accelerating pattern that is typical of FI performance. Now the procedure is changed so that on occasional trials no reinforcer is delivered—the light remains on for about 80 seconds, and then the trial ends in darkness. With further training, the animal will learn that a reinforcer is available after 40 seconds on some trials but not on others. For the first 40 seconds, however, both types of trials look exactly alike, and there is no way to tell whether a reinforcer will be available or not. How do you think the animal will respond on nonreinforced trials? Will it respond faster and faster throughout the 80-second period? Will it cease responding after 40 seconds have elapsed without reinforcement?

Figure 10-5 presents the results from an experiment like the one just described (Roberts,

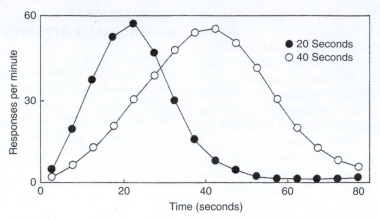

FIGURE 10-5 Pigeons' response rates in S. Roberts's (1981) experiment using the peak procedure. The filled circles show the results from trials with a tone that usually signaled an FI 20-second schedule. The open circles show the results from trials with a light that usually signaled an FI 40-second schedule. From Roberts, S., "Isolation of an internal clock," *Journal of Experimental Psychology: Animal Behavior and Processes, 7*(3), July 1981, 1242–1268, ©American Psychological Association. Adapted with permission.

1981). The open circles show that on trials without reinforcement, response rates started low, increased for a while, reached a maximum at about 40 seconds, and then declined. The location of the peak indicates that the rats were able to estimate the passage of time fairly accurately, since they responded the fastest at just about the time a response might be reinforced. It was no coincidence that the peak occurred at about 40 seconds. On other trials, a tone was presented instead of the light, and the tone usually meant that a reinforcer was available on an FI 20-second schedule. The filled circles in Figure 10-5 show the results from nonreinforced test trials with the tone, which also lasted for about 80 seconds. Again, response rates first increased and then decreased, but on these trials the peak response rate occurred at about 20 seconds. These results show that the rats had learned that the tone signaled a 20-second interval and the light signaled a 40-second interval, and in both cases they could estimate these intervals fairly well. This procedure for studying animal timing abilities is called the **peak procedure** because the peak of the response-rate function tells us how accurately the animals could time the intervals.

How accurately can animals distinguish between two events that have different durations?

Suppose a rat receives food for pressing the left lever after a 5-second tone and for pressing the right lever after an 8-second tone. Even a well-trained rat will make some errors on this task, but if the animal makes the correct response most of the time, we can conclude that the rat can discriminate between the two different durations. Experiments using this type of procedure with both rats and pigeons have shown that they can discriminate between two stimuli if their durations differ by roughly 25% (Church, Getty, & Lerner, 1976; Stubbs, 1968). This finding illustrates a principle of perception called **Weber's law**, which says that the amount a stimulus must be changed before the change is detectable is proportional to the size of the stimulus. Weber's law was first applied to human perception, but it applies equally well to animals. Thus, an animal may be able to discriminate between a 4-second tone and a 5-second tone (which differ by 25%), but not between a 10-second tone and an 11-second tone (which differ by only 10%), even though there is a 1-second difference in both cases.

This research shows that animals are fairly good at judging durations, but it does not tell us exactly how they measure the passage of time.

Some psychologists have proposed that every animal has an "internal clock" that it can use to time the duration of events in its environment (Church, 1978, 2003, 2006; Roberts, 1983). This internal clock is said to include a **pacemaker** that, much like a metronome, pulses at a steady rate and allows the animal to measure durations. Church (1984) and Roberts (1983) have proposed that in some respects an animal's internal clock is analogous to a stopwatch. Like a stopwatch, the internal clock can be used to time different types of stimuli. S. Roberts (1982) trained rats to press one lever after a 1-second tone and another after a 4-second tone. When the stimuli were then changed to 1- and 4-second *lights,* the rats continued to choose correctly without additional training. Like a stopwatch, the internal clock can be stopped and then restarted (e.g., if a stimulus light is turned off for 5 or 10 seconds and then turned back on).

Other theories of animal timing have been developed over the years, including the **behavioral theory of timing** (Killeen, 1991; Killeen & Fetterman, 1988) and the *learning-to-time theory* (Machado & Arantes, 2006; Machado, Malheiro, & Erlhagen, 2009). The details of these theories are complex, but in essence they state that animals can use their own behaviors to measure durations. For example, if a reinforcement schedule requires that the animal wait for 5 seconds and then make a response (a DRL [differential reinforcement of low rates] 5-second schedule; see Chapter 6), the animal might walk to all four corners of the experimental chamber and then make the operant response. In this way, the animal could time the 5-second interval with reasonable accuracy. The behavioral theory of timing also includes an internal clock that supposedly "sets the tempo" of the animal's overt behaviors. However, this internal clock is paced, not by an internal pacemaker, but by the rate at which the animal is currently receiving reinforcers. In short, this theory states that the rate of reinforcement controls the rate of the internal clock, which in turn controls the rate of the animal's behaviors, and the animal uses these behaviors to measure the passage of time. A series of experiments by Fetterman and Killeen (1991)

showed that pigeons' accuracy on timing tasks was determined by the rate of reinforcement, just as their theory predicted.

The experiments we have reviewed show that animals have fairly versatile timing abilities. They can discriminate between stimuli of slightly different durations, and they can transfer this skill from a visual stimulus to an auditory stimulus. They can time the total duration of a stimulus that is temporarily interrupted. They can time the total duration of a compound stimulus that begins as a light and then changes to a tone. An animal's ability to time events is certainly far less accurate than an ordinary wristwatch, but then so is a person's.

Counting

Many of the techniques used to study animals' counting abilities are similar to those used to study timing, and the results are similar as well. Procedures that require animals to count their own responses have shown that they can do so in an approximate way, just as the peak procedure showed that animals can roughly time the absolute durations of stimuli. In an early study on counting by animals, Mechner (1958) used a variation of a fixed-ratio schedule in which a rat had to switch from one lever to another after completing the ratio requirement. For example, if 16 responses were required, on half of the trials, the 16th consecutive response on lever A was reinforced. On the other half of the trials, the rat had to make 16 or more consecutive responses on lever A and then 1 response on lever B to collect the reinforcer. If the rat switched too early (say, after 14 responses), there was no reinforcer, and the rat had to start from the beginning and make another 16 responses on key A before a reinforcer was available. In four different conditions, either 4, 8, 12, or 16 consecutive responses were required. For these four conditions, Figure 10-6 shows one rat's probability of switching to lever B after different run lengths (where a run is a string of consecutive responses on lever A). We can see that as the ratio requirement increased, the average run length also increased in a systematic way.

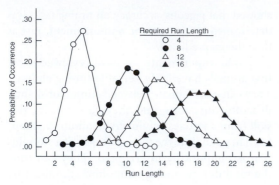

FIGURE 10-6 One rat's probability of switching from lever A to lever B after different run lengths in Mechner's (1958) experiment. The required run length is the number of consecutive responses required on lever A before a switch to lever B would be reinforced. From F. Mechner, "Probability relations within response sequences under ratio reinforcement" *Journal of the Experimental Analysis of Behavior, 1*(2), pages 109–121. Copyright 1958 by the Society for the Experimental Analysis of Behavior, Inc. Reprinted by permission.

When 4 responses were required, the most common run length was 5; when 16 responses were required, the most common run length was 18. Producing run lengths that were, on the average, slightly longer than required was a sensible strategy because the penalty for switching too early was severe. More recent studies with pigeons, using procedures similar to Mechner's, obtained very similar results, and they provided further evidence that number discrimination by animals follows Weber's law (Fetterman & Killeen, 2010; Machado & Rodrigues, 2007).

The counting abilities displayed by the rats and pigeons in these experiments were not exact: On some trials they switched too early, and on others they made more responses on lever A than necessary. In contrast, a person could learn to switch after exactly the right number of responses each time by simply counting responses. Can animals learn to count objects in an exact rather than an approximate way? A few studies suggest that they can, at least with small numbers. Davis and Albert (1986) found that rats were able to learn a discrimination in which three bursts of noise served as the S^+ and either two or four bursts served as S^-. Davis and Bradford (1991)

taught three different groups of rats to eat exactly three, four, or five food pellets per trial by reinforcing this behavior and punishing any attempt to eat more than the correct number of pellets. In another study on counting, Capaldi and Miller (1988) found evidence that the rats learned abstract concepts of number that could transfer from one type of stimulus to another. Some writers have proposed that counting is a skill that animals can learn only with difficulty, but Capaldi and Miller concluded just the opposite, stating that "rats assign abstract number tags to reinforcers readily, easily, and under most, if not all, circumstances" (1988, p. 16). Another study found evidence of a rudimentary counting ability in domestic dogs (West & Young, 2002).

Other evidence for an exact counting ability was presented by Pepperberg (1987), who trained a parrot, Alex, to respond to any number of objects from two through six by actually saying the appropriate number. In training, a number of objects (e.g., keys, small pieces of paper or wood, corks) would be placed on a tray, and Alex was reinforced if he said the correct number. For instance, the experimenter might present three corks and ask, "What's this?" The correct response would be "Three corks." Different objects were used on different trials so that Alex would not simply learn to say "three" whenever he saw corks. After a few months of training, Alex was responding correctly on about 80% of the trials. To show that Alex's counting ability was not limited to the training stimuli, new objects were presented on test trials. In some cases, Alex did not even know the names of the objects (e.g., wooden beads or small bottles), but he was able to give the correct number of objects on about 75% of the test trials with new stimuli. With somewhat less accuracy, Alex could count subsets of heterogeneous objects (e.g., with three keys and two corks, he would be asked either "How many keys?" or "How many corks?"). By arranging the objects on the tray in many different ways, Pepperberg was able to show that Alex was not responding to other cues, such as the length of a row of objects or the overall shape of the group (e.g., a diamond shape that might be formed by four objects). All in all, Pepperberg made a convincing case that

Alex could count up to six objects, whether familiar or novel, with a high degree of accuracy.

Matsuzawa (1985) has reported a similar counting skill in a chimpanzee (although naturally the chimp did not speak, but rather pressed response keys with the numbers 1 through 6 on them). Brannon and Terrace (2000) taught macaques to point to arrays of abstract shapes in order of increasing number: To receive a reward, the monkey had to first point to the array with one shape, then to the arrays with two, three, and four shapes. After learning this task, the monkeys were able to transfer this ability to arrays with between five and nine shapes, even though they had received no training with these larger numbers. These studies, along with Pepperberg's research with Alex, provide the best evidence available for accurate counting by animals.

Serial Pattern Learning

Suppose you are taking a calculus course with an eccentric professor who assigns a certain number of homework problems at the end of each class. He assigns 14 problems in the first class, 7 in the second, 3 in the third, 1 in the fourth, and 0 in the fifth. In the next 10 classes, the numbers of problems assigned are 14, 7, 3, 1, 0, 14, 7, 3, 1, and 0. After 10 or 15 classes, you may detect the repeating pattern of five numbers and thereby be able to predict how many problems will be assigned in each future class.

Hulse and Campbell (1975) wanted to know whether rats can detect such repeating serial patterns. They trained rats to run down a long runway that had food at the end. (The food could not be seen until a rat reached the end of the runway.) For one group of rats, the number of pellets available on each trial in the runway followed the repeating pattern described in the previous paragraph (14 pellets on the first trial, 7 on the second, etc.). With enough training, these rats showed that they had learned something about the cyclical pattern: They ran fast on trials with 14, 7, or 3 pellets, more slowly on trials with 1 pellet, and very slowly on trials with no pellets. The same was true for a second group in which rats were trained

with the reverse pattern (0, 1, 3, 7, and 14 pellets). For a third group, the number of pellets on each trial was chosen randomly (i.e., there was no pattern to be learned), and these rats ran at about the same speed on every trial.

It is clear that the rats in the first two groups had learned something about the serial pattern, but exactly what had they learned? One possibility (Capaldi, Verry, & Davison, 1980) is that they simply learned associations between adjacent items (i.e., that 14 pellets were followed by 7 pellets, 7 pellets by 3 pellets, etc.). Another possibility is that they learned a more abstract rule: The number of pellets steadily decreases over trials until there are none. To support this possibility, Hulse and Dorsky (1979) showed that rats were able to learn a steadily increasing or decreasing sequence in fewer trials than a sequence that decreased, increased, and decreased again—14, 1, 3, 7, and 0 pellets. Their explanation is that the learning was slower with this pattern because a more complex rule is needed to describe it. A third possibility is that the rats learned something about the overall structure of the sequence: that it is five trials long, that three pellets occur in the exact middle of the sequence, and so on. Roitblat, Pologe, and Scopatz (1983) provided evidence for this idea by training rats with the steadily decreasing sequence (14, 7, 3, 1, 0), and then giving occasional test trials with food missing somewhere in the middle of the sequence (e.g., 14, 0, 3, 1, 0). The trial with missing food had no detectable effect on how the rats performed on the remaining trials. The researchers concluded that the rats had learned the overall structure of the sequence, so that an occasional odd trial did not disrupt their performance during the rest of the sequence.

Fountain and his associates have studied how rats and mice can learn to perform impressively long patterns of response sequences (Fountain, 2006; Rowan, Fountain, Kundey, & Miner, 2001). In an octagonal chamber with a retractable lever in each of the eight walls (see Figure 10-7), a rat or mouse receives electrical brain stimulation as a reinforcer for performing the correct sequences. The right side of Figure 10-7 shows some of the sequences different rats were taught (where the

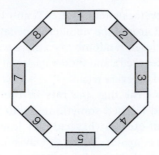

Sequence A: 123-234-345-456-567-678-781-812
Sequence B: 123-234-345-456-567-678-781-81**8**

Sequence C: 121-232-343-454-565-676-787-818
Sequence D: 121-232-343-454-565-676-787-81**2**

FIGURE 10-7 The floor plan of an octagonal chamber with a retractable lever in each of the eight walls. A rat or mouse could receive reinforcement for performing the correct sequence of lever presses. On the right are some of the sequences different animals were taught by Fountain & Rowan (1995), where the numbers refer to the lever positions as labeled in the diagram.

numbers refer to the lever positions as labeled in the diagram). Each sequence required a total of 24 lever presses, which were divided into groups of three lever presses, with a 3-second delay separating each group. After each correct response, two levers were presented (one to the left and one to the right of the last lever pressed), and the rat had to choose one of the two levers. In Sequence A, each group required pressing three levers in a left-to-right pattern. Then, after the 3-second delay, the rat had to go back to the left and start the next three-response pattern. This was an easy sequence for the rats to learn, presumably because of the similar pattern in each group of three responses (Fountain & Rowan, 1995). However, other rats had to learn Sequence B, which was the same except for the very last lever press, which was called a "violation" because it was an exception to the repeating pattern—the correct pattern was left-right-left instead of the usual left-to-right sequence. This proved to be a much harder sequence to learn—the rats made many errors on the final response, where a different response pattern was required. The findings were similar for Sequences C

and D shown in Figure 10-7: Sequence C was learned easily because of its repeating left-right-left pattern, whereas rats given Sequence D made many errors on the final response, which violated the pattern. However, although sequences with violations were difficult to learn, with enough training the rats were able to master them.

Based on results from many variations of this basic procedure, Muller and Fountain (2010) concluded that in learning these response sequences, animals first learn the general rule (the repeating sequence), and only later do they learn the exception to the rule. They also concluded that rats use several different types of cues to help them perform the sequence correctly, including the spatial locations of the levers within the chamber, the spacing of the groups of three responses, and memory for the position of the "violation" within the sequence. It seems that animals have a variety of strategies that they can use to learn complex response patterns.

Chunking

A common idea in human cognitive psychology is that memorizing is easier if a long list of information is divided into portions of more manageable size called **chunks** (Miller, 1956). For example, the telephone number 711-2468 consists of seven digits, which is about all that human short-term memory can hold at once. However, the burden on memory is lightened if "711" reminds you of the name of a chain of convenience stores, and if you remember "2468" as the first four even numbers. In this way, the problem of remembering seven pieces of information is reduced to remembering two chunks of information. Many studies of human memory have shown that organizing a list into chunks can help people remember more information more accurately.

Can animals also recognize chunks of information, and can they use the strategy of chunking to help them learn and remember a long list? Various experiments have shown that they can, including Fountain's experiments described in the last section, in which the long sequences were grouped into "chunks" of three responses. Terrace

(1991) used a different procedure to study how chunking can help pigeons learn and remember. The pigeons' task was basically a list-learning exercise: Five stimuli were presented in random locations on a translucent screen, and a pigeon had to peck the five stimuli in the correct order to obtain a food pellet (see Figure 10-8a). Some of the stimuli were different colors, and others were white shapes on a black background (a horizontal line and a diamond). Terrace wanted to see whether pigeons could learn the list of five stimuli faster if it were divided into two chunks, with only colors in one chunk and only shapes in the other. Five groups of pigeons learned a different list of colors and/or shapes. As Figure 10-8b shows, the list for Group II was nicely divided into two chunks: The first three stimuli were colors and the last two were shapes. The list for Group IV was divided into one large chunk of four colors, followed by the diamond shape. The lists for the other three groups were not organized into chunks: For Group I, the list had only colors, and for Groups III and V, colors and shapes were intermixed.

As Terrace expected, the two groups that had lists divided into chunks (Groups II and IV) required significantly less practice to learn the correct pecking sequence. In addition to the faster acquisition, Groups II and IV also demonstrated faster performance at the end of their training: They could complete the correct five-peck sequence more quickly. As further evidence that the pigeons in these two groups had divided their lists into two chunks, Terrace found that the longest hesitation between pecks occurred at the switch between colors and shapes. For instance, in Group II, the pigeons would peck the three colored stimuli quickly, then hesitate briefly, and then peck the two shapes in rapid succession.

Terrace and Chen (1991) found that once pigeons learned a chunk in one list, they could use this chunk in another list. For example, pigeons in an experimental group that first learned a list with chunks, RED-GREEN-YELLOW-line-diamond, were then quick to learn a second list that started with the same color chunk: RED-GREEN-YELLOW-BROWN-VIOLET. They learned the new list faster than a control group that had not learned the first list. It is especially interesting that once they learned to respond to RED-GREEN-YELLOW as a single chunk, the pigeons could use this chunk in a list which, from an objective standpoint, had no chunks at all.

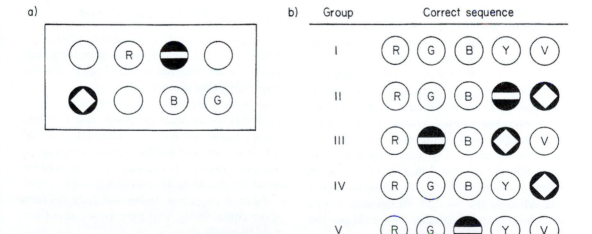

FIGURE 10-8 (a) In Terrace's (1991) experiment, five visual stimuli were arranged randomly in any of eight locations on a rectangular screen, and a pigeon received food only if it pecked the stimuli in exactly the correct sequence. (b) For the five groups of pigeons, the correct sequence is shown. (The letters inside the circles indicate stimuli of different colors: R = red, G = green, B = blue, Y = yellow, V = violet.)

Even if a set of stimuli is not organized into chunks, animals may develop their own chunks if they are free to select items in any order they choose. Dallal and Meck (1990) found evidence for chunking by rats in a 12-arm radial maze. Four arms (in different parts of the maze) had sunflower seeds at the end, four had food pellets, and four had rice puffs. For one group of rats, the locations of the different types of food were changed every trial, so there was no consistent pattern for the rats to learn. For a second group, the locations of the different types of food were the same trial after trial. With practice, the rats in this second group tended to select the arms in chunks based on the different food types. For example, a rat might first go to the four arms with sunflower seeds, then the four with food pellets, and finally the four with rice puffs. A typical rat's performance was usually not so perfectly organized, but rats in the second group showed a strong tendency to group the arms by food type. As a result, their overall performance in the maze was better than that of the group with random food locations—they made fewer repeat visits to arms where they had already consumed the food. Dallal and Meck concluded that by chunking the arms of the maze on the basis of food type, these rats were able to decrease the burdens on their working memories and thereby perform more accurately.

All of these studies involved chunking in laboratory situations, but some animals may use chunking as a learning strategy in their natural environments. Suge and Okanoya (2010) found that when Bengalese finches listen to the songs of others of their species, they perceive them as chunks, not as individual notes. Williams and Staples (1992) studied how young male zebra finches learned songs up to 15 syllables long from older male finches. They found that the older finches tended to divide their songs into chunks of about three syllables; the younger finches would copy these chunks, and eventually they could put the chunks together into a complete song.

Human beings are much better at learning lists than the animals in these experiments. For instance, a child can memorize a list of five items without much effort, but the pigeons in Terrace's

experiment required over 100 sessions to do so. Still, the research on chunking by animals adds to our list of similarities between human and animal memory: (1) If a list is already organized into chunks, both animals and people can learn the list faster. (2) If an already-learned chunk reappears in a new list, the new list will be learned even faster. (3) If a set of items is not already organized, both animals and people may group similar items together, and this will help to improve memory and avoid mistakes.

LANGUAGE AND REASONING

Finding a creative solution to a difficult problem, communicating through language, and engaging in logical reasoning are among the most sophisticated learned behaviors that people can perform. Cognitive psychologists have studied these classes of behavior extensively, almost always with human subjects. Over the years, however, a few psychologists have attempted to determine whether animals are capable of these complex behaviors. Regardless of how this question is ultimately answered, the research with animals should give us a better perspective on the most advanced of human cognitive skills.

Teaching Language to Animals

Most people would probably credit animals with at least some rudimentary problem-solving abilities, since the challenge of surviving in the wild frequently poses obstacles that demand creative solutions. However, many have claimed that the ability to use language is one skill that only human beings possess (e.g., Chomsky, 1972a). For this reason, attempts to teach language to chimpanzees and other animals have received tremendous attention. This section describes some of the most important studies and discusses some of the controversies that have arisen about animals' linguistic abilities.

EARLY STUDIES WITH CHIMPANZEES.   In the first attempts to teach language to chimpanzees, researchers tried to get the animals to speak

(Hayes, 1951; Kellogg & Kellogg, 1933). For the most part, these studies were unsuccessful, although the chimps eventually learned to say a few words. The main problem was that a chimpanzee's vocal apparatus does not permit it to make many human speech sounds. To avoid this problem, Allen and Beatrice Gardner (1969, 1975) decided to try to teach their chimpanzee, Washoe, to use American Sign Language (ASL). Washoe was about 1 year old when the Gardners obtained her, and she lived in an enclosed yard and a small trailer. She was trained by a number of different people, all of whom were moderately proficient in ASL. By relying on a mixture of modeling, manual guidance, and a good deal of patience, the trainers were able to teach Washoe to produce signs for quite a few different words, including nouns (e.g., *flower, toothbrush, hat*), verbs (*go, listen, tickle*), adjectives (*sweet, funny, more*), pronouns (*you, me*), and prepositions (*in, out*). After 4 years with the Gardners, Washoe had learned about 130 signs. This was quite an impressive vocabulary (though still small compared to that of the average 4-year-old child, who knows several thousand words).

After being taught a sign in a few contexts, Washoe sometimes used it in a new context without further training. For instance, she was taught the sign for *more* in combination with a few different signs (including *more tickle* and *more swinging*), and she later began to use the sign to ask for more food and for more of other activities. Although she frequently used signs in various combinations, the order in which she used the signs in a "sentence" was quite inconsistent. For example, she might sign the phrase *food eat* on some occasions and *eat food* on others, with no apparent reason for the different word orders. In contrast, both children and adults tend to use consistent word orders whether they are using spoken or sign language. In short, Washoe had a good vocabulary but poor (perhaps nonexistent) grammar.

Using a very different training situation, David Premack (1971b, 1983) obtained much more encouraging evidence that chimpanzees can learn at least some rules about grammar and word order. Instead of using ASL, Premack constructed a language consisting of different plastic shapes that represented different words. Sentences were created by placing the shapes (which had metal backings) on a magnetic board in a specific order. Premack's pupil, a 6-year-old chimpanzee named Sarah, learned to respond appropriately to many different configurations of these symbols. Sarah's trainers started by teaching her to associate symbols with different objects or events, and they progressed slowly to short sentences and then to longer and more complex ones.

The order of symbols was a critical part of the language Sarah learned, and she demonstrated an impressive ability to respond on the basis of symbol order. For instance, after Sarah learned the symbols for different colors and for the word *on*, she was taught to respond appropriately to the sequences *green on red* versus *red on green:* In the first case she would put a green card on top of a red card, and in the second case she would do the opposite. This shows that her responses were controlled by the order of the symbols, not just by the symbols themselves. Having succeeded at this task, Sarah was then able to respond correctly to new symbol strings such as *blue on yellow* with no further training. Sarah had learned not only that the order of symbols was important but that this same order could be applied to other symbols as well. In a simple way, this example illustrates an understanding of a grammatical rule, that is, an abstract rule about sentence structure that applies to entire classes of words.

In another case where word order was important, Sarah learned to respond to a complex sentence of symbols, *Sarah insert banana pail apple dish,* by putting a banana in a pail and an apple in a dish. To respond correctly, Sarah had to pay attention to word order; otherwise, she would not know what to insert into what. How was Sarah taught such complex tasks? Premack (1971b) explained that his procedure involved "one-to-one substitution" (p. 821)—he started with very simple tasks, and each new type of sentence would differ in only one way from sentence forms Sarah had already learned. Using this technique, Premack and his associates trained Sarah to respond appropriately to a wide range of grammatical forms and concepts, including plurals, yes-no questions, and quantifiers (*all, some, none,* and *several*).

One disappointing feature of Sarah's performance, however, was that she seldom initiated a conversation. Her use of the symbol language was almost exclusively confined to answering questions posed by the experimenters. Furthermore, if one of her trainers placed a question on the board and then left the room, Sarah would usually give either an incorrect response or none at all. This behavior contrasts quite starkly with that of young children, who spontaneously practice and use the words they have learned, even when no one is listening.

CRITICISMS. Despite these accomplishments, some psychologists concluded that the ways these chimpanzees learned to use signs are not really comparable to human language. One researcher who has articulated this view quite forcefully is Herbert Terrace (1979, 1985). Terrace and his associates taught ASL to a chimpanzee called Nim Chimpsky (a name with a curious resemblance to that of Noam Chomsky, the linguist who claimed that only people can learn language). Nim learned about 125 signs for nouns, verbs, adjectives, pronouns, and prepositions. He frequently used these signs in combinations of two or more. With two-sign "sentences," Nim showed some consistency of sign order. For example, of all the two-sign sentences that included the sign for *more,* this sign occurred first in 85% of the cases (*more drink, more tickle,* etc.).

Unfortunately, in Nim's sequences of three or more signs, inconsistency was the rule. For example, in three-sign sequences involving *eat, me, Nim,* and *more,* these signs occurred in almost every possible order (*me more eat, more eat Nim, eat me Nim, Nim me eat,* etc.). As Terrace pointed out, Nim's sequences of signs were different from the short sentences spoken by a typical 2- or 3-year-old child in several ways. First, there was no consistency of word order. Second, there were pointless repetitions of signs, and redundant signs (*me* and *Nim* used in a single sequence). Third, the average length of Nim's sign sequences (corresponding to what psycholinguists call the *mean length of utterance*) leveled off at about 1.5 signs per sequence and never increased again.

In contrast, a child's mean length of utterance steadily increases with age.

Based on his analyses of behavior of Nim, Washoe, Sarah, and other chimps, Terrace took a pessimistic view of what these animals had actually learned. He asserted that the chimps had learned only the most primitive grammatical rules, and that for the most part they would string together signs in a random order. They relied heavily on imitation and on prompting by their trainers; they showed little spontaneous use of language. The complexity of their utterances did not increase with additional training. Terrace (1979) concluded that the "language" these animals had learned lacked many of the essential characteristics of human language.

RESEARCH WITH OTHER SPECIES. One of the most accomplished animal language learners to date has been Kanzi, a bonobo trained by Sue Savage-Rumbaugh and her associates, who are now at the Great Ape Trust in Des Moines, Iowa (Savage-Rumbaugh, 1986; Segerdahl, Fields, & Savage-Rumbaugh, 2005). Kanzi's mother was part of Savage-Rumbaugh's training program that used lexigrams—pictorial symbols that represent words. Even before Kanzi was given any training by the research team, he showed an interest in the lexigrams and started to use them spontaneously. Seeing this, the researchers started to work with him, and since then he has learned over 300 lexigrams and has demonstrated other impressive linguistic abilities (Savage-Rumbaugh, Shanker, & Taylor, 1998). He uses lexigrams in a relatively consistent order (e.g., referring first to an action and then an object), which is evidence of a basic grammar. He exhibits an understanding of many spoken English words in addition to the lexigrams. This has been demonstrated in tests where he wears headphones to listen to recorded words and points to lexigrams that represent each word. He can discriminate among different word orders in spoken sentences and respond appropriately. He has also learned some of the symbols of ASL by watching videos of another animal signing.

Language studies have been conducted with other primates, including gorillas and orangutans (e.g., Bonvillian & Patterson, 1999; Miles, 1999). ASL has been used in some cases and pictorial symbols in others. In many of these studies, the animals were able to learn well over a hundred signs. Patterson and Linden (1981) reported that a gorilla named Koko had mastered more than 400 signs.

There have also been some studies with non-primates. Herman, Richards, and Wolz (1984) trained two bottlenosed dolphins to respond to about two dozen manual gestures by engaging in the appropriate activities. For example, a trainer might make the gestures for *frisbee fetch basket,* and the dolphin would then find the frisbee and put it in the basket. The dolphins could also answer questions about whether a particular object was or was not present in the tank (Herman & Forestell, 1985). Similar work has been done with sea lions (Schusterman & Krieger, 1984). And the parrot Alex, whose counting abilities have already been described, learned to say about 50 English words and use them appropriately to make requests ("Gimme tickle") and answer questions (Trainer: "What's this?"; Alex: "Clothespin"). Alex could also answer questions about the physical properties of objects, describing either an object's shape or color depending on what question his trainer asked (Pepperberg, 1999, 2010). Kaminski, Call, and Fischer (2004) tested a pet collie that was trained by its owners to retrieve different objects and found that it had learned the names of about 200 different objects. In addition, if the collie was asked to retrieve an object with a name it had not learned, the dog would go into the room with the objects, bypass familiar objects, and return with the unfamiliar object. The dog seemed to be able to infer the names of new objects using a process of elimination.

SOME CONCLUSIONS. Terrace was almost surely correct in saying that the linguistic capacities that animals have exhibited are quite limited compared to those of humans. On the positive side, however, this research has shown that animals have at least some measure of language ability. They have demonstrated many of the characteristics of human language:

1. *Use of abstract symbols.* Possibly the most fundamental characteristic of language is that any arbitrary symbol can be used to represent an object or concept. It is also the characteristic that has been most thoroughly demonstrated in animals. As we have seen, animals of several species have shown the ability to use words, signs, or symbols to represent objects, actions, and descriptions.

2. *Productivity.* Much of the power of language stems from the ability to take a finite set of words and combine them in new ways, so that one can communicate and understand new ideas. The ability to use words and symbols in new combinations has been observed in the language of the chimpanzees and other primates. The studies with dolphins and with the parrot Alex have demonstrated an ability to understand new symbol combinations that they heard or saw for the very first time.

3. *Grammar.* The early work by Premack showed that the chimpanzee Sarah could respond, not just to individual symbols, but to the order in which the symbols were presented. This was also found by Herman in his work with dolphins. In terms of language production, the evidence is not impressive. Chimps and bonobos have shown some degree of regularity in word order, but their sentences are short, and the word order they use is not always consistent. There is evidence that other species (pygmy chimpanzees, dolphins, and parrots) can learn at least some basic principles of grammar, such as the use of prepositions and demonstratives (Herman & Uyeyama, 1999; Kako, 1999). Nevertheless, even those who are typically enthusiastic about animal language abilities admit that the grammatical skills of nonhumans seem quite limited (Givón & Rumbaugh, 2009).

4. *Displacement.* The ability to use language to talk about the past or the future, and about objects and events not currently

present, is called displacement. Some studies found that chimpanzees can use their signs to describe behaviors they have just performed or are about to perform (Premack, 1986; Savage-Rumbaugh, 1984). Another study reported that two pygmy chimpanzees, that had learned to use lexigrams without any explicit training by humans, could use them to refer to objects and events not present (Savage-Rumbaugh, McDonald, Sevcik, Hopkins, & Rubert, 1986). However, there is considerable debate about this matter, and other researchers have proposed that animals are "stuck in time" and "stuck in space" (Roberts, 2006)—that they are not capable of temporal or spatial displacement. One study found that whereas 12-month-old human infants could gesture to communicate about a desired object that was not present, chimpanzees did not do so. The researchers concluded that this may be a uniquely human ability (Liszkowski, Schäfer, Carpenter, & Tomasello, 2009).

5. *Use in communication.*   For people, the purpose of language is to communicate with others. Terrace (1979) claimed that the language-trained chimps used their language only to obtain reinforcers, not to communicate information. However, later findings suggested that animals do use their signs to communicate with other animals or with people. Fouts, Fouts, and Schoenfield (1984) reported that five chimpanzees that had been taught ASL signs would use these signs to communicate with one another, even when no human beings were present to prompt or reinforce these behaviors. Greenfield and Savage-Rumbaugh (1993) found that two different species of chimpanzees used the symbols they were taught by humans to express a variety of different functions, such as agreement, requests, and promises. These chimpanzees often displayed the sort of turn-taking in the use of symbols that is typical of human conversations.

In summary, some of the main characteristics of human language have been found, at least at a rudimentary level, in other species. Future research will probably uncover other linguistic abilities in animals. Although no other species has shown the level of language capabilities that people have, it is not quite accurate to say that language is a uniquely human ability.

Reasoning by Animals

Besides language, many other advanced cognitive skills have been studied in animals, including abstract reasoning, problem solving, and the manufacture and use of tools. This section reviews a few of the findings.

OBJECT PERMANENCE.   Related to the preceding topic is the concept of **object permanence**, an understanding that objects continue to exist even when they are not visible. The developmental psychologist Jean Piaget (1926) proposed that during the first 2 years of life, human infants proceed through six different stages, in which their understanding of object permanence becomes more and more complete. Piaget developed a series of tests to determine which of the six stages an infant has reached, and these tests can be adapted quite easily for use with animals. Research with a number of different species, including cats and dogs, has shown that they follow more or less the same sequence of stages as human infants, eventually reaching stage six, in which they will correctly search for an object after an "invisible displacement" (Dore & Dumas, 1987). For example, Figure 10-9 shows the procedure used by Miller, Rayburn-Reeves, and Zentall (2009). A dog watches as a person places a snack in one of the two containers. The bar with the containers is rotated 90 degrees (an "invisible displacement" because the snack cannot be seen), the room is darkened for a few seconds, and then the dog is allowed to choose on e container. The researchers found that most dogs are successful at this task as long as the period of darkness is not too long. This level of competence has been found in several species of primates (Albiach-Serrano, Call, & Barth, 2010) and birds (Pepperberg & Funk, 1990). However, not all species perform

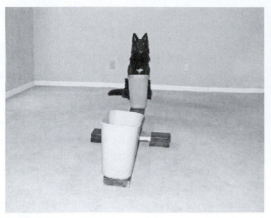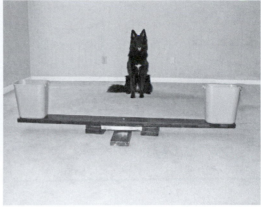

FIGURE 10-9 In this test of object permanence, a dog watches as a person puts a treat in one of the two containers (which are aligned as in the left panel). The bar with the containers is rotated 90 degrees (right panel), the room is darkened for a few seconds, and then the dog is allowed to choose one container. (From Miller, Rayburn-Reeves, & Zentall, 2009). Copyright 2009, with permission from Elsevier.

equally well on these tasks. A study with dolphins found that they were successful with visible object displacements but not invisible displacements (Jaakkola, Guarino, Rodriguez, Erb, & Trone, 2010).

ANALOGIES. An **analogy** is a statement of the form "A is to B as C is to D." To test someone's ability to understand analogies, we can give the person two or more choices for D and ask which is correct. For example, consider the analogy, "Lock is to key as can is to _____." Is *paint brush* or *can opener* a more appropriate answer? On this type of problem, the ability to make judgments about physical similarity is usually not enough. In physical terms, a can opener is not especially similar to a key, a lock, or a can. To solve this analogy, one must understand (1) the relation between lock and key, (2) the relation between can opener and can, and (3) the similarity of the two relations (i.e., that the second item of each pair is used to open the first). In other words, to understand an analogy one must be able to understand a relation (similarity) between two relations.

Gillan, Premack, and Woodruff (1981) tested Sarah, the language-trained chimpanzee, with analogies that involved either perceptual relations or functional relations between objects. The analogy in the previous paragraph involves functional relations because it requires an understanding of the

functions the different objects serve, and it was one of the analogies given to Sarah (see Figure 10-10). An example of a perceptual analogy is the following: Large yellow triangle is to small yellow triangle as large red crescent is to (small red crescent or small yellow crescent)? This analogy also requires an understanding of the relations between objects, but in this case the relations pertain only to the perceptual properties of the objects (their relative sizes).

Sarah was fairly good at solving both types of analogies. In contrast, chimpanzees that had not received language training were never significantly better than chance (50% correct), which led Premack (1983) to conclude that language skills were essential for analogical reasoning. This may not be the case, however, because a recent study found that baboons with no language training could successfully solve perceptual analogies (Fagot & Parron, 2010).

TRANSITIVE INFERENCE. If Alex is shorter than Bill, and if Bill is shorter than Carl, then it follows that Alex is shorter than Carl. This conclusion is justified because inequalities of size are *transitive;* that is, they conform to the following general rule: if $A < B$ and $B < C$, then $A < C$. If we draw the correct conclusion about the heights of Alex and Carl without ever having seen them side by side, we are displaying the capacity for **transitive inference**.

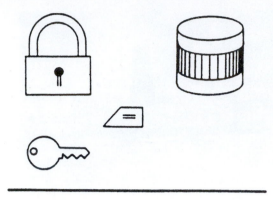

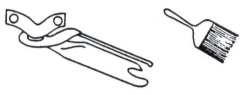

FIGURE 10-10 Pictures presented to the chimpanzee Sarah by Gillan, Premack, and Woodruff (1988). The pictures represent the analogy, "Lock is to key as can is to what?" Two possible answers, can opener and paint brush, were presented below the line, and Sarah chose the correct answer. From Gillan et. al, "Reasoning in the chimpanzee: I. Analogical reasoning," *Journal of Experimental Psychology: Animal Behavior and Processes,* 7(1), Jan 1981, 1–17, © American Psychological Association. Reprinted with permission.

Gillan (1981) tested whether chimpanzees were capable of transitive inference by first training them with containers of different colors, which had food in some situations but not others. For instance, one chimp was taught that blue was better than black, black was better than red, and so on. In the test for transitive inference, a chimp had to choose between two containers that had never been paired before. For instance, when given a choice between blue and red, would the chimp choose blue? Gillan found that the chimps were capable of making such inferences. Later studies have shown that transitive inference can be found in numerous species, including rats (Davis, 1992), mice (DeVito, Kanter, & Eichenbaum, 2010), and pigeons (von Fersen, Wynne, Delius, & Staddon, 1991). A variety of theories have been proposed to try to explain how animals are able to master this task, some of them cognitive in their approach

(Bryson & Leong, 2006) and others based on behavioral principles (Vasconcelos, 2008).

TOOL USE AND MANUFACTURE. You might think that only human beings are capable of making and using tools, but this is not so. Several different species are known to use tools of various types. For example, sea otters hold rocks against their chests while floating in the water and use them to crack open the shells of mollusks. Several birds, including the woodpecker finch and the crow, use sticks or branches to fish out larvae or insects from holes where their beaks will not reach. Examples of tool use among primates are numerous. For instance, chimpanzees use leaves as towels to wipe themselves or as umbrellas in the rain, and they use sticks and rocks as weapons to defend themselves against predators.

Even more impressive than examples of tool use are the rare instances in which animals have been observed to make a tool and then use it for some specific purpose. One example is a chimpanzee that was taught how to hit one stone against another to make a cutting tool, and then to use the tool to cut a cord. Later, the chimp made such cutting tools on his own, learning by trial and error how to smash the stones effectively to get sharp cutting edges (Toth, Schick, Savage-Rumbaugh, Sevcik, & Rumbaugh, 1993). This chimp first learned the skill through observation, but other animals have learned to manufacture tools by themselves. Weir, Chappell, and Kacelnik (2002) found that a female crow learned to bend a straight piece of wire into a hook, and then used the hook to pull a container of food out of a vertical pipe. The crow used her beak and foot to bend the wire, and it was not an accidental behavior: Of 10 trials in which the crow was given a straight piece of wire, she bent the wire and successfully retrieved the food container 9 times. These examples of tool making have generated a great deal of interest, because they suggest that the animals may have some basic understanding of the cause-and-effect relation between modifying an object and then using that object to accomplish some task.

METACOGNITION. Stated simply, **metacognition** is thinking about one's thinking. To be more specific, it is the ability to reflect on one's memories and thought processes and make judgments about them. For instance, people can state how sure they are about something they remember, or about whether they know a particular piece of information. I may tell you that I am positive I know the name of a particular actor, even though I can't think of it at the moment. I may say I think I remember that Sam was at last summer's department picnic, but that I am not really sure. People have the ability to make judgments about the accuracy of their own memories (along with other abilities that would also be classified as metacognition). In recent years, there have been many studies examining whether animals are also capable of metacognition (Kornell, 2009). Different techniques have been used to test for such abilities, and many of them have obtained positive results. For example, to determine whether rhesus could judge the accuracy of their memories, they were given a delayed matching-to-sample task in which they had the option of choosing an "uncertainty response," which allowed them to skip a trial and move on to the next one. The monkeys frequently made the uncertainty response when the trial was a difficult one, but they seldom made the uncertainty response on easy trials. This shows that they could accurately judge when they were likely to make mistakes (Hampton, 2001). One study found that apes would seek more information when on trials where they were uncertain, but not when they already knew the correct choice (Call, 2010). When rhesus monkeys performed a discrimination task with easy and difficult trials, they chose to take larger risks to obtain greater rewards on the easy trials, which suggests that they knew they would make the correct choice (Shields, Smith, Guttmannova, & Washburn, 2005).

The topic of animal metacognition has received a great deal of attention from behavioral and cognitive psychologists because metacognition has been considered to be a sophisticated human capability. Some psychologists are still skeptical about whether these results are convincing demonstrations of metacognition. However, if future research provides more conclusive evidence, this would be a compelling example of continuity between humans and other animals, and it could provide insights into the evolution of human mental abilities (Smith, 2009).

CONCLUSIONS. Human beings cannot boast that they are the only species on earth capable of abstract thinking. Many lines of evidence suggest that other animals can learn a variety of tasks that involve abstract reasoning. It seems likely that more examples of abstract reasoning will be found in other species in future research. Perhaps the moral is that it is always risky to claim, "Here is a problem in abstract reasoning that only humans (or only primates) can solve." The danger is that some clever researcher will find a way to teach a bird or rodent to solve exactly that problem. Although no one would seriously question the vast differences between human and nonhuman intellectual abilities, some of the apparent limitations of animals' reasoning abilities might be attributed to deficiencies in our current training or testing procedures, not to the animals.

PRACTICE QUIZ (2)

1. In the peak procedure, if an animal's responses are sometimes reinforced 20 seconds after the start of a trial, the rate of responding peaks at about _____ from the start of the trial.
2. Two species that have demonstrated the ability to count by using words or symbols to represent numbers are the _____ and the _____.
3. Grouping similar objects together as a strategy for improving memory is called _____.
4. When the chimpanzee Washoe was taught sign language, she learned the signs for many words, but she showed little ability to use _____.
5. _____ is the understanding that objects continue to exist when they are not visible.

Answers

4. grammar, or consistent word order   5. object permanence
1. 20 seconds   2. parrot, chimpanzee   3. chunking

Summary

Two procedures used to study short-term memory in animals are DMTS and the radial-arm maze. In DMTS, performance accuracy declines quickly as the delay between sample and comparison stimuli increases. Studies using radial-arm mazes have shown that rats can generally avoid repeat visits to arms of a maze where they have already collected food, even when a maze has as many as 17 arms. Other studies have found evidence for both maintenance rehearsal and associative rehearsal in animals. Experiments on long-term memory have shown that pigeons can remember several hundred pictures with a high degree of accuracy. Other studies have demonstrated that long-term memory can be improved if an animal is given an appropriate stimulus as a reminder of a previous learning experience.

Various experiments on timing have demonstrated that the duration of a stimulus can control an animal's behavior with reasonable accuracy, and so can the number of stimuli. Animals can also detect repeating serial patterns of stimuli, and they can learn lists of stimuli through chunking.

When researchers have tried to teach language to animals, the responses resemble human language abilities in some respects but not in others. Some chimpanzees have learned to use more than 100 signs or symbols for words, but they seldom use any consistent word order or grammar. Premack obtained better grammar from a chimpanzee by reinforcing only the correct word order (using different plastic shapes to represent words). Other studies have shown that several species (the gorilla, the dolphin, and the parrot) can learn the meanings of gestures, symbols, or spoken words.

Research has shown that animals of various species can exhibit certain types of abstract reasoning. For instance, rats, mice, and pigeons can solve problems of transitive inference. Cats, dogs, and birds can perform tasks involving object permanence. Baboons and chimpanzees have successfully solved tests of analogical reasoning. There is also some evidence that nonhuman primates have the capacity for metacognition.

Review Questions

1. Describe how DMTS and the radial-arm maze can be used to study animal short-term memory. Discuss some of the main findings that have been obtained with these procedures.

2. What are maintenance rehearsal and associative rehearsal? Describe one experiment that appears to demonstrate each type of rehearsal in animals.

3. In experiments on animal timing or counting, what happens when the duration to be timed or the number to be counted is doubled or tripled? What does this show us about animals' timing and counting abilities?

4. Describe two different experiments which show that animals can use chunking as an aid to memory.

5. Discuss the strengths and the limitations of the language abilities of chimpanzees trained to use ASL. What other techniques have been used to teach language to animals, what other species have been used, and what has been found?

6. Describe some tasks that have been used to test animals' reasoning abilities. Give examples of reasoning abilities that are found in many species and of abilities that have been found in just a few species.

CHAPTER

11

Learning by Observation

LEARNING OBJECTIVES

After reading this chapter, you should be able to

- describe several different theories of imitation and discuss their strengths and weaknesses

- explain what is known about observational learning by animals

- explain Bandura's theory about the four factors necessary for successful imitation

- give examples of how observational learning and operant conditioning can

interact to determine an individual's behavior

- give some specific examples of the variety of behaviors that can be learned through observation

- describe several ways in which modeling has been used in behavior therapy

Let there be no mistake about it: A large proportion of human learning occurs, not through classical conditioning or as a result of reinforcement or punishment, but through observation. Two psychologists whose writings and experiments repeatedly emphasized this fact are Albert Bandura and Richard H. Walters. In their classic book, *Social Learning and Personality Development* (1963), Bandura and Walters argued that traditional learning theory was grossly incomplete because it neglected the role of observational learning. As we have seen, traditional learning theory emphasizes the importance of individual experience: An individual performs some behavior and experiences the consequences that follow. The point of Bandura and Walters was that a good deal of learning occurs through vicarious rather than personal experience: We observe the behavior of others, we observe the consequences, and later we may imitate their behavior. In short, Bandura and Walters claim that the traditional approach to learning, which stresses personal experience and practice, is insufficient—it can account for some types of learning but not all.

Bandura and Walters believed that early childhood experiences can have a profound influence on adult personality and that they exerted their influence through the principles of **social learning theory**. By social learning theory, Bandura and Walters meant a combination of (1) the traditional principles of classical and operant conditioning, plus (2) the principles of observational learning, or imitation. Thus, they felt that they were not rejecting the principles of traditional learning theory but rather were adding one more important principle of learning to the list. Later in this chapter, we will examine some of a large body of evidence that shows that observational learning is indeed an important contributor to personality differences among individuals. To begin, however, we will survey a number of different theories about why imitation occurs in the first place.

THEORIES OF IMITATION

Imitation as an Instinct

Some early psychologists suggested that people and other animals have an innate propensity to imitate behaviors they see others perform (McDougall, 1908; Morgan, 1896). William James (1890) stated, "This sort of imitativeness is possessed by man in common with other gregarious animals, and is an instinct in the fullest sense of the term...." (p. 408). This belief that imitation was an innate tendency stemmed in part from evidence that young infants may imitate the movements of an adult. For instance, McDougall (1908) reported that his 4-month-old son would stick out his tongue when an adult in front of the child did the same. In a much more carefully controlled setting, Meltzoff and Moore (1977, 1983) sought to determine whether 12- to 21-day-old infants would imitate any of four gestures made by an adult tester: lip protrusion, mouth opening, tongue protrusion, and sequential finger movement. The tester made one of these gestures at a time and then waited to see whether the infant would copy it. The infant's behavior was videotaped and subsequently scored by people who

did not know which of the four gestures the infant had observed on a given trial. Meltzoff and Moore found a reliable tendency for the infants to imitate the specific behavior that they had just seen. Because of the young ages of these infants, it seems very unlikely that such imitative behaviors had been reinforced by their parents. In fact, all of the parents claimed that they had never seen imitative behavior in their infants, and most felt that it was not possible at such a young age.

The results of Meltzoff and Moore have been replicated several times, so it appears that newborn infants have a tendency to repeat certain gestures made by adults, especially tongue protrusion (Field, Woodson, Greenberg, & Cohen, 1982). Meltzoff (2005) and other developmental psychologists have proposed that the ability of infants to imitate is essential for their learning of language and other important life skills. This may well be true, but it does not necessarily mean that infants are born with a general ability to imitate the actions of others. One hypothesis is that imitation of lip protrusion (and possibly a few other facial expressions) is an inborn fixed-action pattern (as described in Chapter 2), which is triggered when the infant sees someone else make the same gesture (Abravanel & Sigafoos, 1984).

Other research has found little evidence for a general ability to imitate in young children. Children of ages 1 to 2 years were taught to imitate an adult in performing a specific set of gestures (the "baseline matching relations" in Figure 11-1). The children were given toys or other rewards for successful imitation. Once they learned to imitate these gestures, they were tested to see if they would imitate a new set of gestures (the "target matching relations" in Figure 11-1). The children showed very little tendency to imitate the new gestures (Erjavec, Lovett, & Horne, 2009; Horne & Erjavec, 2007). The researchers showed that this failure to imitate was not due to limitations of the children's motor abilities. They concluded that these young children were not yet capable of imitating arbitrary new behaviors, only those that they had been specifically trained to imitate. This research suggests that a general

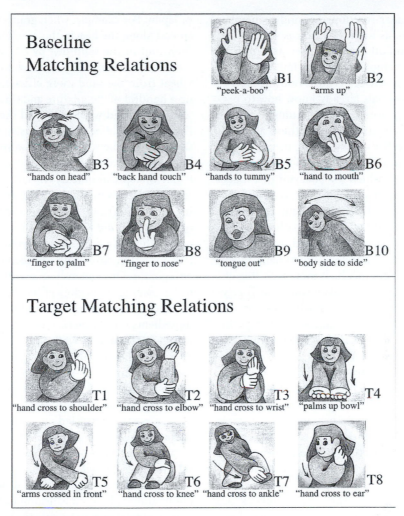

FIGURE 11-1   In a test of generalized imitation, 1- to 2-year-old children who were first taught to imitate an adult making the gestures in the top set later showed little imitation of the new gestures in the bottom set. From M. Erjavec, V.E. Lovett, and P.J. Horne, "Do infants show generalized imitation of gestures?" *Journal of the Experimental Analysis of Behavior, 87*(1), pages 63–87. Copyright 2007 by the Society for the Experimental Analysis of Behavior, Inc. Reprinted with permission.

ability to imitate new behaviors does not appear until later in childhood.

As the quotation from William James shows, he believed that other animals were also capable of learning by imitation. In the past 100 years, hundreds of experiments on imitation by animals have been conducted, with such diverse subjects as primates, cats, dogs, rodents, birds, and fish (see Robert, 1990; Whiten & Ham, 1992). Imitation by animals can occur for a variety of reasons, and

researchers on this topic have identified different types of imitation that differ in their causes, their complexity, and their sophistication (Zentall, 2004).

A very simple form of social influence is **social facilitation**, in which the behavior of one animal prompts similar behaviors from another animal, but the behavior is one that is *already in the repertoire* of the imitator. For instance, an animal may be stimulated to eat by the sight of other animals that are eating. Similarly, animals may copy the fear reactions of another member of their species, as when one deer is startled and starts to run and other nearby deer start running as well. Such examples represent imitation in its most primitive sense, because nothing new is learned: The animals already know how to perform these behaviors (eating, running); they are simply prompted to engage in these activities when they see other animals doing them.

Another category of imitation is **stimulus enhancement**, in which the behavior of a model directs the attention of the learner to a particular stimulus or place in the environment. As a result, a response that might otherwise have been learned through trial and error is acquired more rapidly. For instance, in a laboratory experiment, ravens were tested in pairs in which one raven (the observer) watched another raven (the model) playing with a particular toy. Later, when the observer was alone, it was given a choice of five toys, including the one the model had played with. If two ravens were unrelated, the observer did not show a preference for any toy, but if they were siblings, the observer tended to pick the toy that its sibling had played with (Schwab, Bugnyar, Schloegl, & Kotrschal, 2008). Besides providing an example of stimulus enhancement, this study shows that animals may be selective in whom they imitate. However, in other cases, stimulus enhancement has been found even when the model was not the same species as the learner. Bullock and Neuringer (1977) found that pigeons could learn to produce a two-response chain (pecking two keys in a specific order) by observing a human hand demonstrate the appropriate sequence.

A more advanced type of social learning, **true imitation**, is reserved for cases that cannot be explained by simpler mechanisms such as social facilitation or stimulus enhancement. True imitation occurs when an animal imitates a behavior that it has never performed before, and when it is an unusual behavior pattern for that species, which probably would not have been learned if the animal did not observe another animal performing the behavior. Kawai (1965) described several possible examples of true imitation observed in a troop of monkeys living on an island off the coast of Japan. For example, when grains of wheat were spread along the beach, the monkeys would pick them out of the sand one by one and eat them. However, one monkey learned to separate the wheat from the sand more efficiently by picking up a handful of the mixture and throwing it in the water. The sand would sink and the wheat would float, so it could be collected easily. Soon many of the other monkeys of the troop were imitating this behavior. Kawai reported that several other novel behaviors spread quickly through the troop as a result of observational learning, including washing the sand off sweet potatoes and bathing in the ocean (which the monkeys had never done until one pioneer took up this activity). Examples of true imitation have also been seen in gorillas and orangutans. Orangutans in captivity have imitated many complex behaviors of their human caretakers, such as "sweeping and weeding paths, mixing ingredients for pancakes, tying up hammocks and riding in them, and washing dishes or laundry" (Byrne & Russon, 1998, p. 678). Researchers have reported examples of true imitation in rats, quail, and other species (Akins, Klein, & Zentall, 2002; Heyes, Jaldow, & Dawson, 1994). With pigeons, at least one study reported an example of deferred imitation in which the birds performed a novel response they had observed half an hour earlier (Dorrance & Zentall, 2001).

In summary, the ability to learn through observation is by no means unique to human beings. The tendency to imitate the behavior of others can be observed in many species. There seems to be some truth to the claims of early psychologists that the tendency to imitate is instinctive. The problem with this account, however, is that it tells us nothing about when imitation will occur and when it will not. Other theories of imitation have tried to answer this question.

Imitation as an Operant Response

In an influential book, *Social Learning and Imitation,* Miller and Dollard (1941) claimed that observational learning is not an additional type of learning (besides classical and operant conditioning); rather, it is simply a special case of operant conditioning. We have already seen that discriminative stimuli play a crucial role in operant conditioning both inside and outside the laboratory. For instance, a laboratory animal may learn to make one response in the presence of a red light, another response in the presence of a green light, and yet another response in the presence of a yellow light. (A person driving a car has also learned different responses to these three stimuli.) According to Miller and Dollard, observational learning involves situations where the discriminative stimulus is the behavior of another person, and the appropriate response just happens to be a similar behavior on the part of the observer.

One of Miller and Dollard's many experiments will illustrate their approach. First-grade children participated in this experiment in pairs, with one child being the "leader" and the other the "learner." On each of several trials, the two children would enter a room in which there were two chairs with a large box on top of each. The leader was instructed in advance to go to one of the two boxes, where there might be a piece of candy. The learner could see where the leader went, but not whether the leader obtained any candy. Next, it was the learner's turn to go to one of the two boxes, where he or she might or might not find a piece of candy. Half of the learners were in an *imitation group*—they were reinforced for making the same choice as the leader. The other learners were in the *non-imitation group*—they obtained reinforcement if their choice was opposite that of the leader.

The result of this simple experiment was not surprising: After a few trials, children in the imitation group always copied the response of the leader, and those in the non-imitation group always made the opposite response. Miller and Dollard concluded that, like any other operant response, imitation will occur if an individual is reinforced for imitating. Conversely, non-imitation will occur if non-imitation is reinforced. In both cases, the behavior of some other person is the discriminative stimulus that indicates what response is appropriate. Similar follow-the-leader behavior has been observed in rats and other animals (see Hake, Donaldson, & Hyten, 1983).

According to Miller and Dollard, then, imitative learning fits nicely into the Skinnerian three-term contingency of discriminative stimulus, response, and reinforcement. There is no need to claim that observational learning is a separate class of learning that is different from operant conditioning.

Imitation as a Generalized Operant Response

As Bandura (1969) has pointed out, Miller and Dollard's analysis of imitation applies only to those instances in which a learner (1) observes the behavior of a model, (2) immediately copies the response, and (3) receives reinforcement. Many everyday examples of imitation do not follow this pattern. For instance, suppose a little girl watches her mother make herself a bowl of cereal: The mother takes a bowl out of the cabinet, pours in the cereal, and then adds milk and sugar. The next day, when the mother is not in the kitchen, the girl may decide to make herself a bowl of cereal, and she may do so successfully. Here we have an example of imitation, of learning by observation; but notice that if the girl had never performed this sequence of behaviors before, she obviously could not have been reinforced for these behaviors. This example therefore illustrates a case of learning without prior practice of the response and without prior reinforcement.

Just as the principle of reinforcement cannot explain why a rat makes its first lever press (before receiving any reinforcers for that behavior), it cannot, *by itself,* explain the first occurrence of any response learned by observation. However, the principle of reinforcement can account for some instances of novel behavior if we include the concept of generalization. If the young girl had been previously reinforced for imitating the behaviors of her parents, her imitation of the behaviors involved in making a bowl of cereal might be simply an example of generalization. This explanation seems plausible considering that most parents frequently reinforce their children for imitation. Imitating a parent's behavior of speaking a word or phrase, of solving a puzzle, of holding a spoon correctly, and the like may be reinforced with smiles, hugs, and praise. It would not be surprising if this history of reinforcement led to the imitation of other behaviors.

Generalized imitation has been demonstrated in a number of experiments. For example, children with profound retardation were reinforced for imitating a variety of behaviors performed by the teacher (standing up, nodding yes, opening a door). After establishing imitative responses (which required several sessions), the teacher occasionally performed various new behaviors, and the children would also imitate these behaviors although they never received reinforcers for doing so (Baer, Peterson, & Sherman, 1967). Other studies have also demonstrated generalized imitative behavior in children (Brown, Peace, & Parsons, 2009; Kymissis & Poulson, 1994).

Bandura's Theory of Imitation

Bandura has maintained that the theory of generalized imitation, like the other theories of imitation, is inadequate. His reasons can be illustrated by considering a famous experiment on the imitation of aggressive behaviors by 4-year-olds (Bandura, 1965). The children participated in the experiment individually. Each child first watched a short film (projected onto a TV screen) in which an adult performed four distinctive aggressive behaviors against a Bobo doll (a large inflated doll, see Figure 11-2). For each aggressive behavior, the adult spoke distinctive words. For example, in one segment, the adult sat on the doll and punched it in the face, while saying, "Pow, right in the nose, boom, boom."

Some of the children then saw the adult model being reinforced by another adult: He was given a soft drink, candies, and other snacks and was called a "strong champion." Other children

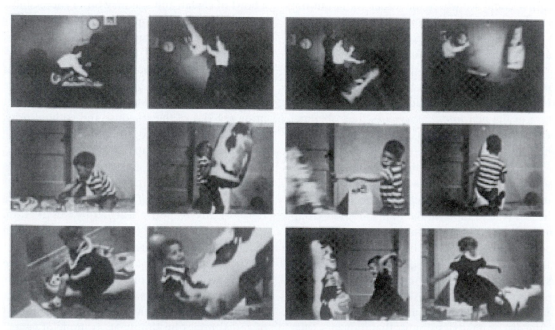

FIGURE 11-2   The top row shows frames from a film in which an adult model exhibits a number of different aggressive behaviors toward a Bobo doll. The two bottom rows show children imitating the model after having watched the film. From Bandura, et. al, "Imitation of film-mediated aggressive models," *Journal of Abnormal Psychology, 66*(1), January 1963, 3–11, © American Psychological Association. Reprinted with permission.

saw the model being punished for his aggressive behavior: The model was scolded for "picking on that clown," was spanked, and was warned not to act that way again. For children in a third group, the film contained no consequences for the model's aggressive behavior.

Immediately after viewing the film, a child was brought into a room that contained a Bobo doll and many other toys. The child was encouraged to play with the toys and was left alone in the room, but was observed through a one-way mirror. Many instances of aggressive behaviors against the Bobo doll were recorded, and most of these resembled those of the adult model in the film (Figure 11-2). In many cases, the children's words were also similar to those used by the model. Boys exhibited significantly more aggression than girls.

So far, these results do not contradict the theory of generalized imitation, but Bandura claimed that two additional findings cannot be explained by this theory. First, the consequences to the model made a difference; that is, children who saw the model being punished exhibited less imitation than children in the other two groups. According to Bandura, the theory of generalized imitation states that children (or adults) imitate others *because imitation has been reinforced in the past,* but it says nothing about how reinforcement or punishment *of the model* should affect the learner. Second, in the final phase of Bandura's study, the experimenter offered to reward the child if he or she would imitate the behavior of the model in the film. With this incentive, children in all three groups produced large and equal amounts of aggressive behavior. Bandura concluded that reinforcement is not necessary for the *learning* of new behaviors through observation, but that the expectation of reinforcement is essential for the *performance* of these new behaviors. Bandura claimed that the theory of generalized imitation makes no provisions for distinguishing between the learning and the performance of imitative behaviors.

As an alternative to the theory of generalized imitation, Bandura (1969, 1986) proposed a theory of his own. Bandura's theory can definitely be classified as a cognitive theory, for it proposes several processes that can never be observed in an individual's behavior. It states that there are four factors that determine whether imitative behavior will occur:

1. *Attentional Processes.* The learner must pay attention to the appropriate features of the model's behavior if imitation is to occur. A young girl may watch her mother make a bowl of cereal, but if she did not pay attention to where the sugar came from and how much to put in, she may be quite unsuccessful in her attempt at imitation.

2. *Retentional Processes.* It is obvious that an individual must retain some of the information that is gained through observation if imitation is to occur at a later time. Bandura states that rehearsal can be important here. Thus the little girl may say to herself, "First the cereal, then the milk, then the sugar." Notice that this information is stated in a fairly abstract way, and Bandura assumes that some abstraction of this type is indeed all that is remembered. Thus the child may not remember exactly where in the refrigerator the milk was, or exactly where on the table her mother placed the bowl, but such specific information is not usually necessary for successful imitation.

A study conducted with 14-month-old infants supports Bandura's view that the information-retained memory is in a fairly abstract form, which might later be expressed in a variety of different overt behaviors (Gergely, Bekkering, & Király, 2002). The infants watched a woman who was sitting at a table bend forward and press her forehead onto a translucent disk, which caused the disk to light up. For one group of infants ("hands-free"), the woman's hands were simply placed on the table, whereas for another group ("hands-occupied"), the woman pretended to be cold and was using both hands to wrap a blanket around her body. One week later, the infants were presented with the translucent disk on the table. Of the infants in the hands-free condition, 69% used their foreheads to turn on the light. Of those in the hands-occupied group, only 21% used their foreheads, and the rest of them used their hands to turn on the light. Apparently, these infants were able to reason that there was no need to use their foreheads if their hands were unoccupied, so they used their hands instead (which was easier and less awkward). As the researchers put it, "79% of them chose not to imitate her because their own hands were free, presumably concluding that the head action was not the most rational" (p. 775). Even at this early age, the infants showed the flexibility to take what they had learned through observation and apply it in a somewhat different (and more sensible) way.

3. *Motor Reproductive Processes.* Of course, the learner must have the appropriate motor skills in order to imitate a model. In other words, the learner must be able to translate general knowledge ("Put a bowl on the table"; "Pour in some cereal") into a coordinated pattern of muscle movements. In the examples of children making cereal or hitting a Bobo doll, this translation of knowledge into action poses no problem, because the children already possessed the required motor skills (handling objects, pouring, kicking, punching, etc.). In other cases of observational learning, however, the motor reproductive processes must not be taken for granted. For example, a model may demonstrate slowly and in a step-by-step manner the sequence of movements involved in juggling three balls, and the learner may retain this information in an abstract form (i.e., he or she may be able to recite the necessary sequences) but may still be unable to produce the appropriate movements without extensive practice. Similarly, imitating behaviors such as doing a cartwheel, landing an airplane, or smoothly plastering a wall may

be impossible because the observer lacks the necessary motor skills. Chapter 12 will have more to say about how these skills are learned.

4. *Incentive and Motivational Processes.* According to Bandura, the first three processes are all that are necessary for an individual to acquire the capability to perform some new behavior, but this capability will not be reflected in the learner's behavior without the appropriate incentive. Bandura states that the individual must have an expectation that the performance of this new behavior will produce some type of reinforcement. Bandura's (1965) study on aggressive behavior provided a clear example of the role of incentive. Children who saw the adult model being punished for his aggressive play with the Bobo doll presumably developed the expectation that such behavior would lead to unpleasant consequences, so they exhibited less imitation than the other groups of children. When the experimenter changed the expectations of the children by offering reinforcement if the children imitated the model, these children exhibited just as much imitation as the other two groups.

Which Theory of Imitation Is Best?

Bandura has claimed that his theory of imitation is better than the theory of generalized imitation because it makes clearer and more specific predictions about when imitation will occur. He argued that two problems with the theory of generalized imitation are (1) that it does not explain why observers will imitate a reinforced model more readily than a punished model and (2) that it does not explain why the children in all three groups were able to imitate when offered a reward for doing so. Not everyone agrees with Bandura's assessment, however. Kymissis and Poulson (1990) have proposed that the theory of generalized imitation can account for all types of imitative behaviors, using only well-established principles of operant conditioning. Based on what we know about generalization, it seems reasonable to make the following, specific prediction from the theory of generalized imitation: Imitation will most likely occur when the current situation is similar to situations in which the observer has been reinforced for imitation in the past. Conversely, imitation will least likely occur when the current situation is similar to situations in which the observer has been punished in the past.

Let us try to apply these two principles to the results of Bandura's (1965) experiment. Why did children frequently fail to imitate the adult model who was punished? A plausible answer from the theory of generalized imitation is that the children learned from past experience that it is not a good idea to imitate someone who has just been punished. The fact that children in all groups exhibited large amounts of imitation when they were offered rewards poses no real problem for theory of generalized imitation either. This result is similar to the Tolman and Honzik (1930) latent learning experiment (Chapter 8), in which rats displayed their ability to run through a maze without errors only after food became available in the goal box. Since that classic experiment, behaviorists have recognized the distinction between learning and performance, and some have concluded that reinforcement is not essential for learning but it is essential for the performance of learned behaviors.

In summary, Bandura's claim that the theory of generalized imitation cannot explain his results is not correct. Both theories can account for the results, but they do so in slightly different ways. Whereas Bandura's theory uses concepts such as attention, retention, and expectation of reward, the theory of generalized imitation relies on behavioral principles such as stimulus discrimination, generalization, and the learning/performance distinction. As in other debates between the cognitive and behavioral approaches, the debate over explanations of imitative behavior is partly about terminology and partly about how much we should speculate about processes that we cannot observe directly.

Mirror Neurons and Imitation

The discovery of mirror neurons in macaque monkeys in the early 1990s and their subsequent discovery in humans have added a new dimension to the discussion about whether observational learning is a unique and special type of learning, different from operant learning. What makes **mirror neurons** unique is that they fire both when an animal makes a certain movement and when the animal *observes someone else make that movement.* They were discovered by accident while researchers were recording from individual neurons in a monkey's premotor cortex, an area of the brain involved in hand movement and grasping. They found neurons that would fire when a monkey reached for a piece food, but also when the experimenter reached for the food (Di Pellegrino, Fadiga, Gallese, & Rizzolatti, 1992). Studies using brain-imaging techniques then identified areas of the human brain that act in a similar way—they become active both when the person makes a movement and when the person observes someone else make the same movement (Rizzolatti, Craighero, & Fadiga, 2002). More recently, individual motor neurons were found in human patients during the course of brain surgery (Keysers & Gazzola, 2010).

Mirror neurons have received a great deal of attention because brain researchers have speculated that they could be involved in a number of important human capabilities. Because mirror neurons respond both when we act and when we see others act, they may help us to understand the actions, intentions, and feelings of other people. Therefore, they may be important for normal social interactions and communication (Oberman & Ramachandran, 2009). Research on children and adults with autism spectrum disorders has found evidence that their mirror neurons may not function in the same ways as those of normal individuals (Bernier & Dawson, 2009). The evidence is preliminary and incomplete, but if it corroborated it could help to explain why people with autism often have difficulties in communication and in understanding the intentions of others.

Not surprisingly, it has also been suggested that mirror neurons are important for observational learning and imitation—they may help to make the connection between seeing someone else perform some action and then being able to perform it ourselves. If so, then the species of animals that are most capable of observational learning should be those that have well-developed mirror neuron systems. It will be interesting to see if future research with other species supports this hypothesis. So far, almost all the research on motor neurons has been conducted with humans and other primates. However, one study with sparrows found neurons in their brains that responded both when the birds sang a specific song and when they heard it (Prather, Peters, Nowicki, & Mooney, 2008).

INTERACTIONS BETWEEN OBSERVATIONAL LEARNING AND OPERANT CONDITIONING

In much of their book, Bandura and Walters (1963) surveyed research findings that showed how the behavior of parents affects a child's personality development. They presented research on such characteristics as dependency, aggressiveness, sexual preferences and behaviors, delinquency, and industriousness. They suggested that there are two main ways a parent can shape a child's personality: by control of rewards and punishments and by serving as a model whom the child can imitate. Bandura and Walters contended that to predict how upbringing will affect a child's personality, both of these factors must be taken into account. They maintained that in some cases direct reinforcement and observational learning can work in concert; in other cases, they may work in opposite directions. We will briefly consider one case of each type.

Achievement Motivation

Bandura and Walters claimed that direct reinforcement and observational learning work together in shaping what we might call self-discipline and a high achievement motivation. These terms encompass such characteristics as an individual's willingness to work and make sacrifices so as to obtain long-term goals, to set high standards for oneself and attempt to achieve them, and to be independent and self-reliant. Bandura and Kupers (1964) conducted an experiment that illustrates how an adult model can influence a child's self-discipline in a situation that allowed the child to reinforce himself or herself for good (or perhaps not so good) behavior. First, a child watched an adult play a bowling game in which the scores could range between 5 and 30. For children in one group, the adult would reward himself by taking a candy from a bowl for every score of 20 or better. For a second group, the adult was more lenient, rewarding himself for any score above 10. As in most studies of this type, the adult left the room before the child began to play the game and the child was secretly observed. The children tended to use the same criteria for rewarding themselves as those they had observed the adult use. Children in a third group, who observed no model, tended to reward themselves no matter what score they obtained.

This study showed that children can learn to apply either strict or lenient standards of self-discipline by observing a model, and Bandura and Walters speculate that numerous learning experiences of a similar type must occur as children observe their parents' behaviors over a period of many years. Of course, besides serving as models, parents may directly reinforce either strict or lenient standards of achievement and self-discipline in their children. One study on 9- to 13-year-old children found that those who grew up in homes where there was a strong emphasis on learning and intellectual activities were more highly motivated to achieve academic success (Gottfried, Fleming, & Gottfried, 1998). Even at the college level, parents can play an important role in their children's levels of achievement. Ratelle, Larose, Guay, and Senécal (2005) found that college students' persistence and competence in a rigorous science program was related to the levels of support and involvement of their parents.

The combined influences of reinforcement and modeling on achievement motivation may operate not only within families but across entire societies. McClelland (1961) noted that folk tales and stories in children's readers from some societies emphasize the achievement of excellence, whereas those from other societies do not. In an ingenious and extensive piece of research, McClelland had readers score the stories of different countries (which were disguised so that the country could not be identified) for achievement-related themes. These stories had all been published during the 1920s. He also developed measures of economic growth in these countries that were based on increases in per capita income and per capita electrical use between 1925 and 1950. McClelland found a significant correlation between the average level of achievement motivation depicted in a country's children's stories and its rate of economic growth during the next 25 years.

Of course, there is nothing in McClelland's research that implies that either achievement motivation or economic growth is desirable. The rapid economic growth of industrialized nations over the past century or so has brought with it the problems of toxic waste, acid rain, nuclear weapons, and other concerns. What the results do suggest, however, is that the values a society emphasizes via its stories, legends, and heroes can have a substantial influence on the level of achievement motivation (and probably other characteristics) in its next generation.

Aggression

Bandura and Walters (1963) presented evidence that parents' behaviors can influence the aggressiveness of their children in conflicting and seemingly paradoxical ways. The apparent paradox is that parents who use the most severe punishment for aggressive behaviors tend to produce more aggressive children (see Hicks-Pass, 2009, for a balanced review of the extensive literature on parental use of physical punishment). On the surface, this seemed to suggest that punishment is ineffective as a deterrent for aggressive behaviors, a finding that conflicts with the ample evidence showing that punishment is an effective procedure for eliminating unwanted behaviors (see Chapter 7).

Bandura and Walters (1959) pointed out that this apparent paradox is resolved when we realize that parents who use physical punishment with their children are providing their children with models of aggressive behavior. They showed that children whose parents punished aggressive behaviors usually avoided aggressive behaviors when their parents were present, but they were aggressive in their interactions outside the home. When parents use threats and physical force to discipline their children, the children often use these same techniques in dealing with peers. The children of parents who make use of force so severe it must be termed *child abuse* are prone to being more aggressive when they become adults (Scarpa, Haden, & Abercromby, 2010). Victims of childhood physical abuse are more likely to resort to physical punishment and child abuse when they become parents (Huesmann, Dubow, & Boxer, 2011; Lefkowitz, Huesmann, & Eron, 1978). All of these results are consistent with the view that when they discipline their children, parents are serving as models as well as controlling agents.

These findings do not mean, however, that parents should feel helpless when they see aggressive behaviors in their children. Chapter 7 described several procedures for reducing unwanted behaviors that do not make use of physical punishment or other aversive stimuli, including differential reinforcement for incompatible behaviors, response cost, and time-out. Research has shown that such techniques can successfully reduce aggressive behaviors and that parents of unusually aggressive children can be trained to use those techniques (Patterson, Chamberlain, & Reid, 1982; Reid, Patterson, & Snyder, 2002). The advantage of these techniques is that besides reducing unwanted behaviors, they provide the child with a model whose reaction is firm yet moderate and nonviolent when displeased with someone else's behavior.

PRACTICE QUIZ (1)

1. Some experiments have found evidence that newborn infants can imitate the _____ of adults.

2. The behavior of one animal prompts another animal to perform the same behavior, but the behavior is one that the second animal has performed before; this is called _____.

3. According to the theory that imitation is a _____ operant response, individuals will imitate the behavior of others if they have been reinforced for imitation in similar situations in the past.

4. Besides attentional and retentional processes, Bandura's theory states that _____ processes and _____ processes are necessary for successful imitation.

5. In Bandura's research, young children were more likely to imitate the aggressive behaviors of an adult if the adult's behaviors were _____ than if the adult's behaviors were _____.

Answers

5. reinforced; punished
4. motor reproductive; incentive and motivational
1. facial expressions   2. social facilitation   3. generalized

EFFECTS OF THE MASS MEDIA

In the modern world, the opportunities for observational learning are not limited to direct personal contact. We are exposed to potential models through TV, radio, movies, the Internet, video games, popular music, and so on. How these cultural influences affect people's behavior is a vast topic. Here, we will take a brief look at just a few effects of the media.

Television Violence and Aggressive Behavior

Bandura' pioneering research on modeling and aggression set the stage for the continuing debate over whether violence on TV makes the people who watch it more violent. This question has been difficult to answer, but now there is substantial evidence that TV viewing can affect the attitudes and behavior of both children and adults. Many studies with children and adolescents have found a positive correlation between the amount of TV they watch and their level of aggressiveness in everyday life (Murray, 2008). However, the results are not always straightforward: A study on fourth- to sixth-grade children in the United States found detrimental effects of TV violence for females and white males, but not for African-American males (Feshbach & Tangney, 2008). Furthermore, a problem with correlational evidence is that correlation does not imply causation; that is, a correlation between two variables does not necessarily mean that the first variable is the cause of the second. Thus, a correlation between TV violence and aggressive behavior in children might or might not mean that watching TV violence causes aggressive behavior. Another possibility is that aggressive tendencies are the cause and watching TV violence is the effect: Perhaps those children who have more aggressive personalities to begin with (for whatever reasons) choose to watch more TV violence than less aggressive children, because the aggressive children find it more enjoyable. Yet another possibility is that both variables, watching TV violence and aggressiveness, could be influenced by some third variable, such as a stressful living situation.

To avoid the weaknesses of correlational evidence, those who study the effects of TV violence have used a number of strategies. One strategy is to conduct a **longitudinal study** in which the relevant variables are measured at different points in time. For example, in a well-known study, Eron, Huesmann, Lefkowitz, and Walder (1972) examined the TV-viewing habits and aggressive tendencies of more than 200 third-grade boys; then they reexamined these same boys 10 years later. They found a moderate correlation between preference for violent TV in the third grade and aggressiveness 10 years later. Conversely, they found no correlation between aggressiveness in third grade and preference for violent TV 10 years later. This pattern of results suggests that watching violent TV can lead to later aggressiveness, not the reverse. Other longitudinal studies have corroborated these findings (Anderson & Bushman, 2002). Furthermore, the effects of TV violence are not limited to young children. One longitudinal study found a substantial correlation between the amount of TV exposure at age 22 and assault and fighting at age 30 (Johnson, Cohen, Smailes, Kasen, & Brook, 2002).

Another strategy in this area of research has been to conduct controlled experiments in which participants are randomly assigned to an experimental group that observes aggressive behavior or to a control group that does not. Studies of this type have generally found increases in aggressiveness after children watch violent TV programs (Christensen & Wood, 2007). A problem with these laboratory experiments, however, is that both the TV viewing and the measurement of aggressiveness take place in very brief time periods and restricted environments, and it is not clear how much applicability they have to real life. To deal with this problem, some researchers have conducted **field experiments** in which the TV viewing and the measurement of aggressive behaviors occur in more realistic settings. For example, children have been exposed to either violent or nonviolent TV programs over a period of several weeks, and their aggressiveness has been assessed in normal activities, such as free-play time at school. In general, the results of field experiments show a modest effect of TV violence on aggressive behavior (Friedrich-Cofer & Huston, 1986).

After analyzing the results of many studies, Hogben (1998) concluded that some types of TV violence are more strongly correlated with viewer aggression than others. Stronger correlations with viewer aggression are found for TV programs in which the violence seems justified (as when the character is fighting for a good cause), and weaker correlations are found when a program emphasizes the unpleasant consequences of violence (the suffering of the victim or punishment of the aggressor). It appears that it is not simply the presence of violence in a TV program but how the violence is portrayed that is important.

Watching TV can, of course, affect children in many other ways as well. Children who sit and watch TV for many hours each day are using up time that might be spent more productively. One extensive correlational study found an inverse relationship between the amount of TV that children watched and their reading comprehension scores on standardized tests, with much lower test scores for children who watched more than 4 hours of TV a day (Neuman, 1988). However, the effects of TV can sometimes be beneficial. Educational programs such as *Sesame Street* can give young children valuable information about letters and words, numbers, and social skills. Some longitudinal research (designed so that cause and effect could be sorted out) has found that children who were regular viewers of *Sesame Street* between the ages of 3 and 5 had higher vocabulary skills 2 years later than those who did not watch this program as often (Fisch & Truglio, 2001; Rice, Huston, Truglio, & Wright, 1990). Watching other shows, such as *Arthur* and *Dora the Explorer,* has been correlated with increased vocabulary and language expressive skills in young children (Linebarger & Walker, 2005).

It should come as no surprise that TV can have many different effects on the viewer. As with most examples of modern technology, it is not the device itself but how it is used that determines whether the effects will be desirable or undesirable.

Video Games and Popular Music

Many parents are concerned about how their children may be affected by playing video games that include violent actions and by music with violent themes and lyrics. Many popular video games portray graphic acts of violence, such as engaging in hand-to-hand combat or shooting and killing realistic human figures. Of course, children know that what takes place in a video game is not real; still, aggression in game playing may lead to a tendency to be more aggressive in real life. Many studies have found that playing violent video games can increase aggressive behaviors in children (Anderson et al., 2008), particularly when the games are most realistic (Krcmar, Farrar, & McGloin, 2011). In fact, playing violent video games may have a greater effect on aggressive behavior in children than watching violence on TV because video games involve active participation. One study found that boys who actually played a violent video game were later more aggressive than boys who simply watched another child playing the game (Polman, de Castro, & van Aken, 2008).

As with TV viewing, playing video games can also have some positive effects. Regular playing of video games with fast action can lead to improved attention and perceptual skills (Donohue, Woldorff, & Mitroff, 2010). Video games designed for health education and physical education in children have had some success, and those that require physical activity to play the game may help promote physical fitness (Papastergiou, 2009). With elderly adults, one study found that playing video games that include physical activity led to less depression (Rosenberg et al., 2010).

There have also been some studies on music lyrics and music videos with violent content. Determining the short-term and long-term effects of exposure to such music is a difficult task. However, some research has found evidence that listening to music with violent lyrics can increase aggressive thoughts and emotions in adolescents (Anderson, Carnagey, & Eubanks, 2003). One study reported a correlation between the amount of music videos children watched on TV and their levels of physical and verbal aggression (Roberts, Christenson, & Gentile, 2003). Not all studies on this topic have found statistically significant effects, but overall the findings suggest that music with violent and antisocial lyrics can have undesirable effects on the attitudes, emotions, and behaviors of children and adolescents.

WHAT CAN BE LEARNED THROUGH OBSERVATION?

Since Bandura and Walters' (1963) influential book was published, hundreds of studies have attempted to demonstrate the effects of observational learning on a person's personality traits, problem-solving skills, aesthetic preferences, and so on. Let us examine a few areas in which the effects of observation and imitation have been investigated.

Phobias

The causes of phobias are complex and still not well understood; they appear to result from learning experiences combined with biological and hereditary factors (Mineka & Sutton, 2006). Various studies have presented indirect evidence suggesting that phobias can be acquired vicariously; most of the studies showed that members of the same family frequently have similar fears (Rachman, 1977). Interviews with children who have dental phobias suggest that these fears are often learned from their parents (Milgrom, Mancl, King, & Weinstein, 1995). During World War II, Grinker and Spiegel (1945) reported case studies of fighter pilots who developed phobias after observing a crewmate's fear reaction during or after a mission. When individuals who suffer from phobias are asked about the origins of their phobias, a substantial number say that they acquired the phobia by watching someone else who was fearful of the same object or situation (Merckelbach, Arntz, & de Jong, 1991).

As you can see, evidence for the vicarious acquisition of phobias is based on correlational evidence, case studies, and retrospective reports, and this is not the strongest type of evidence. However, several experiments with animals have obtained more convincing evidence. For example, Mineka, Davidson, Cook, and Kerr (1984) reported that monkeys rapidly developed a long-lasting fear of snakes by observing another monkey's fearful reactions to a snake. In another study, rats acquired a fear of a tone from cage-mates that had previously been conditioned to fear the tone (Bruchey, Jones, & Monfils, 2010). Thus, in this case, the evidence for observational learning may actually be stronger for animals than for people.

Drug Use and Addictions

Many types of evidence suggest that Bandura's social learning theory can help to account for the acquisition of various addictive behaviors, including smoking, alcoholism, and drug abuse. Note that simple principles of reinforcement and punishment can explain why an addiction is maintained once it has been established. As described in Chapter 2 in the discussion of the Solomon and

Corbit theory, when someone tries to quit smoking or using addictive drugs, there are often aversive withdrawal symptoms that can be escaped (all too conveniently) by further intake of the addictive substance. However, observational learning and social reinforcement can help to explain why such addictions are developed in the first place.

For example, consider the fact that smoking one's first cigarette is usually an aversive event, involving harsh and burning sensations. Why then does a person ever smoke again? One answer is based on observational learning: Even when very young, many children are exposed to parents, older siblings, celebrities, and others who smoke. The consequences of this behavior may appear to be positive: Some people say they started smoking because smokers seemed to be more mature, sophisticated, or attractive. Perhaps these advantages outweigh a little burning in the throat for the beginning smoker. In addition, among teenagers, peers often deliver strong social reinforcers for smoking: They may encourage nonsmokers to begin and ridicule those who do not. These joint factors of observational learning and social reinforcement are frequently cited as major contributors to the onset of smoking, and it has repeatedly been found that the tendency to smoke is correlated with the smoking habits of one's parents, spouse, and peers (Ennet, Bauman, & Koch, 1994; Hunter, Vizelberg, & Berenson, 1991).

The principles of social learning theory also appear to be important in the development of alcoholism and drug abuse. It has been found that about 20% of all heroin addicts have one or more family members who are also addicted (Hekimian & Gershon, 1968). Similarly, a family history of alcohol abuse has been shown to be a predictor of alcohol use in college students (LaBrie, Migliuri, Kenney, & Lac, 2010). Of course, either learning or hereditary factors could cause similar patterns of drug and alcohol use within a family. However, several types of evidence show that similar drug use among family members is not entirely due to heredity. Andrews, Hops, and Duncan (1997) found that adolescents who had good relationships with their parents were more likely to imitate their use of cigarettes, marijuana, and alcohol than those

who had poor relationships. Furthermore, similar drug and alcohol use among peers cannot be due to hereditary factors if the members of a peer group are not related. In fact, researchers have found that drug and alcohol use among adolescents is more highly correlated with the habits of their peers than with the habits of their parents (Windle, 2000), which suggests that observational learning and social reinforcement play an important role.

Cognitive Development

Many developmental psychologists, such as Jean Piaget (1926), have suggested that as children grow, they pass through a number of stages of cognitive ability, and that the passage from one stage to the next depends heavily on growth, maturation, and personal experience. In contrast, social learning theorists claim that observational learning plays a major role in the development and refinement of cognitive skills. As a representative test of cognitive development, let us consider the well-known *conservation task*. In one version of this task, a child is shown three clear cylindrical beakers, as illustrated in Figure 11-3. Beakers A and B are identical, and they contain the same amount of water. The test begins by asking the child which has more water, and the child usually says that A and B have the same amount. Then,

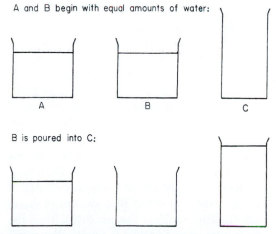

FIGURE 11-3 The steps of a test for conservation of volume. After seeing the contents of B poured into C, the child is asked which container, A or C, has more water.

as the child watches, the contents of B are poured into beaker C, a taller and thinner beaker. The child is then asked whether A or C has more water. Children are said to have mastered the concept of conservation of volume if they say that A and C have the same amount of water. However, children who are younger than about age 7 usually say there is more water in C. They are apparently misled by the higher water level in C. These children are called *nonconservers* because they have not yet learned that liquids retain a constant volume regardless of the shape of the container they are in.

Rosenthal and Zimmerman (1972, 1978) showed that a child's mastery of the conservation task can be enhanced by observational learning. They had children who were nonconservers observe a model (an adult female) perform correctly on the conservation task. In one group, the model gave an explanation for her answer that A and C had the same amount of water (e.g., "Because they were the same in the first place"), and in another group she gave no explanation. In a subsequent test, children in both groups showed improved performance on conservation tasks, and those who heard the model explain her choices improved the most. Some of the children were only 4 to 5 years old, well below the age at which children typically master the conservation task. The children's improved performances generalized to other types of conservation tasks (e.g., a conservation-of-number task, which involves an understanding that the number of objects in a row does not change if the row is made longer by spacing the objects farther apart).

Many other cognitive skills can be improved through observational learning. Children can learn grammatical rules, abstract concepts, and problem-solving skills by observing a model (Rivera & Smith, 1987; Zimmerman & Blom, 1983). Earlier in life, observational learning can help infants learn about retrieving objects that cannot be obtained by simple reaching. In one study, 8- to 18-month-old infants observed an adult who demonstrated how to retrieve an object that was out of direct reach (Esseily, Nadel, & Fagard, 2010). Then the infants were given a chance to retrieve the object themselves. Infants who observed the adult model performed better than those in a control group, especially those 12 months of age or older.

Moral Standards and Behavior

Bandura proposed that a child's judgments about what behaviors are good and what behaviors are bad are largely learned by observation. A child whose parents are impeccably honest in all financial matters may learn to behave the same way. A child who sees and hears his parents cheat on their taxes, steal from their employers, and ignore their bills whenever possible may decide that these are acceptable or even desirable activities. A number of experiments have shown that the behavior of a model can influence the behavior of observers in situations where morally laudable or deplorable behaviors are involved. For instance, it has been found that children are more altruistic after observing an altruistic model (Israely & Guttman, 1983), and that both children and adults are more likely to break rules or laws after observing a model do so (Lefkowitz, Blake, & Mouton, 1955).

Research by D. P. Phillips (1982) provides a striking example of how observing a model can increase a person's likelihood of performing an action that many consider to be both gravely immoral and irrational. Using statistics from the year 1977, Phillips found a significant increase in the number of suicides, motor vehicle deaths, and serious motor vehicle injuries in the several days that followed the suicide of a character in a nationally broadcast soap opera. For each instance of a soap opera suicide, Phillips used the preceding week as a baseline period, and he was careful to correct his data for seasonal fluctuations, to exclude data from holiday periods, and so on. Phillips's explanation of his results is that soap operas are widely watched, that many viewers identify themselves with the characters, and that the suicide of a character leads some (admittedly few) viewers to attempt to imitate this behavior. He interprets the increased motor vehicle accidents as disguised suicides or attempted suicides.

Similar increases in suicides and suicide attempts have been found in the days that follow TV news stories about suicide that are reported in the media (Martin, 1998). However, not all researchers are convinced by these findings, and the topic is still being studied and debated. Hittner (2005) reanalyzed the data from Phillips's studies using different statistical techniques, and he found "only partial support" for imitative suicides after suicides on TV. Still, this research raises some difficult policy issues for the producers of TV dramas and news programs.

MODELING IN BEHAVIOR THERAPY

Largely because of Bandura's influential work, modeling has become an important tool for behavior therapists. Bandura and Walters (1963) suggested that a model can influence an observer's behavior in three main ways, and each of these is used by behavior therapists. First, a model's behavior can facilitate responses the observer already knows how to perform. Second, an observer may learn how to produce totally new behaviors. Third, undesired responses, such as fear reactions to harmless objects or situations (phobias), can be reduced or eliminated through observational learning. The following sections give some samples of the large literature on the different therapeutic applications of modeling.

Facilitation of Low-Probability Behaviors

Modeling has been used in **assertiveness training** for people who are overly submissive in certain situations and want to develop the ability to stand up for their rights. For example, some wives (or husbands) may do whatever their spouses decide is best, regardless of what they think about a decision. Some young adults may be bullied by their parents into occupations or lifestyles they do not really like. Some people have difficulty refusing unreasonable requests made by friends, employers, co-workers, relatives, or strangers. The goal of assertiveness training is to help people deal with these situations more effectively. Frequently the training consists of a combination of modeling, role playing, and behavioral rehearsal, in which the therapist describes a hypothetical

situation, models an appropriate response, asks the client to imitate this response, and evaluates the client's performance. A few sessions of such assertiveness training can have long-term benefits (Goldsmith & McFall, 1975; Zhou, Hou, & Bai, 2008). Kirkland and Caughlin-Carver (1982) found that adults with mental disabilities who received 14 sessions of training showed significant improvement in their ability to refuse unreasonable requests politely, and these improvements were maintained in observations made 12 weeks after the end of training.

In another example where modeling was used to increase low-probability behaviors, O'Connor (1969) used filmed models to increase the sociability of nursery-school children who were socially withdrawn. In a classroom setting, the children would keep to themselves and rarely interact with other children or adults. Children in the experimental group saw a 23-minute film depicting a child of similar age engaging in a series of social interactions. The film began with relatively calm activities, such as two children sharing a book or toy while seated at a table. The film progressed through more involved and energetic social interactions, eventually ending with a scene with six children throwing toys around the room with obvious enjoyment. This method of progressing from simple to more demanding behaviors is called **graduated modeling**, and it is a frequent component in many modeling programs. Children in a control group saw a film of equal length about dolphins that contained no human characters. Immediately after viewing one of the films, the children returned to their classrooms, where observers recorded their behaviors. There was a fivefold increase in the number of social interactions for children in the experimental group, and no increase in the control group.

Acquisition of New Behaviors

Perhaps the best therapeutic example of the training of totally new behaviors through modeling comes from the work of Lovaas (1967) and others who have taught children with autism to speak, as described in Chapter 6. This therapy makes use of a large number of behavioral techniques, such as shaping, prompting, fading, and discrimination training, but the teacher's modeling of speech is indispensable at every stage of therapy. The teacher repeatedly models the desired words and the child is reinforced for successful imitation. Of course, many new behaviors besides speech can be taught through modeling. Modeling (along with other behavioral techniques) has been used to teach children with autism social skills (Nikopoulous & Keenan, 2004), personal hygiene (Lovaas, Freitag, Nelson, & Whalen, 1967), and basic reading skills (Marcus & Wilder, 2009).

Modeling has been used for many different purposes, ranging from training computer skills (Davis & Yi, 2004) to teaching parents how to handle their childrens' tantrums and aggressive behaviors (Marcus, Swanson, & Vollmer, 2001). In a technique known as **behavioral skills training**, modeling is used as a part of a larger program that may include verbal instruction, prompting, guided practice, and feedback. Gunby, Carr, and Leblanc (2010) used behavior skills training to teach abduction-prevention skills to three boys with autism. As part of the instruction component, the boys were taught to recite three simple rules about what to do if a stranger asks them to come with him: Say "no," run, tell (i.e., refuse the stranger's request, run to a safe place, and tell a familiar adult what happened). The modeling of these behaviors was done both with a video and with live models. The boys were then asked to practice these behaviors with a stranger and a familiar adult, and they were given praise and corrective feedback. They were later tested in realistic settings to determine how well they had learned the behaviors. Other applications of behavior skills training have included teaching staff the correct way to give physical assistance to children with physical disabilities (Nabeyama & Sturmey, 2010) and teaching children to avoid playing with firearms (Jostad, Miltenberger, Kelso, & Knudson, 2008). As is typical in behavior modification programs, objective measures of the learners' behaviors before, during, and after training were obtained in all of these studies to ascertain the effectiveness of the training methods.

Elimination of Fears and Unwanted Behaviors

As a treatment for phobias, modeling sometimes offers several advantages over systematic desensitization (see Chapter 3): Modeling can be used with very young patients, who may not be able to follow the therapist's instructions during deep-muscle relaxation training. Modeling can be a more rapid procedure and require less of the therapist's time, especially when films or videos are used. Because of the realistic nature of some modeling procedures, there may be better generalization to real-world situations.

Not surprisingly, Bandura and his colleagues conducted some of the earliest experiments on modeling as a technique for therapy. Bandura, Grusec, and Menlove (1967) attempted to reduce excessive fears of dogs in young children. The children were divided into four groups. The first group received eight 3-minute sessions of graduated modeling in which they observed a child of their own age engage in more and more demanding interactions with a friendly dog. The child approached the dog, petted it, fed it biscuits, walked around with the dog on a leash, and finally climbed into the dog's pen and played with it. In this group, the modeling sequences took place in a party context (with party hats, balloons, cookies, and prizes) to reduce anxiety. A second group of children observed the same modeling sequences without the party context. A third group experienced the party context with the dog present but with no model (to control for exposure to the dog). A fourth group experienced the party context but without the dog and the model. All children then received two posttreatment behavioral tests in which they were asked to imitate the model, one immediately and a second a month later. Figure 11-4 shows the results. Both groups with the model later showed less fear of a dog than the two groups without a model, and there was no significant difference between the party context and the neutral context. For the two groups that watched the model, these improvements remained essentially unchanged a month later.

In a variation called **participant modeling**, the model first performs a behavior related to the phobia and then the patient imitates the behavior of the model. In each step of the treatment, the patient's

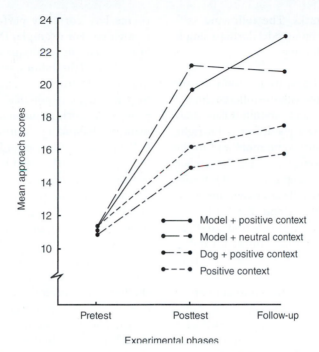

FIGURE 11-4   Results from the four groups in the Bandura et al. (1967) study on the use of modeling in the treatment of children's fear of dogs. Children who observed a model were more likely to approach and interact with a dog. From Bandura, A., Grusec, J.E., Menlove, F.L., "Vicarious extinction of avoidance behavior," *Journal of Personality and Social Psychology, 5*(1), Jan 1967, 16–23, © American Psychological Association. Reprinted with permission.

involvement with the object of the phobia becomes more demanding. For example, Love, Matson, and West (1990) had the mothers of boys with autism serve as models to treat their phobias. For Kenny, who had a fear of going outdoors, his mother first modeled going a few steps outside the front door to retrieve an object. She then used prompting and gentle guidance to encourage Kenny to perform the same behavior. Over time, the distance outside the door was gradually increased until Kenny was able to go out into the yard without crying or other signs of fear. Participant modeling has been successful when used to treat other types of phobias, such as fears of spiders, birds, needles, or dentists, and in some instances a single treatment session is all that is needed to produce long-lasting benefits (Davis, Ollendick, & Öst, 2009; Ollendick & King, 1998).

Modeling can also be used to reduce other unwanted responses. Middleton and Cartledge (1995) used modeling in combination with other behavioral techniques, including reinforcement of incompatible behaviors, to reduce aggressive behaviors in 6- to 9-year-old boys. Meichenbaum and Goodman (1971) used modeling to improve the academic performance of first-grade children with hyperactivity. These children often do poorly in school, partly because they tend to behave erratically or carelessly when working on a challenging task. The goal of Meichenbaum and Goodman was to reduce or eliminate such reckless and error-prone behaviors. They noted that these children exhibit less self-instruction than do average children of their age. For instance, when painting a picture, a typical first-grader might be heard to utter self-instructions such as "Don't spill the paint" or "I want to make a nice, straight line." Meichenbaum and Goodman observed that in children with hyperactivity, either such self-instructions are absent or, if present, they are nevertheless followed by the wrong behavior. Their treatment, therefore, consisted of having a child watch an adult model who gave himself overt self-instructions while performing various tasks. The following self-instructions were used by a model during a simple task of copying a line drawing:

> Okay, what is it I have to do? You want me to copy the picture with the different lines. I have to go slowly and carefully. Okay, draw the line down, down, good; then to the right, that's it; now down some more and to the left. Good, I'm doing fine so far. Remember, go slowly. Now back up again. No, I was supposed to go down. That's okay. Just erase the line carefully…. Good. Even if I make an error I can go on slowly and carefully. I have to go down now. Finished. I did it! (Meichenbaum & Goodman, 1971, p. 117)

Later, the adult would give the child similar instructions as the child worked on the task; eventually, the child was trained to give himself such instructions as he worked. The modeling of self-instruction was also given for more complex tasks. After this training, these children showed significant improvements on a number of standardized tests, and this improvement was maintained in a 1-month follow-up. As with most cases in which a behavior therapist wishes to eliminate one behavior pattern (careless performance in this case), the modeling techniques used by Meichenbaum and Goodman involved teaching an alternative behavior pattern (following one's self-instructions to work carefully) that was incompatible with the unwanted behavior. Other studies have found further evidence that modeling and self-instruction, often used in combination with other techniques, can be effective reducing hyperactivity, aggression, and generalized anxiety in children (Gosch, Flannery-Schroeder, Mauro, & Compton, 2006; Miranda & Presentacion, 2000).

Video Self-Modeling

A variation of modeling called **video self-modeling** has become an increasingly popular technique used by behavior therapists. The goal of this technique is to increase the performance of desired behaviors by having clients watch themselves correctly perform these behaviors in a video. For example, Dowrick and Raeburn (1995) used this technique with children with severe physical disabilities, such as cerebral palsy or muscular dystrophy. First, each child was asked to perform some practical skill that needed improvement, such as maintaining a good posture, walking, balancing, writing, or dressing. This behavior was video-recorded and included the therapist giving the child instructions on how to perform, encouragement, and, when necessary, assistance in completing the task. Next, each child's video was edited to remove all examples of errors and inappropriate behaviors, as well as all segments in which the therapist gave the child assistance. What remained, therefore, was a video in which the child was seen performing the behavior correctly, with no help from anyone else. This is important, because the goal is to teach only correct, unassisted behaviors. After the editing, the children watched themselves on the videos, which were shown to them six times over a 2-week period. The researchers found substantial improvement in most of the children on the self-modeled tasks. They also found that watching the video, not just performing the behaviors in front of a camera, was a crucial part of the treatment.

Video self-modeling has been used to teach better social and communication skills to children with autism spectrum disorders (Shukla-Mehta, Miller, & Callahan, 2010), to decrease stuttering in adults (Cream, O'Brian, Onslow, Packman, & Menzies, 2009), to teach simple cooking skills to people with traumatic brain injuries (McGraw-Hunter, Faw, & Davis, 2006), and to improve the walking skills and mobility of elderly patients (Neef, Bill-Harvey, Shade, Iezzi, & DeLorenzo, 1995). It is becoming an increasing common technique for teaching a variety of skills to both children and adults.

CONCLUSIONS: THE SOPHISTICATED SKILL OF LEARNING BY OBSERVATION

The increasing popularity of modeling as a technique of behavior modification is a reflection of the power of this method of inducing change in behavior. Learning by observation is the most sophisticated type of learning we have considered in this book. Its relative advantages can be appreciated by reviewing the major categories of learning we have examined. We began with habituation, a form of learning so primitive it is found in one-celled organisms. It consists of nothing more than a decrease in the probability of a reflexive response after repeated presentations of the eliciting stimulus. Classical conditioning is considerably more complex, for it typically consists of the transfer of an old response to a new (conditioned) stimulus. Still, no new responses can be taught using classical conditioning, because the form of the response is determined by the learner, not the teacher. With operant conditioning, we finally have a mode of learning in which the teacher can select the response: Any arbitrary response the learner makes can be reinforced, and its probability should increase. And when the techniques of successive approximations and response chaining are added to the principle of reinforcement, the teacher can gradually build up complex behavior patterns that the learner would probably never produce on his or her own. In Chapter 6, it was stated that, in principle, any behavior a learner is capable of performing can be taught using the technique of successive approximations.

What is possible in principle, however, is not always feasible in practice. Teaching a child how to speak, a college student how to write a computer program, or a figure skater how to do a triple jump would be next to impossible if the teacher's intervention was limited to the delivery of reinforcers for successive approximations to the desired goal. However, if the learner is capable of learning through observation, as people and many animals are, the task of teaching such complex behaviors becomes many times easier. The beauty of observational learning is that learners can develop some understanding of the desired behavior well before they actually produce this behavior themselves. To modify a cliché, it is probably not an exaggeration to say that one model is worth a thousand successive approximations.

Closely related to observational learning, though still more advanced, is the human ability to learn new behavior patterns through the spoken or written word. Since most types of formal education rely heavily on these modes of learning, enormous amounts of research have been directed toward the goal of making them more effective. Treatment of this vast topic is well beyond the scope of this book, but the relationship between these types of learning and observational learning should be clear. We have seen that the behavior of even young children can be altered if they (1) watch a live model, (2) watch a filmed model, or (3) listen to a verbal account of the model's behavior. When they are a bit older, children can learn by reading about the behavior of a model and the consequences that followed. In each case, the children are presumably learning about the contingencies of reinforcement—the stimulus–response–reinforcer relationships—that are found in their world. The advantage of education via observation or the spoken or written word is that the individual can learn about these relationships without having to experience them firsthand.

PRACTICE QUIZ (2)

1. In a _____ study, the behaviors of the same individuals are repeatedly measured over long periods of time.
2. Studies have shown that there is a positive correlation between how much violence children watch and their levels of _____ behavior.
3. If a child understands that the amount of water does not change when it is poured into a container of a different shape, the child has learned the concept of _____.
4. Modeling has been used in _____, in which shy or passive individuals learn to avoid letting others take advantage of them by making unreasonable demands or requests.
5. In _____ modeling, the learner imitates the behavior of a model in each step of the treatment.

Answers

4. assertiveness training 5. participant
1. longitudinal 2. aggressive 3. conservation

Summary

One theory of imitation states that it is an instinctive tendency, and there is evidence that animals and even newborn infants can learn by imitation. A second theory states that people imitate when they are reinforced for imitation. A third theory states that imitation is a generalized operant response: People imitate in situations that are similar to those where imitation has been reinforced in the past. Bandura's theory states that four factors determine whether imitative behavior will occur: attentional processes, retentional processes, motor abilities, and incentive and motivational processes. The idea that observational learning is a unique type of learning has been bolstered by the discovery of mirror neurons, which fire both when an individual makes a response and when the individual sees someone else make that response.

Observational learning and operant conditioning can either work together or work in opposite directions. They may work in opposite directions when parents try to use physical punishment for aggressive behavior: Their children may become more aggressive because the parents serve as models of aggression when they use harsh physical punishment. Observational learning can also affect the development of phobias, alcohol and drug use, thinking skills, and moral standards. In modern society, observational learning can occur in many ways other than through direct personal contact, including through TV, video games, popular music, and the Internet.

Many different variations on modeling techniques have been used successfully in behavior therapy, including graduated modeling, participant modeling, and video self-modeling. Through modeling, shy children can learn better social skills, adults can learn to be more assertive, children with autism can be taught to speak, and phobias can be eliminated.

Review Questions

1. Give some examples of imitation by animals. Discuss whether each example represents social facilitation, stimulus enhancement, or true imitation.

2. Explain the theory that imitation is a simple operant response, and the theory that imitation is a generalized operant response. Which theory is better and why?

3. What are the four factors necessary for imitation, according to Bandura's theory? What are Bandura's main criticisms of the generalized operant theory of imitation? Are these criticisms valid? Why or why not?

4. What are mirror neurons, and how might they be related to observational learning?

5. What different types of evidence support the hypothesis that watching violence on TV makes children and young adults more aggressive? Do you find the evidence convincing? Why or why not?

6. Give one specific example to show how modeling has been used in behavior therapy to effect the following: (a) facilitating low-probability behaviors, (b) acquiring new behaviors, and (c) eliminating unwanted behaviors.

12

Learning Motor Skills

LEARNING OBJECTIVES

After reading this chapter, you should be able to

- discuss the roles of reinforcement, knowledge of results, and knowledge of performance in motor-skill learning

- describe how the distribution of practice, observational learning, and transfer from previous training can affect motor-skill learning and performance

- explain Adams's two-stage theory and the evidence that supports it

- explain Schmidt's schema theory and show how it differs from Adams's theory

- compare the response chain approach and the concept of motor programs, and present evidence for the existence of motor programs

Motor skills are an essential ingredient for all types of learned behaviors, but people often take for granted their abilities to perform complex sequences of movement. The bicyclist seldom marvels at her ability to remain upright on two thin wheels. The data-entry clerk seldom wonders how he can coordinate 10 fingers to produce five or more keystrokes a second, usually in the correct order. Likewise, in previous chapters we have generally taken for granted a learner's response-production abilities. This chapter will examine these abilities in some detail.

Scientists have used a variety of strategies to study motor-skill learning, and we can group these strategies into three categories that parallel the three major approaches to the study of learning in general—the behavioral, physiological, and cognitive approaches. Much of the early research on motor-skill learning (beginning with the work of E. L. Thorndike and continuing through the first half of the twentieth century) had a behavioral character. Researchers were interested in discovering the relationships between various independent variables (e.g., the amount of practice, the distribution of practice) and dependent variables (e.g., speed of learning, quality of final performance). Physiologists were interested in the neural mechanisms of movement. They tried to discover what brain, spinal cord, and bodily structures were involved in movement. With the rise of cognitive psychology in the second half of the twentieth century, many theorists adopted the information-processing approach in analyzing motor skills. All three approaches to motor-skill learning have produced many interesting findings, and this chapter will sample some from each category.

THE VARIETY OF MOTOR SKILLS

The skilled movements that people are capable of learning are indeed diverse. Consider the following examples of motor skills: balancing—on a bicycle, on a log, or on an icy sidewalk; shooting a foul shot in basketball; putting a golf ball; pressing a stopwatch as a runner crosses the finish line; slamming on the brakes of an automobile during an emergency; typing; playing the piano or some other musical instrument. Before reading further, pause for a moment and think about these different skills. What features do some of these movements have in common? Along what dimensions do they differ?

One obvious characteristic of a movement is its duration. Some motor skills are called discrete because they are completed shortly after they have begun (pressing a stopwatch, slamming on the brakes). Others are called continuous because they extend for an indefinitely long period of time (balancing). The terms *discrete* and *continuous* represent two ends of a continuum, and many behaviors fall between these two extremes. Most continuous movements can be called **closed-loop movements** because the individual continually receives and can react to feedback about whether the movement is proceeding correctly. Balancing on a log is a good example: If you feel yourself tipping to the right, you can immediately compensate by shifting your weight to the left. In contrast, many discrete movements (e.g., slamming on the brakes) occur so rapidly that a person has no time to react to any possible error. In the terminology of feedback theory, these are called **open-loop movements**, and they are characterized by the fact that once the movement begins, it is too late to make any corrections.

One further difference among motor skills is that some require exactly the same movement every time, whereas others demand that the movement be modified to suit the situation. Compare the skills of shooting a foul shot and putting a golf ball. The movements required in a foul shot are always the same, for the player always stands 15 feet from the basket, which is 10 feet above the floor. If one motion is successful on one foul shot, an exact replica of this movement will be successful on any future foul shot. On the other hand, the movements required to sink a putt can vary considerably from one putt to the next. The ball may be a different distance from the hole and at a different angle, and the slope of the green may be different. The golfer must take all of these factors into account and then produce a stroke that has the appropriate force and direction. Motor-skill researchers have studied both types of tasks: those that require accuracy on a single, repetitive movement and those that demand the flexibility to adapt the movement to fit the occasion.

In studying motor skills, researchers often use unusual tasks, such as turning a knob 90 degrees in 150 milliseconds or tracking a dot on a rotating turntable with a pointer. The reasons motor-skill researchers study these unusual tasks are similar to the reasons operant conditioners study simple responses in a barren Skinner box. First, these tasks are selected to be representative of a wide range of everyday movements—the knob-turning task involves a discrete, open-loop movement, and the tracking task involves a continuous, closed-loop movement. Second, these tasks are selected to be as simple as possible, so that unnecessary complexities will not make the results difficult to interpret. Third, since it is unlikely that participants will have encountered these tasks outside the laboratory, the researcher can witness the acquisition of a new motor skill. If a researcher chose to study a more familiar task, such as steering a car, it could be difficult to sort out the contribution of innate ability, previous driving experience, and practice during the experiment itself.

VARIABLES AFFECTING MOTOR LEARNING AND PERFORMANCE

We will begin our survey of motor-skill research with what can be characterized as the behavioral approach. We will examine some factors that determine how quickly a motor skill is learned and how adroitly it is performed.

Reinforcement and Knowledge of Results

THE LAW OF EFFECT AND MOTOR LEARNING.

E. L. Thorndike, who is best known for his experiments with the puzzle box (Chapter 5), also conducted some of the earliest research on human motor learning (Thorndike, 1927). In one experiment, participants were blindfolded and their goal was to draw a line exactly 3 inches long. One group received reinforcement for each line whose length was within 1/8 inch of 3 inches, plus or minus: Immediately after a participant drew such a line, the experimenter said, "Right," and Thorndike thought of this as reinforcement for making a correct response. If the line did not meet this criterion, the experimenter said, "Wrong." Participants in the second group experienced no consequences for accurate or inaccurate lines. They received as many trials as the first group, but they had no way of knowing which lines were close to 3 inches and which were not. These participants showed no improvement over trials. On the other hand, participants in the reinforcement group showed a substantial increase in accuracy over trials. Thorndike's conclusion was that the Law of Effect is just as important in human motor learning as it was for his animals in the puzzle box. In both cases, reinforcement "stamps in" or strengthens the correct response, so this response is more likely to be repeated in the future.

WHAT CAN BE BETTER THAN REINFORCEMENT?

Trowbridge and Cason (1932) challenged Thorndike's conclusion that reinforcement is the crucial variable in the acquisition of a motor skill. They argued that, although saying "Right" after a response might serve as a reinforcer in some circumstances, in Thorndike's

experiment it was important because it gave the participant information or feedback about the accuracy of each response. In the literature on motor-skill learning, this type of feedback is usually called **knowledge of results (KR)**. In short, Trowbridge and Cason proposed that the information provided by the words "Right" and "Wrong" was what produced the participants' improved accuracy, not the reinforcing and punishing aspects of the words. To test their hypothesis, they repeated Thorndike's experiment, but they used four groups rather than two. Two of their groups were the same as Thorndike's: The group that received practice only was called the *No KR Group,* and the group that was told "Right" or "Wrong" was called the *Qualitative KR Group* (because participants received no quantitative feedback on the size of their errors). In addition, Trowbridge and Cason included a *Quantitative KR Group* in which participants were told the direction and magnitude of each error, to the nearest eighth of an inch. For instance, if a line was 7/8 inch longer than 3 inches, the experimenter would say "Plus seven." If a line was 5/8 inch shorter than 3 inches, the experimenter would say "Minus five." Trowbridge and Cason reasoned that the Quantitative KR Group received more information than the Qualitative KR Group, but not more reinforcement. Finally, a fourth group, the *Irrelevant KR Group,* received useless "feedback" after each trial—a meaningless nonsense syllable.

Each group received 100 trials; the results are shown in Figure 12-1. Neither the No KR nor the Irrelevant KR groups showed any improvement over trials. In the Qualitative KR Group, there was clear improvement: The size of the average error decreased from about 1 inch at the start of the experiment to about 1/2 inch at the end. Figure 12-1 shows, however, that the performance of the Quantitative KR Group was vastly superior to that of the Qualitative KR Group. From this pattern of results, we can conclude that information, not reinforcement, was the crucial factor, and that the more precise, quantitative KR produced much better performance than the less precise, qualitative KR.

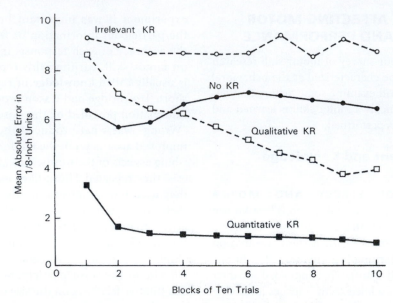

FIGURE 12-1   Results from the four groups of the Trowbridge and Cason (1932) experiment. Copyright © 1932 from "An experimental study of Thorndike's theory of learning" by M.H. Trowbridge and H. Cason, *Journal of General Psychology*. Reproduced by permission of Taylor & Francis Group, LLC, http://www.taylorandfrancis.com.

DIFFERENT WAYS TO DELIVER KNOWLEDGE OF RESULTS.   From the preceding experiment, you might conclude that delivering precise KR on every trial is the best way to teach a motor skill. However, if quantitative KR is given after every trial, the learner may actually become too reliant on this constant feedback and may be less skillful if he or she later has to perform without feedback. Winstein and Schmidt (1990) gave some participants quantitative KR after each trial of a motor-learning experiment, whereas other participants received quantitative KR on only 67% of the trials. During the learning phase, the performance of the group with constant feedback was slightly better. In a test 2 days later, however, *with no feedback given on any trial,* the group that had previously received 67% feedback actually performed better. Similar results have been obtained in other studies. For instance, on a task that required the coordinated movement of both arms, participants who received continuous feedback about their accuracy in the learning phases performed better than participants who were only given intermittent feedback. However, those who received the intermittent feedback performed better on later tests without feedback (Maslovat, Brunke, Chua, & Franks, 2009).

A theory known as the **guidance hypothesis** was developed to account for results like these (Salmoni, Schmidt, & Walter, 1984; Wulf & Shea, 2004). According to the guidance hypothesis, KR provides information that helps the person learn the new motor skill. KR that is given on every trial provides more guidance than KR given on only a portion of the trials, so performance during the acquisition phase is more accurate with 100% KR. However, the participant becomes very dependent on this constant KR and cannot perform well in a later test without KR.

In contrast, participants who do not receive KR on every trial must rely more on their own ability to detect errors in their movements (since they have no other feedback on some trials), so they perform better on a test with KR completely absent. If the guidance hypothesis is correct, it has implications for those who teach motor skills to athletes, musicians, dancers, and so on. The coach should probably give feedback to the athlete or performer on some practice trials, but not on every trial, so that the performer can learn to detect and correct errors in performance without the coach's help. In this way, the performer can continue to perform well when the coach is not there to give feedback.

DELAYING KNOWLEDGE OF RESULTS. In tasks where the individual usually receives continuous immediate feedback, even small delays in this feedback can produce marked deterioration in performance. A number of studies have examined how a person's speech is affected when auditory feedback from the person's voice is delayed by a fraction of a second. (The participant listens to his or her own voice through headphones that delay the transmission of the speech.) The typical result is that participants begin to stutter and to speak more slowly and in a halting manner (Lee, 1950). K. U. Smith (1962) examined peoples' performances on various tracking tasks with delayed feedback. For instance, a participant might have to trace a curving figure with a pencil while watching his or her performance on a television screen that delays the visual feedback of the participant's movements. Not surprisingly, Smith found that performance worsened as delays in feedback got longer.

In contrast to the results just mentioned, delaying KR has little or no detrimental effect on tasks where the learner normally gets KR only after the movement is over. Many studies on delayed KR have used **slow positioning tasks** in which the participant must move a sliding knob or pointer a certain distance, with no time limit. The knob or pointer is usually out of the participant's sight, so the participant must rely on tactile or kinesthetic cues rather than visual ones. In general, if KR is delayed after each trial (by a few seconds, a few minutes, or even longer), there seems to be little effect on the participant's accuracy (I. M. Bilodeau, 1966; Mulder & Hulstijn, 1985a).

We have already seen that delays of only a few seconds can greatly hinder learning in both classical and operant conditioning. The failure to find similar detrimental effects of delayed KR was therefore quite puzzling. This mystery remained unsolved for several decades, but now there appears to be an answer. In one experiment, participants performed a timing task in which they tried to make a response in exactly 1 second (Swinnen, Schmidt, Nicholson, & Shapiro, 1990). One group received immediate quantitative KR, but for a second group, the quantitative KR was delayed for 8 seconds. When tested 2 days later (with no KR), the group that had previously received the delayed KR was actually more accurate than the immediate-KR group.

To explain why performance can be better after delayed KR than after immediate KR, Swinnen and his associates applied the guidance hypothesis. Immediate KR may help to guide participants during acquisition, but the participants may become overly dependent on this immediate feedback and never learn to rely on their own senses to estimate the accuracy of their movements. But the participants with delayed KR had an 8-second period after each trial in which they could try to estimate the accuracy of their movements; therefore, they could improve their skills at detecting their own errors. Another study found that when participants were given delayed KR, they relied instead on various types of intrinsic feedback, such as their hand positions and the estimated duration of their movement (Anderson, Magill, Sekiya, & Ryan, 2005). As further evidence that error estimation is important, Swinnen (1990) showed that if participants are required to make verbal estimates of their errors during the 8-second delay during acquisition, they perform even better in a later test without KR. In contrast, if they are distracted during the 8-second delays (so they do not have time to estimate the accuracy of their movements), their performance on a later test is impaired.

Perhaps so many of the older studies found little effect of delaying KR because the disadvantages of not getting prompt feedback were offset by the opportunity that participants had to practice estimating their errors during the delay. The problem with immediate KR seems to be the same as the problem with getting KR on every trial: An overreliance on immediate KR may lead to improved performance while learning a new motor skill, but it seems to hurt performance in a later test when the participant must perform without external feedback.

Knowledge of Performance

Often it is possible to give a participant many types of feedback besides information on how close the movement came to some goal. Consider, for example, the many useful pieces of information a coach might be able to give a pole-vaulter after each vault in practice. The coach might discuss various details related to the athlete's take-off, approach, pole placement, ascent, limb positions, and the like, and each piece of information might help to improve the athlete's future performances. The delivery of such information about the sequence of components of a complex movement is called **knowledge of performance (KP)**. Hatze (1976) provided one illustration of the usefulness of this type of detailed feedback in a laboratory setting. The participant's task was to stand in front of a target and then to raise his right foot and kick the target as rapidly as possible. For the first 120 trials, the participant received quantitative KR; that is, he was told his time after each trial. The participant's movement time decreased over these trials and leveled off at about 800 milliseconds. After trial 120, the participant was shown a videotape of his performance, and his motions were compared to a stick figure performing the response in the best possible way. After receiving this feedback, the participant immediately began a new phase of improvement, and his movement times decreased to about 500 milliseconds. These results suggest that a comparison between the individual's movements and those of an ideal performer is a particularly effective form of feedback.

KP is commonly used in the training of Olympic athletes. For instance, a discus thrower might be videotaped as he practices; later, his performance can be reviewed and compared to the motions of a computer-generated figure that demonstrates the movements that would maximize the distance the discus is thrown. In addition, there has been an increasing interest in providing athletes with various types of special feedback to determine which are the most effective. In some cases, techniques similar to biofeedback (in which the learner is given amplified or quantitative feedback about his movements;

see Chapter 8) can assist in the acquisition of a novel motor skill (Collins & McPherson, 2006; Mulder & Hulstijn, 1985b).

To investigate what types of feedback are most useful to someone learning a new motor skill, Kernodle and Carlton (1992) had four groups of participants learn to throw a ball with their nondominant hands (i.e., with the left hand for participants who were naturally right-handed throwers, and vice versa). The goal was to throw the ball in a straight line as far as possible. One group received normal KR: They were told the exact distance of each throw. A second group received KP: After each throw, they watched a videotape replay of their throwing motion on that trial. A third group received the same type of KP, but in addition they were told to focus their attention on a particular part of the throwing motion while watching the replay. During the training, they were told to focus on 10 different components of a good throw, such as "Focus on the hips during the throwing phase." A fourth group also received KP, but while watching the replay they were instructed on what to do to improve their motion on the next trial, such as "Stride forward with the right foot toward the target area." All four groups were given 12 training sessions over a 4-week period. This fourth group, which received KP plus instructions on how to improve, showed the greatest improvement, both in the length of their throws and in judges' ratings of their throwing form (see Figure 12-2).

In some cases, KR and KP can yield very different results. Cirstea and Levin (2007) worked with patients to help them recover arm movements they had lost due to strokes. The treatment involved repeatedly trying to point one's arm toward a target. One group of patients received only KR—they were given feedback on how close to the target they were pointing. Another group of patients was given KP—they were given information about the movements of the joints in their arms. The differences in recovery were dramatic: After 10 sessions of therapy, the KP group achieved significant improvements in arm movements and coordination, whereas the KR group showed no overall improvement. The researchers concluded

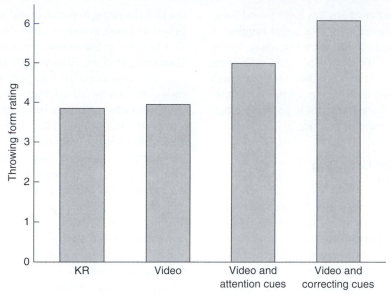

FIGURE 12-2 Judges' rating of movement form for four groups of participants who received four different types of feedback when learning to throw a ball with their nondominant hands. (Based on Kernodle & Carlton, 1992)

that the improvements in the KP patients were due to the detailed feedback they received about their arm movements, over many repetitions.

More research of this type should help to determine what types of feedback are most useful to the learner. The answers will almost surely vary depending on exactly what type of skill is being learned. However, a general conclusion we can draw from this research is that although quantitative KR can be quite helpful in learning a motor skill, more elaborate types of feedback can produce even greater improvements in performance.

Distribution of Practice

What is the most effective way to schedule practice sessions when learning a new skill? For example, suppose a supervisor has 4 hours in which to teach a new employee to operate a semiautomatic machine. Will the employee's performance be best if he or she practices steadily for the 4 hours, or if the employee alternates between 30-minute practice periods and 30-minute rest periods, or with some other distribution of practice and rest?

As a general rule, laboratory studies have found that performance is better if rest periods are interspersed among fairly brief practice periods, than if practice occurs in one continuous block. In short, **distributed practice** is better than **massed practice**. It is interesting to note that Ebbinghaus (1885) obtained a similar result in his research on the memorization of lists of nonsense syllables, a very different type of task. One explanation of this effect is that during continuous practice, a type of fatigue builds up that interferes with performance, and this fatigue dissipates during rest periods, so overall performance is better if frequent rest periods are allowed (Hull, 1943). Indeed, in learning motor skills there is often an improvement in performance immediately after a rest period.

Some researchers have concluded that the advantages of distributed practice are only temporary: Participants who received massed practice did substantially worse during that practice, but after a sufficient rest period, their performance was about as good as that of participants who initially received distributed practice (Adams & Reynolds, 1954; Rider & Abdulahad, 1991).

However, a number of studies have found long-term benefits to practicing in a larger number of short practice sessions compared to fewer, longer practice sessions (Dail & Christina, 2004; Shea, Lai, Black, & Park, 2000). Therefore, although the effects are not always large or permanent, in most cases distributed practice is probably a better strategy than massed practice.

Observational Learning of Motor Skills

As with many other types of learned behaviors, some motor skills can be acquired through observation. Not surprisingly though, simply observing someone else perform a motor skill is not as effective as practicing it yourself. Nevertheless, observational learning can be beneficial, especially when combined with direct practice (Wulf, Shea, & Lewthwaite, 2010). In one experiment, people could make the cursor on a computer screen move either left or right by pressing two different keys; their goal was to keep the cursor on a moving dot on the screen. A group of participants who practiced this task themselves performed better on the test day than participants who watched another person learning the task. However, those who only observed the task performed much better than control participants who neither practiced nor observed the task until the test day. Furthermore, participants who first observed the task and then practiced it themselves performed better than all the other groups on a transfer test in which the movement of the dot was different in the test phase than it was in the previous phase (Shea, Wright, Wulf, & Whitacre, 2000). In short, both individual practice and observation contributed to the participants' acquisition of this new skill. It is also possible for people to learn a sequence of several movements through observational learning, and the performance of those who have the opportunity for observational learning can be as good as or better than that of those who simply practice the sequence themselves (Heyes & Foster, 2002). The benefits of observing someone else demonstrate a new motor skill may be primarily related to the perceptual components of the task (learning to perceive and attend to the appropriate cues), and direct practice may be necessary to develop the motor components of the task (Maslovat, Hodges, Krigolson, & Handy, 2010).

As discussed in Chapter 11, video self-modeling can be an effective way to teach new skills, and this technique has been used in teaching sports and other motor skills. In one example, adults learning to swim received feedback by watching videos of their swimming strokes, and these adults showed more improvement than those who watched videotapes of someone else swimming (Starek & McCullagh, 1999). In another study, children with coordination problems used video self-modeling to help them improve such skills as throwing or catching a ball, batting a ball, and jumping toward a target (Wilson, Thomas, & Maruff, 2002).

Transfer from Previous Training

In motor-skill research, the topic of **transfer of training** is similar to the topic of generalization in animal-learning research. In both cases, the question is how experience with one set of stimuli will affect performance with a new set of stimuli. Early theorists (Osgood, 1949) believed that it should be possible to observe **positive transfer** (in which practice in one task aids the acquisition of a similar task) in some situations and **negative transfer** (in which practice on one task interferes with the acquisition of a similar task) in other situations. From an intuitive standpoint, both possibilities seem reasonable. For instance, it seems likely that learning to drive a car with a three-speed manual transmission should make it easier to learn to drive a car with a four-speed transmission. The topic of negative transfer reminds me of the discussions I had with friends when I was young about how playing baseball early in the day would be detrimental to a golf game later in the day. Our theory was that the flat swing of a baseball bat would interfere with one's ability to produce the relatively upright golf swing shortly afterward.

Quite a few studies have found evidence for positive transfer. As we might expect, the amount of positive transfer from one task to another depends on the similarity of the two tasks. However, there can be positive transfer across different muscle groups and different movement patterns. Latash (1999) had college students practice mirror writing, in which they had to write a sentence while looking in a mirror so that the words read correctly as seen in the mirror. After practicing this task for several days with their normal writing hands, the students showed large transfer effects when they had to switch to their other hands. Palmer and Meyer (2000) found positive transfer when experienced pianists first learned a new piece of music and then were asked to play a variation of the melody that required them to use different hand and finger movements. These researchers concluded that motor learning is not simply a matter of learning specific muscle movements, because experienced learners can transfer their skills to new situations that require them to produce the same general patterns of movements using different muscle groups.

Somewhat surprisingly, it has proven to be quite difficult to find experimental evidence for negative transfer in motor-skill tasks. When it is found, negative transfer is often very fleeting, sometimes lasting only a trial or two (Blais, Kerr, & Hughes, 1993). One demonstration of this phenomenon was provided by Lewis, McAllister, and Adams (1951). The participant's task in this experiment was to use a joystick to move several green lights on a display toward different targets. In the initial phase of the experiment, moving a joystick in one direction caused a green light to move in the same direction (e.g., moving the joystick to the upper left made the light move toward the upper left). In the second (interference) phase, participants in several experimental groups had to perform the task with the joystick controls reversed (moving the joystick to the upper left made the light move to the lower right). Here, too, participants' performances improved with practice. Participants in a control group received no trials with the controls reversed. The test of negative transfer came in the third phase of the experiment, in which the original operation of the joystick was restored. Participants in the experimental groups performed more poorly than they had at the end

of the first phase, and they required several trials to regain their previous performance levels. There was no such drop in the performance of control participants, which shows that the decrements were not simply due to the passage of time without practice.

Another study found strong negative transfer in a task that required moving both hands, but at different rates. For instance, in the initial task, a participant might learn to perform repetitive movements with both hands, but to make two movements of the left hand for every one movement of the right hand. The researchers found strong evidence for negative transfer when participants were required to switch hands—now making two right-hand cycles for every one left-hand movement (Vangheluwe, Suy, Wenderoth, & Swinnen, 2006).

It seems difficult to identify the conditions that will result in negative transfer. We could speculate that negative transfer is most likely to be observed when two tasks demand antagonistic or incompatible responses to a similar stimulus situation. Thus the strong negative transfer found by Lewis and colleagues probably occurred because a particular stimulus (e.g., a green light below its target) required one response in the original task and the opposite response in the interfering task. However, it is often hard to know whether two movements (e.g., swinging a baseball bat and swinging a golf club) should be considered similar or antagonistic. In many cases, two skills may include a mixture of both similar and antagonistic responses. For instance, in one study participants in an experimental group practiced the skills of short tennis and lawn tennis for a few hours each, and a control group practiced lawn tennis only. Then both groups were tested in lawn tennis skills. The researchers found that the experimental participants were better at certain lawn tennis skills and the control participants were better at others, thereby providing evidence for both positive and negative transfer in the same experiment (Coldwells & Hare, 1994).

Ironic Errors in Movement

People sometimes tend to make the very movement they are trying to avoid. If someone hands you a full cup of coffee and says, "Be careful not to spill it on my new rug," it may be harder to avoid spilling a drop than if you are carrying the cup outdoors across the lawn. According to Wegner (1997), this is not just because you are more nervous when carrying the cup over a new rug. Wegner has proposed a theory of **ironic errors**, which states that people have a tendency to make a false movement that they are trying hard to avoid, especially if their attention is distracted by some competing task. Wegner, Ansfield, and Pilloff (1998) tested this theory in an experiment where participants tried to putt a golf ball toward a target. One group of participants was simply told to try to get the ball as close as possible to the target. A second group was told to be particularly careful not to hit the ball past the target. Under conditions of a "mental load" (in which they had to remember a six-digit number while making the putt), those who were specifically instructed not to hit the ball past the target were more likely to do so. In another experiment, these researchers asked people to hold a weight on a string above a target for 30 seconds. A group that was specifically instructed to avoid left or right movements (as opposed to forward or backward movements) tended to make more left or right movements than a group that was simply instructed to hold the weight as steady as possible. This was especially true when participants performed the task under a mental-load condition.

Ironic errors can be frustrating and embarrassing, and they can make us look awkward and clumsy. They can also affect the performance of athletes who are trying to perform at the peak of their abilities. There is evidence that some individuals are more prone to ironic errors than others (Russell & Grealy, 2010). To avoid ironic errors, Janelle (1999) recommends that coaches could use a variety of strategies, such as making sure that athletes are thoroughly familiar with all the possible situations that can arise during a game, so the need to make novel decisions (which would constitute a mental load) is minimized. Further research may show whether these strategies can help to reduce the errors that an athlete is trying hardest to avoid.

PRACTICE QUIZ (1)

1. Movements in which a person continually receives and reacts for feedback are called _____ movements.
2. _____ is telling a person that a movement was right or wrong, and _____ is telling a person how far off target the movement was.
3. Giving a person tips on specific parts of a movement that need improvement is called _____.
4. _____ practice often leads to faster learning of a new motor skill than does _____ practice, but the difference tends to disappear during later performance.
5. Making a movement you are specifically trying to avoid is called a(n) _____.

Answers

1. closed-loop 2. Qualitative KR, quantitative KR 3. KP 4. Distributed, massed 5. ironic error

---

THEORIES OF MOTOR-SKILL LEARNING

So far we have considered some factors that determine how quickly and how well a new skill will be learned, but we have not discussed hypotheses about what takes place inside the individual during such learning episodes. We will now turn to some theories that deal with this question.

Adams's Two-Stage Theory

Jack A. Adams (1971) proposed one of the earliest influential theories of motor learning. To make the discussion of **Adams's two-stage theory** more understandable, it will be helpful to relate some of Adams's terms to the terminology of control systems theory introduced in Chapter 2. One important concept of Adams's theory is the *perceptual trace,* which corresponds to the reference input of control systems theory. According to Adams, when a person begins to learn a new motor skill, the perceptual trace, or reference input, is weak or nonexistent. Consider any simple task in which KR is delivered after the movement is completed, such as Thorndike's line-drawing task. The blindfolded participant knows that the task is to draw a 3-inch line, but the participant does not yet know what it "feels like" to draw a line of this length. Adams proposed that an important part of the learning of such a skill is the development of an appropriate perceptual trace. In the line-drawing task, the perceptual trace is presumably a memory of the sensations produced by the sensory neurons of the hand and arm when a line of the appropriate length was drawn.

A second important concept in Adams's theory is the *motor trace* (which Adams actually called the *memory trace*). The motor trace relates to the workings of the action system of control systems theory. The basic idea is that in addition to learning what it feels like to produce the correct movement, a person must also learn to coordinate his or her muscles so that the movement is indeed produced. For example, a beginning pianist may listen to a recording of a difficult piece again and again, until she has a firm idea of what an excellent rendition sounds like. Having reached this point, however, it may take long hours of painstaking practice before she can even approximate a good rendition on her own. As another example, having hit thousands of golf balls over the years, I believe I can distinguish between the sensations that accompany a good golf swing and those that accompany a bad swing. A good swing involves a certain rhythm of the wrists, arms, hips, and knees that causes the club head to "snap" at the ball, and I can tell the shot is a good one before looking up to see where the ball has gone. My problem is that although I can recognize a good swing when I feel one, my action system does not produce one every time. In fact, I sometimes go through an entire round without ever experiencing the sensations of a good swing.

According to Adams's theory, there are two stages in the learning of a typical motor skill. The first stage is called the *verbal-motor stage*, because in this stage improvement depends on the delivery of feedback, usually in a verbal form. The instructor must supply the learner with KR,

because the learner does not have an accurate perceptual trace and therefore cannot discriminate a good trial from a bad one. The verbal-motor stage is the time when improvement depends on constant feedback from the piano teacher, the pitching coach, or the gymnastics instructor. Without this feedback, the learner cannot tell whether the movement was good, or what was wrong with it. Adams (1976) described the end of the verbal-motor stage in this way:

> The Verbal-Motor Stage has a somewhat indefinite end point, and it will vary from subject to subject, but it comes to an end when knowledge of results has been signifying trivial error for some time and that the response is being successfully made. At this point the subject can switch wholly to the perceptual trace as a reference for responding because it now defines the correct response. The subject can now behave without knowledge of results. (p. 205)

Adams called the second stage the *motor stage*. At this point, the individual can rely on an internal perceptual trace to judge the accuracy of a movement in the absence of external KR. Adams proposed that in addition to maintaining current performance level in the absence of KR, the learner can actually improve performance by refining the precision of the motor trace (i.e., by becoming more skillful in producing the desired movement).

Adams's theory predicts that during the first stage of motor learning, if participants receive KR only intermittently, the perceptual trace will be strengthened on trials when KR is delivered, but it will tend to decay on trials without KR. Sparrow and Summers (1992) found just such a pattern with a slow positioning task in which participants sometimes received KR after every 5th trial and sometimes after every 10th trial. As shown in Figure 12-3, the participants' accuracy improved immediately after a trial with KR; then it gradually deteriorated during the trials without KR.

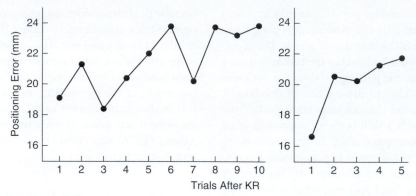

FIGURE 12-3 The magnitude of errors by participants performing a slow positioning task when KR was delivered on every 10th trial (left panel) or on every 5th trial (right panel). As the trials without KR proceeded, the participants' errors tended to increase. An adaptation from Fig 3, p. 202 from Sparrow, W. A., & Summers, J. J., "Performance on trials without knowledge of results (KR) in reduced relative frequency presentations of KR," *Journal of Motor Behavior, 24* (1992) pp. 197–209, reprinted by permission of the publisher, Taylor & Francis Group, www.tandfonline.com.

This experiment shows that KR is essential when a new motor skill is first being learned. However, there is also solid evidence that KR can become unnecessary later in training. The best evidence comes from studies in which KR is withdrawn at some point in the middle of the experiment. For example, Bilodeau, Bilodeau, and Schumsky (1959) had participants practice a discrete movement—moving a lever through an angle of 33 degrees—for 20 trials. One group of participants received quantitative KR on all trials, one group received no KR, and two groups received quantitative KR for two or six trials before it was withdrawn. Figure 12-4 shows that in the group with constant KR, errors steadily decreased to a low level. Not surprisingly, the group with no KR did not improve at all. The results from the groups with two or six trials with KR are more interesting, because they appeared to derive some permanent benefits from the initial KR. There was some deterioration in performance when the KR was removed, but these groups continued to perform better than the group that never received KR. According to Adams's theory, these groups were beginning to develop a perceptual trace. A similar experiment by Newell (1974) suggested that the perceptual trace can get much stronger if participants receive more trials with KR. One group was given 52 trials with KR before it was withdrawn.

This group showed no decreases in accuracy at all when the KR was removed, and its performance equaled that of a group that received continuous KR throughout the experiment. Adams's interpretation is that participants in the 52-trial group had progressed to the motor stage, where an internal perceptual trace replaced external KR as a means of evaluating their performances on each trial.

Adams's theory is also supported by more recent studies showing that delivering KR on only a fraction of the acquisition trials, or delaying KR for a few seconds, can lead to better performance on later tests when participants must perform without KR (Badets & Blandin, 2010; Russell & Newell, 2007). These results, which provide support for the guidance hypothesis (discussed in the section on Reinforcement and Knowledge of Results), can be interpreted using Adams's theory as follows: Participants who received less frequent or delayed KR presumably had more of an opportunity to develop accurate perceptual traces (i.e., to use sensory cues to judge their performances), as external KR was frequently unavailable. On the other hand, participants who received KR on every trial may have had it too easy: They may have failed to develop a keen ability to judge their own performances because the experimenter always provided them with immediate, external KR. These results seem to support Adams's theory that

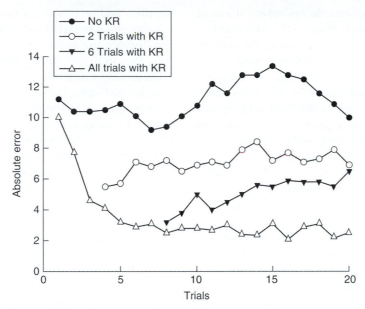

FIGURE 12-4 Results from the four groups in the experiment of Bilodeau, Bilodeau, and Schumsky (1959). Each group received a different number of trials with KR. From Bilodeau et. al., "Some effects of introducing and withdrawing knowledge of results early and late in practice," *Journal of Experimental Psychology, 58*(2), August 1959, 142–144, © American Psychological Association. Adapted with permission.

the development of an accurate perceptual trace is an important part of learning a motor skill.

Once a person has reached the motor stage, feedback from the piano teacher, the pitching coach, or the gymnastics instructor becomes less important. Of course, the instructor can continue to provide helpful feedback to correct minor flaws in one's technique or to make further refinements in one's style. At the same time, however, the learner can also improve through practice on his or her own by relying on internal feedback in place of the coach's feedback. Perhaps the most important contribution of Adams's theory is that it distinguishes between the two types of learning that take place during the acquisition of most motor skills: learning to recognize what it feels like to make an accurate response and learning to produce such a response consistently.

Schmidt's Schema Theory

Adams's two-stage theory represented an important advance in the analysis of motor-skill learning. Yet all theories have their limitations, and a

major limitation of Adams's theory is that it seems to be limited to the acquisition of single, repetitive movements (i.e., to movements of the foul-shot type, where the stimulus conditions and the required movement are exactly the same, trial after trial). The theory says nothing about how people can acquire skills that involve the production of different responses on different trials so as to deal with different stimulus conditions. Consider the tennis player's response to an approaching ball, a bird's response to the diversionary tactics of a flying insect it is chasing, a hiker's response to the irregular terrain of a rocky hillside, or a driver's response to an unfamiliar winding road. In all of these cases and many others, the individual is confronted with new and different stimulus conditions and must generate a response to suit these conditions. It seems clear that more is involved in the acquisition of such skills than the development of a single perceptual trace and a single motor trace. In an effort to go beyond Adams's theory and deal with these more flexible motor skills, Richard Schmidt (1975) developed his schema theory of motor-skill learning.

Schmidt's schema theory retains the most novel part of Adams's theory—the idea that two types of learning take place during the acquisition of most motor skills (learning to recognize the correct response and learning to produce it). However, to deal with more flexible motor skills, such as those discussed earlier, Schmidt proposed that people can acquire general rules (*schemas*) as they practice. Schmidt proposed that people do not retain information about specific past movements and their consequences but rather that they develop what I will call *perceptual schemas* and *motor schemas*. (These are not the terms Schmidt used, but I will use them to be as consistent as possible with the terminology used in describing Adams's theory.)

To make these concepts more concrete, let us consider how a golfer learns to putt a ball the appropriate distance (ignoring the problem of moving the ball in the appropriate direction). The golfer must learn to stroke the ball with different amounts of effort, depending on how far the ball is from the hole. In practice, the golfer may use different amounts of effort on different trials and observe the result (the distance the ball travels). This situation is illustrated in Figure 12-5a. Each point represents a single practice trial: The x-axis represents the golfer's estimate of the effort used in the stroke, and the y-axis represents the golfer's estimate of the distance the ball traveled.

According to Schmidt, these individual data points are soon forgotten, but what the golfer develops and retains is a general rule, or motor schema, about the relationship between effort and the distance the ball moves (as signified by the solid line in Figure 12-5a). Furthermore, motor schemas may consist of more than a single function, because other situational variables can affect the outcome of a particular movement. In the example of putting, one such variable is the slope of the green. Figure 12-5b shows a simplified illustration of the more complex motor schema a golfer might develop by practicing level, uphill, and downhill putts. A skillful golfer's motor schema would be much more complex than this, of course, because the slope of a green can vary continuously, and other factors such as the length of the grass and any moisture on the green must be taken into account. The advantage of such a schema is that it allows the individual to respond to new situations with a reasonable chance of success. Thus, although a golfer may never have practiced a 22-foot putt on a moderately slow green with a downhill slope of 4 degrees, the motor schema allows the golfer to generalize from similar past experiences, so as to produce a reasonably suitable response.

Schmidt's theory states that besides developing such a motor schema, learners also develop perceptual schemas that allow them to use sensory feedback to predict whether the appropriate movement was produced. The perceptual schema is simply a generalized version of the perceptual trace in Adams's theory that is applicable to more

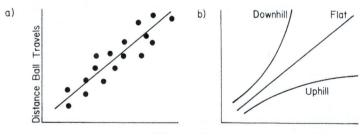

Effort of Putting Stroke

FIGURE 12-5 (a) A hypothetical illustration of how, according to Schmidt's schema theory, a person might learn a general rule or schema about the relationship between the effort of a putting stroke and the distance the golf ball moves. Each data point represents the learner's estimates of effort and distance on one practice trial, and the line represents the general rule the learner supposedly retains from these trials. (b) This figure makes the point that a successful golfer's schema for putting would have to include different rules for downhill, flat, and uphill putts. In reality, the golfer's schema would have to be considerably more complex to account for continuous variations in the slope of the putting surface.

than one situation. Such a perceptual schema presumably allows the performer to predict before seeing the result whether a movement was too strong, too weak, on target or off target, regardless of the exact distance and location of the target. For example, basketball players frequently remark that the shooter is the first person to know whether a shot will go into the basket. All the players can watch the flight of the ball and try to estimate whether it will hit or miss, but only the shooter has the additional sensory feedback provided by the shooting motion itself. The shooter can take advantage of this information by moving in position to grab the rebound if he or she determines that the shot will bounce off the rim.

The ability to deal with open-ended classes of movements, such as putting golf balls and shooting baskets from different parts of the court, makes Schmidt's theory more versatile than Adams's. But what scientific evidence is there that people do in fact learn such motor schemas? To test the theory, several different research strategies have been used. Some studies have tested whether people soon forget the specific examples that they practice but nevertheless retain a general schema (as illustrated in Figure 12-5). For example, Chamberlin and Magill (1992) taught participants a timing task that involved pressing a sequence of three buttons that were a total of 15 cm, 45 cm, or 135 cm apart. For all three distances, the participants' goal was to complete the task in exactly 1.2 seconds, and they received extensive practice with each distance. The participants were then tested 1 day later, and again 1 week later, on both these well-practiced distances and with new distances that they had never tried before (e.g., 30 cm and 90 cm). Chamberlin and Magill found that their participants were just as accurate with the new distances as with the well-practiced distances. This finding is consistent with the prediction of schema theory that people can learn a general rule for movement and not just individual movement patterns.

An important prediction of Schmidt's theory (but not Adams's theory) is that variability in one's practice routine is beneficial, because it contributes to the development of the learner's perceptual and motor schemas. Several experiments have provided support for schema theory's prediction

that variable practice is beneficial. For example, Kerr and Booth (1978) had children toss bean bags at a target without visual feedback, and they were given quantitative KR by the experimenter. One group of children received *specific training* in which they always aimed for a target that was 3 feet away. A second group received *variable training* in which the target was sometimes 2 feet away and sometimes 4 feet away. Both groups later received test trials with the 3-foot target distance, and the group that had received variable training performed more accurately, even though participants had never practiced with the 3-foot distance. Kerr and Booth suggested that the variable training helped the children develop stronger schemas than did the specific training.

To summarize, Schmidt's schema theory provides a framework for understanding how people develop flexible motor skills that allow them to make successful responses when confronted with situations they have never experienced before. Three decades after schema theory was first proposed, Shea and Wulf (2005) evaluated its status. They concluded that one of its strengths is its prediction that variable practice can be more effective than constant practice, an idea that has received substantial empirical support. On the negative side, some research findings pose problems for schema theory, and other theories of motor learning have been proposed to try to accommodate these results (Taktek & Hochman, 2004). Perhaps the fairest way to summarize Schmidt's theory is to say that it represents an important advance, but as the science of motor-skill learning advances, new and more refined theories will almost surely be developed.

What Is the Best Way to Practice?

A good general rule for learning motor skills is that more difficult practice sessions often produce better long-term performance. The advantage of variable training over specific training described in the preceding section is one example of this principle. Discussing this principle in a more general way, Battig (1979) used the term **contextual interference** to refer to any features of the learning situation (the "context") that make performing the task more difficult (i.e., they "interfere" with the learner's performance during the acquisition of a new skill). Battig's theory was that high contextual interference during acquisition ultimately leads to better long-term performance. Some experiments have tested the theory of contextual interference by comparing blocked practice and random practice. In blocked practice, the learner practices the same variation of a skill for a block of trials, then switches to a different variation for another block of trials, and so on. For example, a basketball player might practice 10 shots from a specific spot on the left side of the basket, then 10 shots from one spot in front of the basket, and then 10 shots from one spot on the right side of the basket. In random practice, the task requirements are changed every trial (e.g., the basketball player would randomly switch among the left, front, and right positions after every shot). According to Battig, contextual interference should be higher during random practice, because the movements needed for a successful performance are constantly changing with each practice trial.

Some studies have found the predicted advantage for random practice over blocked practice. Shea and Morgan (1979) taught people to make three different patterns of rapid arm movements in response to three different signals, and their speed in completing the movements was measured. They found that performance during the acquisition phase was worse with random practice, which makes sense according to the theory, because the task demands were more difficult when every trial was different from the last. However, the participants who had random practice performed better than those who had blocked practice when tested 10 minutes later and 10 days later. Similarly, Vera and Montilla (2003) found an advantage for random practice for 6-year-olds learning a throwing task during their physical education class.

Although variable practice is often better than specific practice, and although random practice is often better than blocked practice, there are exceptions to these rules. Some studies comparing blocked and random practice have found no differences in long-term performance (Meira & Tani, 2001; Moreno et al., 2003). In tasks that involve accuracy in several different measures of performance, random practice with one measure may actually lead to worse performance on the other measure. For example, on a task that required accuracy in both the amount of force used and in movement duration, Whitacre and Shea (2000) found that randomly varying the force requirements from trial to trial had a detrimental effect on the participants' timing. It could be that when a task places many demands on the learner, random variations along one dimension may make learning the task overwhelming. Exactly why random practice has an advantage in some situations but not others is not well understood.

LEARNING MOVEMENT SEQUENCES

In this section we will consider motor skills involving sequences of movements that must be performed in a specific order. Some skills of this type are walking, swimming, typing, or playing a musical instrument. Successful performance depends on producing the sequence of movements in the correct order and with the correct timing. For instance, in performing the breast stroke, a swimmer must coordinate the movements of the arms and legs to move through the water efficiently. A pianist must play the notes in the correct sequence, and with the correct tempo. The challenge for motor-skill researchers is to explain why people become more skillful in performing such sequences of movement with practice.

The Response Chain Approach

One major approach to the topic of movement sequences is based on the concept of a response chain, which was discussed in Chapter 5. A response chain was defined as a sequence of behaviors that must occur in a specific order, with a primary reinforcer following the completion of the last behavior of the chain. According to standard analysis, what keeps the behaviors of the chain in their correct sequence is that each response produces a distinctive stimulus that acts as a discriminative stimulus (S^D) for the next response of the chain. It is easy to see how this analysis could be applied to some skilled movement sequences, such as walking. The sight or feeling of having one's right leg in front might serve as a discriminative stimulus to shift one's weight to this leg and bring the left leg forward. The opposite might be true when one's left leg is in front. The main idea is that the visual, tactile, or kinesthetic feedback from one movement serves as a discriminative stimulus for the next movement in the sequence.

Why, according to this analysis, does a person's ability to perform a sequence of movements improve with practice? The answer is that the appropriate stimulus–response associations are strengthened by reinforcement. For instance, to achieve the maximum propulsion in the breast stroke, a swimmer must begin to move his or her hands forward at a particular point during each stroke. If we assume that swimming speed is the reinforcer, then through the process of successive approximations, the swimmer should eventually learn exactly what cues signal that the forward movement of the hands should begin.

The response chain analysis of movement sequences is compatible with theories such as those of Adams and Schmidt, which emphasize the role of feedback in the control of movement. Yet although the response chain approach provides a satisfactory analysis for many response sequences, several types of evidence now suggest that it cannot account for all examples of behavioral sequences.

Motor Programs

The strongest line of attack against the response chain approach to movement sequencing is based on evidence for the existence of **motor programs**. Those who favor the concept of motor programs suggest that the response chain approach is incorrect because some movement sequences do not depend on continual sensory feedback for their proper execution. Keele (1973) described the concept of a motor program as follows:

> If neither visual nor kinesthetic feedback is needed for the execution of patterns of movement, then the movement patterns must be represented centrally in the brain, or perhaps in some cases in the spinal cord. Such representation is called a motor

program. As a motor program is executed, neural impulses are sent to the appropriate muscles in proper sequence, timing, and force, as predetermined by the program, and the neural impulses are largely uninfluenced by the resultant feedback. (p. 124)

To clarify the distinction between a response chain and a motor program, let us consider a concrete example of a movement sequence—the typing of the word *the*. A response chain analysis might proceed as follows: Upon seeing the word *the* in the text to be typed, a typist responds by striking the *t* key with the left forefinger. This movement produces sensory feedback (kinesthetic feedback from the finger and perhaps auditory feedback from the keyboard) that serves as a discriminative stimulus to make the next response—striking the *h* key with the right forefinger. Sensory feedback from this response serves as a stimulus for the final response of striking the *e* key with the left middle finger.

Advocates of the motor program approach might agree that this analysis is correct for a beginning typist, but that after typing *the* many times, a skilled typist may develop a motor program for producing this response sequence. The idea is that when the skilled typist sees the word *the,* this motor program is activated and sends a series of commands to the muscles of the left forefinger, the right forefinger, and the left middle finger. These commands are timed so that the three movements are performed in the correct sequence, but this timing does not depend on sensory feedback from each successive movement in the sequence. One obvious advantage of the motor program is an increase in speed: The typist can begin to produce the second keystroke before receiving sensory feedback from the first keystroke.

EVIDENCE FOR MOTOR PROGRAMS.   One of the first advocates of the concept of a motor program was Karl Lashley (1951), who described several types of evidence that a response chain analysis cannot explain all movement sequences. For one thing, Lashley argued that human reaction times are too slow to support the idea that sensory feedback from one response can serve as the stimulus for the next response in a rapid sequence.

Lashley pointed out that musicians can produce as many as 16 finger movements per second. His point is that this rate could never be achieved if the musician had to wait for sensory feedback from one movement before beginning the next. Similar arguments have been made for the skill of typing (Shaffer, 1978). However, recent studies have suggested that human reaction times can sometimes be faster than previously believed possible, so this argument for motor programs is not quite as convincing as it once seemed (Bruce, 1994).

A second argument made by Lashley was that skilled movements and sequences of movements are still possible for individuals who have lost sensory feedback. He reported the case of a man who had lost all sensation in the area of the knee as a result of a gunshot wound. Despite the loss of sensation, the man could move and position his leg as accurately as an uninjured person (Lashley, 1917). Other evidence that complex movements can continue in the absence of sensory feedback comes from animal studies in which sensory nerve fibers are severed before they enter the spinal cord. For example, Taub and Berman (1968) surgically removed all sensory feedback from both forelimbs of several monkeys. After this surgery, the monkeys were still able to use these limbs to walk and climb (even when blindfolded, which removed the possible influence of visual feedback). The monkeys could coordinate the movements of their senseless forelimbs with their normal hindlimbs. This research provides evidence that sensory feedback is not always necessary for skilled movements.

Further evidence for movement sequencing without sensory feedback has been found in other species. In research on various songbirds, Nottebohm (1970) determined that young birds will not develop the normal song of their species unless they (1) have the opportunity to hear other members of their species sing, and (2) can hear themselves sing as they first learn the song. However, if the birds are deafened after they have learned the song, they can continue to sing the song with only minor deterioration of their performance. One interpretation is that auditory feedback is necessary while a motor program for the song is being developed, but once it is developed, auditory feedback is no longer necessary.

Lashley's third argument for motor programs concerns the types of errors frequently found in rapid-movement sequences. He noted that many typing mistakes are errors of anticipation or transposition. For instance, I sometimes type *hte* when I intend to type *the*. It is difficult to explain this sort of error with a response chain analysis. If the stimulus for striking the *h* key was the sensory feedback from the movement of striking the *t* key, the second movement should never precede the first. Instead, Lashley would argue that the separate movements were sequenced by a motor program, but that the synchronization of the movements became distorted somewhere along the line from command to execution. In short, Lashley suggested that any errors that indicate the individual was planning ahead support the notion of a motor program but are inconsistent with the response chain approach.

A fourth type of evidence, not known to Lashley, is that the amount of time needed to begin a sequence of movements depends on the number of separate movements that are part of the sequence. For instance, a person needs more time to begin a sequence that involves four discrete motions than one that involves only two motions (Ulrich, Giray, & Schaffer, 1990). The explanation usually offered for this effect is that the person is constructing a motor program for all of the motions at the beginning, and it takes more time to preprogram four movements than two movements. If the participant was only planning the first movement before beginning, why would it take longer to plan this single movement in one case than in the other? Starting times are slower for longer movement sequences even when such sequences have been practiced extensively (Fischman & Lim, 1991).

An experiment on handwriting found evidence of this last type (Portier, Van Galen, & Meulenbroek, 1990). Participants were taught to write six different patterns, each composed of three letter-like characters. Participants wrote with a pen that was connected to sophisticated recording equipment that could detect the exact location of the pen at each instant. Not surprisingly, with practice, participants got faster at writing the patterns.

However, writing speed increased substantially for the second and third characters of each pattern, whereas writing speed for the first character did not increase very much. Why should it take participants so long to write the first character, which had a relatively simple shape? The experimenters concluded that this was because participants were not simply learning to write the three individual characters; they were developing motor programs for each pattern as a whole. The first character presumably took longer to write because participants were simultaneously planning the rest of the pattern.

As in many other areas of learning, physiological research is beginning to provide insights into the neural basis of motor programs. Research with the marine snail *Aplysia* has identified groups of neurons that appear to control motor programs that coordinate various movements (Friedman & Weiss, 2010; Perrins & Weiss, 1996). With humans, Jennings (1995) used a reaction-time task to compare the performance of normal adults and those suffering from Parkinson's disease, which causes impairments in motor coordination. The task involved pressing three keys in the correct sequence as quickly as possible, after receiving a signal that indicated which sequence to produce. Participants with Parkinson's disease actually made the first response of the sequence faster than normal participants, but they were slower to make the second and third responses. This observation, plus other details about their performances, led Jennings to conclude that patients with this disease tend to start the first movement in the sequence before the entire motor program has been planned; as a result, they have difficulty completing a smooth, coordinated sequence of movements. By using what is known about the neurophysiology of Parkinson's disease, Jennings was able to make some preliminary hypotheses about how different parts of the brain may contribute to the execution of motor programs.

GENERALIZED MOTOR PROGRAMS. In his development of the schema theory, Schmidt (1988, 2003) introduced the concept of a **generalized motor program**. The idea is that a motor program may include the neural mechanisms that both send a series of commands in a specified sequence and have the ability to adjust the exact movements that are part of that sequence to suit the current circumstances. Even in seemingly repetitive sequences of movements, such as typing the word *the,* different movements will be required on different occasions. The spacing between keys and the force and amount of movement required to operate them can vary considerably from one keyboard to the next. Nevertheless, an experienced typist will have little difficulty transferring his or her skills from one keyboard to another. The individual can also adapt reasonably well to a keyboard that is 6 inches below the waist or 12 inches above the waist, although the relationships among forearms, wrists, and fingers will be considerably different. For a motor program to be useful in such variable conditions, it cannot simply specify one fixed pattern of muscle movements. Instead, Schmidt suggested that motor programs provide a general framework (or schema) about the proper timing and sequencing of movements, but the details of the movement sequence can (and must) be adapted to suit the current situation. A motor program that can be adapted to a variety of different situations is called a *generalized motor program.*

A good example of this adaptability is the observation that people's handwriting styles retain their individuality whether they are writing 1/4-inch letters on a piece of paper or 5-inch letters on a blackboard. The concept of a generalized motor program offers some suggestions about how this adaptability is possible. The idea is that individuals can generalize from their past experience with different stimulus conditions, different movements, and the results of those movements so as to select a new movement to meet the requirements of a new situation. Thus, in handwriting, an individual has presumably already learned what muscle movements are needed to draw a 1/4-inch oval, a 5-inch oval, or one of any other size (within limits). According to Schmidt, once these relationships are learned, the production of letters of any size requires only the selection of the appropriate parameters within an existing motor program.

Shapiro, Zernicke, Gregor, and Diestel (1981) obtained evidence for generalized motor programs by having participants walk or run on a treadmill, at speeds ranging from 3 to 6 kilometers per hour for walking, and from 8 to 12 kilometers per hour for running. The researchers recorded the amounts of time the participants took to perform several different movement components during each stride (e.g., the amount of time the knee was flexed before the lower leg was extended to move forward). Their key finding was that the percentage of time devoted to the different parts of a stride remained constant regardless of a person's walking speed. For example, the knee-flexion component remained at about 10% of each stride at all walking speeds. Similarly, the different movement components occupied a constant percentage of each stride when the participants were running, but they were different percentages than for walking—the knee-flexion component remained constant at about 30% of each stride when running. The researchers called this result *relative time invariance,* and they hypothesized that people have two different generalized motor programs—one for walking and one for running. The motor program presumably keeps the relative timing of the different parts of each stride constant regardless of the speed of locomotion. Later research found additional evidence for relative time invariance in other movement sequences, such as handwriting and typing (Longstaff & Heath, 1997; Shea & Wulf, 2005).

Dynamic Pattern Theory

Although the concept of generalized motor programs is accepted by many researchers, others have proposed an alternative approach called **dynamic pattern theory** (Jantzen, Steinberg, & Kelso, 2009; Kelso, 1997). Proponents of dynamic pattern theory do not believe that the ability of people to perform rapid and adaptable sequences of movements necessarily means that the movements are controlled by a generalized motor program. The debate is a complex one, but we can examine two key points of difference between generalized motor programs and dynamic pattern theory. First, those who favor

dynamic pattern theory argue that the evidence for relative time invariance in movement sequences (e.g., as found in walking and running) could be the result of the physical properties of the body (such as the length and weight of one's limbs and flexibility of one's joints), not the product of a generalized motor program. As an example, try walking across the room at a slow, leisurely pace. Next, try walking across the room at a rapid pace. If you do not normally have problems walking, you should be able to walk at both paces without difficulty. But now try walking across the room at the slow pace with each left stride and at the rapid pace with each right stride. You should find this quite awkward, because you will be constantly speeding up and slowing down your forward momentum. This simple demonstration suggests that the rhythmic nature of walking may occur, not because the strides are paced by a motor program, but simply because it is physically easier to move forward at a constant velocity. According to dynamic pattern theory, this same sort of reasoning may account for relative time invariance in other movement sequences.

Second, dynamic pattern theory emphasizes the important role of feedback from the body and the environment during a movement sequence. To be fair, we should note that those who favor the motor program approach have long known that feedback can play some role in motor programs. For example, Summers (1981) suggested that walking is usually controlled by a motor program, but when a person's foot unexpectedly strikes an object, sensory feedback tells the person he or she is about to fall: "To avoid falling the person must consciously attend to his movements and make a rapid correction to the motor program" (p. 49). However, critics of the motor program concept argue that continual sensory feedback plays such a critical role in skilled movements that it raises doubts about whether these movement sequences are "preprogrammed" by a motor program. For example, Crump and Logan (2010) had skilled typists type on four different keyboards: (1) a regular computer keyboard, (2) a keyboard with the keys removed, exposing rubber buttons that could be typed on, (3) the keyboard consisting of a rubber mat that could be typed

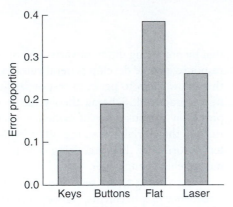 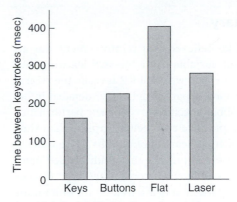

FIGURE 12-6 Error rates (left) and time between keystrokes (right) of skilled typists when typing on keyboards that provided different amounts of tactile feedback.

SOURCE: Adaptation of Figure 1 from Crump, M. C., & Logan, G. D. (2010). Warning: This keyboard will deconstruct—the role of the keyboard in skilled typewriting," *Psychonomic Bulletin & Review, 17*(3), 2010. Reprinted with kind permission from Spring Science+Business Media B.V.

on, and (4) a laser projection of a keyboard on a desktop. The idea was to examine the effects of using keyboards that provided less sensory feedback than normal. The researchers argued that if typing is controlled by motor programs that do not require sensory feedback, performance should be roughly the same on all four keyboards. That is not what they found, however. As shown in Figure 12-6, the typists made many more errors on the keyboards that provided less sensory feedback. Their typing speeds were also significantly slower on these keyboards. Crump and Logan concluded that continuous tactile feedback plays a crucial role in allowing skilled typists to maintain their high levels of performance.

The question of how skilled movement sequences are produced is still being studied, and it may turn out that the theory of generalized motor programs and dynamic pattern theory are both partly correct. As we have seen, several types of evidence strongly favor the idea that some well-practiced movement sequences are preplanned, as the theory of motor programs claims. However, those who favor dynamic pattern theory have made some valid points about the important roles played by the physical environment and ongoing sensory feedback during the execution of skilled movement sequences.

Practice Quiz (2)

1. According to Adams's theory, in the _____ stage, a person needs external feedback in order to improve a motor skill, but not in the _____ stage.
2. In Schmidt's theory, when a person learns how different movements produce different results, this is called a _____.
3. _____ theory deals with movements that are the same every time, whereas _____ theory deals with movements that must be varied for each new situation.
4. According to the _____, feedback from one movement in a sequence serves as stimulus for the next movement in the sequence.
5. In a _____, feedback from each movement is not necessary for a person to produce a coordinated sequence of movements.

Answers

1. verbal-motor, motor 2. motor schema
3. Adams's two-stage, Schmidt's schema
4. response chain approach 5. motor program

Summary

Thorndike believed that reinforcement was an important variable in motor-skill learning, but later research showed that KR is really the critical variable. Giving participants more detailed information about specific parts of their performance (KP) can produce even better learning than simple KR. People learn motor skills more quickly with distributed practice than with massed practice, but the difference is not always large. Studies in which participants are trained on one motor task and then tested on a somewhat different task have found evidence for both positive and negative transfer.

Adams's two-stage theory states that motor-skill learning first involves a verbal-motor stage in which feedback from a teacher or coach is essential, and later a motor stage in which the learner can continue to improve without external feedback. Studies in which KR is either delivered on a percentage basis or withdrawn at different points during training have provided support for Adams's theory. Schmidt's schema theory states that by practicing different variations of the same response, people develop general rules (schemas) that allow them to perform responses they have never practiced. Schema theory has been supported by various types of evidence, such as the finding that variable training often leads to better performance than practicing exactly the same movement over and over.

According to the response chain theory, in a sequence of movements, sensory feedback from one movement serves as a stimulus for the next response in the chain. Lashley presented several types of evidence against this theory, such as errors of anticipation that suggest a person is planning ahead. The theory of motor programs maintains that well-practiced sequences of movements can become a single unit that can be executed without sensory feedback from each individual response. In contrast, dynamic pattern theory emphasizes the roles of physical constraints and ongoing sensory feedback in the performance movement sequences.

Review Questions

1. Describe a study showing that KR is an important variable in motor-skill learning. What happens when KR is delayed and when it is given on only a percentage of the trials?
2. What is KP? Describe a few different types of KP that have been found to be useful in helping people learn new motor skills.
3. Give an example of positive transfer in a motor task, and give an example of negative transfer. Try to give a reasonable explanation why the transfer is positive in the first case but negative in the second.
4. What are the two stages of Adams's theory of motor-skill learning? What is Schmidt's schema theory and how does it differ from the theory of Adams? Describe some research that supports each theory.
5. Think of the difference between a person just learning to type and a skilled typist. Explain how the response chain approach may describe the behavior of the new typist, but how the skilled typist may rely on motor programs.
6. Describe several different types of evidence that have been used to argue for the existence of motor programs. Which do you find most convincing and why?

13

Choice

LEARNING OBJECTIVES

After reading this chapter, you should be able to

- describe the matching law and explain how it has been applied to different choice situations

- describe optimization theory and discuss studies that compare its predictions to those of the matching law

- describe momentary maximization theory and explain how it differs from optimization theory

- define the self-control choice situation, and give examples from the laboratory and from everyday life

- discuss techniques people can use to improve their self-control

- explain the phenomenon of the "tragedy of the commons" and discuss ways that it can be avoided

It is not much of an exaggeration to say that all behavior involves choice. Even in the most barren experimental chamber, an animal can choose among performing the operant response, exploring, sitting, standing, grooming, sleeping, and so on. Outside the laboratory, the choices are much more numerous. At any moment, an organism can choose to either continue with its current behavior or switch to another. Because both people and animals are constantly making choices, understanding choice is an essential part of understanding behavior itself.

One of the most remarkable characteristics of the behavior of animals in choice situations is its orderliness and predictability. Much of my own research deals with choice behavior, and when I give students or visitors a tour of the laboratory, they frequently ask, "Can these pigeons and rats really understand the complex choices you present to them and respond in anything but a haphazard way?" The answer is that they certainly can, and in fact the choice behavior of animals in laboratory experiments is often so orderly that it can be described by simple mathematical equations. One such equation is the matching law, developed by Richard Herrnstein. The next several sections describe the matching law, illustrate how it has been applied to many types of experimental results, and discuss some theories about why matching behavior is such a prevalent result in experiments on choice.

THE MATCHING LAW

Herrnstein's Experiment

Herrnstein (1961) used a pigeon chamber with two response keys located a few inches apart on one wall, a red key on the left and a white key on the right. Beneath and midway between the two keys was an opening in the wall where grain could be presented as a reinforcer. The experiment consisted of a series of conditions in which each key was associated with its own variable-interval (VI) schedule of reinforcement. For example, in one condition, pecks at the left key were reinforced on a VI 135-second schedule, and pecks at the right key were reinforced on a VI 270-second schedule. (Technically, this schedule is called a concurrent VI 135-second VI 270-second schedule. In general, any situation in which two or more reinforcement schedules are presented simultaneously can be called a **concurrent schedule**.) The schedules on the two keys were completely independent; that is, each key had its own VI timer. As in a typical VI schedule, once a reinforcer was stored, the VI timer for that key would be stopped until that reinforcer was collected. In this condition, the birds received approximately 27 reinforcers per hour from the left key and 13 reinforcers per hour (half as many) from the right key.

Herrnstein's main question was this: After the birds have learned all that they can about this choice situation, how will they distribute their responses? He therefore gave them many days of training with the same two VI schedules and then measured their responses. As in most VI schedules, the birds made many responses for each reinforcer they received. What is of interest, however, is that in this condition, where about two thirds of the reinforcers came from the left key, the birds made approximately two thirds of their responses on the left key. That is, the proportion of

responses on the left key equaled, or *matched,* the proportion of reinforcers delivered by the left key.

In another condition of Herrnstein's experiment, two birds received only about 15% of their reinforcers from the left key; on average, the birds made about 15% of their responses on this key. Once again, the percentage of left-key responses approximately matched the percentage of left-key reinforcers. Based on results like these, Herrnstein proposed the following general principle, now known as the **matching law**:

$$\frac{B_1}{B_1 + B_2} = \frac{R_1}{R_1 + R_2} \qquad (13\text{-}1)$$

B_1 is the number of responses of type 1 (e.g., left-key responses), and B_2 is the number of responses of type 2 (e.g., right-key responses). Similarly, R_1 is the number of reinforcers obtained by making response 1, and R_2 is the number of reinforcers obtained by making response 2. Equation 13-1 states that in a two-choice situation, the proportion of responses directed toward one alternative should equal the proportion of reinforcers delivered by that alternative.

Figure 13-1 plots the results from all of the conditions of Herrnstein's experiment. The *x*-axis represents the percentage of left-key reinforcers and the *y*-axis the percentage of left-key responses. According to the matching law, the data points should fall along the diagonal line, because this is where these two percentages are equal. As can be seen, all the points are close to the line. We can conclude, therefore, that the matching law provided a good description of the pigeons' behavior, except for the sort of random variations found in any psychological experiment.

Other Experiments on Matching

In Herrnstein's experiment, each pair of VI schedules was used for many sessions before he collected the final data. Davison and Baum (2000, 2002) also presented pigeons with pairs of VI schedules, but they changed the schedules much more

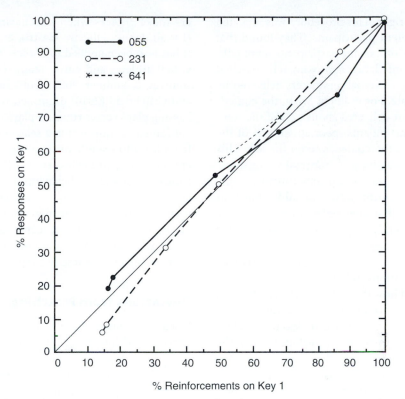

FIGURE 13-1   Results from three pigeons in Herrnstein's (1961) experiment on concurrent VI schedules. Each data point shows the results from a different condition. The diagonal line shows the predictions of the matching law (Equation 13-1), which predicts that response percentages will match reinforcement percentages. (From R.J. Hernstein, "Relative and absolute strength of response as a function of frequency of reinforcement" *Journal of the Experimental Analysis of Behavior, 4*(3), pages 267–272. Copyright 1961 by the Society for the Experimental Analysis of Behavior, Inc. Reprinted with permission.)

rapidly. Each daily session included seven periods (separated by brief time-outs), and each period had a different pair of VI schedules. Even though each period lasted only 7 minutes, the pigeons' choices quickly shifted in the direction predicted by the matching law (with more extreme preferences when the differences between the VI schedules were more extreme). These studies and others (Kyonka & Grace, 2010; Palya & Allan, 2003) show that when the environment introduces rapid changes in the choice alternatives, animals can adapt with rapid changes in their choice responses.

The matching law has been applied with reasonable success in a wide range of experiments with both animals and humans (e.g., Davison & McCarthy, 1988; Hoch & Symons, 2007; Schneider & Lickliter, 2010). One experiment examined the social interactions of college students (Conger & Killeen, 1974). Groups of four students sat around a table and had a 30-minute discussion about drug abuse. However, three members of the group were not real participants but confederates working for the experimenter. The tasks of the confederates to the left and right of the real participant were to deliver verbal reinforcers to the participant on two different VI schedules. For instance, whenever the confederate on the left received a signal (a light only he could see), he would reinforce the next statement of the participant by saying something like "That's a good point." The same was true for the confederate on the right. Conger and Killeen later had observers view the videos of these discussions and measure the amount of time the participants spent talking to the confederates on their left and right. This procedure was repeated with five different participants. They found that the percentage of time the participants spent talking to each confederate approximately matched the percentage of verbal reinforcers delivered by that confederate. For example, when the confederate on the left delivered about 82% of the reinforcers, the participants spent about 78% of the time talking to the confederate on the left. This approximate matching is impressive considering the brief duration of the experiment and the many possible **confounding variables** (such as the possibility that one confederate might have appeared inherently more friendly or more likable than the other).

The matching law has been applied to many real-world situations. Billington and DiTommaso (2003) showed how the matching law can be used to analyze classroom behavior. According to the matching law, the percentage of class time a child spends off-task versus on-task will depend on the relative amounts of reinforcement each provides. A teacher who wants to increase on-task behavior must find ways either to reduce the reinforcers for off-task behavior (which might be difficult) or to increase the reinforcers for on-task behavior (by providing praise, encouragement, special privileges, and so on). In other applications, the matching law has been used to analyze conflicts between career and family (Redmon & Lockwood, 1986) and to describe how consum-

ers make choices when purchasing food items (Foxall, James, Oliveira-Castro, & Ribier, 2010). It has also been applied to choices made by individual athletes and entire teams (Romanowich, Bourret, & Vollmer, 2007). For example, Stilling and Critchfield (2010) examined the numbers of passing plays versus running plays used by different football teams during a season (which varied from team to team because of differences in talent, coaching strategies, etc.). They treated the choice of plays as the behaviors and yards gained as the reinforcers, and they found an approximate matching relation—the percentage of passing plays used by the different teams varied in accordance with the relative amounts of yardage the teams gained from these two types of plays.

Deviations from Matching

Not all experiments have produced results that are consistent with Equation 13-1. W. M. Baum (1974, 1979) listed three ways that the results of experiments have deviated from strict matching, each of which is depicted graphically in Figure 13-2. The most common of these deviations is **undermatching**, in which response proportions are consistently less extreme (i.e., closer to .5) than reinforcement proportions. In the idealized example of undermatching shown in Figure 13-2, when the proportion of left reinforcers is .8, the proportion of left responses is only .6. When the

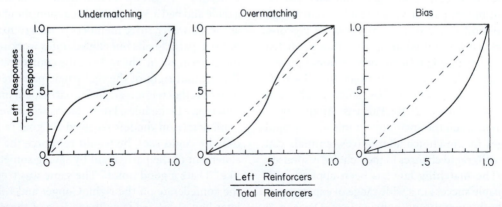

FIGURE 13-2 In each panel, the broken diagonal line shows where data points would fall if a subject's behavior conformed perfectly to the matching law (Equation 13-1). The solid curves illustrate three types of deviation from perfect matching.

proportion of left reinforcers is .3, the proportion of left responses is .45. In other words, undermatching describes the case where a subject's preferences are closer to indifference than they should be according to the matching law.

One explanation of undermatching is that it can occur if subjects develop a habit of rapidly switching back and forth between the two options, a pattern that could be accidentally reinforced if food was delivered immediately after a switch. For instance, if a bird pecks left, then right, then receives a reinforcer, the left-right sequence could be accidentally reinforced even though only the right response was necessary for that particular reinforcer. To reduce the chance that switching behavior might be inadvertently reinforced, Herrnstein included a 1.5-second **changeover delay**, which was, in essence, a penalty for switching between keys. With this changeover delay, no food could be delivered during the first 1.5 seconds after a pigeon switched from one key to the other. This meant that a pigeon had to make two or more consecutive responses on the same key before collecting a reinforcer, thereby making the adventitious reinforcement of switching behavior less likely.

Another hypothesis about undermatching is that animals may occasionally attribute a reinforcer to the wrong response (Davison & Jenkins, 1985). For instance, in the short time between making a response and collecting the reinforcer, a pigeon may forget which key it pecked. Other explanations of undermatching have also been proposed, and there is no general agreement about why it occurs (Myers & Myers, 1977; Sutton, Grace, McLean, & Baum, 2008).

The opposite of undermatching is **overmatching**, in which a subject's response proportions are more extreme than the reinforcement proportions. For example, in the illustration of overmatching in Figure 13-2, a reinforcer proportion of .8 produces a response proportion of .9, and a reinforcer proportion of .3 produces a response proportion of .15. Overmatching is not as common as matching or undermatching, but it has been observed in situations where there is a substantial penalty for switching between schedules. For example, W. M. Baum (1982) found overmatching when pigeons had to walk around a barrier and over a hurdle to switch from one key to the other. As the effort involved in switching keys was increased, the pigeons switched between keys less and less and spent most of their time responding on the better VI schedule, which resulted in overmatching.

In the third type of deviation from matching, **bias**, a subject consistently spends more time on one alternative than predicted by the matching equation. Figure 13-2 illustrates the sort of results that might be obtained if a subject has a bias for the right key. When 80% of the reinforcers come from the left key, the subject makes only 50% of its responses on the left key. When 30% of the reinforcers come from the left key, the subject makes only 10% of its responses on the left key. Regardless of the reinforcer percentage, the subject makes more responses on the right key than predicted by the matching law. Many factors can produce a bias, such as a preference for a particular side of the chamber, for a particular response key (if one key requires a bit less effort than the other), or for a particular color (if the two response keys have different colors). In some cases, the reason for bias is easy to explain. In a study of college basketball players' choices between 2-point and 3-point shots, researchers found that the matching law described the players' shot selections quite well, except that there was a consistent bias for 3-point shots (Alferink, Critchfield, Hitt, & Higgins, 2009). The explanation for this bias is straightforward and obvious—3-point shots are worth more than 2-point shots.

Varying the Quality and Amount of Reinforcement

All of the experiments described so far have dealt with two alternatives that deliver exactly the same reinforcer (e.g., food or verbal approval) but at different rates. However, if different types of reinforcers are used, the matching law can be used to measure an individual's preferences for these different reinforcers. For instance, H. L. Miller (1976) presented pigeons with pairs of VI schedules that provided different types of grain as reinforcers. When the two reinforcers were wheat and buck-wheat, Miller found a strong preference (bias) for the wheat. However, he suggested that the matching equation could take this bias into account if it were modified in the following way:

$$\frac{B_1}{B_1 + B_2} = \frac{Q_1 R_1}{Q_1 R_1 + Q_2 R_2} \quad (13\text{-}2)$$

where Q_1 and Q_2 stand for the qualities of the reinforcers available on the two keys. This equation states that a pigeon's behavior is determined by both the rate of reinforcement and the quality of reinforcement delivered by the different schedules. Miller arbitrarily assigned a value of 10 to Q_b, the quality of buckwheat, and he found that Equation 13-2 provided a good description of the results if Q_w, the quality of wheat, was given a value of about 14. He interpreted this number as meaning that each wheat reinforcer was worth about 1.4 times as much as each buckwheat re-inforcer. Miller made similar calculations for conditions where the alternatives were hemp and buckwheat, and he estimated that Q_h, the quality of hemp, was about 9.1, or slightly less than that of buckwheat. Based on these numbers, Miller predicted that he should observe a preference (bias) of 14 to 9.1 when the pigeons had to choose between wheat and hemp, and this is approximately what he found. This experiment nicely demonstrates how the matching law can be used to scale animals' preferences for different types of reinforcers. The matching law has been used in other studies to measure preferences among reinforcers of different qualities, with subjects as different as humans (Neef, Mace, Shea, & Shade, 1992) and cows (Foster, Temple, Robertson, Nair, & Poling, 1996).

Besides the rate of reinforcement and the quality of reinforcement, another variable that can affect preference is the amount or size of each reinforcer. If one key delivers two food pellets as a reinforcer and the other key delivers only one, this should certainly affect a subject's choices. Baum and Rachlin (1969) suggested that when amount

of reinforcement is the independent variable, it can be used in place of rate of reinforcement in the matching equation:

$$\frac{B_1}{B_1 + B_2} = \frac{A_1}{A_1 + A_2} \quad (13\text{-}3)$$

where A_1 and A_2 are the amounts of reinforcement delivered by the two alternatives. In some cases, Equation 13-3 has been quite accurate (Catania, 1963), but other studies have found substantial undermatching or overmatching (Davison & Hogsden, 1984; Dunn, 1982).

An Application to Single Schedules

It may appear that the matching law, which makes predictions for choice situations, has nothing to say about cases where there is only one reinforcement schedule. However, Herrnstein (1970, 1974) developed a way to use the matching law to make predictions about behavior on single reinforcement schedules. Imagine that a pigeon's pecking on a response key delivers food on a VI schedule. Although pecking the key is the only way the pigeon can obtain food reinforcers, Herrnstein assumed that there are always some "built-in" reinforcers available (we might call them "Premackian re-inforcers") for performing other behaviors such as grooming, exploring, and resting. Herrnstein suggested that whereas the experimenter can control the number of food reinforcers, the built-in reinforcers for nonpecking behaviors are out of the experimenter's control, and they occur at a fairly constant rate.

Although these background reinforcers are not food, in order to perform the necessary calculations, we need to measure them in the same units as the food reinforcers. Let us suppose that all behaviors other than pecking provide the pigeon with built-in reinforcers having a value equivalent to 30 food reinforcers per hour. Similarly, although the pigeon's various behaviors, such as grooming and exploring, are quite different from key pecking, we need to measure them on a common scale. A useful strategy is to measure all behaviors in units of time, thereby translating Equation 13-1 to the following:

$$\frac{T_1}{T_1 + T_2} = \frac{R_1}{R_1 + R_2} \quad (13\text{-}4)$$

Let T_1 represent the time spent key pecking and T_2 the total time spent in all other behaviors, so that $T_1 + T_2$ equals the total session time. R_1 is the rate at which food reinforcers are delivered by the VI schedule, and R_2 is the equivalent reinforcing value of all the built-in reinforcers (which equals 30 in our example).

We are now ready to make predictions for different VI schedules. If the pigeon is exposed to a VI schedule that delivers 30 reinforcers per hour, Equation 13-4 predicts that the bird will spend half of its time pecking and half of its time engaging in other behaviors (because R_1 and R_2 both equal 30). If the bird is now presented with a VI schedule that delivers 90 reinforcers per hour, Equation 13-4 states that it should spend 75% of its time pecking (because the food re-

inforcers represent 75% of all the reinforcers in this situation). Similar predictions can be made for any size of VI schedule the experimenter might arrange. The solid curve in Figure 13-3 shows the predictions for all reinforcement rates between 0 and 500 food reinforcers per hour, for a pigeon that can peck at a rate of two keypecks per second. As the rate of reinforcement increases, Equation 13-4 predicts that response rates will climb toward the animal's full-time rate of 120 pecks per minute. Of course, these predictions are based on specific assumptions about the pigeon's pecking rate and the values of all nonpecking behaviors. Suppose we took this same pigeon and put it in a more interesting chamber where R_2 was equal to 60 (perhaps because this second chamber had a window through which the subject could watch another pigeon). With the increased value of nonpecking behaviors, Equation 13-4 now predicts that the bird will spend less time pecking on all VI schedules, as shown by the broken line in Figure 13-3.

Herrnstein (1970) applied this analysis to the results of an experiment by Catania and Reynolds (1968) in which six pigeons responded on several different VI schedules (presented

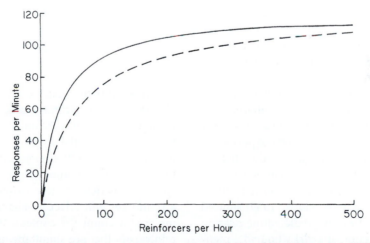

FIGURE 13-3 The two curves depict some representative predictions from Herrnstein's (1970) equation for single reinforcement schedules (Equation 13-4). This equation predicts how response rates should change as reinforcement rates are varied. The solid curve represents a case where there are relatively few reinforcers for behavior other than pecking ($R_2 = 30$ in Equation 13-4). The broken curve represents a case where there are more reinforcers for behaviors other than pecking ($R_2 = 60$), so the subject's rate of pecking should be slower.

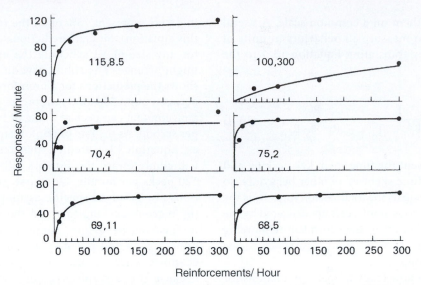

FIGURE 13-4 Each panel shows the results from one of six pigeons in the Catania and Reynolds (1968) experiment. Each point shows the reinforcement rate and response rate on one VI schedule. For each subject, the curve shows the predictions of Equation 13-4, using the best-fitting estimates of the bird's full-time pecking rate and of R_2. The numbers in each panel are the best-fitting estimates of these two quantities. The pattern of results for each subject is well described by Equation 13-4. (From R.J. Hernstein, "On the law of effect," *Journal of the Experimental Analysis of Behavior, 13*(2), pages 243–266. Copyright 1970 by the Society for the Experimental Analysis of Behavior, Inc. Reprinted with permission.)

one at a time, for several sessions each). Figure 13-4 shows the results of the Catania and Reynolds study (data points), and the curves are the predictions of Equation 13-4. The close correspondence between predictions and data points in Figure 13-4 is impressive. De Villiers and Herrnstein (1976) performed similar analyses of several dozen experiments involving a variety of species, operant responses, and reinforcers. In nearly all cases, the correspondence between the predictions of the matching law and the results was about as good as it was for the Catania and Reynolds (1968) experiment. Herrnstein's analysis of single-schedule behavior has also been applied to human behavior in natural settings (Beardsley & McDowell, 1992). For example, Martens and Houk (1989) showed that Equation 13-4 nicely predicted the relation between the behavior of a girl who had a mental disability and the amount of reinforcement delivered by her teacher.

Since Herrnstein (1970) first presented his analysis of single-schedule performance, other researchers have suggested changes or alternatives to the simple mathematical rule described by Equation 13-4 (Dallery, McDowell, & Lancaster, 2000; Navakatikyan, 2007). Some of these theories are mathematically more complex, and they may also provide more accurate descriptions of actual behavior (e.g., McDowell & Caron, 2010). Nevertheless, the matching law does have some clear implications for real-world behavior. Herrnstein's theory can be stated quite simply: An operant response must compete with all other possible behaviors for the individual's time. As the reinforcement for the operant response increases, the individual will devote more and more time to this behavior. One important implication of this viewpoint is that it is impossible to predict how a reinforcer will affect a behavior without taking into account the context, that is, the other reinforcers that are simultaneously available for other behaviors. This principle is illustrated in Figure 13-3, which shows two different predictions for each VI schedule, depending on the amount of reinforcement available for nonpecking behaviors. As a real-world parallel, try to predict how a young child's behavior would be altered by giving him a new reinforcer—a yo-yo, for example. To make any sensible prediction, we need to know something about the context. If the yo-yo is given on an average rainy day in August, the child may play with the yo-yo for hours, because he may be bored with all his other toys and indoor activities. On the other hand, if the yo-yo is given on Christmas and the context includes a host of new toys—trucks, video games, puzzles—the amount of time spent playing with the yo-yo will probably be small. The rich supply of other reinforcers will attract most of the child's time.

Other examples where the total reinforcement context plays a major role are easy to imagine. Many people claim that they tend to eat more when they are bored. This presumably happens not because the reinforcing value of food actually increases when one is bored, but rather because there are few reinforcers available to compete with eating. As another example of a situation where the reinforcement context is meager, imagine that you are sitting in a reception area waiting for an appointment with someone who is running behind schedule (e.g., your mechanic or your optometrist). There is little to do but wait, and if you are like me, you may find yourself reading magazines you would not ordinarily spend your time on, such as 2-year-old issues of *Newsweek, Good Housekeeping,* or *Optometry Today.* What little reinforcement value these outdated magazines offer takes on added significance in the absence of any alternative sources of reinforcement.

THEORIES OF CHOICE BEHAVIOR

In many areas of science, it is important to distinguish between *descriptions* and *explanations.* For example, the statement that water increases in volume when it freezes is simply a description—it does not explain why this expansion occurs. Such descriptive statements can be extremely useful in their own right, for they can help us to predict and control future events (e.g., avoiding the bursting of outdoor water pipes by draining them before they freeze). On the other hand, a statement

that attributes this expansion to the crystalline structure that hydrogen and oxygen molecules form when in a solid state can be called an explanation: It is a theory about the molecular events that underlie this phenomenon.

The matching equation can be viewed as either simply a description of choice behavior or a theory about the mechanisms of choice behavior. We have seen that as a description of behavior in certain choice situations, the matching equation is fairly accurate. We will now consider the possibility that the matching law is an explanatory theory, and we will compare it to a few other theories that have been presented as possible explanatory theories of choice.

Matching Theory and Melioration Theory

In his earlier writings, Herrnstein (1970, 1974) suggested that the matching equation is also a general explanatory theory of choice behavior. The theory is quite simple: It states that animals exhibit matching behavior because they are built to do so. That is, in any choice situation, an animal might measure the value of the reinforcement it receives from each alternative (where "value" encompasses such factors as the rate, size, and quality of the reinforcers), and the animal then might distribute its behavior in proportion to the values of the various alternatives. According to such a theory, matching is not just a description of behavior in concurrent VI schedules. It is a general principle that explains how animals make choices in all situations, in the laboratory and in the wild.

Later, Herrnstein decided that this theory needed some modification. One problem concerns cases where an animal must choose between two ratio schedules (such as variable-ratio [VR] 20 and VR 100). The matching equation predicts that the animal will make all of its responses on one of the two alternatives, but it does not specify which. Whether the animal makes 100% of its responses on the VR 20 schedule or 100% of its responses on the VR 100 schedule, it will receive 100% of its reinforcers from that schedule, and so the matching equation will be satisfied. However, studies with both animals and people have found that they always choose the smaller VR schedule in such situations, never the larger (Herrnstein & Loveland, 1984; Shah, Bradshaw, & Szabadi, 1989). This is not surprising, because the smaller VR schedule requires less work per reinforcer.

To deal with this matter, Herrnstein and Vaughan (1980; Vaughan, 1981, 1985) developed a refinement of the matching law that they called **melioration**. To meliorate is to "make better." In essence, the principle of melioration states that animals will invest increasing amounts of time and/or effort into whichever alternative is better. This principle sounds simple enough, but let us see how it can be put into practice.

It is easy to show that Equation 13-1 is equivalent to the following equation:

$$\frac{R_1}{B_1} = \frac{R_2}{B_2} \tag{13-5}$$

This equation emphasizes the fact that at the point of matching, the ratio of reinforcers received to responses produced is equal for both alternatives. We might say that the "cost" of each reinforcer is the same for both alternatives. The principle of melioration states that if these ratios are not equal, the animal will shift its behavior toward whichever alternative currently has the higher reinforcer:response ratio, until it reaches a point where the two ratios are equal. For example, suppose the two schedules are VI schedules, and a pigeon receives twice as many reinforcers per hour from Key 1 as from Key 2 (i.e., $R_1 = 2$ times R_2). Melioration theory predicts that an animal's responses will shift to Key 1 until it makes twice as many responses on that alternative (i.e., $B_1 = 2$ times B_2). At that point, Equation 13-5 is satisfied, so there should be no further shifts in behavior (except for inevitable random variations). In short, the principle of melioration predicts that matching behavior will occur in concurrent VI schedules.

The situation is different with two VR schedules, however. For example, if the two schedules are VR 30 and VR 120, then their respective reinforcer:response ratios are 1:30 and 1:120. These ratios will not change no matter how the animal distributes its behavior, so the principle of melioration predicts that the animal's behavior will continue to shift toward the VR 30 key until there is no more behavior to shift (until it is responding exclusively at that key). The predictions are the same for any pair of VR schedules: The individual should eventually respond exclusively on the schedule with the more favorable reinforcer:response ratio. In summary, the principle of melioration correctly predicts matching behavior in a choice between two VI schedules, and it predicts exclusive preference for the better of two VR schedules.

Herrnstein and Prelec (1991) proposed that the principle of melioration is a general rule of choice that people use when making everyday decisions in such matters as personal relationships, shopping, gambling, and business investments. A practical problem, however, is that the principles of matching and melioration do not always lead to the optimal choices (see Herrnstein, 1990). To put it simply, matching behavior proportions to reinforcer proportions is not always the best strategy. For this reason, matching theory and melioration theory are viewed as competitors for optimization theory, which states that people tend to make decisions that maximize their satisfaction.

Optimization Theory

As discussed in Chapter 8, some psychologists have proposed that optimization theory is a general explanatory theory of choice for both humans and nonhumans. It is easy to see that optimization theory predicts exclusive preference for the better of two VR schedules—this behavior maximizes reinforcement and minimizes effort. Some psychologists have proposed that optimization theory can also explain why matching occurs on concurrent VI schedules (Silberberg, Thomas, & Berendzen, 1991). Supporters of optimization theory propose that although the matching law may provide a satisfactory *description* of behavior in these situations, optimization theory actually provides an *explanation* of matching behavior.

OPTIMIZATION AS AN EXPLANATION OF MATCHING. To examine this logic, imagine a pigeon on a concurrent VI 30-second (left-key) VI 120-second (right-key) schedule. Rachlin, Green, Kagel, and Battalio (1976) conducted a series of computer simulations to determine how different ways of distributing responses between the two keys would affect the total rate of reinforcement. The results of these simulations are presented in Figure 13-5. If a pigeon made all of its responses on the left key, it would obtain about 120 reinforcers per hour (which is shown by the point at the extreme right in Figure 13-5). If the bird responded only on the right key, it would collect about 30 per hour (the point at the extreme left in Figure 13-5). By making some responses on each key, however, the bird could collect many of the reinforcers from both schedules. The computer simulations of Rachlin and colleagues projected that a pigeon could obtain the highest possible rate of reinforcement by making 80% of its responses to the left key, which is also the point of matching behavior. Speaking more generally, Rachlin and his colleagues have proposed that with any typical

concurrent VI schedules, matching behavior will maximize the rate of reinforcement. Of course, it should take a pigeon some time to determine what manner of responding is optimal. According to optimization theory, an animal in this type of situation will try different ways of distributing its behaviors (e.g., 50% left, 80% left, 90% left), and the animal will eventually settle on the response distribution that maximizes the overall rate of reinforcement. With concurrent VI schedules, it just so happens that the maximum rate of reinforcement can be obtained by matching.

TESTS OF OPTIMIZATION VERSUS MATCHING. A common strategy when comparing scientific theories is to find a situation for which the theories make distinctly different predictions, and then to conduct the appropriate experiment to see what actually happens. Quite a few experiments have examined choice situations for which the matching law makes one prediction and optimization theory makes a very different prediction. A number of experiments by Herrnstein and his colleagues obtained results that favored the matching law over optimization theory (Herrnstein & Vaughan, 1980; Heyman & Herrnstein, 1986).

An experiment with pigeons that I conducted was also designed to compare the two theories (Mazur, 1981). In many ways, my experiment was similar to Herrnstein's (1961) original experiment on matching. Pigeons could peck at either of two keys, one red and one green. Occasionally, a peck on one of the keys would cause the key lights to go off, and food was presented for 3 seconds. One main difference in my procedure, however, was that a single VI schedule randomly assigned the food deliveries to the two keys, whereas Herrnstein used two separate VI schedules. This was an important difference, because whenever food was assigned to one key, the VI clock stopped until the food was collected. This meant that a pigeon had to respond on both keys frequently to keep the VI clock moving. Therefore, the optimal strategy was for the pigeon to make half of its responses on each key, switching back and forth frequently, because this kept the clock

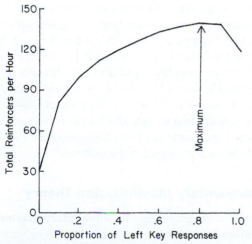

FIGURE 13-5 Predictions of the computer simulations of Rachlin, Green, Kagel, and Battalio (1976) for a concurrent VI 30-second (left-key) VI 120-second (right-key) schedule. According to the predictions, a subject on this schedule would maximize the rate of reinforcement by making 80% of its responses on the left key.

moving and kept the food deliveries coming. In one condition, where the pigeons received about 32 food deliveries per hour on each key, they did perform optimally, making about 50% of their responses on each key (which was also matching, of course).

A second condition provided the critical test between optimization and matching. In this condition, 90% of the food deliveries for the red key were replaced with "dark-key periods"—the keys went dark for 3 seconds, but no food was delivered. Despite this change, the optimal strategy was still to switch back and forth between the two keys frequently, making about 50% of one's responses on each key. This strategy would ensure that the VI timer would be running most of the time. However, the matching law predicted that the pigeons should now make many more responses on the green key, since this key now provided about 10 times as many food reinforcers. This is what happened: The pigeons shifted most of their responses to the green key, and at the end of the condition they made an average of 86% of their responses on the green key (which delivered about 92% of the reinforcers). However, because they responded so little on the red key, the VI clock was often stopped, and as a result, the pigeons lost about 29% of their potential reinforcers. In other conditions, the pigeons lost 75% or more of their potential reinforcers.

The procedure of this experiment may seem a bit complex, but the results can be stated simply: Although optimization theory predicted that the birds should always make about 50% of their responses on each key, the birds consistently showed a preference for whichever key delivered more reinforcers, as predicted by the matching law. But by doing so, they slowed down the VI clock and lost many potential reinforcers, which is exactly the opposite of what optimization theory predicted should happen.

Psychologists have used a variety of other experimental procedures to compare the predictions of the matching law and optimization theory. For example, in choice situations involving both a VI schedule and a VR schedule, optimization theory predicts that animals should make most of their responses on the VR schedule, because most of the responses on any VI schedule are wasted, whereas every response on a VR schedule brings the animal closer to reinforcement. Several experiments with animals failed to support this prediction, but the results were consistent with the predictions of the matching law (DeCarlo, 1985; Vyse & Belke, 1992). Similar results were obtained in a study with college students working for money: The students spent more time on the VI schedule than predicted by optimization theory, and their choices were closer to the predictions of the matching law (Savastano & Fantino, 1994).

Several other experiments, some with animals and some with humans, have failed to support the predictions of optimization theory (e.g., Ettinger, Reid, & Staddon, 1987; Jacobs & Hackenberg, 2000). However, some experiments have supported optimization theory (MacDonall, Goodell, & Juliano, 2006; Sakagami, Hursh, Christensen, & Silberberg, 1989). With some evidence favoring each theory, some psychologists continue to favor optimization theory, whereas others favor matching (or melioration) theory.

Because they deal with an individual's overall distribution of responses over long periods of time (e.g., over an entire experimental session), matching theory, melioration theory, and optimization theory can all be classified as molar theories (see Chapter 6). Some researchers now believe that more complete explanations of choice behavior will be found in molecular theories, which attempt to predict moment-to-moment behavior and which assume that short-term consequences have large effects on choice. One molecular theory of choice is presented in the next section.

Momentary Maximization Theory

In its most general sense, **momentary maximization theory** states that at each moment, an organism will select whichever alternative has the highest value *at that moment*. The value of an alternative will usually depend on many factors: the size and quality of the reinforcer, the individual's state of deprivation, and so on. Although both momentary maximization theory and optimization theory state that animals attempt to maximize the value of their choices, the two theories frequently make different predictions because the best choice in the short run is not always the best choice in the long run. As a simple example, consider a dieter who must choose between orange gelatin and a strawberry sundae for dessert. The strawberry sundae may appear more attractive at the moment, but the gelatin might be the more beneficial alternative for the dieter in the long run. Choices that involve a conflict between short-term and long-term benefits will be examined in detail later in the chapter; this issue is raised now only to show that the strategies of momentary maximization and overall optimization may lead to very different decisions.

To understand what sorts of predictions the momentary maximization hypothesis makes for concurrent VI schedules, try playing the following hypothetical gambling game. Imagine that you are allowed to play this game for nine trials. You are seated in front of a panel with two small doors, and on each trial you are allowed to open one of the two doors. There may be a dollar behind the door (which you win) or there may be no money. The following rules determine whether a dollar is deposited behind a door or not: There is a modified roulette wheel for each door, which is spun before each trial begins. The probability of winning is .1 on the roulette wheel for door 1, and .2 on the wheel for door 2. Therefore, on trial 1 of the game, there may be a dollar behind both doors, behind one door, or behind neither door, depending on the outcome of spinning the wheel for each door. Which door do you choose on trial 1?

Two additional rules apply for the next eight trials:

1. Once a dollar is deposited behind a door, it will remain there until you collect it. Thus, if a dollar is deposited behind door 1 on trial 4, it will remain there until you choose door 1, say, on trial 7.
2. There will never be more than one dollar behind a door at one time. For instance, if a dollar is deposited behind door 1 on trial 4

and you do not collect it until trial 7, the spinning of the wheel is irrelevant on trials 5, 6, and 7, since no more dollars will be deposited behind door 1. However, the spinning of the wheel for door 2 will continue to be important on these trials, since it might pay off on any trial. In other words, door 2 is not affected by what is happening at door 1, and vice versa.

Before reading further, write down what door you would choose on each of the nine trials.

For a situation like this, momentary maximization theory predicts that the player will choose whichever alternative has the higher probability of reinforcement on each trial. On the first two trials, door 2 has the higher probability of reinforcement, and so it should be chosen. However, it can be shown (using some elementary rules of probability theory that will not be explained here) that after two choices of door 2, p_2 will equal .2 but p_1 will equal .271 (because there are now three trials on which a dollar might have been deposited at door 1). A momentary maximizer would therefore choose door 1 on trial 3. After checking door 1 on trial 3, it is best to go back to door 2 on trial 4, because now p_2 is again greater than p_1. The pattern followed by a momentary maximizer on the nine trials would be 2, 2, 1, 2, 2, 1, 2, 2, 1. Check to see whether your choices followed the momentary maximizing strategy.

This hypothetical gambling game is quite similar to concurrent VI schedules. The two roulette wheels are similar to two independent VI timers, and like VI clocks, the roulette wheels will only store one reinforcer at a time. Therefore, you can probably see what momentary maximizing theory predicts about a subject's behavior on concurrent VI schedules: It predicts that there should be an orderly and cyclical pattern to an animal's moment-by-moment choices. Of course, advocates of momentary maximizing theory (Shimp, 1966, 1969; Silberberg, Hamilton, Ziriax, & Casey, 1978) recognize that animals have limited memorial and decision-making capacities, and they do not expect perfect momentary maximizing behavior to occur. (After all, even people have difficulty determining the probabilities in situations like the gambling game described.) What these theorists do predict, however, is that animals will show at least some tendency to choose the alternative that has the higher probability of reinforcement. For example, after an animal has made several consecutive responses on the better of two VI schedules, it should show a tendency to switch to the other VI (as a reinforcer may have been stored on this VI during the interim). According to momentary maximizing theory, matching behavior is simply an incidental by-product of an animal's orderly moment-by-moment choices. In contrast, molar theories of choice do not predict that an animal's moment-to-moment behavior will exhibit any orderly patterns, because these theories assume that an animal's behavior is controlled by variables (e.g., total reinforcement rate) that do not change from moment to moment.

When animals exhibit matching behavior, are there orderly moment-by-moment patterns in their behavior? It seems that sometimes there are, but not always. Some studies have found evidence for the sort of moment-by-moment changes predicted by momentary maximizing theory (Shimp, 1966; Silberberg, Hamilton, Ziriax, & Casey, 1978), but others have not (Heyman, 1979; Nevin, 1969). For example, Nevin (1979) analyzed his data in several different ways in search of orderly sequences of responses, but he found none. At the molar level, however, the data were quite orderly: The pigeons' overall choice proportions were well described by the matching law. Nevin concluded that the momentary maximizing theory does not provide the correct explanation of why animals match, because matching behavior sometimes occurs even when animals' choices appear to be random from moment to moment.

Hinson and Staddon (1983) used a different method of analysis and came to a different conclusion. Instead of looking at sequences of responses, as was done in all previous studies, Hinson and Staddon continuously recorded the time since a pigeon sampled (pecked at) each of two VI keys. They reasoned that time is the critical independent variable, since on VI schedules it is the passage of time and not the number of responses that actually determines the availability of a reinforcer. They showed that their pigeons could follow a momentary maximizing strategy if they used a fairly simple rule: If schedule 1 delivers, for example, *three times* as many reinforcers as schedule 2, you should check schedule 2 if the time since you last checked it is more than *three times longer* than the time since you last checked schedule 1. Hinson and Staddon showed that their pigeons' behaviors were by no means perfect from the standpoint of momentary maximization theory, but a majority of their responses did follow this rule.

More recently, many other studies have found additional evidence that animals' moment-to-moment choices are influenced by a variety of short-term factors, such as the time since their last response (Brown & Cleaveland, 2009) or which response has just delivered a reinforcer (Aparicio & Baum, 2009; Lau & Glimcher, 2005). These results do not necessarily support momentary maximizing theory, but they do show that animals' moment-to-moment choices are clearly affected by molecular events, not just the molar reinforcement contingencies.

Other Theories of Choice

As a result of the intense interest in choice behavior among those who study operant conditioning, quite a few different theories have been proposed besides those that we have already examined. Some of these theories involve fairly complex mathematics, and we will not go into their details here. However, we can take a brief look at some of the major trends in this area of research.

Not all molecular theories of choice assume that animals follow the principle of momentary maximization. As one example of different type of molecular theory, Baum and his colleagues have proposed that on concurrent VI schedules, animals follow a pattern that they call *fix and sample*

(Aparicio & Baum, 2006; Baum, Schwendiman, & Bell, 1999). Their analysis of moment-to-moment responding has found that animals respond mostly on the better alternative (they "fix" on that alternative), but they occasionally make short visits to the other alternative (they "sample" that alternative). Their visits to the better alternative are very long if it delivers a large percentage of the reinforcers (e.g., 90%), but they are not as long if it delivers only slightly more reinforcers than the other alterative (e.g., 60%). Baum has presented evidence that this pattern of fixing and sampling at the molecular level leads to matching (or sometimes undermatching or overmatching) at the molar level.

Other theories of choice might be called *hybrid* theories, because they assume that both molar and molecular variables affect choice. For example, Fantino's *delay-reduction theory* (Fantino, 1969; Fantino & Silberg, 2010) includes the basic idea of the matching law, but in addition it assumes that animals' choices are directed toward whichever alternative produces a greater reduction in the delay to the next reinforcer. In other words, this theory includes both a molar component (matching of response proportions to reinforcement proportions) and a molecular component (control by the shorter delay to reinforcement). Other theories of this type include Killeen's (1982) incentive theory and Grace's (1994) contextual choice model. Another trend in the research on choice has been an increasing interest in the dynamics of choice—how choice behavior adapts to a change in the reinforcement alternatives (Baum, 2010; Navakatikyan & Davison, 2010). Considerable work is now being conducted to evaluate the strengths and weaknesses of different mathematical theories of choice.

Regardless of which theory of choice proves to be most accurate, no one can dispute the more general assertion of molecular theories that short-term factors have a large effect on choice behavior. The next section shows that when a small but immediate reinforcer is pitted against a large but delayed reinforcer, the small, immediate reinforcer is frequently chosen.

PRACTICE QUIZ (1)

1. According to the matching law, if an animal receives 75% of its reinforcers from one schedule, it will make _____ of its responses on that schedule.
2. If an animal receives 20% of its reinforcers from one schedule, but makes 30% of its responses on that schedule, this is called _____.
3. Even when a pigeon pecks on a single key that delivers food as a reinforcer, this can be viewed as a choice between food reinforcers and _____.
4. In experiments designed to compare the predictions of optimization theory and the matching law, the results have usually supported the _____.
5. According to _____ theory, an individual will choose whichever alternative has the highest value at that moment.

Answers

1. 75% 2. undermatching 3. background reinforcers (or built-in reinforcers for other activities) 4. matching law 5. momentary maximization theory

SELF-CONTROL CHOICES

Every day, people make many choices that involve a conflict between their short-term and long-term interests. Consider the situation of a college student who has a class that meets early Monday morning, and in this course it is important to attend each lecture. On Sunday evening, the student sets her alarm clock so that she can awaken early enough to get to class on time. The student has chosen going to class (and the improved chances for a good grade this will bring) over an hour of extra sleep. This sounds like a prudent choice, but unfortunately the student has plenty of time to change her mind. When the alarm clock rings on Monday morning, the warmth and comfort of the bed are more appealing than going to class, and the student turns off the alarm and goes back to sleep. Later in the day, she will probably regret her choice and vow not to miss class again.

This example is a typical **self-control choice** situation, that is, one involving a choice between a small, proximal reinforcer and a larger but more distant reinforcer. The small reinforcer is the extra hour of sleep, and the larger, delayed reinforcer is the better grade that will probably result from going to class. An important characteristic of self-control situations is that one's preferences may exhibit systematic changes over time. On Sunday evening, the young woman in our example evidently preferred going to class (and its long-term benefits) over an extra hour of sleep, since she set the alarm for the appropriate time. The next morning, her preference had changed, and she chose the extra hour of sleep. Later that day, she regrets this choice and decides to make a different decision in the future.

In case you are not convinced that self-control situations are commonplace, consider the following everyday decisions. You should be able to identify the small, more immediate reinforcer and larger, delayed reinforcer in each case:

1. To smoke a cigarette or not to smoke.
2. To keep the thermostat at 65°F during the winter months or set it at a higher temperature and face a larger fuel bill at the end of the month.
3. When on a diet, to choose between low-fat yogurt or ice cream for dessert.
4. To shout at your roommate in anger or control your temper and avoid saying something you do not really mean.
5. To save money for some big item you want (e.g., a car) or spend it on parties each weekend.

For each example, you should also be able to see how one's preference might change over time. It is easy to say you will begin a diet—tomorrow. On Monday or Tuesday, it is easy to decide you will have a frugal weekend and begin saving for that car. It is much harder, however, to keep these commitments when the time comes to make your final choice. Herrnstein and Mazur (1987) argued that this tendency to switch preferences over time in self-control choices is one of the strongest pieces of evidence against optimization theory. If people followed the strategy that optimized their satisfaction in the long run, they would consistently choose one alternative or the other.

Delay Discounting

Self-control choices illustrate quite dramatically how the strength or value of a reinforcer decreases as its delay increases. This effect is called **delay discounting**. To get an idea of how delay discounting works, imagine that you have won a prize in a lottery, and you can choose to receive either $1,000 in one year or a smaller amount of money today. Before reading further, take a moment to answer the questions in Figure 13-6. There are no right or wrong answers; just try to answer as if these choices were real.

When given a series of hypothetical choices like those in Figure 13-6, most people start by choosing Option A, but at some point their preference switches to Option B. For instance,

A. $1000 today	or	B. $1000 in 1 year
A. $950 today	or	B. $1000 in 1 year
A. $900 today	or	B. $1000 in 1 year
A. $800 today	or	B. $1000 in 1 year
A. $700 today	or	B. $1000 in 1 year
A. $600 today	or	B. $1000 in 1 year
A. $500 today	or	B. $1000 in 1 year
A. $400 today	or	B. $1000 in 1 year
A. $300 today	or	B. $1000 in 1 year
A. $200 today	or	B. $1000 in 1 year
A. $100 today	or	B. $1000 in 1 year
A. $50 today	or	B. $1000 in 1 year

FIGURE 13-6 Hypothetical questions that can be used to estimate delay discounting. For each question, imagine that you really had to make such a choice, and pick either A or B.

suppose that a college student selected Option A when it was $700 today, but for the next question ($600 today), he chose Option B ($1000 in a year). Because his preference switched between $700 and $600, we can conclude that somewhere in between these two values there is an **indifference point**—a combination of delays and amounts that the student finds equally preferable. For this student, we could estimate that receiving $650 today would be about equal in value to receiving $1,000 in 1 year (because $650 is half-way between $700 and $600).

In numerous studies, people have answered hypothetical questions such as those in Figure 13-6, and their answers have been used to estimate how the value of a reinforcer like money decreases with delay. One main finding is that the rates of delay discounting are different for different people. For example, Green, Fry, and Myerson (1994) compared three different age groups and found that the rates of delay discounting were fastest for 12-year-old children, slower for 20-year-old college students, and slowest for adults in their 60s. In other words, the older people were more willing to wait for the larger, delayed reward than were the younger people. Other studies have found faster rates of delay discounting for smokers than for nonsmokers (Bickel, Odum, & Madden, 1999; Mitchell, 1999), and it is also faster for individuals with addictions to drugs or alcohol (de Wit, 2009). Rates of delay discounting can also be measured for other reinforcers besides money. For example, when Odum and Rainaud (2003) gave adults hypothetical choices involving delayed versus immediate food or alcohol, they obtained similar delay discounting functions, except that the rate of discounting for food or alcohol was faster than for money. Many factors can affect the rate of delay discounting, and it varies both from person to person and from situation to situation (Odum & Baumann, 2010).

The concept of delay discounting is not hard to understand, but we need to take this idea one step further to explain why a person's choices change as time passes. Why does a student set the alarm in the evening for an early morning class, but then stay in bed the next morning and skip class? Why does a person resolve to start saving money for a car, but then spend excessive money on entertainment when the weekend arrives? In other words, why do people's preferences change over time in these situations? To answer questions like these, Howard Rachlin (1970, 1974) and George Ainslie (1975) independently developed similar ideas about self-control, which are known as the **Ainslie–Rachlin theory**.

The Ainslie–Rachlin Theory

The example of the student who must choose between sleep and an important class can be used to illustrate the features of this theory. Relying on the concept of delay discounting, the theory assumes that the value of a reinforcer decreases as the delay between making a choice and receiving the reinforcer increases. The upper panel of Figure 13-7 shows that the value of a good grade is high at the end of the term, but on the Sunday and Monday

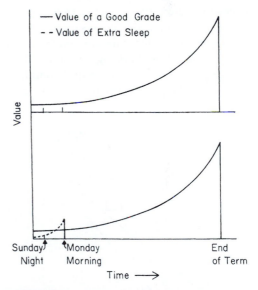

FIGURE 13-7 An application of the Ainslie–Rachlin model to the hypothetical example described in the text. The top panel shows how the subjective value of a good grade increases as the time of its delivery gets closer. The bottom panel shows that the value of a bit of extra sleep also increases as the time of its delivery gets closer. Because of these changes in value, a person may prefer the good grade at some times (e.g., Sunday evening) and the extra sleep at other times (say, Monday morning).

in question, its value is much lower because it is so far in the future. In the lower panel, the value of an hour of extra sleep at different points in time is also shown, and the same principle of delay discounting applies to this reinforcer: With greater delays between choice and the delivery of the reinforcer, its value decreases. The second and (very reasonable) assumption of the theory is that an individual will choose whichever reinforcer has the higher value at the moment a choice is made. Notice that the way the curves are drawn in Figure 13-7, the value of the good grade is higher on Sunday evening, which explains why the student sets the alarm with the intention of going to class. On Monday morning, however, the value of an hour of extra sleep has increased substantially because of its proximity. Because it is now greater than that of the good grade, the student chooses the more immediate reinforcer.

If you find the curves in Figure 13-7 difficult to understand, it may help to draw an analogy between time and distance. Figure 13-8 is a sketch of a long street with two buildings on the left. The buildings are analogous to the two reinforcers in a self-control situation. Building 2 is clearly larger, but for a person standing at point A, building 1 would subtend a greater visual angle. We might

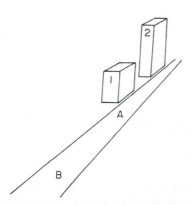

FIGURE 13-8 For a person standing at point A, building 1 subtends a larger visual angle than building 2. The opposite is true for a person standing at point B. This situation is somewhat analogous to a self-control situation if we replace physical distance with time and think of the large, distant building as a large, delayed reinforcer and the small, closer building as a small, more immediate reinforcer.

say that from the perspective of point A, building 1 appears larger (although people obviously have the ability to take their distances into consideration, and so would not be fooled by this illusion). On the other hand, if the person walked to point B, both buildings would appear smaller, but now the visual angle subtended by building 2 would be the larger of the two. Thus, by stepping back from both buildings, a person can get a better perspective on their relative sizes. Similarly, by examining two reinforcers (say, an extra hour of sleep and a better grade) from a distance (e.g., the night before a class), a person "gets a better perspective" on the values of the two reinforcers, and is more likely to choose the "larger" one.

As you can probably see, the student's problem is that she is free to change her mind on Monday morning, when the proximity of the extra hour of sleep gives her a distorted perspective on its value. If she had some way of making her decision of Sunday evening a binding one, she would have a better chance of obtaining the larger, delayed reinforcer. One technique that exploits this possibility is called **precommitment**: The individual makes a decision in advance, which is difficult or impossible to change at a later time. For example, on Sunday evening the student might ask a friend from the same class to come and get her on the way to class Monday morning and not to take "no" for an answer. This would not make it impossible for the student to change her mind, but it would make it more difficult and more embarrassing to stay in bed. In short, the student could make a precommitment to go to class by having a friend pick her up. The technique of precommitment is a useful way to avoid making an impulsive choice, and the next section shows that it can work for animals as well as people.

Animal Studies on Self-Control

A good deal of the research supporting the Ainslie–Rachlin theory has involved animal subjects, and this research shows how it is often possible to design simple laboratory analogs of complex real-world situations. Probably the major difference between the self-control situations described in the previous section and the following animal research is the time scale involved. With pigeons, rats, and other animals, a delay of a few seconds can often make the difference between self-control and impulsiveness.

A study by Green, Fischer, Perlow, and Sherman (1981) demonstrated the sort of preference reversals we would expect if the Ainslie–Rachlin theory is correct. Pigeons received many trials each day, and on each trial a bird made its choice by pecking just once at one of two keys. A peck at the red key delivered 2 seconds of grain, and a peck at the green key delivered 6 seconds of grain. There was, however, a short delay between a peck and the delivery of the reinforcer. For example, in one condition there was a 2-second delay for the 2-second reinforcer and a 6-second delay for the 6-second reinforcer. In this condition, the birds showed impulsive behavior on nearly every trial, choosing the 2-second reinforcer. This choice did not speed up future trials, because the trials occurred every 40 seconds regardless of which choice was made. This behavior is certainly inconsistent with optimization theory, because the optimal solution would be to choose the 6-second reinforcer on every trial. By consistently choosing the smaller but more immediate reinforcer, the birds lost about two thirds of their potential access to grain. Similar results have been obtained with rats when both food and water were used as reinforcers (Green & Estle, 2003).

In another condition, the experimenters simply added 18 seconds to the delay for *each* reinforcer, so the delays were now 20 seconds and 24 seconds. When they had to choose so far in advance, the birds' behaviors were more nearly optimal; that is, they chose the 6-second reinforcer on more than 80% of the trials. This shift in preference when both reinforcers are farther away is exactly what the Ainslie–Rachlin model predicts.

Ainslie (1974) conducted an ingenious experiment showing that at least some pigeons can learn to make use of the strategy of precommitment to avoid impulsive choices. The pigeons had to choose between 2 seconds of food delivered immediately and 4 seconds of food delivered after a short delay. Not surprisingly, when faced with

these options, pigeons chose the immediate food more than 95% of the time. However, a few seconds before each choice trial, the pigeons had the opportunity to peck a green key, and pecking at this key served as a precommitment to the larger, delayed reinforcer. When the key was green, both reinforcers were several seconds away, so the 2-second reinforcer should not be so tempting. By making one peck on the green key, a pigeon made an irreversible choice of the 4-second reinforcer—when the actual trial began, the bird had no opportunity to choose the immediate 2 seconds of food. Three of Ainslie's 10 pigeons learned to use the precommitment option, pecking the green key on more than half of the trials. In a similar experiment that used a slightly different procedure, four of five pigeons chose the precommitment option on a majority of the trials (Rachlin & Green, 1972).

In summary, the precommitment procedure seems to work because the individual can make an irreversible choice when neither reinforcer is immediately available—when the individual has "a better perspective" on the relative sizes of the reinforcers (as illustrated in Figures 13-7 and 13-8). When the alternatives in a self-control situation are punishers rather than reinforcers, they have the reverse effect on choice. In one study, rats tended to choose a large, delayed shock over a smaller but more immediate one. However, when they could make a precommitment a few seconds before the trial began to the smaller but more immediate shock, they frequently did so (Deluty, Whitehouse, Mellitz, & Hineline, 1983). This study provides one more example of how reinforcers and punishers have symmetrical but opposite effects on behavior.

Other research with animals has examined factors that may make them more or less likely to choose a more preferred but delayed reinforcer. Grosch and Neuringer (1981) gave pigeons choices between two different types of grain: A pigeon could either wait 15 seconds and then eat a preferred grain or peck a key and receive a less preferred type of grain immediately. The pigeons must have had a strong preference for the delayed reinforcer, because Grosch and Neuringer found that they would wait for this reinforcer on about 80% of the trials. The experimenters then made one small change in the procedure: The two types of food were now placed where they were visible to the pigeons (behind a transparent barrier) throughout the waiting period. With the food in plain sight, the pigeons became much more impulsive, and they waited for the preferred type of grain on only about 15% of the trials. The sight of the food evidently provided too much of a temptation to resist. In another study, Grosch and Neuringer found that stimuli associated with the food reinforcers had a similar effect. In this case, no food was visible during the waiting interval, but the food hoppers were lit with the same colored lights that normally accompanied the presentation of food. Like the presence of food itself, the colored lights made the pigeons more likely to choose the immediate, less desirable grain.

Grosch and Neuringer (1981) also found that their pigeons were more likely to wait for the delayed reinforcer if they had the opportunity to engage in some specific activity during the delay. We have seen that with the food in sight, the pigeons would wait for the preferred grain on only about 15% of the trials. Grosch and Neuringer then taught the birds to peck at a key in the rear of the chamber, which at first delivered food on an FR 20 schedule. Not surprisingly, the birds found it easier to wait for preferred grain when they could spend the delay working on the FR 20 schedule. More surprising was the fact that when the rear key no longer delivered any reinforcers, the birds continued to peck at it during the delays for the rest of the experiment with no signs of extinction.

These studies illustrate a few of the factors that have been found to affect the self-control choices of animal subjects. The next section shows that these same factors affect children's choices.

Factors Affecting Self-Control in Children

The experiments of Grosch and Neuringer were patterned after a series of experiments conducted by Walter Mischel and his colleagues with children. In one experiment (Mischel & Ebbesen, 1970), preschool children (tested one at a time) were given a choice between waiting 15 minutes for a preferred reinforcer (e.g., pretzels) versus receiving a less preferred reinforcer (e.g., cookies) immediately. During the 15-minute wait, a child could terminate the trial at any time and get the less preferred snack. Like the pigeons of Grosch and Neuringer, the children found it considerably more difficult to wait when the reinforcers were visible (in an open cake tin in front of the child). In another study, Mischel, Ebbesen, and Zeiss (1972) told some children that they could "think about the marshmallow and the pretzel for as long as you want." Other children were given no such instructions. The children who were encouraged to think about the reinforcers chose to terminate the trial and obtain the less preferred reinforcer more frequently. Mischel and co-workers also found that children were more likely to wait for the preferred reinforcer when given an activity to engage in during the delay (some children were given a toy).

Just as with adults (as discussed in the section on delay discounting), there are substantial individual differences among children in their self-control abilities: Some children will wait for quite a while for a delayed reinforcer and others will not. Some of these differences may be due to genetic factors (Beaver, Ferguson, & Lynn-Whaley, 2010). Individual differences in self-control can be found in children as young as 2. It seems that some 2- or 3-year-olds have already learned the strategy of diverting their attention away from the desired objects as a way of avoiding an impulsive choice (Cournoyer & Trudel, 1991; Silverman & Ragusa, 1990). Researchers have found that the tendency to wait for a large delayed reinforcer is related to a child's age, IQ, and other factors (Mischel, 1981, 1983). One study reported that the quality of a toddler's interactions with his or her mother is related to self-control ability 4 years later. Children who had "responsive, cognitively stimulating parent–toddler interactions" (p. 317) at age 2 tended to be less impulsive at age 6 (Olson, Bates, & Bayles, 1990).

Mischel (1966) found that a child's behavior in a self-control situation can be influenced by observational learning. Fourth and fifth graders were asked to participate in a study of consumer behavior. Each child first observed an adult make choices between such items as a set of plastic chess pieces and a set of wooden pieces, with the latter not available for 2 weeks. The child then made similar choices, but with items appropriate for children. The youngster was told to take his or her decisions seriously because he or she would actually receive one of the choices. Some children observed an adult who consistently chose the immediate reinforcer while making statements such as, "Chess figures are chess figures. I can get much use out of the plastic ones right away" (p. 103). Other children observed an adult who chose the delayed reinforcers while noting their better quality and remarking, "I usually find that life is more gratifying when one is willing to wait for good things" (p. 103). The children's choices were greatly affected by the adult model's behavior. Furthermore, the model had a long-lasting influence, for most children continued to follow the example of the model they observed when tested 4 weeks later in a different setting. Like so many other behaviors, self-control choices are heavily influenced by observational learning.

Modeling is only one way to teach children to tolerate a delay. Schweitzer and Sulzer-Azaroff (1988) taught a group of impulsive preschoolers to wait for a larger, delayed reinforcer by beginning with very short delays and progressively increasing the delays as the training proceeded. Similar procedures have been used for children with hyperactivity and attention-deficit disorder (Bloh, 2010) and for adults with developmental disabilities (Dixon, Rehfeldt, & Randich, 2003). Other techniques for training in self-control have also been developed (Dixon & Cummings, 2001; Eisenberger & Adornetto, 1986). But no matter how self-control is learned, acquiring the ability to wait for delayed reinforcers at an early age may have long-lasting effects. Mischel, Shoda, and Rodriguez (1989) found that self-control ability at age 4 was correlated with a variety of personality characteristics during adolescence, including the abilities to concentrate on a task, to pursue goals, to resist temptation, and to tolerate frustration.

We should view these findings with caution because they are based on correlational evidence, but it is easy to imagine how learning to tolerate delays might help a child develop these other desirable traits.

Techniques for Improving Self-Control

Behavior therapists can offer quite a few suggestions to clients who wish to avoid impulsive behaviors in such varied realms as dieting, maintaining an exercise program, studying regularly, saving money, and avoiding excessive drinking or smoking. Let us look at some of these strategies and see how they relate to the Ainslie–Rachlin model and to the research just described.

We have already seen how a student can make a precommitment to attend an early morning class by arranging to have a classmate meet her and insist that she go. The strategy of precommitment can be used in many other self-control situations. People who wish to lose weight are advised to shop for food when they are not hungry and to purchase only foods that are low in calories and require some preparation before they can be eaten. The role of precommitment in this case should be obvious. A dieter cannot impulsively eat some high-calorie snack if there are no such snacks in the house. If a food item requires, say, an hour of cooking, this delay between the time of choice and the time of eating may decrease the value of the food enough so that the dieter can resist that option. People who habitually spend money impulsively are advised to make a list before they go shopping, to take only enough money to buy what they need, to destroy their credit cards, and to avoid going to a shopping mall without some definite purpose in mind (Paulsen, Rimm, Woodburn, & Rimm, 1977). Similarly, people prone to excessive gambling can bring only a limited amount of money to the casino, or use debit cards that set limits on how much they can lose before being forced to stop (Nower & Blaszczynski, 2010). All of these strategies make it more difficult for the person to buy something on the spur of the moment because it seems appealing at the time.

Another variation of the precommitment strategy is to give yourself deadlines to make sure that you complete work assignments on time. Ariely and Wertenbroch (2003) gave college students the opportunity to commit themselves to deadlines for turning in three assignments. They found that students who set up deadlines for themselves to space out the three assignments were more likely to turn the assignments in on time and do a better job on them.

As Figure 13-7 suggests, impulsive behaviors occur when the value of a delayed reinforcer is too small to compete with the currently high value of an immediate reinforcer. It follows that any strategy which either increases the value of the delayed alternative or decreases the value of the immediate alternative should make the choice of the delayed reinforcer more likely. One useful strategy, therefore, is to make an additional, more immediate reinforcer contingent on the choice of the large, delayed reinforcer. For instance, a dieter may make an agreement with himself that he will watch his favorite evening television program only on those days when he forgoes dessert. A college student who wishes to improve her study habits may allow herself to go out with friends for a snack only after she has studied in the library for two solid hours. Psychologists have labeled this type of strategy **self-reinforcement** because it is the individual who delivers his or her own reinforcers for the appropriate behaviors. Although self-reinforcement can work, a frequent problem is that it is easy to "cheat"—to give yourself the reinforcer even when you have failed to perform the appropriate behavior. For this reason, it is advisable to enlist the help of a friend or family member. The dieter's wife might make sure he only watches his television program if he did not have dessert. The college student may go to the library with a conscientious roommate who makes sure she has spent 2 hours studying (rather than reading magazines or talking with friends) before they go out for a snack.

The complementary strategy is to make the value of the impulsive option lower by attaching some form of punishment to it. J. A. Ross (1974) reports a case in which this technique was used

to cure a woman of a nail-biting problem. The woman was unhappy with the way her nails looked after she chewed on them, but as with many nail biters, she found the behavior pleasurable in the short run (for reasons that are unclear). As part of her treatment, the woman gave the therapist a deposit of $50, and the woman was told that the money would be donated to an organization she intensely disliked if her nails did not grow a certain length each week.

Another strategy for improving self-control relies on the use of rule-governed behavior (see Chapter 6). The basic idea is that people can be taught to use verbal rules to guide their choices toward the larger, delayed reinforcer. For example, Benedick and Dixon (2009) taught individuals with developmental disabilities to exhibit significantly more self-control simply by having them read out loud a card stating that it was better to pick the larger, delayed option.

Other strategies have a more cognitive flavor, in that they attempt to train people to use specific thought processes to improve their self-control. Whereas Mischel et al. (1972) found that children were more impulsive when they were told to think about both reinforcers (immediate and delayed), it has been suggested that selectively thinking about the large, delayed reinforcer can forestall an impulsive action (Ainslie, 1975; Watson & Tharp, 1997). For instance, a person on a diet may be advised to visualize the attractive, healthy body he or she is striving for before sitting down to eat. A similar tactic is to tape on the refrigerator door a picture of an attractive person in a swimsuit to remind you of your long-term goal each time you have the urge for a snack. A person trying to save money to buy a large item (e.g., a camera) might tape a picture of the item to the inside of his wallet, to be seen whenever he reaches for some money. The idea behind all of these tactics is that a picture or visual image somehow bridges the gap between the present and the long-term goal, thereby increasing the subjective value of that goal. There is even evidence that giving people training to improve their short-term memories can lead to greater self-control, presumably because it enhances their ability to think about future rewards (Bickel, Yi, Landes, Hill, & Baxter, 2011).

We have surveyed some of the major strategies recommended by behavior therapists for improving self-control. All of these strategies show that there is more to self-control than simple determination and willpower. People who blame their impulsive behaviors on a lack of willpower may actually be lacking only the knowledge of how to apply the appropriate strategies.

OTHER CHOICE SITUATIONS

To conclude this chapter on choice behavior, we will examine a few other situations where people's or animals' decisions seem paradoxical. In some cases, their decisions appear to be inconsistent; in others, they are self-defeating. We will examine how psychologists have tried to analyze these situations.

Risk Taking

In many everyday decisions, the outcomes are not certain. If you invest in a company, you cannot be certain whether its stock will increase or decrease in value. If you leave home without your umbrella, you cannot be certain that it will not rain. If you go to a party, you cannot be certain whether you will enjoy yourself. An interesting fact about choices involving uncertain consequences is that sometimes people seem to prefer a risky alternative, and sometimes they prefer a safe alternative instead. The same has been found for animals. Researchers have tried to understand why individuals are sometimes risk-prone (preferring a risky alternative) and sometimes risk-averse (preferring a safer alternative).

In one experiment on this topic, Caraco, Martindale, and Whittam (1980) presented juncos (small birds) choices of the following type. Every trial, a junco could go to one of two feeding sites. If it went to one feeding site, it would receive one millet seed every time. If it went to the other feeding site, the bird had a 50% chance of finding two seeds, and a 50% chance of finding none. Caraco and colleagues found that if

the trials followed one another rapidly (so there were plenty of opportunities to obtain food), the birds preferred the single, guaranteed millet seed. However, if the trials were separated by longer delays (so there were fewer opportunities to obtain food), the birds preferred the 50% chance of getting two seeds. Caraco concluded that these strategies maximize a junco's chances of survival in the wild. When food is plentiful, there is no need to take a risk, because choosing small but certain food sources will guarantee that the bird has enough to eat. When food is scarce and the safe food sources do not provide enough food, the bird will choose riskier options with larger possible payoffs because the bird has nothing to lose—getting lucky with the risky option is the bird's only chance of survival.

Some research with other species has obtained results that support Caraco's theory (Ito, Takatsuru, & Saeki, 2000), but other studies have not (Case, Nichols, & Fantino, 1995). Humans who need to earn a certain amount of money also tend to be risk-prone when their resources are scarce and risk-averse when their resources are plentiful (Pietras, Locey, & Hackenberg, 2003; Pietras, Searcy, Huitema, & Brandt, 2008). March and Shapira (1992) suggested that both individuals (e.g., politicians) and groups (e.g., companies) are likely to take large risks when their survival (in a political campaign, in the marketplace) is at stake. However, they also proposed that besides being concerned merely with survival, individuals and groups also have aspiration levels (goals they wish to achieve), and their level of risk taking may depend on how close they are to their goals. For instance, a company may take large risks if its profits for the year are far below its goal, but if its profits are close to the goal, it may behave more conservatively. If the company's profits have exceeded the goal by a comfortable margin, the company may start to take greater risks once again. March and Shapira also proposed that other factors affect the level of risk taking by an individual or group, such as past habits, previous successes or failures, and self-confidence.

Considering all of these factors, it is no wonder that it can be difficult to predict how a person will behave in a risky situation. When it comes to games of chance, however, the choices of many people are all too predictable. Many people enjoy gambling—in casinos, in office pools, in state lotteries. Betting a few dollars a week may be harmless, but for some people, gambling becomes excessive, and they create financial ruin for themselves and their families because of their gambling losses. Excessive betting on lotteries or in casinos makes little financial sense, because the average gambler has to lose money (since state lotteries and casinos always make a profit). Why do people gamble, sometimes heavily, despite the fact that the odds are against them in the long run? Rachlin (1990) suggested that the preference for gambling is based on the possibility of obtaining an immediate reward. Consider the "instant lottery" games found in some states, in which you have a chance of winning money immediately (usually a fairly small amount) each time you buy a ticket. If you buy a ticket every day, you may sometimes go for weeks before you get a winner. But there is always a chance that you will win the very next time you play. Rachlin proposed that buying a lottery ticket is an attractive option for some people for the same reason that VR or VI schedules produce steady and persistent responding in the laboratory: In both cases, there is a chance that a reinforcer will be delivered almost immediately.

To summarize, we have now examined several choice situations in which the immediacy of a reinforcer is a crucial factor. In self-control choices, people and animals often choose a small, immediate reinforcer over a delayed reinforcer that would be better for them in the long run. Similarly, the possibility of winning a prize the very next time you place a bet makes gambling attractive, even though you are likely to lose money in the long run. The next section describes some additional situations in which people may choose short-term gains at the expense of larger long-term losses.

The Tragedy of the Commons

When a person makes an impulsive choice in a self-control situation, the person is acting against his or her long-term interests. The following situations are similar, except here; by acting in their short-term interests, people make choices that are detrimental to society as a whole.

In an article entitled "The Tragedy of the Commons," Garrett Hardin (1968) described a situation that has far too many parallels in modern society. In many villages of colonial America, the commons was a grassland owned by the village, where residents could allow their cows to graze freely. The commons was therefore a public resource that benefited everyone as long as the number of grazing animals did not grow too large. This might not happen for decades or for centuries, but according to Hardin, it was inevitable that eventually there would be more animals than the commons could support. Then, because of overgrazing, the grass becomes scarce, erosion occurs, and the commons is destroyed, to the detriment of everyone.

Why did Hardin believe this unhappy scenario was inevitable? His reasoning was that it is to each herder's benefit to have as many cows as possible, for this will maximize one's income. Now suppose an individual must decide whether to add one more cow to the herd. What are the benefits and costs to consider? The benefits are the profits to be earned from this cow, which go entirely to the owner of the cow. The cost is the extra strain imposed on the commons, but one additional cow will not make much of a difference, and besides, this cost is shared by everyone who uses the commons. Hardin therefore concluded that the herder will experience a net gain by adding the additional cow to the herd, and by adding a second cow, and so on.

> But this is the conclusion reached by each and every rational herdsman sharing a commons. Therein is the tragedy. Each man is locked into a system that compels him to increase his herd without limit—in a world that is limited. Ruin is the destination toward which all men rush, each pursuing his own best interest in a society that believes

in the freedom of the commons. Freedom in a commons brings ruin to all. (Hardin, 1968, p. 1244)

The **tragedy of the commons** is a play that has been acted out many times in our civilization. The buffalo herds on the American plains were hunted nearly to the point of extinction. Excessive fishing has ruined many of the world's richest fishing areas. Whalers are killing off whales at a rate that could lead to their extinction, which, besides being deplorable in its own right, will of course put the whalers out of business. With every acre of forest land that is turned into a highway or a shopping mall, there is less wilderness for everyone to enjoy.

Most problems of pollution have a similar structure. A company that must pollute the air in order to manufacture its product cheaply keeps the profits of its enterprise to itself; the air pollution is shared by everyone. Before we condemn big business, however, we should realize that individual people frequently make equally selfish decisions. Every person who drives to work in a large city (rather than walking, riding a bike, or taking public transportation) contributes to the air pollution of that city. The reason that many people behave selfishly in this situation is obvious: The driver alone receives the benefits of convenience and comfort that come from driving one's own car. If the driver chose to walk, the reduction in air pollution would be so slight as to be undetectable.

Another instance of the commons tragedy can be seen in the annual trade deficit of the United States, a consequence of the large amounts of foreign products that Americans buy. Most people know that the trade deficit hurts the economy and that it would be eliminated if people bought fewer foreign goods. Nevertheless, when an individual consumer is deciding which product to purchase, alleviating the trade deficit usually seems far less important than getting the best buy, regardless of whether the product is domestic or foreign.

Although there are many examples of the tragedy of the commons in modern life, Hardin (1968) and Platt (1973) have suggested several ways in which the tragedy can be averted. These suggestions will probably sound familiar, because in recent years our society has focused a good deal of attention on the problems of pollution, the extinction of wildlife, and the like, as well as on potential solutions. What is interesting, however, is the strong resemblance these remedies bear to the strategies that individuals can use to avoid impulsiveness in a self-control situation.

We saw that one powerful technique for improving self-control is the precommitment strategy in which an individual takes some action in advance that makes it difficult or impossible to make an impulsive choice later. Similarly, a society can decide to make it difficult or impossible for individuals to act selfishly. For example, a society can pass legislation that simply makes it illegal to dump dangerous chemicals where they might seep into the water supply, to pollute the air, or to kill a member of an endangered species.

Less coercive strategies for self-control situations are those that either attach a punisher to the small, immediate alternative or attach an additional (often immediate) reinforcer to the large, delayed alternative. These strategies do not make an impulsive choice impossible, only less likely. In a similar fashion, a city with traffic and pollution problems can punish the behavior of driving one's own car by prohibiting parking on city streets and by making it expensive to park in garages. On the basis of what we know about punishment, however, it would be advisable to couple such punishment with reinforcement for a desirable alternative behavior. For instance, the city should do all that it can to make public transportation convenient, reliable, safe, and inexpensive.

Finally, we should not underestimate the capacity of human beings to attend to and be influenced by the long-term consequences of their behaviors for society. Just as a picture on the refrigerator can remind a dieter of his or her long-term goal, educational programs and advertising campaigns can encourage individuals to alter their behaviors for the long-term benefits of the community. A good example is the personal sacrifices civilians were willing to make for the war effort during World War II, not to mention the soldiers who gave their lives in the name of freedom. In some fishing communities, overfishing is avoided by informal agreements among individuals to limit their catches for the good of all (Leal, 1998). From a logical perspective, such behaviors may seem puzzling: Why should people behave in a way that is helpful to others but is harmful to them personally? One solution to this puzzle is simply to assert that, at least in certain circumstances, behaviors that benefit others can be inherently reinforcing for many people (just as eating, reading a novel, or exercising can be inherently reinforcing). Admittedly, this is not much of an explanation. But given the many examples of selfish behaviors we have been forced to consider, it is refreshing to remember that people will often make sacrifices when the only personal benefit from their behavior is the knowledge that they are promoting the common good.

PRACTICE QUIZ (2)

1. An individual who chooses a _____ reinforcer over a _____ reinforcer is said to be making an impulsive choice.
2. Making a choice of a large, delayed reinforcer in advance, so that later it is difficult to choose a smaller, more immediate reinforcer, is called _____.
3. In a self-control choice situation where the actual reinforcers are visible during a delay, both children and animals are more likely to choose the _____ reinforcer.
4. The rate of delay discounting is usually _____ for children than for adults.
5. If a person chooses an option with an uncertain outcome over one with a guaranteed outcome, the person is said to be _____.

Answers

1. small, immediate; large, delayed   2. precommitment   3. smaller, more immediate   4. faster   5. risk-prone

---

Summary

The matching law states that the proportion of responses on each schedule tends to match the proportion of reinforcers delivered by that schedule. This law has been demonstrated with many different species of subjects, including people. However, three different types of deviations from exact matching are often found: undermatching, overmatching, and bias. The matching law has also been applied to other variables, such as reinforcer quality and amount. It has also been applied to response rates on single reinforcement schedules by assuming that the individual must choose between the reinforcers delivered by the schedule and other, extraneous reinforcers.

Herrnstein proposed that matching is a fundamental property of behavior, and later he developed a related theory called melioration. A very different theory, optimization theory, states that individuals will distribute their responses in whatever way will maximize the reinforcement they receive. Some studies that compared the predictions of the matching law and optimization theory have favored the matching law; that is, subjects exhibited approximate matching even when this behavior decreased the overall amount of reinforcement. Momentary maximization theory states that, at each moment, an individual chooses whichever behavior has the highest value at that moment. Some experiments have found such moment-to-moment patterns in choice behavior that are predicted by this theory, but others have not.

In a self-control choice situation, an individual must choose between a small, fairly immediate reinforcer and a larger, more delayed reinforcer. Individuals frequently choose the small, immediate reinforcer, even though the larger reinforcer would be better in the long run.

Studies with animals and children have demonstrated several factors that can affect choice in these situations. Making a precommitment to choose the larger, delayed reinforcer is an effective self-control strategy, as are adding additional reinforcers to the long-term alternative, adding punishers to the short-term alternative, or using cognitive strategies to focus attention on the long-term consequences of one's choices.

The effects of delay can also be seen in other choice situations, such as in risk-prone behavior (e.g., gambling when the odds are against winning). The tragedy of the commons occurs when individuals make decisions that benefit them in the short run but are harmful to society as a whole in the long run. Strategies similar to those used to improve self-control may also be helpful in such cases.

Review Questions

1. What is the matching law? Describe Herrnstein's experiment on matching, and discuss three ways that behavior can deviate from perfect matching.

2. Explain how the matching law can account for behavior on a single VI schedule as the rate of reinforcement is increased to higher and higher levels.

3. Summarize the main differences between the matching law, optimization theory, and momentary maximizing theory. What has research found about the strengths and weaknesses of these competing theories?

4. Describe the Ainslie–Rachlin theory, and use an everyday example to show how it accounts for the reversals in preference that occur in self-control choices.

5. Describe several techniques a person could use to help him avoid eating foods that are high in fat and cholesterol.

6. What is the tragedy of the commons? Give a few modern-day examples of this problem and describe some strategies that can be used to overcome the problem.

GLOSSARY

a-process In the opponent-process theory, an initial fast-acting emotional response to a stimulus, which is later followed by the b-process, leading to the opposite emotion.

ABAB design A design for behavioral treatment where each "A" phase is a baseline phase in which the patient's behavior is recorded but no treatment is given, and each "B" phase is a treatment phase.

absolute theory of stimulus control A theory about how animals learn about reinforced and non-reinforced stimuli. The theory states that animals simply learn about the two stimuli separately but learn nothing about the relation between the two.

acquisition phase The period in the learning process when an individual is learning a new behavior.

Adams's two-stage theory A theory of motor-skill learning that consists of a verbal-motor stage in which improvement depends on the delivery of feedback from the teacher, followed by a motor stage in which the learner can continue to improve without the teacher's feedback.

adjunctive behaviors Stereotyped behaviors that arise when food or some other reinforcer is delivered at regular intervals.

Ainslie–Rachlin theory A theory of self-control choices that explains why an individual's preference can shift from a larger, delayed reinforcer to a smaller, more immediate reinforcer as the time of reinforcer delivery approaches.

analogy A statement in the form "A is to B as C is to D." To test the ability to understand analogies, the subject is given two or more choices for D and asked which is correct.

animal cognition Also called comparative cognition, a field of psychology that compares the cognitive processes and abilities of different species, including humans.

arborization The branching of the dendrites of neurons, a process that occurs especially rapidly before birth and during the first year of a child's life.

assertiveness training A form of therapy for people who are overly submissive in certain situations and want to develop the ability to stand up for their rights. It frequently consists of a combination of modeling, role playing, and behavioral rehearsal.

Associationists Philosophers who developed early theories about how people learn to associate separate thoughts or ideas as a result of their experiences.

associative rehearsal A type of rehearsal that strengthens the information in long-term memory.

autism A severe disorder that affects somewhat less that 1% of all children, usually appearing when a child is a few years old. Major symptoms are extreme social withdrawal and failure to learn language.

automatic reinforcement Reinforcement of a behavior derived from the sensory stimulation that occurs as a result of performing the behavior itself.

aversive counterconditioning A treatment for alcoholism and other addictions in which the addictive substance is paired with an aversive stimulus, such as an illness-inducing drug, designed to condition an aversive response to the addictive substance.

avoidance A type of negative reinforcement in which performing a response prevents an aversive stimulus from occurring in the first place.

avoidance paradox The puzzle about how the nonoccurrence of an aversive event can serve as a reinforcer for an avoidance response.

axon A long branch-like part of a neuron that transmits electrical pulses, or action potentials, when the neuron is stimulated. Enlarged structures at the ends of the axons, the axon terminals, release chemical transmitters that stimulate the dendrites of other neurons.

b-process In the opponent-process theory, an emotional response that is the opposite of the a-process. The b-process is supposedly activated only in response to the activity of the a-process, and it is more sluggish both to rise and to decay.

backward chaining A strategy, used for teaching response chains, in which the teacher starts with the last response in the chain and works backward.

backward conditioning A classical conditioning procedure in which the conditioned stimulus is presented after the unconditioned stimulus.

Bandura's theory of imitation A theory that four factors are needed for imitation to occur: attentional processes, retentional processes, motor reproductive processes, and incentive and motivational processes.

behavior decelerator Any procedure that leads to a slowing, reduction, or elimination of an unwanted behavior.

behavior-systems analysis The view that different reinforcers evoke different systems or collections of species-typical behaviors, which can account for the types of behaviors seen in autoshaping, classical conditioning, and some operant conditioning situations.

behavioral contrast A phenomenon in which responding in the presence of one stimulus changes as a result of a change in the reinforcement conditions during another stimulus.

behavioral economics A field that uses principles from both behavioral psychology and economics to predict people's choices and behaviors.

behavioral momentum An operant behavior's resistance to change when the reinforcement conditions change (e.g., when free reinforcers are delivered or when the schedule changes to extinction).

behavioral skills training A method for teaching new behaviors that include techniques such as modeling, verbal instruction, prompting, guided practice, and feedback.

behavioral theory of timing A theory of animal timing proposed by Killeen and Fetterman that states that animals use their own behaviors to measure durations. The theory states that the rate of reinforcement controls the rate of the internal clock, which in turn controls the rate of the animal's behaviors, and the animal uses these behaviors to measure the passage of time.

behaviorism An approach to psychology and the field of learning that emphasizes the study of external events (observable stimuli and responses) and avoids speculation about processes inside the organism.

bias In choice behavior, a deviation from matching in which a subject consistently allocates more time or responding to one alternative than predicted by the matching equation.

biofeedback A procedure that provides a person with amplified feedback about some bodily function, usually presented with the intention of increasing the individual's control over that bodily function to treat some medical problem.

blocking In classical conditioning, the finding that there is little or no conditioning to a stimulus if it is presented along with a previously conditioned stimulus on conditioning trials.

British Associationists British philosophers who proposed early theories about how the ideas in memory are formed from a person's experiences.

cell body The part of a neuron that contains the nucleus, which regulates the basic metabolic functions of the cell.

central instance In research of concept formation, an example from a natural category that people tend to judge as a "good," or "typical," example.

cerebellum A part of the brain, located in the back of the head beneath the cerebral cortex, that is important for many skilled movements.

chained schedule A set of two or more reinforcement schedules that must be completed in a specific sequence before the reinforcer is delivered. Each schedule is signaled by a different stimulus.

changeover delay In choice behavior, a requirement that a certain amount of time must pass after a subject switches from one response to another before any reinforcer can be delivered.

chunk A group of items that the learner combines into a single unit (e.g., a group of letters that form a word), which makes learning easier than if all the items had to be learned individually.

classical conditioning The procedure of repeatedly pairing an initially neutral stimulus (the conditioned stimulus) and an unconditioned stimulus, through which the conditioned stimulus develops the capacity to elicit a conditioned response.

closed-loop movement In feedback theory, a movement during which the performer continually receives feedback about whether the movement is proceeding correctly and can adjust his or her behavior in response to this feedback.

cognitive map According to Tolman, a mental map of its environment that an animal develops by exploring or observing its surroundings (as when a rat learns a maze).

cognitive psychology An approach to psychology which, unlike behaviorism, makes use of theories about processes that take place inside the head (memory, attention, rehearsal, etc.) that cannot be observed directly.

cognitive theory of avoidance The theory that avoidance responses will occur when the individual has expectations that (1) an aversive event will occur if no response is made and (2) the aversive event will be avoided if a response is made. Avoidance responding will continue until one or both of these expectations are violated.

comparative cognition A field of psychology that compares the cognitive processes and abilities of different species, including humans.

comparator In control systems theory, a device that compares its goal state (the reference input) and the current situation (the actual input) and signals that action is necessary if the two are not equal.

comparator theory A theory of classical conditioning that states that the strength of a conditioned response depends on a comparison of the likelihood of an unconditioned stimulus in the presence of the conditioned stimulus versus its absence.

complex idea A term used by James Mill, a British Associationist, to describe what happens when two or more simple ideas are combined.

compound CS In classical conditioning, the simultaneous presentation of two or more conditioned stimuli.

concurrent schedule A situation in which two or more reinforcement schedules are available at the same time, each requiring its own responses and delivering its own reinforcers.

conditional discrimination task A discrimination task in which the subject must choose between one of two stimuli, and the correct response depends on which of two other stimuli was presented previously.

conditioned compensatory response In classical conditioning, a conditioned response that is the opposite of the unconditioned response.

conditioned emotional response (CER) A classical conditioning procedure in which the

conditioned stimulus signals that an aversive event is coming. The measure of conditioning is the suppression of ongoing behavior (e.g., pressing a lever to obtain food) when the conditioned stimulus is presented, so this procedure is also called *conditioned suppression.*

conditioned inhibitor (CS⁻) In classical conditioning, a conditioned stimulus that prevents the occurrence of a conditioned response or reduces the size of the conditioned response from what it would otherwise be. It is also called an *inhibitory CS.*

conditioned opponent theory A theory of classical conditioning that states that the later portions of an unconditioned response (which are often opposite in form to the early portions) become associated with the conditioned stimulus. The theory accounts for conditioned responses that appear to be the opposite of the unconditioned response.

conditioned reflex Another name for a conditioned response.

conditioned reinforcer A previously neutral stimulus that has acquired the capacity to strengthen responses because it has been repeatedly paired with a primary reinforcer.

conditioned response (CR) The response that is elicited by a conditioned stimulus after classical conditioning has taken place.

conditioned stimulus (CS) An initially neutral stimulus that develops the capacity to elicit a conditioned response after it is paired with an unconditioned stimulus.

confounding variable A variable that is not of interest to the researcher but might nevertheless affect the results of an experiment, thereby making the results difficult or impossible to interpret.

context-shift effect The finding that if one learns information in a particular context, recall of that information will be better if one is tested in the same context than if the testing occurs in a different context.

contextual interference Any features of the learning situation which make learning a new task more difficult, but which may lead to better performance in the long run.

contextual stimuli The sights, sounds, and smells of a creature's environment.

contiguity   One of Aristotle's principles of association, which states that two ideas will be associated if they tend to occur together in space or time. In modern psychology, contiguity between stimuli is an important factor in classical conditioning, and contiguity between a response and its consequences is important in operant conditioning.

contingency contract   A written agreement used in behavior therapy that lists the duties (behaviors) required of each party and the privileges (reinforcers) that will result if the duties are performed.

contingency-shaped behavior   Behavior that is controlled by the schedule of reinforcement or punishment (as opposed to rule-governed behavior, which is controlled by a verbal or mental rule about how to behave).

continuous reinforcement (CRF)   A reinforcement schedule that delivers a reinforcer after every occurrence of a specific response.

contrast   One of Aristotle's principles of association, which states that the thought of one concept often leads to the thought of the opposite concept.

control group   In experimental research, a group of subjects that receives no special training or treatment and whose performance is compared to that of the experimental group.

control systems theory   A branch of science that analyzes goal-directed behaviors in both living creatures and inanimate objects.

CS preexposure effect   The finding that classical conditioning proceeds more slowly if the conditioned stimulus is repeatedly presented by itself before it is paired with the unconditioned stimulus.

CS–US interval   In classical conditioning, the amount of time between the start of the conditioned stimulus and the start of the unconditioned stimulus.

cue exposure treatment   In the treatment of drug addictions, exposing the individual to stimuli that are normally associated with the drug, so that conditioned drug cravings can be extinguished.

cumulative recorder   A simple mechanical device that records responses in a way that plots time on the horizontal axis and cumulative responses on the vertical axis. It allows the observer to see at a glance the moment-to-moment patterns of a subject's behavior.

delay discounting   A decrease in the strength or value of reinforcer as its delay increases.

delayed matching to sample (DMTS)   A procedure used to measure short-term memory, or working memory. First, a sample stimulus is presented, followed by a delay with no stimuli; then two comparison stimuli are presented, and a choice of the comparison that matches the sample is reinforced.

demand curve   A graph that plots the demand for product as a function of its price.

dendrite   A branch-like structure on the receptive side of a neuron that is sensitive to transmitters released by the axon terminals of other neurons.

dependent variable   In psychological research, the behavior of a subject that is measured by the experimenter to see how it is affected by changes in the independent variable.

differential reinforcement of alternative behavior (DRA)   A technique for reducing unwanted behaviors by using extinction combined with reinforcement of more desirable behaviors.

differential reinforcement of high rates (DRH) schedule   A reinforcement schedule in which a reinforcer is delivered if a certain number of responses have occurred within a fixed amount of time.

differential reinforcement of low rates (DRL) schedule   A reinforcement schedule in which a reinforcer is delivered if a certain amount of time has elapsed between two responses.

directed forgetting   A procedure for studying memory and forgetting in which the learner (either human or animal) is taught that on some trials it is important to remember a stimulus and on other trials it is safe to forget the stimulus.

discrimination   In either classical or operant conditioning, learning to respond to one stimulus but not to another similar stimulus.

discrimination hypothesis   An explanation of the partial reinforcement effect, which states that the rate of decrease in responding depends on how quickly the subject can discriminate the change from reinforcement to extinction.

discriminative stimulus In operant conditioning, a stimulus that indicates whether or not responding will lead to reinforcement.

disinhibition In classical conditioning, the reappearance of a conditioned response to a stimulus that has undergone extinction that can occur if a novel stimulus is presented shortly before the extinguished stimulus.

distributed practice In motor-skill learning, a training procedure in which fairly brief practice periods alternate with rest periods, which may lead to better learning than massed practice.

drive-reduction theory A theory proposed by Hull that any decrease in a biological drive (the hunger drive, the sex drive, etc.) will serve as a reinforcer.

duplex idea A term developed by James Mill, a British Associationist, to describe what happens when complex ideas are combined.

dynamic pattern theory A theory that emphasizes the importance of feedback from the body and the environment during movement sequences. It also asserts that regularities in movement sequences may be the result of the physical properties of the body rather than the product of a generalized motor program.

elastic demand In economics, demand for a product that exhibits large changes as the price increases or decreases.

electrical stimulation of the brain (ESB) A mild, pulsating electrical current which, when delivered to certain parts of the brain, acts as a powerful reinforcer.

equipotentiality premise The hypothesis that a stimulus or response that is difficult to condition in one context should also be difficult to condition in all other contexts.

errorless discrimination learning A procedure for teaching discriminations developed by Herbert Terrace; errorless discrimination learning begins with stimuli that are easy for the subject to discriminate and progresses to more difficult ones, so the subject makes very few errors during the course of learning.

escape A type of negative reinforcement in which performing a response leads to the termination of an aversive stimulus.

escape extinction A procedure used to eliminate an unwanted behavior that has been previously reinforced by escape from an unpleasant situation, in which escape is prevented if the unwanted behavior occurs.

ethologist A scientist who studies how animals behave in their natural environments.

evaluative conditioning A form of second-order classical conditioning with human subjects in which neutral stimuli are paired with a positive or negative stimuli; then the subjects are asked to rate how much they like or dislike the stimuli.

excitatory CS (CS$^+$) In classical conditioning, a conditioned stimulus that regularly elicits a conditioned response.

exemplar theory A theory of concept learning that states that one's ability to categorize objects depends on one's memory of specific examples.

extinction In classical conditioning, presenting the conditioned stimulus without the unconditioned stimulus. In operant conditioning, no longer presenting the reinforcer when the operant response is made. In both cases, responding decreases and eventually disappears.

fading A behavior modification procedure in which a prompt for a desired behavior is gradually withdrawn, thereby teaching the learner to produce the behavior without the prompt.

feature detector A neuron that responds to a specific type of visual stimulus.

feature theory A theory of concept learning that states that one judges whether a given instance is a member of a category by checking for specific features.

field experiment A study that is conducted in a realistic setting as opposed to a laboratory setting.

first-order CS In classical conditioning, a stimulus that has been conditioned by pairing it directly with the unconditioned stimulus.

fixed action pattern An innate sequence of behaviors that is elicited by a specific stimulus and, once started, continues to its end whether or not the behaviors are appropriate in the current situation.

fixed-interval (FI) schedule A reinforcement schedule in which the first response after a fixed amount of time has elapsed is reinforced.

fixed-ratio (FR) schedule   A reinforcement schedule that delivers a reinforcer after a fixed number of responses.

flooding   A treatment for phobias in which a patient is presented with a highly feared object or situation, which is not removed until the patient's fear diminishes.

forgetting curve   A graph showing how performance on a memory task declines with the passage of time since learning.

forward chaining   A strategy used to teach a response chain in which the teacher starts by reinforcing the first response of the chain, then gradually adds the second response, the third response, and so on.

free-operant avoidance   Another name for the Sidman avoidance task.

free-operant procedure   A procedure developed by Skinner in which, unlike a discrete trial procedure, the operant response can occur at any time and can occur repeatedly for as long as the subject remains in the experimental chamber.

functional analysis   A method in which stimuli and/or reinforcers are systematically varied so that a therapist can determine which are maintaining a patient's behavior.

functional magnetic resonance imaging (fMRI)   A brain-imaging technique that can show, in real time, which parts of a person's brain are currently most active.

generalization   The transfer of a learned response from one stimulus to another, similar stimulus.

generalization decrement hypothesis   An explanation of the partial reinforcement effect, which states that responding during extinction will be rapid if the stimuli present during extinction are different from those that occurred during reinforcement, but slow if the stimuli are similar to those that occurred during reinforcement.

generalization gradient   A graphic representation of generalization in which the *x*-axis plots some dimension along which the test stimuli are varied and the *y*-axis shows the strength of conditioned responding to the different stimuli.

generalized motor program   A motor program that can be adapted to a variety of different situations.

generalized reinforcer   A conditioned reinforcer that has been associated with a large number of different primary reinforcers.

graduated modeling   A type of modeling in which the model's behaviors steadily progress from simple to more difficult behaviors.

guidance hypothesis   In motor-skill learning, a theory that if knowledge of results (KR) is given on every trial during learning, the learner becomes overly dependent on this KR and will not perform well in a later test without KR.

habituation   A decrease in the strength of a reflexive response after repeated presentation of the stimulus that elicits the response.

human universals   Abilities or behaviors that are found in all known human cultures.

Humphreys's paradox   Another name for the partial reinforcement effect, or the seemingly paradoxical finding that a response that is only intermittently reinforced is more resistant to extinction than a response that is reinforced every time it occurs.

independent variable   In scientific research, a variable that the experimenter manipulates to determine how this affects the dependent variable.

indifference point   In choice behavior, a pair of alternatives that an individual finds equally preferable, or chooses equally often.

inelastic demand   In economics, demand for a product that shows relatively little change as the price increases or decreases.

instinctive drift   In operant conditioning, innate behaviors that are related to the type of reinforcer being used that cause an animal's performance to drift away from the reinforced behavior and toward instinctive behaviors.

interim behavior   A behavior pattern that occurs in the early parts of each interval when food or some other primary reinforcer is delivered at regular intervals.

intermediate-size problem   A discrimination problem in which the subject learns to choose the middle stimulus along some dimension (e.g., a medium-sized circle) and is then tested when this stimulus is no longer the medium one (e.g., it is now the smallest of three circles).

interneuron Any neuron that occurs in a chain of synapses that begins with a sensory neuron and ends with a motor neuron.

interresponse time (IRT) reinforcement theory The theory that responding is faster on variable-ratio schedules than on variable-interval schedules because long IRTs (long pauses between responses) are more frequently reinforced on variable-interval schedules.

intervening variable A theoretical concept that cannot be observed directly, but is used in science to predict the relationship between independent and dependent variables.

intradimensional training A type of discrimination training in which responses in the presence of one stimulus are reinforced, but responses in the presence of a different stimulus from the same physical continuum are not reinforced.

ironic error In motor-skill learning, a false movement that a person is trying hard to avoid but has a tendency to make, especially if attention is distracted by some competing task.

kinesis A tropism in which the direction of the movement is random in relation to the stimulus.

knowledge of performance (KP) In motor-skill learning, detailed feedback given to the learner, such as information about which parts of the movement were performed well and how other parts of the movement could be improved.

knowledge of results (KR) In motor-skill learning, feedback given to the learner about how close his or her movement came to the goal.

latent learning Tolman's term for the hidden learning that occurs on trials when no reinforcer is delivered, but can only be seen in the subject's behavior once trials with reinforcement begin.

Law of Effect Thorndike's version of the principle of reinforcement, which states that responses that are followed by pleasant or satisfying stimuli will be strengthened and will occur more often in the future.

learned helplessness Seligman's term for the impaired ability to learn an avoidance response that occurs after a subject has been exposed to inescapable aversive stimuli.

learned optimism Seligman's term for the ability to think about potentially bad situations in positive ways.

learning set An improvement in the rate of learning across a series of discrimination problems, which occurs even though the positive and negative stimuli are different from one problem to the next.

long-delay conditioning A type of classical conditioning in which the onset of the conditioned stimulus precedes that of the unconditioned stimulus by at least several seconds and continues until the unconditioned stimulus is presented.

long-term memory A part of memory that has a very large capacity and can retain information for months, years, or longer, although some information is lost through interference or forgetting.

long-term potentiation An increase in the strengths of connections between neurons caused by electrical stimulation, which can last for weeks or months.

longitudinal study In psychological research, a method in which the same individuals are repeatedly observed at different points in time to look for possible changes in their behavior.

maintenance rehearsal A type of rehearsal that retains information in short-term memory but does not necessarily strengthen information in long-term memory.

massed practice In motor-skill learning, a training procedure in which practice takes place in one continuous block, without rest periods, which may lead to worse learning than distributed practice.

matching law Herrnstein's general principle of choice behavior that states that in a two-choice situation, the percentage of responses directed toward one alternative will equal the percentage of reinforcers delivered by that alternative.

matching to sample A procedure in which reinforcement is delivered if the subject chooses the comparison stimulus that matches a sample stimulus.

melioration A principle proposed by Herrnstein and Vaughan that states that matching behavior in choice situations is the result of a process in which the individual invests increasing amounts of time and effort into whichever alternative delivers a higher ratio of reinforcers per response.

metacognition The ability to reflect on one's memories and thought processes and make judgments about them.

mirror neurons Neurons that respond both when an individual makes a certain movement and when the individual observes someone else make that movement.

molar theory A theory of behavior that focuses on the long-term relationships between behaviors and their consequences.

molecular theory A theory of behavior that focuses on the moment-by-moment relationships between behaviors and their consequences.

momentary maximization theory A theory of choice behavior that states that at each moment, a creature will select whichever alternative has the highest value at that moment, even though it may not be the best choice in the long run.

motor program A brain or spinal cord mechanism, first proposed by Lashley, which controls a sequence of movements and does not rely on sensory feedback from one movement to initiate the next movement in the sequence.

multiple schedule A procedure in which two or more reinforcement schedules are presented one at a time in an alternating pattern, and each schedule is signaled by a different discriminative stimulus.

narrowing A technique of stimulus control that involves gradually reducing the range of situations in which an unwanted behavior is allowed to occur.

nativism The hypothesis that some ideas are innate (inborn) and do not depend on an individual's past experience.

need-reduction theory A theory proposed by Hull that all primary reinforcers are stimuli that reduce some biological need, and all stimuli that reduce a biological need will act as reinforcers.

negative contrast A type of behavioral contrast in which there is a decrease in responding in the presence of one stimulus due to an increase in the reinforcement conditions for another stimulus.

negative punishment A behavior reduction procedure, more commonly called omission, in which a desired stimulus is removed or omitted if the behavior occurs.

negative reinforcement A behavior-strengthening procedure in which an aversive stimulus is removed or omitted if the behavior occurs.

negative transfer In motor-skill learning, when practice of one task interferes with learning or performance on another task.

neurofeedback A type of biofeedback in which a person receives feedback about some brainwave pattern, for the purpose of changing or controlling that pattern.

neurogenesis The growth of new neurons.

nondifferential training A simple type of discrimination training in which the positive stimulus is presented on every trial, and there are no trials with negative stimuli.

nonsense syllable A meaningless syllable consisting of two consonants separated by a vowel, first used in memory experiments by Hermann Ebbinghaus.

object permanence An understanding that objects continue to exist even when they are not visible. Researchers have studied how and when young children develop the concept of object permanence and whether different species of animals can also develop this concept.

occasion setter In classical conditioning, a stimulus that does not itself elicit a response, but its presence causes another stimulus to elicit a conditioned response.

omission A behavior reduction procedure in which a desired stimulus is removed or omitted if the unwanted behavior occurs.

one-factor theory A theory of avoidance that states that avoidance of an aversive stimulus, such as a shock, can in itself serve as a reinforcer, and that the classical conditioning component of two-factor theory is not necessary.

open-loop movement In feedback theory, a movement that occurs so rapidly that there is no time to make any corrections once the movement begins.

opponent-process theory Solomon and Corbit's theory that states that many emotional responses include an initial emotional reaction followed by an after-reaction of the opposite emotion.

optimization theory A theory of choice behavior that states that people tend to make decisions that maximize their satisfaction.

organizational behavior management A field of applied behavior analysis that uses the principles of behavioral psychology to improve human performance in the workplace.

orienting response An innate reaction to a sudden or unexpected stimulus in which an animal stops its current activity to look at or listen to the novel stimulus.

overcorrection A behavior reduction procedure in which the individual is required to make several repetitions of an alternate, more desirable behavior if an undesired behavior occurs.

overexpectation effect A decrease in the strength of responding to two conditioned stimuli that have been trained separately that occurs if they are presented as a compound CS and followed by the usual unconditioned stimulus.

overlearning Continuing to practice a response after performance is apparently perfect, which often results in stronger or more accurate performance in a delayed test.

overmatching A deviation from matching in which response percentages are consistently more extreme than reinforcement percentages in a choice situation.

overshadowing In classical conditioning, the finding that there is less conditioning to a weak conditioned stimulus if it is presented along with a more intense conditioned stimulus.

pacemaker In theories of animal timing, a hypothetical internal process that pulses at a steady rate and allows the animal to measure durations.

partial reinforcement effect The finding that responses are more rapidly extinguished after continuous reinforcement than after a schedule of intermittent reinforcement.

participant modeling A type of modeling in which the learner imitates the behavior of the model in each step of the treatment.

peak procedure A procedure for studying animal timing abilities in which the time of its peak response rate shows how accurately the animal can time the intervals.

peak shift After discrimination training with a reinforced stimulus and an unreinforced stimulus, a shift in the peak of a generalization gradient from the reinforced stimulus in a direction away from the unreinforced stimulus.

percentile schedule of reinforcement A reinforcement schedule in which a given response is reinforced if it is better than a certain percentage of the last several responses the learner has made.

peripheral instance In research of concept formation, an example from a natural category that people tend to judge as a "bad" or "atypical" example.

plasticity The nervous system's ability to change as a result of experience or stimulation.

positive contrast A type of behavioral contrast in which there is an increase in responding in the presence of one stimulus due to a decrease in the reinforcement conditions for another stimulus.

positive reinforcement A behavior-strengthening procedure in which the occurrence of a behavior is followed by a desired stimulus, or reinforcer.

positive transfer In motor-skill learning, when practice of one task improves learning or performance on a similar task.

positron emission tomography (PET) A brain-imaging technique that can show which parts of a person's brain are currently most active.

postreinforcement pause A pause in responding that usually occurs after each reinforcer in fixed-ratio schedules.

precommitment A technique for improving self-control in which the individual makes a choice in advance that is difficult or impossible to change at a later time.

Premack's principle The theory that more probable behaviors will act as reinforcers for less probable behaviors, and that less probable behaviors will act as punishers for more probable behaviors.

prepared association An association between stimuli, or between stimuli and responses, in which members of a particular species have an innate tendency to learn quickly and easily.

presence–absence training   A type of discrimination training in which the presence or absence of a specific stimulus indicates whether responding will be reinforced.

primary reinforcer   A stimulus that naturally strengthens any response it follows (e.g., food, water, sexual pleasure, and comfort).

proactive interference   When previously learned material impairs the learning of new material.

progressive relaxation (or deep muscle relaxation)   A technique for inducing a state of bodily calm and relaxation by having the person alternately tense and relax specific groups of muscles.

prompt   In behavior modification, a stimulus that makes a desired response very likely to occur, and is gradually removed (faded out) as training proceeds.

prospective coding   A memory strategy in which subjects remember what response needs to be made next, rather than remembering what events have occurred previously.

prototype theory   A theory of concept learning that states that one's ability to categorize objects depends forming a prototype or ideal example, to which new examples are compared.

punishment   A behavior reduction procedure in which the occurrence of a behavior is followed by an aversive stimulus.

puzzle box   A type of experimental chamber used by Thorndike in which an animal had to make a certain response in order to open the door and obtain food that was available outside.

radial-arm maze   A maze for animals in which eight or more arms radiate from a central starting area, and each of the arms may contain food at the end.

rapid reacquisition   Learning in a second acquisition phase that follows extinction that occurs more quickly than in the initial acquisition phase.

ratio strain   A general weakening of responding that is found when a fixed-ratio schedule requires a very large number of responses.

reaction chain   An innate sequence of behaviors in which the progression from one behavior to the

next depends on the presence of the appropriate external stimulus. Portions of the sequence may be skipped or omitted depending on which stimuli are presented and which are not.

receptor   A specialized neuron that responds to sensory stimulation, either from the traditional "five senses" or from internal bodily sensations such as muscle tension and balance.

reciprocal contingency   A procedure that ensures that two behaviors occur in a fixed proportion by requiring the individual to perform fixed amounts of the two behaviors in alternation.

reflex   An innate movement that can be reliably elicited by presenting the appropriate stimulus.

rehearsal   An active processing of stimuli or events after they have occurred, which can keep information active in short-term memory and promote its transfer into long-term memory.

reinforcement relativity   An idea promoted by Premack that there are no absolute categories of reinforcers and reinforceable responses, but that more probable behaviors can reinforce less probable behaviors.

reinforcement schedule   A rule that states under what conditions a reinforcer will be delivered.

reinforcer   A stimulus that strengthens behavior if it is delivered after the behavior occurs.

relational theory of stimulus control   The theory that animals can learn to respond to relationships between stimuli (e.g., larger, redder, or brighter). The opposite is the absolute theory of stimulus control, which assumes that animals cannot learn such relationships.

Rescorla–Wagner model   A mathematical theory of classical conditioning that states that, on each trial, the amount of excitatory or inhibitory conditioning depends on the associative strengths of all the conditioned stimuli that are present and on the intensity of the unconditioned stimulus.

resistance to extinction   The degree to which a response continues when it is no longer reinforced.

response blocking   A behavior reduction procedure in which the individual is physically prevented from making an unwanted response. In extinction of avoidance responding, response blocking can teach the individual that the avoidance response is no longer necessary.

response chain A sequence of learned behaviors that must occur in a specific order, with a primary reinforcer delivered only after the final response. Each stimulus in the middle of a response chain is assumed to serve as a conditioned reinforcer for the previous response and a discriminative stimulus for the next response of the chain.

response cost A behavior reduction procedure in which the individual is penalized by the loss of reinforcers if an undesired behavior occurs.

response deprivation theory A theory of reinforcement which states that any contingency that deprives an animal of its preferred level of a behavior will cause that behavior to act as a reinforcer for less restricted behaviors.

response–reinforcer correlation theory The theory that responding is faster on variable-ratio schedules than on variable-interval schedules, because faster responding leads to more reinforcers on variable-ratio schedules but not on variable-interval schedules.

resurgence The reappearance of a previously reinforced response that occurs when a more recently reinforced response is extinguished.

retroactive interference When the presentation of new material interferes with the memory of something that was learned earlier.

retrospective coding A memory strategy in which subjects choose later responses by remembering what stimuli have occurred previously.

rule-governed behavior Behavior that is controlled by a verbal or mental rule about how to behave (as opposed to contingency-shaped behavior, which is controlled by the schedule of reinforcement or punishment).

S-R association A hypothetical association between brain areas representing the conditioned stimulus and a response, which might develop during classical conditioning and thereby give the conditioned stimulus the capacity to elicit a conditioned response.

S-S association A hypothetical association between brain areas representing two different stimuli, which might develop if the two stimuli are paired.

savings Ebbinghaus's measure of the strength of memory, which showed how much less time was required to relearn a previously learned list of nonsense syllables.

Schmidt's schema theory A theory of motor-skill learning that applies to open-ended classes of movements, where a person may need to make a response that has never been practiced. The theory states that as people practice a task, they acquire general rules (schemas) about how to recognize the correct response and how to produce it.

second-order conditioning A classical conditioning procedure in which a conditioned response is transferred from one stimulus to another by pairing a neutral stimulus with a previously conditioned stimulus.

self-control choice A choice between a small, more immediate reinforcer and a larger but more delayed reinforcer.

self-reinforcement A behavior modification technique in which the individual delivers his or her own reinforcers for appropriate behavior.

sensory preconditioning A classical conditioning procedure in which two neutral stimuli are repeatedly paired before either is paired with an unconditioned stimulus.

shaping (or method of successive approximations) A procedure for teaching a new behavior in which closer and closer approximations to the desired behavior are reinforced.

short-delay conditioning A classical conditioning procedure in which the conditioned stimulus begins a second or so before the unconditioned stimulus.

short-term memory A type of memory that can only hold information for a matter of seconds and has a very limited capacity.

shuttle box An experimental chamber with two rectangular compartments. An animal may be required to move from one compartment to the other to escape or avoid an aversive stimulus, such as shock.

Sidman avoidance task An avoidance procedure in which shocks occur at regular intervals if the subject does not respond, but a response postpones the next shock for a fixed period of time.

sign stimulus   A stimulus that initiates a fixed action pattern.

sign-tracking theory   A theory of classical conditioning that states that animals tend to orient themselves toward, approach, and explore any stimuli that are good predictors of important events, such as the delivery of food.

similarity   One of Aristotle's principles of association, which states that the thought of one concept often leads to the thought of similar concepts.

simple cell   A type of neuron in the visual cortex, discovered by Hubel and Wiesel, which fires most rapidly when a line is presented at a specific angle in a specific part of the visual field.

simple systems approach   In physiological research, the strategy of studying primitive creatures, which have smaller and less complex nervous systems.

simultaneous conditioning   A type of classical conditioning in which the conditioned stimulus and unconditioned stimulus begin at the same moment.

simultaneous discrimination procedure   A discrimination procedure in which the positive and negative stimuli are presented together and the subject must choose between them.

single neuron doctrine of perception   The theory that there are individual neurons in the brain that respond to specific, complex stimuli in the individual's environment.

slow positioning task   A motor-learning task in which the subject must move an object toward a target, usually out of sight, with no time limit.

social facilitation   A type of imitation in which the behavior of one individual prompts a similar behavior from another individual, but that behavior was already in the repertoire of the imitator.

social learning theory   A theory developed by Bandura and Walters that states that people learn both through the traditional principles of classical and operant conditioning and through observational learning.

sometimes opponent process (SOP)   A general theory of classical conditioning developed by Allan Wagner, which speculates about why some conditioned responses are similar in form and others are opposite in form to the unconditioned response.

species-specific defense reaction (SSDR)   An innate defensive reaction that occurs when an animal encounters any kind of new or sudden stimulus in the wild. SSDRs usually fall into the categories of freezing, fleeing, or fighting.

spinal reflex arc   Neural pathways that produce the reflexive withdrawal of one's hand from a painful stimulus consisting of pain-sensitive neurons in the hand with axons that extend into the spinal cord, interneurons, and motor neurons that activate the muscles of the arm.

spontaneous recovery   In classical or operant conditioning, the reappearance of a response that has undergone extinction after a passage of time without further conditioning trials.

stimulus control   The general topic of how behaviors can be controlled by the stimuli that precede them.

stimulus enhancement   A type of imitation in which a model directs the learner's attention to a particular object or place in the environment, so that the learner acquires a new behavior more quickly than through trial and error.

stimulus equivalence   A situation in which an individual learns to respond to all stimuli in a category as if they are interchangeable even though the individual has been taught only a few relations between these stimuli, not all the possible relations.

stimulus satiation   A behavior reduction procedure in which the reinforcer is presented in such great quantities that it loses its effectiveness.

stimulus substitution theory   Pavlov's theory of classical conditioning, which states that the conditioned stimulus becomes a substitute for the unconditioned stimulus and elicits the same response.

stop-action principle   A principle of reinforcement that states that the precise movements being performed at the moment of reinforcer delivery will be strengthened and be more likely to occur in the future.

subject effect   The finding that when people know they are participating in an experiment, their behaviors may change or improve, even if they are in a control group and receive no special treatment.

successive discrimination procedure A discrimination procedure in which the positive and negative stimuli are presented at separate times.

superstition experiment Skinner's classic experiment in which food was delivered to pigeons every 15 seconds no matter what they were doing, and most pigeons developed distinctive behaviors that they performed repeatedly between food presentations.

superstitious behavior A behavior that occurs because, by accident or coincidence, it has previously been followed by a reinforcer.

synapse A small gap between the axon terminal of one neuron and the dendrite of another neuron into which transmitters are released.

systematic desensitization A behavioral treatment for phobias that involves slowly presenting the patient with increasingly strong fear-provoking stimuli while keeping the patient in a very relaxed state.

taxis A tropism in which the eliciting stimulus determines the direction of the creature's movement.

temporal coding hypothesis The hypothesis that in classical conditioning, the individual learns about the timing of the CS and US, not just an association between them.

terminal behavior A behavior pattern that occurs near the end of each interval when food or some other primary reinforcer is delivered at regular intervals.

three-term contingency A contingency involving a discriminative stimulus, a response, and a reinforcer or punisher. The contingency states that in the presence of a specific discriminative stimulus, a specific response will lead to specific consequences.

time-out A behavior reduction procedure in which one or more desirable stimuli are temporarily removed if the individual performs some unwanted behavior.

token economy A behavior modification system, often used with groups of people, in which each person can earn tokens by performing specific behaviors and can later exchange these tokens for a variety of primary reinforcers.

tolerance A decrease in the effects of a drug that is observed after repeated use of the drug.

trace conditioning A classical conditioning procedure in which the conditioned stimulus and the unconditioned stimulus are separated by some time interval in which neither stimulus is present.

tragedy of the commons A situation in which people, acting in their individual short-term interests, make choices that are detrimental to society as a whole.

transfer of training In motor-skill learning, how experience on one task affects performance on another task.

transitive inference Learning a rule about the relation between three stimuli, such as the following: "If A < B, and B < C, then A < C."

transmitter A chemical released into the synapse by the axon terminals of a neuron, to which cell bodies and dendrites of other neurons are sensitive.

transposition A case in which a subject receives reinforcers for choosing one of two stimuli in a discrimination task (e.g., choosing a 2-inch circle rather than a 1-inch circle), but later chooses a more extreme stimulus along the same dimension rather than the previously reinforced stimulus (e.g., choosing a 3-inch circle rather than the 2-inch circle).

trans-situationality The theory that once a stimulus is determined to be a reinforcer in one situation, it will also serve as a reinforcer in other situations.

tropism An innate movement of a creature's entire body in response to a specific stimulus. The two major categories of tropisms are kineses and taxes.

true imitation Imitation of a behavior pattern that is very unusual or improbable for the species, so that it would seldom be learned through trial and error.

two-factor theory (or two-process theory) The theory that both classical conditioning (learning to fear a stimulus) and operant conditioning (escape from the fear-eliciting stimulus) are required for avoidance responding.

unconditioned response (UR) In classical conditioning, an innate response that is elicited by an unconditioned stimulus.

unconditioned stimulus (US) In classical conditioning, a stimulus that naturally elicits a specific response (an unconditioned response).

undermatching A deviation from matching in which response percentages are consistently less extreme than reinforcement percentages in a choice situation.

variable-interval (VI) schedule A reinforcement schedule in which reinforcers become available after variable and unpredictable time intervals. Once a reinforcer becomes available, a single response is required to collect it.

variable-ratio (VR) schedule A reinforcement schedule that delivers a reinforcer after a variable and unpredictable number of responses.

video self-modeling A behavior modification technique in which clients watch videos of themselves correctly performing the desired behaviors.

virtual reality therapy A type of systematic desensitization in which a patient wears a headset that displays realistic visual images that change with every head movement, simulating a three-dimensional environment.

visual cortex An area of the cerebral cortex, located in the back of the head, just beneath the skull, which processes visual information.

Weber's law A principle of perception that states that the just noticeable difference (the smallest difference between two stimuli that can be detected) is proportional to the sizes of the stimuli.

working memory A type of memory that holds information for a short period of time, has a limited capacity, and is assumed to guide whatever tasks an individual is currently performing.

REFERENCES

Abramowitz, A. J., & O'Leary, S. G. (1990). Effectiveness of delayed punishment in an applied setting. *Behavior Therapy, 21,* 231–239.

Abramowitz, J. S., & Foa, E. B. (2000). Does major depressive disorder influence outcome of exposure and response prevention for OCD? *Behavior Therapy, 31,* 795–800.

Abravanel, E., & Sigafoos, A. D. (1984). Exploring the presence of imitation during early infancy. *Child Development, 55,* 381–392.

Acebes, F., Solar, P., Carnero, S., & Loy, I. (2009). Blocking of conditioning of tentacle lowering in the snail (*Helix aspersa*). *Quarterly Journal of Experimental Psychology, 62,* 1315–1327.

Adams, C. D., & Kelley, M. L. (1992). Managing sibling aggression: Overcorrection as an alternative to time-out. *Behavior Therapy, 23,* 707–717.

Adams, J. A. (1971). A closed-loop theory of motor learning. *Journal of Motor Behavior, 3,* 111–150.

Adams, J. A. (1976). *Learning and memory: An introduction.* Homewood, IL: Dorsey Press.

Adams, J. A., & Reynolds, B. (1954). Effect of shift in distribution of practice conditions following interpolated rest. *Journal of Experimental Psychology, 47,* 32–36.

Ader, R. (2001). Psychoneuroimmunology. *Current Directions in Psychological Science, 10,* 94–98.

Ader, R., & Cohen, N. (1975). Behaviorally conditioned immunosuppression. *Psychosomatic Medicine, 37,* 333–340.

Ader, R., Felten, D., & Cohen, N. (1990). Interactions between the brain and the immune system. *Annual Review of Pharmacology and Toxicology, 30,* 561–602.

Aeschleman, S. R., Rosen, C. C., & Williams, M. R. (2003). The effect of non-contingent negative and positive reinforcement operations on the acquisition of superstitious behaviors. *Behavioural Processes, 61,* 37–45.

Ainslie, G. (1974). Impulse control in pigeons. *Journal of the Experimental Analysis of Behavior, 21,* 485–489.

Ainslie, G. (1975). Specious reward: A behavioral theory of impulsiveness and impulse control. *Psychological Bulletin, 82,* 463–496.

Akins, C. K., Klein, E. D., & Zentall, T. R. (2002). Imitative learning in Japanese quail (*Coturnix japonica*) using the bidirectional procedure. *Animal Learning and Behavior, 30,* 275–281.

Albert, M., Ricker, S., Bevins, R. A., & Ayres, J. J. B. (1993). Extending continuous versus discontinuous conditioned stimuli before versus after unconditioned stimuli. *Journal of Experimental Psychology: Animal Behavior Processes, 19,* 255–264.

Alberts, E., & Ehrenfreund, D. (1951). Transposition in children as a function of age. *Journal of Experimental Psychology, 41,* 30–38.

Albiach-Serrano, A., Call, J., & Barth, J. (2010). Great apes track hidden objects after changes in the objects' position and in subject's orientation. *American Journal of Primatology, 72,* 349–359.

Alferink, L. A., Critchfield, T. S., Hitt, J. L., & Higgins, W. J. (2009). Generality of the matching law as a descriptor of basketball shot selection. *Journal of Applied Behavior Analysis, 42,* 592–605.

Allen, J. D., & Butler, J. A. (1990). The effect of interplay interval on adjunctive behavior in humans in a game-playing situation. *Physiology and Behavior, 47,* 719–725.

Allison, J. (1993). Response deprivation, reinforcement, and economics. *Journal of the Experimental Analysis of Behavior, 60,* 129–140.

Alvero, A. M., Bucklin, B. R., & Austin, J. (2001). An objective review of the effectiveness and essential characteristics of performance feedback in organizational settings. *Journal of Organizational Behavior Management, 21,* 3–29.

Amari, A., Grace, N. C., & Fisher, W. W. (1995). Achieving and maintaining compliance with the ketogenic diet. *Journal of Applied Behavior Analysis, 28,* 341–342.

Amundson, J. C., & Miller, R. R. (2008). Associative interference in Pavlovian conditioning: A function of similarity between the interfering and target associative structures. *Quarterly Journal of Experimental Psychology, 61,* 1340–1355.

Anderson, C. A., & Bushman, B. J. (2002). Media violence and the American public revisited. *American Psychologist, 57,* 448–450.

Anderson, C. A., Carnagey, N. L., & Eubanks, J. (2003). Exposure to violent media: The effects of songs with violent lyrics on aggressive thoughts and feelings. *Journal of Personality and Social Psychology, 84,* 960–971.

Anderson, C. A., Sakamoto, A., Gentile, D. A., Ihori, N., Shibuya, S. Y., Naito, M., et al. (2008). Longitudinal effects of violent video games on aggression in Japan and the United States. *Pediatrics, 122,* 1067–1072.

Anderson, D. I., Magill, R. A., Sekiya, H., & Ryan, G. (2005). Support for an explanation of the guidance effect in motor skill learning. *Journal of Motor Behavior, 37,* 231–238.

Andrews, E. A., & Braveman, N. S. (1975). The combined effects of dosage level and interstimulus interval on the formation of one-trial poison-based aversions in rats. *Animal Learning and Behavior, 3,* 287–289.

Andrews, J. A., Hops, H., & Duncan, S. C. (1997). Adolescent modeling of parent substance use: The moderating effect of the relationship with the parent. *Journal of Family Psychology, 11,* 259–270.

Anger, D. (1956). The dependence of interresponse times upon the relative reinforcement of different interresponse times. *Journal of Experimental Psychology, 52,* 145–161.

Antonov, I., Kandel, E. R., & Hawkins, R. D. (2010). Presynaptic and postsynaptic mechanisms of synaptic plasticity and metaplasticity during intermediate-term memory formation in Aplysia. *Journal of Neuroscience, 30,* 5781–5791.

Aparicio, C. F., & Baum, W. M. (2006). Fix and sample with rats in the dynamics of choice. *Journal of the Experimental Analysis of Behavior, 86,* 43–63.

Aparicio, C. F., & Baum, W. M. (2009). Dynamics of choice: Relative rate and amount affect local preference at three different time scales. *Journal of the Experimental Analysis of Behavior, 91,* 293–317.

Arcediano, F., Escobar, M., & Miller, R. R. (2005). Bidirectional associations in humans and rats. *Journal of Experimental Psychology: Animal Behavior Processes, 31,* 301–318.

Ariely, D., & Wertenbroch, K. (2003). Procrastination, deadlines, and performance: Self-control by precommitment. *Psychological Science, 13,* 216–224.

Aristotle. (ca. 350 B.C.). *De memoria et reminiscentia.* In J. A. Smith (Trans.) & W. D. Ross (Ed.), *The works of Aristotle* (Vol. 3). Oxford: Clarendon Press. (English translation published 1931.)

Armsworth, C. G., Bohan, D. A., Powers, S. J., Glen, D. M., & Symondson, W. O. C. (2005). Behavioural responses by slugs to chemicals from a generalist predator. *Animal Behaviour, 69,* 805–811.

Ash, D. W., & Holding, D. H. (1990). Backward versus forward chaining in the acquisition of a keyboard skill. *Human Factors, 32,* 139–146.

Athens, E. S., Vollmer, T. R., & St. Peter Pipkin, C. C. (2007). Shaping academic task engagement with percentile schedules. *Journal of Applied Behavior Analysis, 40,* 475–488.

Ayllon, T. (1963). Intensive treatment of psychotic behavior by stimulus satiation and food reinforcement. *Behaviour Research and Therapy, 1,* 53–62.

Ayllon, T., & Haughton, E. (1964). Modification of symptomatic verbal behavior of mental patients. *Behaviour Research and Therapy, 2,* 87–97.

Ayres, J. J. B., Bombace, J. C., Shurtleff, D., & Vigorito, M. (1985). Conditioned suppression tests of context-blocking hypothesis: Testing in the absence of the preconditioned context. *Journal of Experimental Psychology: Animal Behavior Processes, 11,* 1–14.

Ayres, J. J. B., Haddad, C., & Albert, M. (1987). One-trial excitatory backward conditioning as assessed by conditioned suppression of licking in rats: Concurrent observations of lick suppression and defensive behaviors. *Animal Learning and Behavior, 15,* 212–217.

Azrin, N. H. (1956). Effects of two intermittent schedules of immediate and nonimmediate punishment. *Journal of Psychology, 42,* 3–21.

Azrin, N. H. (1960). Effects of punishment intensity during variable-interval reinforcement. *Journal of the Experimental Analysis of Behavior, 3,* 123–142.

Azrin, N. H., & Holz, W. C. (1966). Punishment. In W. K. Honig (Ed.), *Operant behavior: Areas of research and application.* Upper Saddle River, NJ: Prentice Hall, 380–447.

Azrin, N. H., Holz, W. C., & Hake, D. F. (1963). Fixed–ratio punishment. *Journal of the Experimental Analysis of Behavior, 6,* 141–148.

Azrin, N. H., Vinas, V., & Ehle, C. T. (2007). Physical activity as reinforcement for classroom calmness of ADHD children: A preliminary study. *Child & Family Behavior Therapy, 29,* 1–8.

Babb, S. J., & Crystal, J. D. (2003). Spatial navigation on the radial maze with trial-unique intramaze cues and restricted extramaze cues. *Behavioural Processes, 64,* 103–111.

Baddeley, A. (2010). Long-term and working memory: How do they interact? In L. Bäckman & L. Nyberg (Eds.), *Memory, aging and the brain: A Festschrift in honour of Lars-Göran Nilsson* (pp. 7–23). New York: Psychology Press.

Badets, A., & Blandin, Y. (2010). Feedback schedules for motor-skill learning: The similarities and differences between physical and observational practice. *Journal of Motor Behavior, 42,* 257–268.

Baer, D. M., Peterson, R. F., & Sherman, J. A. (1967). The development of imitation by reinforcing behavioral similarity to a model. *Journal of the Experimental Analysis of Behavior, 10,* 405–416.

Baeyens, F., Eelen, P., Van den Bergh, O., & Crombez, G. (1992). The content of learning in human evaluative conditioning: Acquired valence is sensitive to US revaluation. *Learning and Motivation, 23,* 200–224.

Bailey, C. H., & Kandel, E. R. (2004). Synaptic growth and the persistence of long-term memory: A molecular perspective. In M. S. Gazzaniga (Ed.), *The cognitive neurosciences* (3rd ed., pp. 647–663). Cambridge, MA: MIT Press.

Bailey, C. H., & Kandel, E. R. (2009). Synaptic and cellular basis of learning. *Handbook of neuroscience for the behavioral sciences* (Vol. 1, pp. 528–551). Hoboken, NJ: Wiley.

Baker, M. (2001). *The atoms of language.* New York: Basic Books.

Baker, T. B., Piper, M. E., McCarthy, D. E., Majeskie, M. R., & Fiore, M. C. (2004). Addiction motivation reformulated: An affective processing model of negative reinforcement. *Psychological Review, 111,* 33–51.

Baker, T. B., & Tiffany, S. T. (1985). Morphine tolerance as habituation. *Psychological Review, 92,* 78–108.

Balaban, M. T., Rhodes, D. L., & Neuringer, A. (1990). Orienting and defense responses to punishment: Effects on learning. *Biological Psychology, 30,* 203–217.

Balaz, M. A., Kasprow, W. J., & Miller, R. R. (1982). Blocking with a single compound trial. *Animal Learning and Behavior, 10,* 271–276.

Baldwin, E. (1993). The case for animal research in psychology. *Journal of Social Issues, 49,* 121–131.

Balleine, B. W. (2009). Taste, disgust, and value: Taste aversion learning and outcome encoding in instrumental conditioning. In T. R. Schachtman & S. Reilly (Eds.), *Conditioned taste aversion: Behavioral and neural processes* (pp. 262–280). New York: Oxford University Press.

Balsam, P. D., Drew, M. R., & Yang, C. (2002). Timing at the start of associative learning. *Learning and Motivation, 33,* 141–155.

Balsam, P. D., & Gallistel, C. R. (2009). Temporal maps and informativeness in associative learning. *Trends in Neurosciences, 32,* 73–78.

Bandura, A. (1965). Influence of models' reinforcement contingencies on the acquisition of imitative responses. *Journal of Personality and Social Psychology, 1,* 589–595.

Bandura, A. (1969). *Principles of behavior modification.* New York: Holt, Rinehart & Winston.

Bandura, A. (1986). *Social foundations of thought and action.* Upper Saddle River, NJ: Prentice Hall.

Bandura, A., Grusec, J. E., & Menlove, F. L. (1967). Vicarious extinction of avoidance behavior. *Journal of Personality and Social Psychology, 5,* 16–23.

Bandura, A., & Kupers, C. J. (1964). The transmission of patterns of self-reinforcement through modeling. *Journal of Abnormal and Social Psychology, 69,* 1–9.

Bandura, A., Ross, D., & Ross, S. A. (1963). Imitation of film-mediated aggressive models. *Journal of Abnormal and Social Psychology, 66,* 3–11.

Bandura, A., & Walters, R. H. (1959). *Adolescent aggression.* New York: Ronald Press.

Bandura, A., & Walters, R. H. (1963). *Social learning and personality development.* New York: Holt, Rinehart & Winston.

Barlow, H. B. (1972). Single units and sensation: A neural doctrine for perceptual psychology? *Perception, 1,* 371–394.

Barnes, D., & Keenan, M. (1993). Concurrent activities and instructed human fixed-interval performance. *Journal of the Experimental Analysis of Behavior, 59,* 501–520.

Baron, A., Kaufman, A., & Fazzini, D. (1969). Density and delay of punishment of free-operant avoidance. *Journal of the Experimental Analysis of Behavior, 12,* 1029–1037.

Baron, A., & Leinenweber, A. (1994). Molecular and molar analyses of fixed-interval performance. *Journal of the Experimental Analysis of Behavior, 61,* 11–18.

Batsell, W. R., Trost, C. A., Cochran, S. R., Blankenship, A. G., & Batson, J. D. (2003). Effects of postconditioning inflation on odor 1 taste compound conditioning. *Learning and Behavior, 31,* 173–184.

Battig, W. F. (1979). The flexibility of human memory. In L. S. Cermakl & F. I. M. Craik (Eds.), *Levels of processing in human memory.* Hillsdale, NJ: Erlbaum, 23–44.

Battig, W. F., & Montague, W. E. (1969). Category norms for verbal items in 56 categories: A replication and extension of the Connecticut category norms. *Journal of Experimental Psychology Monograph* (3, Pt. 2).

Baum, M. (1966). Rapid extinction of an avoidance response following a period of response prevention in the avoidance apparatus. *Psychological Reports, 18,* 59–64.

Baum, M. (1976). Instrumental learning: Comparative studies. In M. P. Feldman & A. Broadhurst (Eds.), *Theoretical and experimental bases of the behavior therapies.* New York: Wiley.

Baum, W. M. (1973). The correlation-based law of effect. *Journal of the Experimental Analysis of Behavior, 20,* 137–153.

Baum, W. M. (1974). On two types of deviation from the matching law: Bias and undermatching. *Journal of the Experimental Analysis of Behavior, 22,* 231–242.

Baum, W. M. (1979). Matching, undermatching, and overmatching in studies of choice. *Journal of the Experimental Analysis of Behavior, 32,* 269–281.

Baum, W. M. (1982). Choice, changeover, and travel. *Journal of the Experimental Analysis of Behavior, 38,* 35–49.

Baum, W. M. (1993). Performances on ratio and interval schedules of reinforcement: Data and theory. *Journal of the Experimental Analysis of Behavior, 59,* 245–264.

Baum, W. M. (2001). Molar versus molecular as a paradigm clash. *Journal of the Experimental Analysis of Behavior, 75,* 338–341.

Baum, W. M. (2010). Dynamics of choice: A tutorial. *Journal of the Experimental Analysis of Behavior, 94,* 161–174.

Baum, W. M., & Rachlin, H. C. (1969). Choice as time allocation. *Journal of the Experimental Analysis of Behavior, 12,* 861–874.

Baum, W. M., Schwendiman, J. W., & Bell, K. E. (1999). Choice, contingency discrimination, and foraging theory. *Journal of the Experimental Analysis of Behavior, 71,* 355–373.

Baxter, G. A., & Schlinger, H. (1990). Performance of children under a multiple random-ratio random-interval schedule of reinforcement. *Journal of the Experimental Analysis of Behavior, 54,* 263–271.

Beardsley, S. D., & McDowell, J. J. (1992). Application of Herrnstein's hyperbola to time allocation of naturalistic human behavior maintained by naturalistic social reinforcement. *Journal of the Experimental Analysis of Behavior, 57,* 177–185.

Beatty, W. W., & Shavalia, D. A. (1980). Rat spatial memory: Resistance to retroactive interference at long retention intervals. *Animal Learning and Behavior, 8,* 550–552.

Beaver, K. M., Ferguson, C. J., & Lynn-Whaley, J. (2010). The association between parenting and levels of self-control: A genetically informative analysis. *Criminal Justice and Behavior, 37,* 1045–1065.

von Bekesy, G. (1964). Sweetness produced electrically on the tongue and its relation to taste theories. *Journal of Applied Physiology, 19,* 1105–1113.

von Bekesy, G. (1966). Taste theories and the chemical stimulation of single papillae. *Journal of Applied Physiology, 21,* 1–9.

Belke, T. W., & Pierce, W. D. (2009). Body weight manipulation, reinforcement value and choice between sucrose and wheel running: A behavioral economic analysis. *Behavioural Processes, 80,* 147–156.

Benedick, H., & Dixon, M. R. (2009). Instructional control of self-control in adults with co-morbid developmental disabilities and mental illness. *Journal of Developmental and Physical Disabilities, 21,* 457–471.

Bennett, H. J. (2005). *Waking up dry: A guide to help children overcome bedwetting.* Elk Grove, IL: American Academy of Pediatrics.

Bentall, R. P., & Lowe, C. F. (1987). The role of verbal behavior in human learning: III. Instructional effects in children. *Journal of the Experimental Analysis of Behavior, 47,* 177–190.

Berger, T. W., & Weisz, D. J. (1987). Rabbit nictitating membrane responses. In I. Gormezano, W. F. Prokasy, & R. F. Thompson (Eds.), *Classical conditioning* (3rd ed.). Hillsdale, NJ: Erlbaum, 217–253.

Bernier, R., & Dawson, G. (2009). The role of mirror neuron dysfunction in autism. In J. A. Pineda (Ed.), *Mirror neuron systems: The role of mirroring processes in social cognition* (pp. 261–286). Totowa, NJ: Humana Press.

Bernstein, I. L., Webster, M. M., & Bernstein, I. D. (1982). Food aversions in children receiving chemotherapy for cancer. *Cancer, 50,* 2961–2963.

Besson, A., Privat, A. M., Eschalier, A., & Fialip, J. (1999). Dopaminergic and opioidergic mediations of tricyclic antidepressants in the learned helplessness paradigm. *Pharmacology, Biochemistry, and Behavior, 64,* 541–548.

Bickel, W. K., DeGrandpre, R. J., & Higgins, S. T. (1995). The behavioral economics of concurrent drug reinforcers: A review and reanalysis of drug self-administration research. *Psychopharmacology, 118,* 250–259.

Bickel, W. K., Marsch, L. A., & Carroll, M. E. (2000). Deconstructing relative reinforcing efficacy and situating the measures of pharmacological reinforcement with behavioral economics: A theoretical proposal. *Psychopharmacology, 153,* 44–56.

Bickel, W. K., Odum, A. L., & Madden, G. J. (1999). Impulsivity and cigarette smoking: Delay discounting in current, never, and ex-smokers. *Psychopharmacology, 146,* 447–454.

Bickel, W. K., & Vuchinich, R. (Eds.). (2000). *Reframing health behavior change with behavioral economics*. Mahwah, NJ: Erlbaum.

Bickel, W. K., Yi, R., Landes, R. D., Hill, P. F., & Baxter, C. (2011). Remember the future: Working memory training decreases delay discounting among stimulant addicts. *Biological Psychiatry, 69,* 260–265.

Billington, E. J., & DiTommaso, N. M. (2003). Demonstrations and applications of the matching law in education. *Journal of Behavioral Education, 12,* 91–104.

Bilodeau, E. A., Bilodeau, I. M., & Schmusky, D. A. (1959). Some effects of introducing and withdrawing knowledge of results early and late in practice. *Journal of Experimental Psychology, 58,* 142–144.

Bilodeau, I. M. (1966). Information feedback. In E. A. Bilodeau (Ed.), *Acquisition of skill*. New York: Academic Press, 255–296.

Black, A. H. (1965). Cardiac conditioning in curarized dogs: The relationship between heart rate and skeletal behavior. In W. F. Prokasy (Ed.), *Classical conditioning: A symposium*. New York: Appleton-Century-Crofts, 20–47.

Blais, C., Kerr, R., & Hughes, K. (1993). Negative transfer or cognitive confusion. *Human Performance, 6,* 197–206.

Blakely, E., & Schlinger, H. (1988). Determinants of pausing under variable-ratio schedules: Reinforcer magnitude, ratio size, and schedule configuration. *Journal of the Experimental Analysis of Behavior, 50,* 65–73.

Blakemore, C., & Cooper, G. F. (1970). Development of the brain depends on the visual environment. *Nature, 228,* 477–478.

Blatter, K., & Schultz, W. (2006). Rewarding properties of visual stimuli. *Experimental Brain Research, 168,* 541–546.

Bleak, J. L., & Frederick, C. M. (1998). Superstitious behavior in sport: Levels of effectiveness and determinants of use in three collegiate sports. *Journal of Sport Behavior, 21,* 1–15.

Bliss, T. V. P., & Lomo, T. (1973). Long-lasting potentiation of synaptic transmission in the dentate area of the anaesthetized rabbit following stimulation of the perforant path. *Journal of Physiology, 232,* 331–356.

Bloh, C. (2010). Assessing self-control training in children with attention deficit hyperactivity disorder. *Behavior Analyst Today, 10,* 357–363.

Blough, D. S. (1959). Delayed matching in the pigeon. *Journal of the Experimental Analysis of Behavior, 2,* 151–160.

Blough, D. S. (1982). Pigeon perception of letters of the alphabet. *Science, 218,* 397–398.

Bolles, R. C. (1970). Species-specific defense reactions and avoidance learning. *Psychological Review, 77,* 32–48.

Bonardi, C., & Jennings, D. (2009). Learning about associations: Evidence for a hierarchical account of occasion setting. *Journal of Experimental Psychology: Animal Behavior Processes, 35,* 440–445.

Bonvillian, J. D., & Patterson, F. P. (1999). Early sign-language acquisition: Comparisons between children and gorillas. In S. Parker, R. W. Mitchell, H. Miles, S. Parker, R. W. Mitchell, & H. Miles (Eds.), *The mentalities of gorillas and orangutans: Comparative perspectives* (pp. 240–264). New York: Cambridge University Press.

Bootzin, R. R. (1972). Stimulus control treatment for insomnia. *Proceedings of the 80th Annual Convention of the American Psychological Association, 7,* 395–396.

Bouton, M. E. (2000). A learning theory perspective on lapse, relapse, and the maintenance of behavior change. *Health Psychology, 19,* 57–63.

Bouton, M. E., Woods, A. M., & Pineño, O. (2004). Occasional reinforced trials during extinction can slow the rate of rapid reacquisition. *Learning and Motivation, 35,* 371–390.

Bowd, A. D., & Shapiro, K. J. (1993). The case against laboratory animal research in psychology. *Journal of Social Issues, 49,* 133–142.

Bradfield, L., & McNally, G. P. (2008). Unblocking in Pavlovian fear conditioning. *Journal of*

Experimental Psychology: Animal Behavior Processes, 34, 256–265.

Bradshaw, C. M. (2010). Reinforcement, impulsivity and behavioural economics. In C. L. Cooper, J. Field, U. Goswami, R. Jenkins, B. J. Sahakian, C. L. Cooper, & B. J. Sahakian (Eds.), *Mental capital and wellbeing* (pp. 101–110). Hoboken, NJ: Wiley-Blackwell.

Brannon, E. M., & Terrace, H. S. (2000). Representation of the numerosities 1-9 by Rhesus Macaques (*Macaca mulata*). *Journal of Experimental Psychology: Animal Behavior Processes, 26,* 31–49.

Breland, K., & Breland, M. (1961). The misbehavior of organisms. *American Psychologist, 16,* 681–684.

Brogden, W. J. (1939). Sensory pre-conditioning. *Journal of Experimental Psychology, 25,* 323–332.

Brooks, D. C., & Bouton, M. E. (1993). A retrieval cue for extinction attenuates spontaneous recovery. *Journal of Experimental Psychology: Animal Behavior Processes, 19,* 77–89.

Brooks, D. C., Palmatier, M. I., Garcia, E. O., & Johnson, J. L. (1999). An extinction cue reduces spontaneous recovery of a conditioned taste aversion. *Animal Learning and Behavior, 27,* 77–88.

Brown, D. E. (1991). *Human universals.* New York: McGraw-Hill.

Brown, E., & Cleaveland, J. (2009). An application of the active time model to multiple concurrent variable-interval schedules. *Behavioural Processes, 81,* 250–255.

Brown, F. J., Peace, N., & Parsons, R. (2009). Teaching children generalized imitation skills: A case report. *Journal of Intellectual Disabilities, 13,* 9–17.

Brown, G. E., Hughes, G. D., & Jones, A. A. (1988). Effects of shock controllability on subsequent aggressive and defensive behaviors in the cockroach (*Periplaneta americana*). *Psychological Reports, 63,* 563–569.

Brown, J. F., Spencer, K., & Swift, S. (2002). A parent training programme for chronic food refusal:

A case study. *British Journal of Learning Disabilities, 30,* 118–121.

Brown, K. L., Calizo, L. H., & Stanton, M. E. (2008). Dose-dependent deficits in dual interstimulus interval classical eyeblink conditioning tasks following neonatal binge alcohol exposure in rats. *Alcoholism: Clinical and Experimental Research, 32,* 277–293.

Brown, P. L., & Jenkins, H. M. (1968). Auto-shaping of the pigeon's key-peck. *Journal of the Experimental Analysis of Behavior, 11,* 1–8.

Brown, R., & Herrnstein, R. J. (1975). *Psychology.* Boston, MA: Little, Brown.

Brown, T. (1820). *Lectures on the philosophy of the human mind* (Vols. 1 and 2). Edinburgh, UK: James Ballantyne.

Bruce, D. (1994). Lashley and the problem of serial order. *American Psychologist, 49,* 93–103.

Bruchey, A. K., Jones, C. E., & Monfils, M. H. (2010). Fear conditioning by-proxy: Social transmission of fear during memory retrieval. *Behavioural Brain Research, 214,* 80–84.

Bruzek, J. L., Thompson, R. H., & Peters, L. C. (2009). Resurgence of infant caregiving responses. *Journal of the Experimental Analysis of Behavior, 92,* 327–343.

Bryson, J. J., & Leong, J. C. S. (2006). Primate errors in transitive "inference": A two tier learning model. *Animal Cognition, 10,* 1–15.

Bucher, B., & Fabricatore, J. (1970). Use of patient-administered shock to suppress hallucinations. *Behavior Therapy, 1,* 382–385.

Bucklin, B. R., & Dickinson, A. M. (2001). Individual monetary incentives: A review of different types of arrangements between performance and pay. *Journal of Organizational Behavior Management, 21,* 45–137.

Budzynski, T. H., Stoyva, J. M., Adler, C. S., & Mullaney, M. A. (1973). EMG biofeedback and tension headache: A controlled outcome study. In L. Birk (Ed.), *Biofeedback: Behavioral medicine.* New York: Grune & Stratton, 37–50.

Bullock, C. E., & Hackenberg, T. D. (2006). Second-order schedules of token reinforcement with pigeons: Implications for unit price. *Journal of the Experimental Analysis of Behavior, 85,* 95–106.

Bullock, C. E., & Myers, T. M. (2009). Stimulus-food pairings produce stimulus-directed touch-screen responding in cynomolgus monkeys (*Macaca fascicularis*) with or without a positive response contingency. *Journal of the Experimental Analysis of Behavior, 92,* 41–55.

Bullock, D., & Neuringer, A. (1977). Social learning by following: An analysis. *Journal of the Experimental Analysis of Behavior, 25,* 127–135.

Burger, J. M., & Lynn, A. L. (2005). Superstitious behavior among American and Japanese professional baseball players. *Basic and Applied Social Psychology, 27,* 71–76.

Bush, R. R., & Mosteller, F. (1955). *Stochastic models for learning.* New York: Wiley.

Buske-Kirschbaum, A., Kirschbaum, C., Stierle, H., Jabaij, L., & Hellhammer, D. (1994). Conditioned manipulation of natural killer (NK) cells in humans using a discriminative learning protocol. *Biological Psychology, 38,* 143–155.

Butler, R. A. (1953). Discrimination learning by rhesus monkeys to visual-exploration motivation. *Journal of Comparative and Physiological Psychology, 46,* 95–98.

Byrne, R. W., & Russon, A. E. (1998). Learning by imitation: A hierarchical approach. *Behavioral and Brain Sciences, 21,* 667–721.

Call, J. (2010). Do apes know that they could be wrong? *Animal Cognition, 13,* 689–700.

Campolattaro, M. M., Schnitker, K. M., & Freeman, J. H. (2008). Changes in inhibition during differential eyeblink conditioning with increased training. *Learning and Behavior, 36,* 159–165.

Cancado, C. R. X., & Lattal, K. A. (2011). Resurgence of temporal patterns of responding. *Journal of the Experimental Analysis of Behavior, 95,* 271–287.

Canli, T., & Donegan, N. H. (1995). Conditioned diminution of the unconditioned response in rabbit eyeblink conditioning: Identifying neural substrates in the cerebellum and brainstem. *Behavioral Neuroscience, 109,* 874–892.

Capaldi, E. J. (1966). Partial reinforcement: A hypothesis of sequential effects. *Psychological Review, 73,* 459–477.

Capaldi, E. J., & Miller, D. J. (1988). Counting in rats: Its functional significance and the independent cognitive processes which comprise it. *Journal of Experimental Psychology: Animal Behavior Processes, 14,* 3–17.

Capaldi, E. J., Verry, D. R., & Davison, T. L. (1980). Memory, serial anticipation pattern learning and transfer in rats. *Animal Learning and Behavior, 8,* 575–585.

Caraco, T., Martindale, S., & Whittam, T. S. (1980). An empirical demonstration of risk-sensitive foraging preferences. *Animal Behavior, 28,* 820–830.

Carew, T. J., Hawkins, R. D., & Kandel, E. R. (1983). Differential classical conditioning of a defensive withdrawal reflex in *Aplysia californica. Science, 219,* 397–400.

Carmagnani, A., & Carmagnani, E. F. (1999). Biofeedback: Present state and future possibilities. *International Journal of Mental Health, 28,* 83–86.

Carroll, M. E. (1993). The economic context of drug and non-drug reinforcers affects acquisition and maintenance of drug-reinforced behavior and withdrawal effects. *Drug and Alcohol Dependence, 33,* 201–210.

Case, D. A., Nichols, P., & Fantino, E. (1995). Pigeons' preference for variable-interval water reinforcement under widely varied water budgets. *Journal of the Experimental Analysis of Behavior, 64,* 299–311.

Castellucci, V., Pinsker, H., Kupfermann, I., & Kandel, E. R. (1970). Neuronal mechanisms of habituation and dishabituation of the gill-withdrawal reflex in *Aplysia. Science, 167,* 1745–1748.

Catania, A. C. (1963). Concurrent performances: A baseline for the study of reinforcement magnitude. *Journal of the Experimental Analysis of Behavior, 6,* 299–300.

Catania, A. C., Matthews, B. A., & Shimoff, E. (1982). Instructed versus shaped human verbal behavior: Interactions with nonverbal responding. *Journal of the Experimental Analysis of Behavior, 38,* 233–248.

Catania, A. C., & Reynolds, G. S. (1968). A quantitative analysis of the responding maintained by interval schedules of reinforcement. *Journal of the Experimental Analysis of Behavior, 11,* 327–383.

Cavalier, A. R., Feretti, R. P., & Hodges, A. E. (1997). Self-management within a classroom token economy for students with learning disabilities. *Research in Developmental Disabilities, 18,* 167–178.

Chamberlin, C. J., & Magill, R. A. (1992). The memory representation of motor skills: A test of schema theory. *Journal of Motor Behavior, 24,* 309–319.

Champion, R. A., & Jones, J. E. (1961). Forward, backward, and pseudoconditioning of the GSR. *Journal of Experimental Psychology, 62,* 58–61.

Chaney, J. M., Mulins, L. L., Uretsky, D. L., Pace, T. M., Werden, D., & Hartman, V. L. (1999). An experimental examination of learned helplessness in older adolescents and young adults with long-standing asthma. *Journal of Pediatric Psychology, 24,* 259–270.

Chen, J., Lin, W., Wang, W., Shao, F., Yang, J., Wang, B., et al. (2004). Enhancement of antibody production and expression of c-Fos in the insular cortex in response to a conditioned stimulus after a single-trial learning paradigm. *Behavioural Brain Research, 154,* 557–565.

Chen, W. R., Lee, S. H., Kato, K., Spencer, D. D., Shepherd, G. M., & Williamson, A. (1996). Long-term modifications of synaptic efficacy in the human inferior and middle temporal cortex. *Proceedings of the National Academy of Sciences, 93,* 8011–8015.

Cherukupalli, R. (2010). A behavioral economics perspective on tobacco taxation. *American Journal of Public Health, 100,* 609–615.

Chomsky, N. (1959). Review of Skinner's verbal behavior. *Language, 35,* 26–58.

Chomsky, N. (1972a). *Language and the mind.* New York: Harcourt Brace Jovanovich.

Chomsky, N. (1972b). Psychology and ideology. *Cognition, 1,* 11–46.

Chouinard, P. A., & Goodale, M. A. (2010). Category-specific neural processing for naming pictures of animals and naming pictures of tools: An ALE meta-analysis. *Neuropsychologia, 48,* 409–418.

Christensen, C. J., Silberberg, A., Hursh, S. R., Huntsberry, M. E., & Riley, A. L. (2008). Essential value of cocaine and food in rats: Tests of the exponential model of demand. *Psychopharmacology, 198,* 221–229.

Christensen, P., & Wood, W. (2007). Effects of media violence on viewers' aggression in unconstrained social interaction. In R. W. Preiss, B. Gayle, N. Burrell, M. Allen, & J. Bryant (Eds.), *Mass media effects research: Advances through meta-analysis* (pp. 145–168). Mahwah, NJ: Lawrence Erlbaum Associates Publishers.

Christian, K. M., & Thompson, R. F. (2003). Neural substrates of eyeblink conditioning: Acquisition and retention. *Learning and Memory, 10,* 427–455.

Church, R. M. (1978). The internal clock. In S. H. Hulse, H. Fowler, & W. K. Honig (Eds.), *Cognitive processes in animal behavior.* Hillsdale, NJ: Erlbaum, 277–310.

Church, R. M. (1984). Properties of the internal clock. In J. Gibbon & L. Allen (Eds.), *Timing and time perception* (Vol. 438). New York: Annals of the New York Academy of Sciences, 566–582.

Church, R. M. (2003). A concise introduction to scalar timing theory. In W. H. Meck (Ed.), *Functional and neural mechanisms of interval timing.* Boca Raton, FL: CRC Press, 55–81.

Church, R. M. (2006). Behavioristic, cognitive, biological, and quantitative explanations of timing. In E. A. Wasserman & T. R. Zentall (Eds.), *Comparative cognition: Experimental explorations of animal intelligence* (pp. 249–269). New York: Oxford University Press.

Church, R. M., Getty, D. J., & Lerner, N. D. (1976). Duration discrimination by rats. *Journal of Experimental Psychology: Animal Behavior Processes, 4,* 303–312.

Church, R. M., LoLordo, V. M., Overmier, J. B., Solomon, R. L., & Turner, L. H. (1966). Cardiac responses to shock in curarized dogs. *Journal of Comparative and Physiological Psychology, 62,* 1–7.

Ciborowski, T. (1997). "Superstition" in the collegiate baseball player. *Sport Psychologist, 11,* 305–317.

Cicero, S. D., & Tryon, W. W. (1989). Classical conditioning of meaning: II. A replication and triplet associative extension. *Journal of Behavior Therapy and Experimental Psychiatry, 20,* 197–202.

Cipani, E., Brendlinger, J., McDowell, L., & Usher, S. (1991). Continuous vs. intermittent punishment: A case study. *Journal of Developmental and Physical Disabilities, 3,* 147–156.

Cirstea, M. C., & Levin, M. F. (2007). Improvement of arm movement patterns and endpoint control depends on type of feedback during practice in stroke survivors. *Neurorehabilitation and Neural Repair, 21,* 398–411.

Cisek, P., & Kalaska, J. F. (2004). Neural correlates of mental rehearsal in dorsal premotor cortex. *Nature, 431,* 993–996.

Clare, L., Wilson, B. A., Carter, G., Roth, I., & Hodges, J. R. (2002). Relearning face-name associations in early Alzheimer's disease. *Neuropsychology, 16,* 538–547.

Clayton, N. S., Yu, K. S., & Dickinson, A. (2001). Scrub jays (*Aphelocoma coerulescens*) form integrated memories of the multiple features of caching episodes. *Journal of Experimental Psychology: Animal Behavior Processes, 27,* 17–29.

Cohen, P. S., & Campagnoni, F. R. (1989). The nature and determinants of spatial retreat in the pigeon between periodic grain presentations. *Animal Learning and Behavior, 17,* 39–48.

Cohen, P. S., & Looney, T. A. (1973). Schedule-induced mirror responding in the pigeon. *Journal of the Experimental Analysis of Behavior, 19,* 395–408.

Coldwells, A., & Hare, M. E. (1994). The transfer of skill from short tennis to lawn tennis. *Ergonomics, 37,* 17–21.

Cole, M. R. (1999). Molar and molecular control in variable-interval and variable-ratio schedules. *Journal of the Experimental Analysis of Behavior, 71,* 319–328.

Cole, M. R., & Chappell-Stephenson, R. (2003). Exploring the limits of spatial memory in rats, using very large mazes. *Learning and Behavior, 31,* 349–368.

Cole, R. P., Barnet, R. C., & Miller, R. R. (1995). Effect of relative stimulus validity: Learning or performance deficit. *Journal of Experimental Psychology: Animal Behavior Processes, 21,* 293–303.

Collins, D., & McPherson, A. (2006). The psychophysiology of biofeedback and sport performance. In E. O. Acevedo & P. Ekkekakis (Eds.), *Psychobiology of physical activity* (pp. 241–250). Champaign, IL: Human Kinetics.

Colwill, R. M. (1996). Detecting associations in Pavlovian conditioning and instrumental learning in vertebrates and in invertebrates. In C. F. Moss & S. J. Shettleworth (Eds.), *Neuroethological studies of cognitive and perceptual processes*. Boulder, CO: Westview Press.

Colwill, R. M., & Rescorla, R. A. (1985). Postconditioning devaluation of a reinforcer affects instrumental responding. *Journal of Experimental Psychology: Animal Behavior Processes, 11,* 120–132.

Colwill, R. M., & Rescorla, R. A. (1986). Associative structures in instrumental learning. In G. H. Bower (Ed.), *The psychology of learning and motivation* (Vol. 20). New York: Academic Press, 55–104.

Colwill, R. M., & Rescorla, R. A. (1988). Associations between the discriminative stimulus and the reinforcer in instrumental learning. *Journal of Experimental Psychology: Animal Behavior Processes, 14,* 155–164.

Compton, D. M., Dietrich, K. L., & Johnson, S. D. (1995). Animal rights activism and animal welfare concerns in the academic setting: Levels of activism and the perceived importance of research with animals. *Psychological Reports, 76,* 23–31.

Condon, C. D., & Weinberger, N. M. (1991). Habituation produces frequency-specific plasticity of receptive fields in the auditory cortex. *Behavioral Neuroscience, 105,* 416–430.

Conger, R., & Killeen, P. (1974). Use of concurrent operants in small group research. *Pacific Sociological Review, 17,* 399–416.

Conn, P. M., & Parker, J. V. (2008). *The animal research war.* New York: Palgrave Macmillan.

Cook, R. G., Brown, M. F., & Riley, D. A. (1985). Flexible memory processing by rats: Use of prospective and retrospective information in the radial maze. *Journal of Experimental Psychology: Animal Behavior Processes, 11,* 453–469.

Cook, R. G., Levison, D. G., Gillett, S. R., & Blaisdell, A. P. (2005). Capacity and limits of associative memory in pigeons. *Psychonomic Bulletin & Review, 12,* 350–358.

Costa, D. S. J., & Boakes, R. A. (2009). Context blocking in rat autoshaping: Sign-tracking versus goal-tracking. *Learning and Motivation, 40,* 178–185.

Cournoyer, M., & Trudel, M. (1991). Behavioral correlates of self-control at 33 months. *Infant Behavior and Development, 14,* 497–503.

Cream, A., O'Brian, S., Onslow, M., Packman, A., & Menzies, R. (2009). Self-modelling as a relapse intervention following speech-restructuring treatment for stuttering. *International Journal of Language & Communication Disorders, 44,* 587–599.

Creer, T. L., Chai, H., & Hoffman, A. (1977). A single application of an aversive stimulus to eliminate chronic cough. *Journal of Behavior Therapy and Experimental Psychiatry, 8,* 107–109.

Crossman, E. K. (1968). Pause relationships in multiple and chained fixed-ratio schedules. *Journal of the Experimental Analysis of Behavior, 11,* 117–126.

Crossman, E. K., Bonem, E. J., & Phelps, B. J. (1987). A comparison of response patterns on fixed-, variable-, and random-ratio schedules. *Journal of the Experimental Analysis of Behavior, 48,* 395–406.

Crowell, C. R., Hinson, R. E., & Siegel, S. (1981). The role of conditional drug responses in tolerance to the hypothermic effect of ethanol. *Psychopharmacology, 72,* 147–153.

Crown, E. D., Ferguson, A. R., Joynes, R. L., & Grau, J. W. (2002). Instrumental learning within the spinal cord: IV. Induction and retention of the behavioral deficit observed after noncontingent shock. *Behavioral Neuroscience, 116,* 1032–1051.

Crump, M. C., & Logan, G. D. (2010). Warning: This keyboard will deconstruct—the role of the keyboard in skilled typewriting. *Psychonomic Bulletin & Review, 17,* 394–399.

Cunningham, C. E., & Linscheid, T. R. (1976). Elimination of chronic infant ruminating by electric shock. *Behavior Therapy, 1,* 231–234.

Cunningham, T. R., & Austin, J. (2007). Using goal setting, task clarification, and feedback to increase the use of the hands-free technique by hospital operating room staff. *Journal of Applied Behavior Analysis, 40,* 673–677.

Cuthill, I. C. (2007). Ethical regulation and animal science: Why animal behaviour is not so special. *Animal Behaviour, 74,* 15–22.

Dail, T. K., & Christina, R. W. (2004). Distribution of practice and metacognition in learning and long-term retention. *Research Quarterly for Exercise and Sport, 75,* 148–155.

Dallal, N. L., & Meck, W. H. (1990). Hierarchical structures: Chunking by food type facilitates spatial memory. *Journal of Experimental Psychology: Animal Behavior Processes, 16,* 69–84.

Dallery, J., Glenn, I. M., & Raiff, B. R. (2007). An Internet-based abstinence reinforcement treatment for cigarette smoking. *Drug and Alcohol Dependence, 86,* 230–238.

Dallery, J., McDowell, J. J., & Lancaster, L. S. (2000). Falsification of matching theory's account of single-alternative responding: Herrnstein's *K* varies with sucrose concentration. *Journal of the Experimental Analysis of Behavior, 73,* 23–43.

D'Amato, M. R. (1973). Delayed matching and short-term memory in monkeys. In G. H. Bower (Ed.), *The psychology of learning and motivation* (Vol. 7). New York: Academic Press, 227–269.

Darwin, C. (1872). *The expression of emotion in man and animals.* New York: Philosophical Library.

da Silva, S. P., Maxwell, M. E., & Lattal, K. A. (2008). Concurrent resurgence and behavioral history. *Journal of the Experimental Analysis of Behavior, 90,* 313–331.

Daum, I., Schugens, M. M., Ackermann, H., Lutzenberger, W., Dichgans, J., & Birbaumer, N. (1993). Classical conditioning after cerebellar lesions in humans. *Behavioral Neuroscience, 107,* 748–756.

Davey, G. C. L., & McKenna, I. (1983). The effect of postconditioning revaluation of CS1 and CS2 following Pavlovian second-order electrodermal conditioning in humans. *Quarterly Journal of Experimental Psychology, 35B,* 125–133.

Davies, S. N., Lester, R. A. J., Reymann, K. G., & Collingridge, G. L. (1989). Temporally distinct pre- and post-synaptic mechanisms maintain long-term potentiation. *Nature, 338,* 500–503.

Davis, F. D., & Yi, M. Y. (2004). Improving computer skill training: Behavior modeling, symbolic mental rehearsal, and the role of knowledge structures. *Journal of Applied Psychology, 89,* 509–523.

Davis, H. (1992). Transitive inference in rats (*Rattus norvegicus*). *Journal of Comparative Psychology, 106,* 342–349.

Davis, H., & Albert, M. (1986). Numerical discrimination by rats using sequential auditory stimuli. *Animal Learning and Behavior, 14,* 57–59.

Davis, H., & Bradford, S. A. (1991). Numerically restricted food intake in the rat in a free-feeding situation. *Animal Learning and Behavior, 19,* 215–222.

Davis, J. R., & Russell, R. H. (1990). Behavioral staff management: An analogue study of acceptability and its behavioral correlates. *Behavioral Residential Treatment, 5,* 259–270.

Davis, M. (1989). Neural systems involved in fear-potentiated startle. *Annals of the New York Academy of Sciences, 563,* 165–183.

Davis, M., Gendelman, D. S., Tischler, M. D., & Gendelman, P. M. (1982). A primary acoustic startle circuit: Lesion and stimulation studies. *Journal of Neuroscience, 2,* 791–805.

Davis, T., Ollendick, T. H., & Öst, L. (2009). Intensive treatment of specific phobias in children and adolescents. *Cognitive and Behavioral Practice, 16,* 294–303.

Davison, M., & Baum, W. M. (2000). Choice in a variable environment: Every reinforcer counts. *Journal of the Experimental Analysis of Behavior, 74,* 1–24.

Davison, M., & Baum, W. M. (2002). Choice in a variable environment: Effects of blackout duration and extinction between components. *Journal of the Experimental Analysis of Behavior, 77,* 65–89.

Davison, M., & Hogsden, I. (1984). Concurrent variable-interval schedule performance: Fixed versus mixed reinforcer durations. *Journal of the Experimental Analysis of Behavior, 41,* 169–182.

Davison, M., & Jenkins, P. E. (1985). Stimulus discriminability, contingency discriminability, and schedule performance. *Animal Learning and Behavior, 13,* 77–84.

Davison, M., & McCarthy, D. (1988). *The matching law.* Hillsdale, NJ: Erlbaum.

DeCarlo, L. T. (1985). Matching and maximizing with variable-time schedules. *Journal of the Experimental Analysis of Behavior, 43,* 75–81.

Declercq, M., De Houwer, J., & Baeyens, F. (2008). Evidence for an expectancy-based theory of avoidance behaviour. *Quarterly Journal of Experimental Psychology, 61,* 1803–1812.

Delius, J. D. (1992). Categorical discrimination of objects and pictures by pigeons. *Animal Learning and Behavior, 20,* 301–311.

Deluty, M. Z., Whitehouse, W. G., Mellitz, M., & Hineline, P. N. (1983). Self-control and commitment involving aversive events. *Behaviour Analysis Letters, 3,* 213–219.

Denniston, J. C., & Miller, R. R. (2007). Timing of omitted events: An analysis of temporal control of inhibitory behavior. *Behavioural Processes, 74,* 274–285.

de Quirós Aragón, M. B., Labrador, F. J., & de Arce, F. (2005). Evaluation of a group cue exposure treatment for opiate addicts. *The Spanish Journal of Psychology, 8,* 229–237.

Derenne, A. (2010). Shifts in postdiscrimination gradients with a stimulus dimension based on bilateral facial symmetry. *Journal of the Experimental Analysis of Behavior, 93,* 485–494.

Derenne, A., & Baron, A. (2002). Preratio pausing: Effects of an alternative reinforcer on fixed- and variable-ratio responding. *Journal of the Experimental Analysis of Behavior, 77,* 273–282.

Desimone, R., Albright, T. D., Gross, C. G., & Bruce, C. (1984). Stimulus-selective properties of inferior temporal neurons in the macaque. *Journal of Neuroscience, 4,* 2051–2062.

de Villiers, P. A., & Herrnstein, R. J. (1976). Toward a law of response strength. *Psychological Bulletin, 83,* 1131–1153.

DeVito, L. M., Kanter, B. R., & Eichenbaum, H. (2010). The hippocampus contributes to memory expression during transitive inference in mice. *Hippocampus,* 208–217.

de Wit, H. (2009). Impulsivity as a determinant and consequence of drug use: A review of underlying processes. *Addiction Biology, 14,* 22–31.

Diamond, P., & Vartiainen, H. (Eds.). (2007). *Behavioral economics and its applications.* Princeton, NJ: Princeton University Press.

DiCara, L. V. (1970). Learning in the autonomic nervous system. *Scientific American, 222,* 30–39.

Dielenberg, R. A., & McGregor, I. S. (1999). Habituation of the hiding response to cat odor in rats (*Rattus norvegicus*). *Journal of Comparative Psychology, 113,* 376–387.

DiGian, K. A., & Zentall, T. R. (2007). Pigeons may not use dual coding in the radial maze analog task. *Journal of Experimental Psychology: Animal Behavior Processes, 33,* 262–272.

Dimberg, U., & Ohman, A. (1983). The effects of directional facial cues on electrodermal conditioning to facial stimuli. *Psychophysiology, 20,* 160–167.

Dimberg, U., & Öhman, A. (1996). Behold the wrath: Psychophysiological responses to facial stimuli. *Motivation and Emotion, 20,* 149–182.

Dinsmoor, J. A. (2001). Stimuli inevitably generated by behavior that avoids electric shock are inherently reinforcing. *Journal of the Experimental Analysis of Behavior, 75,* 311–333.

Di Pellegrino, G., Fadiga, L., Gallese, V., & Rizzolatti, G. (1992). Understanding motor events: A neurophysiological study. *Experimental Brain Research, 91,* 176–180.

Dixon, M. R., & Cummings, A. (2001). Self-control in children with autism: Response allocation during delays to reinforcement. *Journal of Applied Behavior Analysis, 34,* 491–495.

Dixon, M. R., Rehfeldt, R. A., & Randich, L. (2003). Enhancing tolerance for delayed reinforcers: The role of intervening activities. *Journal of Applied Behavior Analysis, 36,* 263–266.

Dodwell, P. C., & Bessant, D. E. (1960). Learning without swimming in a water maze. *Journal of Comparative and Physiological Psychology, 53,* 422–425.

Domjan, M. (1983). Biological constraints on instrumental and classical conditioning: Implications for general process theory. In G. H. Bower (Ed.), *The psychology of learning and motivation* (Vol. 17). New York: Academic Press, 215–277.

Domjan, M. (2008). Adaptive specializations and generality of the laws of classical and instrumental conditioning. In R. Menzel (Ed.), *Learning theory and behavior* (pp. 327–340). Oxford: Elsevier.

Domjan, M., & Best, M. R. (1980). Interference with ingestional aversion learning produced by preexposure to the unconditioned stimulus: Associative and nonassociative aspects. *Learning and Motivation, 11,* 522–537.

Donegan, N. H., & Wagner, A. R. (1987). Conditioned diminution and facilitation of the UR: A sometimes opponent-process interpretation. In I. Gormezano, W. F. Prokasy, & R. F. Thompson (Eds.), *Classical conditioning*. Hillsdale, NJ: Erlbaum, 339–369.

Donohue, S. E., Woldorff, M. G., & Mitroff, S. R. (2010). Video game players show more precise multisensory temporal processing abilities. *Attention, Perception, & Psychophysics, 72,* 1120–1129.

Dopson, J. C., Pearce, J. M., & Haselgrove, M. (2009). Failure of retrospective revaluation to influence blocking. *Journal of Experimental Psychology: Animal Behavior Processes, 35,* 473–484.

Dore, F. Y., & Dumas, C. (1987). Psychology of animal cognition: Piagetian studies. *Psychological Bulletin, 102,* 219–233.

Dorrance, B. R., & Zentall, T. R. (2001). Imitative learning in Japanese quail depends on the motivational state of the observer at the time of observation. *Journal of Comparative Psychology, 115,* 62–67.

Dougan, J. D., McSweeney, F. K., & Farmer-Dougan, V. A. (1986). Behavioral contrast in competitive and noncompetitive environments. *Journal of the Experimental Analysis of Behavior, 46,* 185–197.

Doughty, A. H., Cash, J. D., Finch, E. A., Holloway, C., & Wallington, L. K. (2010). Effects of training history on resurgence in humans. *Behavioural Processes, 83,* 340–343.

Dowrick, P. W., & Raeburn, J. M. (1995). Self-modeling: Rapid skill training for children with physical disabilities. *Journal of Developmental and Physical Disabilities, 7,* 25–37.

Draganski, B., Gaser, C., Busch, V., Schuierer, G., Bogdahn, U., & May, A. (2004). Neuroplasticity: Changes in grey matter induced by training. *Nature, 427,* 311–312.

Dragoi, V., & Staddon, J. E. R. (1999). The dynamics of operant conditioning. *Psychological Review, 106,* 20–61.

Droit-Volet, S. (2002). Scalar timing in temporal generalization in children with short and long stimulus durations. *Quarterly Journal of Experimental Psychology, 55A,* 1193–1209.

Drummond, D. C., Tiffany, S. T., Glautier, S., & Remington, B. (Eds.). (1995). *Addictive behaviour: Cue exposure research and theory*. New York: Wiley.

Dube, W. V., Ahearn, W. H., Lionello-DeNolf, K. M., & McIlvane, W. J. (2009). Behavioral momentum: Translational research in intellectual and developmental disabilities. *Behavior Analyst Today, 10,* 238–253.

Ducharme, J. M., & Van Houten, R. (1994). Operant extinction in the treatment of severe maladaptive behavior. *Behavior Modification, 18,* 139–170.

Duffy, L., & Wishart, J. G. (1987). A comparison of two procedures for teaching discrimination skills to Down's syndrome and non-handicapped children. *British Journal of Educational Psychology, 57,* 265–278.

Dugdale, N., & Lowe, F. C. (2000). Testing for symmetry in the conditional discriminations of language-trained chimpanzees. *Journal of the Experimental Analysis of Behavior, 73,* 5–22.

Dunn, R. M. (1982). Choice, relative reinforcer duration, and the changeover ratio. *Journal of the Experimental Analysis of Behavior, 38,* 313–319.

Durand, K., Lecuyer, R., & Frichtel, M. (2003). Representation of the third dimension: The use of perspective cues by 3- and 4-month-old infants. *Infant Behavior and Development, 26,* 151–166.

Dushanova, J., & Donoghue, J. (2010). Neurons in primary motor cortex engaged during action observation. *European Journal of Neuroscience, 31,* 386–398.

Easterbrook, M. A., Kisilevsky, B. S., Muir, D. W., & Laplante, D. P. (1999). Newborns discriminate schematic faces from scrambled faces. *Canadian Journal of Experimental Psychology, 53,* 231–241.

Ebbinghaus, H. (1885). *Memory.* Leipzig, Germany: Duncker.

Eelen, P., & Vervliet, B. (2006). Fear conditioning and clinical implications: What can we learn from the past? *Fear and learning: From basic processes to clinical implications* (pp. 17–35). Washington, DC: American Psychological Association.

Eibl-Eibesfeldt, I. (1975). *Ethology* (2nd ed.). New York: Holt, Rinehart & Winston.

Eikelboom, R., & Stewart, J. (1982). Conditioning of drug-induced physiological responses. *Psychological Review, 89,* 507–528.

Eisenberger, R., & Adornetto, M. (1986). Generalized self-control of delay and effort. *Journal of Personality and Social Psychology, 51,* 1020–1031.

Ekman, P. (1973). Cross-cultural studies of facial expression. In P. Ekman (Ed.), *Darwin and facial expression.* New York: Academic Press, 91–168.

Ekman, P. (2003). *Emotions revealed: Recognizing faces and feelings to improve communication and emotional life.* New York: Times Books/ Henry Holt.

Ellingson, S. A., Miltenberger, R. G., Stricker, J. M., Garlinghouse, M. A., Roberts, J., Galensky, T. L., et al. (2000). Analysis and treatment of finger sucking. *Journal of Applied Behavior Analysis, 33,* 41–52.

Ellison, G. D. (1964). Differential salivary conditioning to traces. *Journal of Comparative and Physiological Psychology, 57,* 373–380.

Elsmore, T. F., Fletcher, G. V., Conrad, D. G., & Sodetz, F. J. (1980). Reduction of heroin intake in baboons by an economic constraint. *Pharmacology, Biochemistry and Behavior, 13,* 729–731.

Engelmann, M. (2009). Competition between two memory traces for long-term recognition memory. *Neurobiology of Learning and Memory, 91,* 58–65.

Enkel, T., Spanagel, R., Vollmayr, B., & Schneider, M. (2010). Stress triggers anhedonia in rats bred for learned helplessness. *Behavioural Brain Research, 209,* 183–186.

Ennet, S. T., Bauman, K. E., & Koch, G. G. (1994). Variability in cigarette smoking within and between adolescent friendship cliques. *Addictive Behaviors, 19,* 295–305.

Epstein, L. H., Paluch, R. A., Kilanowski, C. K., & Raynor, H. A. (2004). The effect of reinforcement or stimulus control to reduce sedentary behavior in the treatment of obesity. *Health Psychology, 4,* 371–380.

Epstein, R. (1983). Resurgence of a previously reinforced behavior during extinction. *Behaviour Analysis Letters, 3,* 391–397.

Epstein, R. (1996). *Cognition, creativity, and behavior: Selected essays.* Westport, CT: Praeger.

Epstein, R., & Medalie, S. D. (1983). Spontaneous use of a tool by a pigeon. *Behaviour Analysis Letters, 3,* 241–247.

Epstein, S. M. (1967). Toward a unified theory of anxiety. In B. A. Maher (Ed.), *Progress in experimental personality research* (Vol. 4). New York: Academic Press, 2–89.

Erjavec, M., Lovett, V. E., & Horne, P. J. (2009). Do infants show generalized imitation of gestures? II. The effects of skills training and multiple exemplar matching training. *Journal of the Experimental Analysis of Behavior, 91,* 355–376.

Eron, L. D., Huesmann, L. R., Lefkowitz, M. M., & Walder, L. O. (1972). Does television violence cause aggression? *American Psychologist, 27,* 253–263.

Esseily, R. R., Nadel, J. J., & Fagard, J. J. (2010). Object retrieval through observational learning in 8- to 18-month-old infants. *Infant Behavior and Development, 33,* 695–699.

Estes, W. K. (1950). Toward a statistical theory of learning. *Psychological Review, 57,* 94–107.

Etscorn, F., & Stephens, R. (1973). Establishment of conditioned taste aversions with a 24-hour CS-US interval. *Physiological Psychology, 1,* 251–253.

Ettinger, R. H., Reid, A. K., & Staddon, J. E. R. (1987). Sensitivity to molar feedback functions: A test of molar optimality theory. *Journal of Experimental Psychology: Animal Behavior Processes, 13,* 366–375.

Evans, N., & Levinson, S. C. (2009). The myth of language universals: Language diversity and its importance for cognitive science. *Behavioral and Brain Sciences, 32,* 429–448.

Fagan, A., Eichenbaum, H., & Cohen, N. (1985). Normal learning set and facilitation of reversal learning in rats with combined fornix-amygdala lesions: Implications for preserved learning abilities in amnesia. *Annals of the New York Academy of Sciences, 444,* 510–512.

Fagot, J., & Parron, C. (2010). Relational matching in baboons (*Papio papio*) with reduced grouping requirements. *Journal of Experimental Psychology: Animal Behavior Processes, 36,* 184–193.

Falk, J. L. (1961). Production of polydipsia in normal rats by an intermittent food schedule. *Science, 133,* 195–196.

Fanselow, M. S. (1997). Species-specific defense reactions: Retrospect and prospect. In M. E. Bouton & M. S. Fanselow (Eds.), *Learning, motivation, and cognition: The functional behaviorism of Robert C. Bolles.* Washington, DC: American Psychological Association, 321–341.

Fantino, E. (1969). Choice and rate of reinforcement. *Journal of the Experimental Analysis of Behavior, 12,* 723–730.

Fantino, E. (2008). Choice, conditioned reinforcement, and the Prius effect. *The Behavior Analyst, 31,* 95–111.

Fantino, E., & Silberberg, A. (2010). Revisiting the role of bad news in maintaining human observing behavior. *Journal of the Experimental Analysis of Behavior, 93,* 157–170.

Fehr, A., & Beckwith, B. E. (1989). Water misting: Treating self-injurious behavior in a multiply handicapped, visually impaired child. *Journal of Visual Impairment and Blindness, 83,* 245–248.

von Fersen, L., Wynne, C. D., Delius, J. D., & Staddon, J. E. R. (1991). Transitive inference formation in pigeons. *Journal of Experimental Psychology: Animal Behavior Processes, 17,* 334–341.

Ferster, C. B., & Skinner, B. F. (1957). *Schedules of reinforcement.* New York: Appleton-Century-Crofts.

Feshbach, S., & Tangney, J. (2008). Television viewing and aggression: Some alternative perspectives. *Perspectives on Psychological Science, 3,* 387–389.

Fetterman, J. G., & Killeen, P. R. (1991). Adjusting the pacemaker. *Learning and Motivation, 22,* 226–252.

Fetterman, J. G., & Killeen, P. R. (2010). Categorical counting. *Behavioural Processes, 85,* 28–35.

Field, T. M., Woodson, R., Greenberg, R., & Cohen, D. (1982). Discrimination and imitation of facial expressions by neonates. *Science, 218,* 179–181.

Fields, L., Travis, R., Roy, D., Yadlovker, E., De Aguiar-Rocha, L., & Sturmey, P. (2009). Equivalence class formation: A method for teaching statistical interactions. *Journal of Applied Behavior Analysis, 42,* 575–593.

Fisch, S., & Truglio, R. (Eds.). (2001). *"G" is for "growing": Thirty years of Sesame Street research.* Mahwah, NJ: Lawrence Erlbaum.

Fischer, H., Wright, C. I., Whalen, P. J., McInerney, S. C., Shin, L. M., & Rauch, S. L. (2003). Brain habituation during repeated exposure to fearful and neutral faces: A functional MRI study. *Brain Research Bulletin, 59,* 387–392.

Fischer, S. M., Iwata, B. A., & Worsdell, A. S. (1997). Attention as an establishing operation and as reinforcement during functional analyses. *Journal of Applied Behavior Analysis, 30,* 335–338.

Fischman, M. G., & Lim, C. H. (1991). Influence of extended practice on programming time, movement time, and transfer in simple target-striking responses. *Journal of Motor Behavior, 23,* 39–50.

Fisher, W. W., Adelinis, J. D., Thompson, R. H., Worsdell, A. S., & Zarcone, J. R. (1998). Functional analysis and treatment of destructive behavior maintained by termination of "don't" (and symmetrical "do") requests. *Journal of Applied Behavior Analysis, 31,* 339–356.

Fisher, W. W., Lindauer, S. E., Alterson, C. J., & Thompson, R. H. (1998). Assessment and treatment of destructive behavior maintained by stereotypic object manipulation. *Journal of Applied Behavior Analysis, 31,* 513–527.

Flannery, R. B. (2002). Treating learned helplessness in the elderly dementia patient: Preliminary inquiry. *American Journal of Alzheimer's Disease and Other Dementias, 17,* 345–349.

Foster, T. M., Temple, W., Robertson, B., Nair, V., & Poling, A. (1996). Concurrent-schedule performance in dairy cows: Persistent undermatching. *Journal of the Experimental Analysis of Behavior, 65,* 57–80.

Fountain, S. B. (2006). The structure of sequential behavior. In E. A. Wasserman & T. R. Zentall (Eds.), *Comparative cognition: Experimental explorations of animal intelligence* (pp. 439–458). New York: Oxford University Press.

Fountain, S. B., & Rowan, J. D. (1995). Sensitivity to violations of "run" and "trill" structures in rat serial-pattern learning. *Journal of Experimental Psychology: Animal Behavior Processes, 21,* 78–81.

Fouts, R., Fouts, D., & Schoenfield, D. (1984). Sign language conversation interaction between chimpanzees. *Sign Language Studies, 42,* 1–12.

Fox, D. K., Hopkins, B. L., & Anger, W. K. (1987). The long-term effects of a token economy on safety performance in open-pit mining. *Journal of Applied Behavior Analysis, 20,* 215–224.

Fox, L. (1962). Effecting the use of efficient study habits. *Journal of Mathetics, 1,* 75–86.

Foxall, G. R., James, V. K., Oliveira-Castro, J. M., & Ribier, S. (2010). Product substitutability and the matching law. *Psychological Record, 60,* 185–216.

Foxall, G. R., & Schrezenmaier, T. C. (2003). The behavioral economics of consumer brand choice: Establishing a methodology. *Journal of Economic Psychology, 24,* 675–695.

Fraenkel, G. S., & Gunn, D. L. (1940). *The orientation of animals: Kineses, taxes, and compass reactions.* Oxford: Oxford University Press.

Friedman, A. K., & Weiss, K. R. (2010). Repetition priming of motoneuronal activity in a small motor network: Intercellular and intracellular signaling. *Journal of Neuroscience, 30,* 8906–8919.

Friedrich-Cofer, L., & Huston, A. C. (1986). Television violence and aggression: The debate continues. *Psychological Bulletin, 100,* 364–371.

Galbicka, G. (1994). Shaping in the 21st century: Moving percentile schedules into applied settings. *Journal of Applied Behavior Analysis, 27,* 739–760.

Galbicka, G., & Branch, M. N. (1981). Selective punishment of interresponse times. *Journal of the Experimental Analysis of Behavior, 35,* 311–322.

Galbicka, G., & Platt, J. R. (1984). Interresponse-time punishment: A basis for shock-maintained behavior. *Journal of the Experimental Analysis of Behavior, 41,* 291–308.

Gallistel, C. R., & Gibbon, J. (2002). *The symbolic foundations of conditioned behavior.* Mahwah, NJ: Lawrence Erlbaum Associates Publishers.

Gámez, A. M., & Rosas, J. M. (2005). Transfer of stimulus control across instrumental responses is attenuated by extinction in human instrumental conditioning. *International Journal of Psychology and Psychological Therapy, 5,* 207–222.

Gámez, A. M., & Rosas, J. M. (2007). Associations in human instrumental conditioning. *Learning and Motivation, 38,* 242–261.

Garcia, J., Ervin, F. R., & Koelling, R. A. (1966). Learning with prolonged delay of reinforcement. *Psychonomic Science, 5,* 121–122.

Garcia, J., & Koelling, R. (1966). Relation of cue to consequence in avoidance learning. *Psychonomic Science, 4,* 123–124.

Gardner, R. A., & Gardner, B. T. (1969). Teaching sign language to a chimpanzee. *Science, 165,* 664–672.

Gardner, R. A., & Gardner, B. T. (1975). Early signs of language in child and chimpanzee. *Science, 187,* 752–753.

Gaultney, J. F., & Gingras, J. L. (2005). Fetal rate of behavioral inhibition and preference for novelty during infancy. *Early Human Development, 81,* 379–386.

Gelfo, F., De Bartolo, P., Giovine, A., Petrosini, L., & Leggio, M. G. (2009). Layer and regional effects of environmental enrichment on the pyramidal neuron morphology of the rat. *Neurobiology of Learning and Memory, 9,* 353–365.

Gergely, G., Bekkering, H., & Király, I. (2002). Rational imitation in preverbal infants. *Nature, 415,* 775.

Gerwig, M., Guberina, H., Eßer, A. C., Siebler, M., Schoch, B., Frings, M., et al. (2010). Evaluation of multiple-session delay eyeblink conditioning comparing patients with focal cerebellar lesions and cerebellar degeneration. *Behavioural Brain Research, 212,* 143–151.

Gifford, E. V., & Shoenberger, D. (2009). Rapid smoking. *General principles and empirically supported techniques of cognitive behavior therapy* (pp. 513–519). Hoboken, NJ: Wiley.

Gilboy, S. (2005). Students' Optimistic Attitudes and Resiliency program: Empirical validation of a prevention program developing hope and optimism. *Dissertation Abstracts International, 66*(6-B), 3434.

Gillan, D. J. (1981). Reasoning in the chimpanzee: II. Transitive inference. *Journal of Experimental Psychology: Animal Behavior Processes, 7,* 150–164.

Gillan, D. J., Premack, D., & Woodruff, G. (1981). Reasoning in the chimpanzee: I. Analogical reasoning. *Journal of Experimental Psychology: Animal Behavior Processes, 7,* 1–17.

Givón, T. T., & Rumbaugh, S. (2009). Can apes learn grammar? A short detour into language evolution. In J. Guo, E. Lieven, N. Budwig, S. Ervin-Tripp, K. Nakamura, & Ş. Özçalişkan (Eds.), *Crosslinguistic approaches to the psychology of language: Research in the tradition of Dan Isaac Slobin* (pp. 299–309). New York: Psychology Press.

Glaister, B. (1985). A case of auditory hallucination treated by satiation. *Behaviour Research and Therapy, 23,* 213–215.

Glanzman, D. L. (1995). The cellular basis of classical conditioning in *Aplysia californica*—it's less simple than you think. *Trends in Neuroscience, 18,* 30–36.

Glasscock, S. G., Friman, P. C., O'Brien, S., & Christopherson, E. R. (1986). Varied citrus treatment of ruminant gagging in a teenager with Batten's disease. *Journal of Behavior Therapy and Experimental Psychiatry, 17,* 129–133.

Gleeson, S., Lattal, K. A., & Williams, K. S. (1989). Superstitious conditioning: A replication and extension of Neuringer (1970). *Psychological Record, 39,* 563–571.

Gleitman, H. (1971). Forgetting of long-term memories in animals. In W. K. Honig & P. H. R. James (Eds.), *Animal memory*. New York: Academic Press, 1–44.

Glover, H. (1992). Emotional numbing: A possible endorphin-mediated phenomenon associated with post-traumatic stress disorders and other allied psychopathologic states. *Journal of Traumatic Stress, 5,* 643–675.

Gluck, M. A. (1991). Stimulus generalization and representation in adaptive network models of category learning. *Psychological Science, 2,* 50–55.

Glynn, S. M. (1990). Token economy approaches for psychiatric patients: Progress and pitfalls over 25 years. *Behavior Modification, 14,* 383–407.

Goebel, M. U., Meykadeh, N., Kou, W., Schedlowski, M., & Hengge, U. R. (2008). Behavioral conditioning of antihistamine effects in patients with allergic rhinitis. *Psychotherapy and Psychosomatics, 77,* 227–234.

Goldsmith, J. B., & McFall, R. M. (1975). Development and evaluation of an interpersonal skill-training program for psychiatric inpatients. *Journal of Abnormal Psychology, 84,* 51–58.

Gonzalez, R. C., Gentry, G. V., & Bitterman, M. E. (1954). Relational discrimination of intermediate size in the chimpanzee. *Journal of Comparative and Physiological Psychology, 47,* 385–388.

Gordon, K. C., Dixon, L. J., Willett, J. M., & Hughes, F. M. (2009). Behavioral and cognitive-behavioral therapies. In J. H. Bray & M. Stanton (Eds.), *The Wiley-Blackwell handbook of family psychology* (pp. 226–239). Hoboken, NJ: Wiley-Blackwell.

Gordon, W. C., Smith, G. J., & Katz, D. S. (1979). Dual effects of response blocking following avoidance learning. *Behavior Research and Therapy, 17,* 479–487.

Gore, S. A., Foster, J. A., DeiLillo, V. G., Kirk, K., & West, D. S. (2003). Television viewing and snacking. *Eating Behaviors, 4,* 399–405.

Gosch, E. A., Flannery-Schroeder, E., Mauro, C. F., & Compton, S. N. (2006). Principles of cognitive-behavioral therapy for anxiety disorders in children. *Journal of Cognitive Psychotherapy, 20,* 247–262.

Gottfried, A. E., Fleming, J. S., & Gottfried, A. W. (1998). Role of cognitively stimulating home environment in children's academic intrinsic motivation: A longitudinal study. *Child Development, 69,* 1448–1460.

Gottfried, J. A., O'Doherty, J., & Dolan, R. J. (2002). Appetitive and aversive olfactory learning in humans studied using event-related functional magnetic resonance imaging. *Journal of Neuroscience, 22,* 10829–10837.

Gottlieb, D. A., & Rescorla, R. A. (2010). Within-subject effects of number of trials in rat conditioning procedures. *Journal of Experimental Psychology: Animal Behavior Processes, 36,* 217–231.

Gould, E., Beylin, A., Tanapat, P., Reeves, A., & Shors, T. J. (1999). Learning enhances adult neurogenesis in the hippocampal formation. *Nature Neuroscience, 2,* 260–265.

Gould, E., Reeves, A. J., Graziano, M. S., & Gross, C. G. (1999). Neurogenesis in the neocortex of adult primates. *Science, 286,* 548–552.

Grace, R. C. (1994). A contextual choice model of concurrent-chains choice. *Journal of the Experimental Analysis of Behavior, 61,* 113–129.

Grant, D. S. (1975). Proactive interference in pigeon short-term memory. *Journal of Experimental Psychology: Animal Behavior Processes, 1,* 207–220.

Grant, D. S. (1981). Short-term memory in the pigeon. In N. E. Spear & R. R. Miller (Eds.), *Information processing in animals: Memory mechanisms.* Hillsdale, NJ: Erlbaum, 227–256.

Grau, J. W., Crown, E. D., Ferguson, A. R., Washburn, S. N., Hook, M. A., & Miranda, R. C. (2006). Instrumental learning within the spinal cord: Underlying mechanisms and implications for recovery after injury. *Behavioral and Cognitive Neuroscience Reviews, 5,* 191–239.

Green, L., & Estle, S. J. (2003). Preference reversals with food and water reinforcers in rats. *Journal of the Experimental Analysis of Behavior, 79,* 233–242.

Green, L., Fischer, E. B., Perlow, S., & Sherman, L. (1981). Preference reversal and self control: Choice as a function of reward amount and delay. *Behavior Analysis Letters, 1,* 43–51.

Green, L., Fry, A. F., & Myerson, J. (1994). Discounting of delayed rewards: A life-span comparison. *Psychological Science, 5,* 33–36.

Green, L., & Holt, D. D. (2003). Economic and biological influences on key pecking and treadle pressing in pigeons. *Journal of the Experimental Analysis of Behavior, 80,* 43–58.

Green, L., Kagel, J. H., & Battalio, R. C. (1987). Consumption-leisure tradeoffs in pigeons: Effects of changing marginal rates by varying amount of reinforcement. *Journal of the Experimental Analysis of Behavior, 47,* 17–28.

Greenfield, P. M., & Savage-Rumbaugh, E. S. (1993). Comparing communicative competence in child and chimp: The pragmatics of repetition. *Journal of Child Language, 20,* 1–26.

Grinker, R., & Spiegel, J. (1945). *Men under stress.* London: Churchill.

Grosch, J., & Neuringer, A. (1981). Self-control in pigeons under the Mischel paradigm. *Journal of the Experimental Analysis of Behavior, 35,* 3–21.

Gruber, B. L., & Taub, E. (1998). Thermal and EMG biofeedback learning in nonhuman primates. *Applied Psychophysiology and Biofeedback, 23,* 1–12.

Guess, D., & Sailor, W. (1993). Chaos theory and the study of human behavior: Implications for special education and developmental disabilities. *Journal of Special Education, 27,* 16–34.

Gunby, K. V., Carr, J. E., & Leblanc, L. A. (2010). Teaching abduction-prevention skills to children with autism. *Journal of Applied Behavior Analysis, 43,* 107–112.

Guthrie, E. R., & Horton, G. P. (1946). *Cats in a puzzle box.* New York: Holt, Rinehart & Winston.

Gutman, A. (1977). Positive contrast, negative induction, and inhibitory stimulus control in the rat. *Journal of the Experimental Analysis of Behavior, 27,* 219–233.

Guttman, N., & Kalish, H. I. (1956). Discriminability and stimulus generalization. *Journal of Experimental Psychology, 51,* 79–88.

Hackenberg, T. R. (2009). Token reinforcement: A review and analysis. *Journal of the Experimental Analysis of Behavior, 91,* 257–286.

Hagopian, L. P., & Thompson, R. H. (1999). Reinforcement of compliance with respiratory treatment in a child with cystic fibrosis. *Journal of Applied Behavior Analysis, 32,* 233–236.

Hake, D. F., Donaldson, T., & Hyten, C. (1983). Analysis of discriminative control by social behavioral stimuli. *Journal of the Experimental Analysis of Behavior, 39,* 7–23.

Hall, G., & Pearce, J. M. (1983). Changes in stimulus associability during acquisition: Implications for theories of acquisition. In M. L. Commons, R. J. Herrnstein, & A. R. Wagner (Eds.), *Quantitative analyses of behavior: Vol. 3. Acquisition.* Cambridge, MA: Ballinger, 221–239.

Halweg, K., & Markman, H. J. (1988). The effectiveness of behavioral marriage therapy: Empirical status of behavioral techniques in preventing and alleviating marital distress. *Journal of Consulting and Clinical Psychology, 56,* 440–447.

Hampton, J. A. (2006). Concepts as prototypes. In B. H. Ross (Ed.), *The psychology of learning and motivation: Advances in research and theory* (Vol. 46, pp. 79–113). San Diego, CA: Elsevier Academic Press.

Hampton, R. (2001). Rhesus monkeys know when they remember. *Proceedings of the National Academy of Sciences of the United States of America, 98,* 5359–5362.

Hanley, G. P., Iwata, B. A., Roscoe, E. M., Thompson, R. H., & Lindberg, J. S. (2003). Response-restriction analysis: II. Alteration of activity preferences. *Journal of Applied Behavior Analysis, 36,* 59–76.

Hanson, H. M. (1959). Effects of discrimination training on stimulus generalization. *Journal of Experimental Psychology, 58,* 321–334.

Hardin, G. (1968). The tragedy of the commons. *Science, 162,* 1243–1248.

Hare, R. D. (2006). The effects of delay and schedule of punishment on avoidance of a verbal response class. *Dissertation Abstracts International: Section B. The Sciences and Engineering, 67,* 581.

Harlow, H. F. (1949). The formation of learning sets. *Psychological Review, 56,* 51–65.

Hart, J., Berndt, R. S., & Caramazza, A. (1985). Category-specific naming deficit following cerebral infarction. *Nature, 316,* 439–440.

Haslam, C., Moss, Z., & Hodder, K. (2010). Are two methods better than one? Evaluating the effectiveness of combining errorless learning with vanishing cues. *Journal of Clinical and Experimental Neuropsychology, 32,* 973–985.

Hatze, H. (1976). Biomechanical aspects of a successful motion optimization. In P. V. Komi (Ed.), *Biomechanics V-B.* Baltimore, MD: University Park Press, 5–12.

Hawkins, R. D., Carew, T. J., & Kandel, E. R. (1983). Effects of interstimulus interval and contingency on classical conditioning in *Aplysia. Society for Neuroscience Abstracts, 9,* 168.

Hawkins, R. D., Cohen, T. E., & Kandel, E. R. (2006). Dishabituation in *Aplysia* can involve either reversal of habituation or superimposed sensitization. *Learning and Memory, 13,* 397–403.

Hawkins, R. D., Greene, W., & Kandel, E. R. (1998). Classical conditioning, differential conditioning, and second-order conditioning of the *Aplysia* gill-withdrawal reflex in a simplified mantle organ preparation. *Behavioral Neuroscience, 112,* 636–645.

Hayes, C. (1951). *The ape in our house.* New York: Harper.

Hearst, E., & Jenkins, H. M. (1974). *Sign tracking: The stimulus-reinforcer relation and directed action.* Austin, TX: Monograph of the Psychonomic Society.

Heidegger, T., Krakow, K., & Ziemann, U. (2010). Effects of antiepileptic drugs on associative LTP-like plasticity in human motor cortex. *European Journal of Neuroscience, 32,* 1215–1222.

Hekimian, L. J., & Gershon, S. (1968). Characteristics of drug abusers admitted to a psychiatric hospital. *Journal of the American Medical Association, 205,* 125–130.

Heller, R. F., & Strang, H. R. (1973). Controlling bruxism through automated aversive conditioning. *Behavior Research and Therapy, 11,* 327–329.

Hembree, E. A., Rauch, S. A. M., & Foa, E. B. (2003). Beyond the manual: The insider's guide to prolonged exposure therapy for PTSD. *Cognitive and Behavioral Practice, 10,* 22–30.

Hendry, D. P., & Van-Toller, C. (1964). Fixed-ratio punishment with continuous reinforcement. *Journal of the Experimental Analysis of Behavior, 7,* 293–300.

Herman, L. M., & Forestell, P. H. (1985). Reporting presence or absence of named objects by a language-trained dolphin. *Neuroscience & Biobehavioral Reviews, 9,* 667–681.

Herman, L. M., Richards, D. G., & Wolz, J. P. (1984). Comprehension of sentences by bottlenosed dolphins. *Cognition, 16,* 1–90.

Herman, L. M., & Uyeyama, R. K. (1999). The dolphin's grammatical competency: Comments on Kako (1999). *Animal Learning and Behavior, 27,* 18–23.

Heron, W. T., & Skinner, B. F. (1940). The rate of extinction in maze-bright and maze-dull rats. *Psychological Record, 4,* 11–18.

Herrnstein, R. J. (1961). Relative and absolute strength of response as a function of frequency of reinforcement. *Journal of the Experimental Analysis of Behavior, 4,* 267–272.

Herrnstein, R. J. (1966). Superstition: A corollary of the principles of operant conditioning. In W. K. Honig (Ed.), *Operant behavior: Areas of research and application.* New York: Appleton-Century-Crofts, 33–51.

Herrnstein, R. J. (1969). Method and theory in the study of avoidance. *Psychological Review, 76,* 49–69.

Herrnstein, R. J. (1970). On the law of effect. *Journal of the Experimental Analysis of Behavior, 13,* 243–266.

Herrnstein, R. J. (1974). Formal properties of the matching law. *Journal of the Experimental Analysis of Behavior, 21,* 159–164.

Herrnstein, R. J. (1979). Acquisition, generalization, and reversal of a natural concept. *Journal of Experimental Psychology: Animal Behavior Processes, 5,* 116–129.

Herrnstein, R. J. (1990). Rational choice theory: Necessary but not sufficient. *American Psychologist, 45,* 356–367.

Herrnstein, R. J., & de Villiers, P. A. (1980). Fish as a natural category for people and pigeons. In G. H. Bower (Ed.), *The psychology of learning and motivation* (Vol. 14). New York: Academic Press, 59–95.

Herrnstein, R. J., & Hineline, P. N. (1966). Negative reinforcement as shock-frequency reduction. *Journal of the Experimental Analysis of Behavior, 9,* 421–430.

Herrnstein, R. J., & Loveland, D. H. (1964). Complex visual concept in the pigeon. *Science, 146,* 549–551.

Herrnstein, R. J., Loveland, D. H., & Cable, C. (1976). Natural concepts in pigeons. *Journal of Experimental Psychology: Animal Behavior Processes, 2,* 285–302.

Herrnstein, R. J., & Mazur, J. E. (1987). Making up our minds: A new model of economic behavior. *The Sciences, 27,* 40–47.

Herrnstein, R. J., & Prelec, D. (1991). Melioration: A theory of distributed choice. *Journal of Economic Perspectives, 5,* 137–156.

Herrnstein, R. J., & Vaughan, W. (1980). Melioration and behavioral allocation. In J. E. R. Staddon (Ed.), *Limits to action: The allocation of individual behavior.* New York: Academic Press, 143–176.

Heyes, C. M., & Foster, C. L. (2002). Motor learning by observation: Evidence from a serial reaction time task. *Quarterly Journal of Experimental Psychology, 55A,* 593–607.

Heyes, C. M., Jaldow, E., & Dawson, G. R. (1994). Imitation in rats: Conditions of occurrence in a bidirectional control procedure. *Learning and Motivation, 25,* 276–287.

Heyman, G. M. (1979). A Markov model description of changeover probabilities on concurrent variable-interval schedules. *Journal of the Experimental Analysis of Behavior, 31,* 41–51.

Heyman, G. M. (2009). *Addiction: A disorder of choice.* Cambridge, MA: Harvard University Press.

Heyman, G. M., & Herrnstein, R. J. (1986). More on concurrent interval-ratio schedules: A replication and review. *Journal of the Experimental Analysis of Behavior, 46,* 331–351.

Hicks-Pass, S. (2009). Corporal punishment in America today: Spare the rod, spoil the child? A systematic review of the literature. *Best Practices in Mental Health: An International Journal, 5,* 71–88.

Higgins, S. T., Morris, E. K., & Johnson, L. M. (1989). Social transmission of superstitious behavior in preschool children. *Psychological Record, 39,* 307–323.

Hilgard, E. R. (1936). The nature of the conditioned response: I. The case for and against stimulus-substitution. *Psychological Review, 43,* 366–385.

Hineline, P. N. (2001). Beyond the molar-molecular distinction: We need multiscaled analyses. *Journal of the Experimental Analysis of Behavior, 75,* 342–347.

Hinson, J. M., & Staddon, J. E. R. (1983). Hill-climbing by pigeons. *Journal of the Experimental Analysis of Behavior, 39,* 25–47.

Hiroto, D. S., & Seligman, M. E. P. (1975). Generality of learned helplessness in man. *Journal of Personality and Social Psychology, 31,* 311–327.

Hittner, J. B. (2005). How robust is the Werther effect? A re-examination of the suggestion-imitation model of suicide. *Mortality, 10,* 193–200.

Hobbes, T. (1651). *Leviathan, or the matter, forme and power of a commonwealth ecclesiasticall and civill.* London: Andrew Crooke.

Hoch, J., & Symons, F. J. (2007). Matching analysis of socially appropriate and destructive behavior in developmental disabilities. *Research in Developmental Disabilities, 28,* 238–248.

Hoehler, F. K., Kirschenbaum, D. S., & Leonard, D. W. (1973). The effects of overtraining and successive extinctions upon nictitating membrane conditioning in the rabbit. *Learning and Motivation, 4,* 91–101.

Hogben, M. (1998). Factors moderating the effect of televised aggression on viewer behavior. *Communication Research, 25,* 220–247.

Holland, P. C. (1986). Temporal determinants of occasion setting in feature-positive discriminations. *Animal Learning and Behavior, 14,* 111–120.

Holland, P. C. (1991). Transfer of control in ambiguous discriminations. *Journal of Experimental Psychology: Animal Behavior Processes, 17,* 231–248.

Holland, P. C., & Rescorla, R. A. (1975). The effect of two ways of devaluing the unconditioned stimulus after first- and second-order appetitive conditioning. *Journal of Experimental Psychology: Animal Behavior Processes, 1,* 355–363.

Hollister, J. M., Mednick, S. A., Brennan, P. A., & Cannon, T. D. (1994). Impaired autonomic nervous system habituation in those at genetic risk for schizophrenia. *Archives of General Psychiatry, 51,* 552–558.

Holz, W. C., & Azrin, N. H. (1961). Discriminative properties of punishment. *Journal of the Experimental Analysis of Behavior, 4,* 225–232.

Homme, L. E., deBaca, P. C., Devine, J. V., Steinhorst, R., & Rickert, E. J. (1963). Use of the Premack principle in controlling the behavior of nursery school children. *Journal of the Experimental Analysis of Behavior, 6,* 544.

Honig, W. K., & Stewart, K. E. (1988). Pigeons can discriminate locations presented in pictures. *Journal of the Experimental Analysis of Behavior, 50,* 541–551.

Honig, W. K., & Stewart, K. E. (1993). Relative numerosity as a dimension of stimulus control: The peak shift. *Animal Learning and Behavior, 21,* 346–354.

Horne, P. J., & Erjavec, M. (2007). Do infants show generalized imitation of gestures. *Journal of the Experimental Analysis of Behavior, 87,* 63–87.

Houts, A. C. (2003). Behavioral treatment for enuresis. In A. E. Kazdin (Ed.), *Evidence-based psychotherapies for children and adolescents.* New York: Guilford Press , 389–406.

Hubel, D. H., & Wiesel, T. N. (1963). Receptive fields of cells in striate cortex of very young, visually inexperienced kittens. *Journal of Neurophysiology, 26,* 994–1002.

Hubel, D. H., & Wiesel, T. N. (1965). Binocular interaction in striate cortex of kittens reared with artificial squint. *Journal of Neurophysiology, 28,* 1041–1059.

Hubel, D. H., & Wiesel, T. N. (1970). The period of susceptibility to the physiological effects of unilateral eye closure in kittens. *Journal of Physiology, 206,* 419–436.

Hubel, D. H., & Wiesel, T. N. (1979). Brain mechanisms in vision. *Scientific American, 241,* 150–162.

Huber, L., & Aust, U. (2006). A modified feature theory as an account of pigeon visual categorization. In E. A. Wasserman & T. R. Zentall (Eds.), *Comparative cognition: Experimental explorations of animal intelligence* (pp. 325–342). New York: Oxford University Press.

Huesmann, L. R., Dubow, E. F., & Boxer, P. (2011). The transmission of aggressiveness across generations: Biological, contextual, and social learning processes. In P. R. Shaver & M. Mikulincer (Eds.), *Human aggression and violence: Causes, manifestations, and consequences* (pp. 123–142). Washington, DC: American Psychological Association.

Hull, C. L. (1943). *Principles of behavior.* New York: Appleton-Century-Crofts.

Hulse, S. H., & Campbell, C. E. (1975). "Thinking ahead" in rat discrimination learning. *Animal Learning and Behavior, 3,* 305–311.

Hulse, S. H., & Dorsky, N. P. (1979). Serial pattern learning by rats: Transfer of a formally defined stimulus relationship and the significance of nonreinforcement. *Animal Learning and Behavior, 7,* 211–220.

Humphreys, L. G. (1939). The effect of random alternation of reinforcement on the acquisition and extinction of conditioned eyelid reactions. *Journal of Experimental Psychology, 25,* 141–158.

Hunter, S. M., Vizelberg, I. A., & Berenson, G. S. (1991). Identifying mechanisms of adoption of tobacco and alcohol use among youth: The Bogalusa heart study. *Social Networks, 13,* 91–104.

Hur, J., & Osborne, S. (1993). A comparison of forward and backward chaining methods used in teaching corsage making skills to mentally retarded adults. *British Journal of Developmental Disabilities, 39,* 108–117.

Hursh, S. R. (1991). Behavioral economics of drug self-administration and drug abuse policy.

Journal of the Experimental Analysis of Behavior, 56, 377–393.

Hursh, S. R., & Silberberg, A. (2008). Economic demand and essential value. *Psychological Review, 115,* 186–198.

Huttenlocher, P. R. (1990). Morphometric study of human cerebral cortex development. *Neuropsychologia, 28,* 517–527.

Israely, Y., & Guttman, J. (1983). Children's sharing behavior as a function of exposure to puppet-show and story models. *Journal of Genetic Psychology, 142,* 311–312.

Ito, M., Takatsuru, S., & Saeki, D. (2000). Choice between constant and variable alternatives by rats: Effects of different reinforcer amounts and energy budgets. *Journal of the Experimental Analysis of Behavior, 73,* 79–92.

Jaakkola, K., Guarino, E., Rodriguez, M., Erb, L., & Trone, M. (2010). What do dolphins (*Tursiops truncatus*) understand about hidden objects? *Animal Cognition, 13,* 103–120.

Jacobs, B. L. (2002). Adult brain neurogenesis and depression. *Brain, Behavior, and Immunity, 16,* 602–609.

Jacobs, E. A., & Hackenberg, T. D. (2000). Human performance on negative slope schedules of points exchangeable for money: A failure of molar maximization. *Journal of the Experimental Analysis of Behavior, 73,* 241–260.

Jacobson, J. W., Mulick, J. A., & Green, G. (1998). Cost-benefit estimates for early intensive behavioral intervention for young children with autism—general model and single state case. *Behavioral Interventions, 13,* 201–226.

Jacobson, N. S. (1977). Problem solving and contingency contracting in the treatment of marital discord. *Journal of Consulting and Clinical Psychology, 45,* 92–100.

Jacobson, N. S., & Dallas, M. (1981). Helping married couples improve their relationships. In W. E. Craighead, A. E. Kazdin, & M. J. Mahoney (Eds.), *Behavior modification: Principles, issues and applications.* Boston, MA: Houghton Mifflin.

Jäkel, F., Schölkopf, B., & Wichmann, F. A. (2008). Generalization and similarity in exemplar models of categorization: Insights from machine learning. *Psychonomic Bulletin & Review, 15,* 256–271.

James, W. (1890). *The principles of psychology.* New York: Holt, Rinehart & Winston.

Janelle, C. M. (1999). Ironic mental processes in sport: Implications for sport psychologists. *Sport Psychologist, 13,* 201–220.

Jantzen, K. J., Steinberg, F. L., & Kelso, J. (2009). Coordination dynamics of large-scale neural circuitry underlying rhythmic sensorimotor behavior. *Journal of Cognitive Neuroscience, 21,* 2420–2433.

Jarvik, M. E., Goldfarb, T. L., & Carley, J. L. (1969). Influence of interference on delayed matching in monkeys. *Journal of Experimental Psychology, 81,* 1–6.

Jenkins, H. M., & Harrison, R. H. (1960). Effects of discrimination training on auditory generalization. *Journal of Experimental Psychology, 59,* 246–253.

Jenkins, H. M., & Harrison, R. H. (1962). Generalization gradients of inhibition following auditory discrimination learning. *Journal of the Experimental Analysis of Behavior, 5,* 435–441.

Jenkins, H. M., & Moore, B. R. (1973). The form of the autoshaped response with food or water reinforcers. *Journal of the Experimental Analysis of Behavior, 20,* 163–181.

Jennings, P. J. (1995). Evidence of incomplete motor programming in Parkinson's disease. *Journal of Motor Behavior, 27,* 310–324.

Jin, N. G., Tian, L.-M., & Crow, T. (2009). 5-HT and GABA modulate intrinsic excitability of type I interneurons in Hermissenda. *Journal of Neurophysiology, 102,* 2825–2833.

Jitsumori, M. (2006). Category structure and typicality effects. In E. A. Wasserman & T. R. Zentall (Eds.), *Comparative cognition: Experimental explorations of animal intelligence* (pp. 343–362). New York: Oxford University Press.

Jitsumori, M., Siemann, M., Lehr, M., & Delius, J. D. (2002). A new approach to the formation of equivalence classes in pigeons. *Journal of the Experimental Analysis of Behavior, 78,* 397–408.

Joanisse, M. F., Zevin, J. D., & McCandliss, B. D. (2007). Brain mechanisms implicated in the preattentive categorization of speech sounds revealed using fMRI and a short-interval habituation trial paradigm. *Cerebral Cortex, 17,* 2084–2093.

John, E. R. (1967). *Mechanisms of memory.* New York: Academic Press.

Johnson, C. M., Redmon, W. K., & Mawhinney, T. C. (2001). *Handbook of organizational performance: Behavior analysis and management.* New York: Haworth Press.

Johnson, H. E., & Garton, W. H. (1973). Muscle re-education in hemiplegia by use of electromyographic device. *Archives of Physiological and Medical Rehabilitation, 54,* 320–325.

Johnson, J. G., Cohen, P., Smailes, E. M., Kasen, S., & Brook, J. S. (2002). Television viewing and aggressive behavior during adolescence and adulthood. *Science, 295,* 2468–2471.

Johnson, S. P., & Aslin, R. N. (1995). Perception of object unity in 2-month-old infants. *Developmental Psychology, 31,* 739–745.

Johnson, S. P., Welsh, T. M., Miller, L. K., & Altus, D. E. (1991). Participatory management: Maintaining staff performance in a university housing cooperative. *Journal of Applied Behavior Analysis, 24,* 119–127.

Jones, R. S., & Eayrs, C. B. (1992). The use of errorless learning procedures in teaching people with a learning disability: A critical review. *Mental Handicap Research, 5,* 204–214.

Jostad, C. M., Miltenberger, R. G., Kelso, P., & Knudson, P. (2008). Peer tutoring to prevent firearm play: Acquisition, generalization, and long-term maintenance of safety skills. *Journal of Applied Behavior Analysis, 41,* 117–123.

Joynes, R. L., & Grau, J. W. (2004). Instrumental learning within the spinal cord: III. Prior exposure to noncontingent shock induces a behavioral deficit that is blocked by an opioid antagonist. *Neurobiology of Learning and Memory, 82,* 35–51.

Justice, T. C., & Looney, T. A. (1990). Another look at "superstitions" in pigeons. *Bulletin of the Psychonomic Society, 28,* 64–66.

Kako, E. (1999). Elements of syntax in the systems of three language-trained animals. *Animal Learning and Behavior, 27,* 1–14.

Kamin, L. J. (1968). Attention-like processes in classical conditioning. In M. R. Jones (Ed.), *Miami symposium on the prediction of behavior: Aversive stimulation.* Miami, FL: University of Miami Press, 9–33.

Kaminski, J., Call, J., & Fischer, J. (2004). Word learning in a domestic dog: Evidence for "fast mapping." *Science, 304,* 1682–1683.

Kandel, E. R. (1979). Small systems of neurons. *Scientific American, 241,* 66–76.

Kangas, B. D., Vaidya, M., & Branch, M. N. (2010). Titrating-delay matching-to-sample in the Pigeon. *Journal of the Experimental Analysis of Behavior, 94,* 69–81.

Kanner, L., Rodriguez, A., & Ashenden, B. (1972). How far can autistic children go in matters of social adaptation. *Journal of Autism and Childhood Schizophrenia, 2,* 9–33.

Kant, I. (1781/1881). *Kritik der reinen Vernunft.* Riga [*Critique of pure reason*]. (F. Max Muller, Trans.). London: Henry G. Bohn.

Kastak, C. R., & Schusterman, R. J. (2002). Sea lions and equivalence: Expanding classes by exclusion. *Journal of the Experimental Analysis of Behavior, 78,* 449–465.

Kawai, M. (1965). Newly acquired pre-cultural behavior of the natural troop of Japanese monkeys on Koshima Islet. *Primates, 6,* 1–30.

Kazdin, A. E. (1977). *The token economy: A review and evaluation.* New York: Plenum.

Kazdin, A. E. (1980). *Behavior modification in applied settings* (Rev. ed.). Homewood, IL: Dorsey Press.

Keele, S. W. (1973). *Attention and human performance*. Pacific Palisades, CA: Goodyear Publishing.

Keith, J. R., & McVety, K. M. (1988). Latent place learning in a novel environment and the influences of prior training in rats. *Psychobiology, 16*, 146–151.

Kelley, T. M. (2004). Positive psychology and adolescent mental health: False promise or true breakthrough? *Adolescence, 39*, 257–278.

Kellogg, W. N., & Kellogg, L. A. (1933). *The ape and the child: A study of environmental influence upon early behavior*. New York: McGraw-Hill.

Kelly, D. M., Kamil, A. C., & Cheng, K. (2010). Landmark use by Clark's nutcrackers (*Nucifraga Columbiana*): Influence of disorientation and cue rotation on distance and direction estimates. *Animal Cognition, 13*, 175–188.

Kelso, J. A. S. (1997). *Dynamic patterns: The self-organization of brain and behavior*. Cambridge, MA: MIT Press.

Kern, R. S., Liberman, R. P., Kopelowicz, A., Mintz, J., & Green, M. F. (2002). Applications of errorless learning for improving work performance in persons with schizophrenia. *American Journal of Psychiatry, 159*, 1921–1926.

Kernodle, M. W., & Carlton, L. G. (1992). Information feedback and the learning of multiple-degree-of-freedom activities. *Journal of Motor Behavior, 24*, 187–196.

Kerr, R., & Booth, B. (1978). Specific and varied practice of motor skill. *Perceptual and Motor Skills, 46*, 395–401.

Keysers, C., & Gazzola, V. (2010). Social neuroscience: Mirror neurons recorded in humans. *Current Biology, 20*, R353–R354.

Khallad, Y., & Moore, J. (1996). Blocking, unblocking, and overexpectation in autoshaping with pigeons. *Journal of the Experimental Analysis of Behavior, 65*, 575–591.

Killeen, P. R. (1982). Incentive theory: II. Models for choice. *Journal of the Experimental Analysis of Behavior, 38*, 217–232.

Killeen, P. R. (1991). Behavior's time. *The Psychology of Learning and Motivation, 27*, 295–334.

Killeen, P. R., & Fetterman, J. G. (1988). A behavioral theory of timing. *Psychological Review, 95*, 274–295.

Kim, J., Matthews, N. L., & Park, S. (2010). An event-related fMRI study of phonological verbal working memory in schizophrenia. *PLoS ONE, 5*(8), ArtID e12068.

Kimble, G. A. (1961). *Hilgard and Marquis' conditioning and learning* (2nd ed.). New York: Appleton-Century-Crofts.

King, G. D. (1974). Wheel running in the rat induced by a fixed-time presentation of water. *Animal Learning and Behavior, 2*, 325–328.

Kirkland, K., & Caughlin-Carvar, J. (1982). Maintenance and generalization of assertive skills. *Education & Training of the Mentally Retarded, 17*, 313–318.

Kirkpatrick, K., & Church, R. M. (2004). Temporal learning in random control procedures. *Journal of Experimental Psychology: Animal Behavior Processes, 30*, 213–228.

Kirkpatrick-Steger, K., Wasserman, E. A., & Biederman, I. (1996). Effects of spatial rearrangement of object components on picture recognition in pigeons. *Journal of the Experimental Analysis of Behavior, 65*, 465–475.

Klatt, K. P., & Morris, E. K. (2001). The Premack principle, response deprivation, and establishing operations. *The Behavior Analyst, 24*, 173–180.

Klein, M., Shapiro, E., & Kandel, E. R. (1980). Synaptic plasticity and the modulation of the calcium current. *Journal of Experimental Biology, 89*, 117–157.

Knight, D. C., Waters, N. S., King, M. K., & Bandettini, P. A. (2010). Learning-related diminution of unconditioned SCR and fMRI signal responses. *NeuroImage, 49*, 843–848.

Knowlton, B. J., & Thompson, R. F. (1992). Conditioning using a cerebral cortical conditioned stimulus is dependent on the cerebellum and brain stem circuitry. *Behavioral Neuroscience, 106*, 509–517.

Kohler, W. (1939). Simple structural function in the chimpanzee and the chicken. In W. D. Ellis (Ed.), *A source book of gestalt psychology*. New York: Harcourt Brace, 217–227.

Kokaia, Z., & Lindvall, O. (2003). Neurogenesis after ischaemic brain insults. *Current Opinion in Neurobiology, 13,* 127–132.

Kolb, B., & Gibb, R. (2008). Principles of neuroplasticity and behavior. In D. T. Stuss, G. Winocur, I. H. Robertson, D. T. Stuss, G. Winocur, & I. H. Robertson (Eds.), *Cognitive neurorehabilitation: Evidence and application* (2nd ed., pp. 6–21). New York: Cambridge University Press.

Konarski, E. A. (1987). Effects of response deprivation on the instrumental performance of mentally retarded persons. *American Journal of Mental Deficiency, 91,* 537–542.

Konen, C. S., & Kastner, S. (2008). Two hierarchically organized neural systems for object information in human visual cortex. *Nature Neuroscience, 11,* 224–231.

Konorski, J. (1948). *Conditioned reflexes and neuron organization*. New York: Cambridge University Press.

Konorski, J. (1967). *Integrative activity of the brain: An interdisciplinary approach*. Chicago, IL: University of Chicago Press.

Konorski, J., & Miller, S. (1937). On two types of conditioned reflex. *Journal of Genetic Psychology, 16,* 264–272.

Koob, G. F., Caine, S. B., Parsons, L., Markou, A., & Weiss, F. (1997). Opponent process model and psychostimulant addiction. *Pharmacology, Biochemistry and Behavior, 57,* 513–521.

Koob, G. F., & Le Moal, M. (2006). *Neurobiology of addiction*. Amsterdam, Netherlands: Elsevier.

Koob, G. F., & Le Moal, M. (2008). Addiction and the brain antireward system. *Annual Review of Psychology, 59,* 29–53.

Kornell, N. (2009). Metacognition in humans and animals. *Current Directions in Psychological Science, 18,* 11–15.

Kosugi, D., Ishida, H., Murai, C., & Fujita, K. (2009). Nine- to 11-month-old infants' reasoning about causality in anomalous human movements. *Japanese Psychological Research, 51,* 246–257.

Koychev, I., El-Deredy, W., Haenschel, C., & Deakin, J. F. W. (2010). Visual information processing deficits as biomarkers of vulnerability to schizophrenia: An event-related potential study in schizotypy. *Neuropsychologia, 48,* 2205–2214.

Krcmar, M., Farrar, K., & McGloin, R. (2011). The effects of video game realism on attention, retention and aggressive outcomes. *Computers in Human Behavior, 27,* 432–439.

Krebs, J. R., & Davies, N. B. (Eds.). (1978). *Behavioral ecology: An evolutionary approach*. Sunderland, MA: Sinauer.

Kremer, E. F. (1978). The Rescorla-Wagner model: Losses in associative strength in compound conditioned stimuli. *Journal of Experimental Psychology: Animal Behavior Processes, 4,* 22–36.

Kuo, Z. Y. (1921). Giving up instincts in psychology. *Journal of Philosophy, 18,* 645–664.

Kushner, M. (1968). The operant control of intractable sneezing. In C. D. Spielberger, R. Fox, & D. Masterson (Eds.), *Contributions to general psychology*. New York: Ronald Press, 326–365.

Kymissis, E., & Poulson, C. L. (1990). The history of imitation in learning theory: The language acquisition process. *Journal of the Experimental Analysis of Behavior, 54,* 113–127.

Kymissis, E., & Poulson, C. L. (1994). Generalized imitation in preschool boys. *Journal of Experimental Child Psychology, 58,* 389–404.

Kyonka, E. G. E., & Grace, R. C. (2010). Rapid acquisition of choice and timing and the provenance of the terminal-link effect. *Journal of the Experimental Analysis of Behavior, 94,* 209–225.

LaBrie, J. W., Migliuri, S., Kenney, S. R., & Lac, A. (2010). Family history of alcohol abuse associated with problematic drinking among college students. *Addictive Behaviors, 35,* 721–725.

Lalli, J. S., Livezey, K., & Kates, K. (1996). Functional analysis and treatment of eye poking with response blocking. *Journal of Applied Behavior Analysis, 29,* 129–132.

Lamb, R. J., Morral, A. R., Kirby, K. C., Iguchi, M. Y., & Galbicka, G. (2004). Shaping smoking cessation using percentile schedules. *Drug and Alcohol Dependence, 76,* 247–259.

Lane, I. M., Wesolowski, M. D., & Burke, W. H. (1989). Teaching socially appropriate behavior to eliminate hoarding in a brain-injured adult. *Journal of Behavior Therapy and Experimental Psychiatry, 20,* 79–82.

Lashley, K. S. (1917). The accuracy of movement in the absence of excitation from the moving organ. *American Journal of Physiology, 43,* 169–194.

Lashley, K. S. (1950). In search of the engram: Physiological mechanisms in animal behavior. In J. F. Danielli & R. Brown (Eds.), *Symposium of the Society for Experimental Biology.* Cambridge, MA: Cambridge University Press, 454–482.

Lashley, K. S. (1951). The problem of serial order in behavior. In L. A. Jeffress (Ed.), *Cerebral mechanisms in behavior.* New York: Wiley, 112–146.

Lashley, K. S., & Wade, M. (1946). The Pavlovian theory of generalization. *Psychological Review, 53,* 72–87.

Latash, M. L. (1999). Mirror writing: Learning, transfer, and implications for internal inverse models. *Journal of Motor Behavior, 31,* 107–111.

Lau, B., & Glimcher, P. W. (2005). Dynamic response-by-response models of matching behavior in rhesus monkeys. *Journal of the Experimental Analysis of Behavior, 84,* 555–579.

Laucht, M., Esser, G., & Schmidt, M. H. (1994). Contrasting infant predictors of later cognitive functioning. *Journal of Child Psychology and Psychiatry and Allied Disciplines, 35,* 649–662.

Lawrence, D. H., & DeRivera, J. (1954). Evidence for relational transposition. *Journal of Comparative and Physiological Psychology, 47,* 465–471.

Lazareva, O. F., Miner, M., Wasserman, E. A., & Young, M. E. (2008). Multiple-pair training enhances transposition in pigeons. *Learning and Behavior, 36,* 174–187.

Lazareva, O. F., & Wasserman, E. A. (2010). Category learning and concept learning in birds. In D. Mareschal, P. C. Quinn, & S. G. Lea (Eds.), *The making of human concepts* (pp. 151–172). New York: Oxford University Press.

Lazareva, O. F., Wasserman, E. A., & Young, M. E. (2005). Transposition in pigeons: Reassessing Spence (1937) with multiple discrimination training. *Learning and Behavior, 33,* 22–46.

Leader, G., Loughnane, A., McMoreland, C., & Reed, P. (2009). The effect of stimulus salience on overselectivity. *Journal of Autism and Developmental Disorders, 39,* 330–338.

Leal, D. R. (1998). Community-run fisheries: Avoiding the "tragedy of the commons." *Population and Environment: A Journal of Interdisciplinary Studies, 19,* 225–245.

Leander, J. D., Lippman, L. G., & Meyer, M. E. (1968). Fixed interval performance as related to subject's verbalization of the reinforcement contingency. *Psychological Record, 18,* 469–474.

Lee, B. S. (1950). Effects of delayed speech feedback. *Journal of the Acoustical Society of America, 22,* 824–826.

Lee, V. L. (1996). Superstitious location changes by human beings. *Psychological Record, 46,* 71–86.

Lefkowitz, M., Blake, R. R., & Mouton, J. S. (1955). Status factors in pedestrian violation of traffic signals. *Journal of Abnormal and Social Psychology, 51,* 704–706.

Lefkowitz, M. M., Huesmann, L. R., & Eron, L. D. (1978). Parental punishment: A longitudinal analysis of effect. *Archives of General Psychiatry, 35,* 186–191.

LeFrancois, J. R., & Metzger, B. (1993). Low-response-rate conditioning history and fixed-interval responding in rats. *Journal of the Experimental Analysis of Behavior, 59,* 543–549.

LeGray, M. W., Dufrene, B. H., Sterling-Turner, H., Olmi, D. J., & Bellone, K. (2010). A comparison of function-based differential reinforcement interventions for children engaging in disruptive classroom behavior. *Journal of Behavioral Education, 19,* 185–204.

Leknes, S., Brooks, J. C. W., Wiech, K., & Tracey, I. (2008). Pain relief as an opponent process: A psychophysical investigation. *European Journal of Neuroscience, 28,* 794–801.

Lemere, F., & Voegtlin, W. L. (1950). An evaluation of the aversion treatment of alcoholism. *Quarterly Journal of Studies on Alcohol, 11,* 199–204.

Lemere, F., Voegtlin, W. L., Broz, W. R., O'Hallaren, P., & Tupper, W. E. (1942). The conditioned reflex treatment of chronic alcoholism: VIII. A review of six years' experience with this treatment of 1526 patients. *Journal of the American Medical Association, 120,* 269–270.

Lenneberg, E. H. (1967). *Biological foundations of language.* New York: Wiley.

Lerch, J. P., Yiu, A. P., Martinez-Canabal, A., Pekar, T., Bohbot, V. D., Frankland, P. W., et al. (2011). Maze training in mice induces MRI-detectable brain shape changes specific to the type of learning. *NeuroImage, 54,* 2086–2095.

Lerman, D. C., Iwata, B. A., Shore, B. A., & DeLeon, I. G. (1997). Effects of intermittent punishment on self-injurious behavior: An evaluation of schedule thinning. *Journal of Applied Behavior Analysis, 30,* 198–201.

Lerman, D. C., & Vorndran, C. M. (2002). On the status of knowledge for using punishment: Implications for treating behavior disorders. *Journal of Applied Behavior Analysis, 35,* 431–464.

Lett, B. T. (1973). Delayed reward learning: Disproof of the traditional theory. *Learning and Motivation, 4,* 237–246.

Lett, B. T. (1979). Long-delay learning: Implications for learning and memory theory. In N. S. Sutherland (Ed.), *Tutorial essays in psychology* (Vol. 2). Hillsdale, NJ: Erlbaum, 1–38.

Leuner, B., & Gould, E. (2010). Structural plasticity and hippocampal function. *Annual Review of Psychology, 61,* 111–140.

Levis, D. J. (1989). The case for a return to a two-factor theory of avoidance: The failure of non-fear interpretations. In S. B. Klein & R. R. Mowrer (Eds.), *Contemporary learning theories: Pavlovian conditioning and the status of traditional learning theory.* Hillsdale, NJ: Erlbaum, 227–277.

Lewis, D., McAllister, D. E., & Adams, J. A. (1951). Facilitation and interference in performance on the modified Mashburn apparatus: I. The effects of varying the amount of original learning. *Journal of Experimental Psychology, 41,* 247–260.

Lewis, M. C., & Gould, T. J. (2007). Reversible inactivation of the entorhinal cortex disrupts the establishment and expression of latent inhibition of cued fear conditioning in C57BL/6 mice. *Hippocampus, 17,* 462–470.

Lieving, G. A., & Lattal, K. A. (2003). Recency, repeatability, and reinforcer retrenchment: An experimental analysis of resurgence. *Journal of the Experimental Analysis of Behavior, 80,* 217–233.

Linden, M., Habib, T., & Radojevic, V. (1996). A controlled study of the effects of EEG biofeedback on cognition and behavior of children with attention deficit disorder and learning disabilities. *Biofeedback and Self-Regulation, 21,* 35–49.

Linebarger, D. L., & Walker, D. (2005). Infants' and toddlers' television viewing and language outcomes. *American Behavioral Scientist, 48,* 624–645.

Liszkowski, U., Schäfer, M., Carpenter, M., & Tomasello, M. (2009). Prelinguistic infants, but not chimpanzees, communicate about absent entities. *Psychological Science, 20,* 654–660.

Little, K. D., Lubar, J. F., & Cannon, R. (2010). Neurofeedback: Research-based treatment for ADHD. In R. A. Carlstedt & R. A. Carlstedt (Eds.), *Handbook of integrative clinical psychology, psychiatry, and behavioral medicine: Perspectives, practices, and research* (pp. 807–821). New York: Springer.

Liu, S. S., Differential conditioning and stimulus generalization of the rabbit's nictitating membrane response. *Journal of Comparative and Physiological Psychology, 77,* 136–141

LoBue, V., & DeLoache, J. S. (2008). Detecting the snake in the grass: Attention to fear-relevant stimuli by adults and young children. *Psychological Science, 19,* 284–289.

Lochbaum, M. R. (1999). Affective and cognitive performance due to exercise training: An examination of individual difference variables. *Dissertation Abstracts International: Section B: The Sciences and Engineering, 59*(10-B), 5611.

Lockard, R. B. (1971). Reflections on the fall of comparative psychology: Is there a message for us all? *American Psychologist, 26,* 168–179.

Locke, J. (1690). *An essay concerning humane understanding: In four books.* London: Thomas Bassett.

Locurto, C. M., Terrace, H. S., & Gibbon, J. (Eds.). (1981). *Autoshaping and conditioning theory.* New York: Academic Press.

Loeb, J. (1900). *Comparative physiology of the brain and comparative psychology.* New York: Putnam's.

Logue, A. W. (1979). Taste aversion and the generality of the laws of learning. *Psychological Bulletin, 86,* 276–296.

Logue, A. W. (1988). A comparison of taste-aversion learning in humans and other vertebrates: Evolutionary pressures in common. In R. C. Bolles & M. D. Beecher (Eds.), *Evolution and learning.* Hillsdale, NJ: Erlbaum, 97–116.

Logue, A. W., Ophir, I., & Strauss, K. E. (1981). The acquisition of taste aversions in humans. *Behavior Research and Therapy, 19,* 319–333.

Longstaff, M. G., & Heath, R. A. (1997). Space-time invariance in adult handwriting. *Acta Psychologica, 97,* 201–214.

Lovaas, O. I. (1967). A behavior therapy approach to the treatment of childhood schizophrenia. In J. P. Hill (Ed.), *Minnesota symposium on child psychology.* Minneapolis, MN: University of Minnesota Press, 108–159.

Lovaas, O. I. (1977). *The autistic child.* New York: Wiley.

Lovaas, O. I. (1987). Behavioral treatment and normal educational and intellectual functioning in young autistic children. *Journal of Consulting and Clinical Psychology, 55,* 3–9.

Lovaas, O. I., Freitag, L., Nelson, K., & Whalen, C. (1967). The establishment of imitation and its use for the development of complex behavior in schizophrenic children. *Behavior Research and Therapy, 5,* 171–181.

Love, S. R., Matson, J. L., & West, D. (1990). Mothers as effective therapists for autistic children's phobias. *Journal of Applied Behavior Analysis, 23,* 379–385.

Lovibond, P. F. (2006). Fear and avoidance: An integrated expectancy model. In M. G. Craske, D. Hermans, & D. Vansteewegen (Eds.), *Fear and learning: Basic science to clinical application* (pp. 117–132). Washington, DC: American Psychological Association.

Lowe, C. F. (1979). Determinants of human operant behaviour. In M. D. Zeiler & P. Harzem (Eds.), *Advances in the analysis of behaviour: Vol. 1. Reinforcement and the organization of behaviour.* Chichester, England: Wiley, 159–192.

Lowe, C. F., Beasty, A., & Bentall, R. P. (1983). The role of verbal behavior in human learning: Infant performance on fixed-interval schedules. *Journal of the Experimental Analysis of Behavior, 39,* 157–164.

Lowe, C. F., Harzem, P., & Bagshaw, M. (1978). Species differences in the temporal control of behavior: Human performance. *Journal of the Experimental Analysis of Behavior, 29,* 351–361.

Loy, I., & Hall, G. (2002). Taste aversion after ingestion of lithium chloride: An associative analysis. *Quarterly Journal of Experimental Psychology B: Comparative and Physiological Psychology, 55B,* 365–380.

Lubow, R. E. (1974). High-order concept formation in the pigeon. *Journal of the Experimental Analysis of Behavior, 21,* 475–483.

Lubow, R. E. (2009). Conditioned taste aversion and latent inhibition: A review. In T. R. Schachtman & S. Reilly (Eds.), *Conditioned taste aversion: Behavioral and neural processes* (pp. 37–57). New York: Oxford University Press.

Lubow, R. E., & Moore, A. U. (1959). Latent inhibition: The effect of nonreinforced preexposure to the conditional stimulus. *Journal of Comparative and Physiological Psychology, 52,* 415–419.

Lucas, G. A., Deich, J. D., & Wasserman, E. A. (1981). Trace autoshaping: Acquisition, maintenance, and path dependence at long trace intervals. *Journal of the Experimental Analysis of Behavior, 36,* 61–74.

Lucchelli, F., Muggia, S., & Spinnler, H. (1997). Selective proper name anomia: A case involving only contemporary celebrities. *Cognitive Neuropsychology, 14,* 881–900.

MacCorquodale, K., & Meehl, P. E. (1954). Edward C. Tolman. In W. K. Estes, S. Koch, K. MacCorquodale, P. Meehl, C. G. Mueller, Jr., W. N. Schoenfeld, & W. S. Verplanck (Eds.), *Modern learning theory*. New York: Appleton-Century-Crofts, 177–266.

MacDonall, J. S., Goodell, J., & Juliano, A. (2006). Momentary maximizing and optimal foraging theories of performance on concurrent VR schedules. *Behavioural Processes, 72,* 283–299.

Machado, A., & Arantes, J. (2006). Further tests of the Scalar Expectancy Theory (SET) and the Learning-to-Time (LeT) model in a temporal bisection task. *Behavioural Processes, 72,* 195–206.

Machado, A., Malheiro, M. T., & Erlhagen, W. (2009). Learning to time: A perspective. *Journal of the Experimental Analysis of Behavior, 92,* 423–458.

Machado, A., & Rodrigues, P. (2007). The differentiation of response numerosities in the pigeon. *Journal of the Experimental Analysis of Behavior, 88,* 153–178.

Mackintosh, N. J. (1975). A theory of attention: Variations in the associability of stimuli with reinforcement. *Psychological Review, 82,* 276–298.

Mackintosh, N. J., & Dickinson, A. (1979). Instrumental (Type II) conditioning. In A. Dickinson & R. A. Boakes (Eds.), *Mechanisms of learning and motivation*. Hillsdale, NJ: Erlbaum, 143–169.

Macnish, R. (1859). *The anatomy of drunkenness*. Glasgow, Scotland: W. R. McPuhn.

Madden, G. J., Smethells, J. R., Ewan, E. E., & Hursh, S. R. (2007). Tests of behavioral-economic assessments of relative reinforcer efficacy: Economic substitutes. *Journal of the Experimental Analysis of Behavior, 87,* 219–240.

Maes, J. R., & Vossen, J. M. (1993). Competition between contextual and punctate stimuli for inhibitory control in a Pavlovian discrimination procedure. *Learning and Motivation, 24,* 194–218.

Maier, S. F., & Seligman, M. E. P. (1976). Learned helplessness: Theory and evidence. *Journal of Experimental Psychology: General, 105,* 3–46.

Maki, W. S., & Hegvik, D. K. (1980). Directed forgetting in pigeons. *Animal Learning and Behavior, 8,* 567–574.

Malagodi, E. F. (1967). Fixed-ratio schedules of token reinforcement. *Psychonomic Science, 8,* 469–470.

Malott, M. K. (1968). Stimulus control in stimulus-deprived chickens. *Journal of Comparative and Physiological Psychology, 66,* 276–282.

Manabe, K., Murata, M., Kawashima, T., Asahina, K., & Okutsu, K. (2009). Transposition of line-length discrimination in African penguins (*Spheniscus demersus*). *Japanese Psychological Research, 51,* 115–121.

March, J. G., & Shapira, Z. (1992). Variable risk preferences and the focus of attention. *Psychological Review, 99,* 172–183.

Marcus, A., & Wilder, D. A. (2009). A comparison of peer video modeling and self video modeling to teach textual responses in children with autism. *Journal of Applied Behavior Analysis, 42,* 335–341.

Marcus, B. A., Swanson, V., & Vollmer, T. R. (2001). Effects of parent training on parent and child behavior using procedures based on functional analyses. *Behavioral Interventions, 16,* 87–104.

Marks, I. M., & Gelder, M. (1967). Transvestism and fetishism: Clinical and psychological changes during faradic aversion. *British Journal of Psychiatry, 113,* 711–739.

Marsh, H. L., & MacDonald, S. E. (2008). The use of perceptual features in categorization by orangutans (*Pongo abelli*). *Animal Cognition, 11,* 569–585.

Marshall, W. L. (2006). Ammonia aversion with an exhibitionist: A case study. *Clinical Case Studies, 5,* 15–24.

Martens, B. K., & Houk, J. L. (1989). The application of Herrnstein's law of effect to disruptive and on-task behavior of a retarded adolescent girl. *Journal of the Experimental Analysis of Behavior, 51,* 17–27.

Martin, G. (1998). Media influence to suicide: The search for solutions. *Archives of Suicide Research, 4,* 51–66.

Martin, G., & Pear, J. (2010). *Behavior modification: What it is and how to do it* (9th ed.). Upper Saddle River, NJ: Prentice Hall.

Maslovat, D., Brunke, K. M., Chua, R., & Franks, I. M. (2009). Feedback effects on learning a novel bimanual coordination pattern: Support for the Guidance Hypothesis. *Journal of Motor Behavior, 41,* 45–54.

Maslovat, D., Hodges, N. J., Krigolson, O. E., & Handy, T. C. (2010). Observational practice benefits are limited to perceptual improvements in the acquisition of a novel coordination skill. *Experimental Brain Research, 204,* 119–130.

Matson, J. L., & Duncan, D. (1997). Aggression. In N. N. Singh (Ed.), *Prevention and treatment of severe behavior problems: Models and methods in developmental disabilities*. Pacific Grove, CA: Brooks/Cole, 217–236.

Matsuzawa, T. (1985). Use of numbers by a chimpanzee. *Nature, 315,* 57–59.

Matthews, B. A., Catania, A. C., & Shimoff, E. (1985). Effects of uninstructed verbal responding on nonverbal responding: Contingency descriptions versus performance descriptions. *Journal of the Experimental Analysis of Behavior, 43,* 155–164.

Matthews, B. A., Shimoff, E., Catania, A. C., & Sagvolden, T. (1977). Uninstructed human responding: Sensitivity to ratio and interval contingencies. *Journal of the Experimental Analysis of Behavior, 27,* 453–467.

Matute, H. (1994). Learned helplessness and superstitious behavior as opposite effects of uncontrollable reinforcement in humans. *Learning and Motivation, 25,* 216–232.

Matute, H. (1995). Human reactions to uncontrollable outcomes: Further evidence for superstitions rather than helplessness. *Quarterly Journal of Experimental Psychology. B: Comparative and Physiological Psychology, 48B,* 142–157.

Matzel, L. D., Brown, A. M., & Miller, R. R. (1987). Associative effects of US preexposure: Modulation of conditioned responding by an excitatory training context. *Journal of Experimental Psychology: Animal Behavior Processes, 13,* 65–72.

Matzel, L. D., Held, F. P., & Miller, R. R. (1988). Information and expression of simultaneous and backward associations: Implications for contiguity theory. *Learning and Motivation, 19,* 317–344.

Mawhinney, V. T., Bostow, D. E., Laws, D. R., Blumenfeld, G. J., & Hopkins, B. L. (1971). A comparison of students studying-behavior produced by daily, weekly, and three-week testing schedules. *Journal of Applied Behavior Analysis, 4,* 257–264.

Mazmanian, D. S., & Roberts, W. A. (1983). Spatial memory in rats under restricted viewing conditions. *Learning and Motivation, 14,* 123–139.

Mazur, J. E. (1975). The matching law and quantifications related to Premack's principle. *Journal of Experimental Psychology: Animal Behavior Processes, 1,* 374–386.

Mazur, J. E. (1981). Optimization theory fails to predict performance of pigeons in a two-response situation. *Science, 214,* 823–825.

Mazur, J. E. (1983). Steady-state performance on fixed-, mixed-, and random-ratio schedules. *Journal of the Experimental Analysis of Behavior, 39,* 293–307.

McAfee, R. B., & Winn, A. R. (1989). The use of incentives/feedback to enhance workplace safety:

A critique of the literature. *Journal of Safety Research, 20,* 7–19.

McClelland, D. C. (1961). *The achieving society.* Princeton, NJ: Van Nostrand.

McCormick, D. A., & Thompson, R. F. (1984). Neuronal responses of the rabbit cerebellum during acquisition and performance of a classically conditioned nictitating membrane-eyelid response. *Journal of Neuroscience, 4,* 2811–2822.

McDevitt, M. A., & Williams, B. A. (2010). Dual effects on choice of conditioned reinforcement frequency and conditioned reinforcement value. *Journal of the Experimental Analysis of Behavior, 93,* 147–155.

McDonnell, J., & McFarland, S. (1988). A comparison of forward and concurrent chaining strategies in teaching laundromat skills to students with severe handicaps. *Research in Developmental Disabilities, 9,* 177–194.

McDougall, W. (1908). *An introduction to social psychology.* London: Methuen.

McDowell, J. J., & Caron, M. L. (2010). Matching in an undisturbed natural human environment. *Journal of the Experimental Analysis of Behavior, 93,* 415–433.

McEachin, J. J., Smith, T., & Lovaas, O. I. (1993). Long-term outcome for children with autism who received early intensive behavioral treatment. *American Journal of Mental Retardation, 97,* 359–372.

McEchron, M. D., Tseng, W., & Disterhoft, J. F. (2003). Single neurons in CA1 hippocampus encode trace interval duration during trace heart rate (fear) conditioning. *Journal of Neuroscience, 23,* 1535–1547.

McFarland, D. S. (1971). *Feedback mechanisms in animal behavior.* New York: Academic Press.

McGraw-Hunter, M. M., Faw, G. D., & Davis, P. K. (2006). The use of video self-modelling and feedback to teach cooking skills to individuals with traumatic brain injury: A pilot study. *Brain Injury, 20,* 1061–1068.

McIlvane, W. J., Kledaras, J. B., Iennaco, F. M., McDonald, S. J., & Stoddard, L. T. (1995). Some possible limits on errorless discrimination reversals in individuals with severe mental retardation. *American Journal of Mental Retardation, 99,* 430–436.

McKean, K. J. (1994). Academic helplessness: Applying learned helplessness theory to undergraduates who give up when faced with academic setbacks. *College Student Journal, 28,* 456–462.

McNally, G. P., & Westbrook, R. F. (2006). A short intertrial interval facilitates acquisition of context-conditioned fear and a short retention interval facilitates its expression. *Journal of Experimental Psychology: Animal Behavior Processes, 32,* 164–172.

McNamara, H. J., Long, J. B., & Wike, E. L. (1956). Learning without response under two conditions of external cues. *Journal of Comparative and Physiological Psychology, 49,* 477–480.

McSweeney, F. K., & Weatherly, J. N. (1998). Habituation to the reinforcer may contribute to multiple-schedule behavioral contrast. *Journal of the Experimental Analysis of Behavior, 69,* 199–221.

Mechner, F. (1958). Probability relations within response sequences under ratio reinforcement. *Journal of the Experimental Analysis of Behavior, 1,* 109–121.

Meehl, P. E. (1950). On the circularity of the law of effect. *Psychological Bulletin, 47,* 52–75.

Meichenbaum, D. H., & Goodman, J. (1971). Training impulsive children to talk to themselves: A means of developing self-control. *Journal of Abnormal Psychology, 77,* 115–126.

Meira, C. M., & Tani, G. (2001). The contextual interference effect in acquisition of dart-throwing skill tested on a transfer test with extended trials. *Perceptual and Motor Skills, 92,* 910–918.

Melchiori, L. E., de Souza, D. G., & de Rose, J. C. (2000). Reading, equivalence, and recombination of units: A replication with students with different learning histories. *Journal of Applied Behavior Analysis, 33,* 97–100.

Meltzoff, A. N. (2005). Imitation and other minds: The "lie me" hypothesis. In S. Hurley & N. Chater (Eds.), *Perspectives on imitation: From neuroscience to social science* (Vol. 2, pp. 1–52). London: MIT Press.

Meltzoff, A. N., & Moore, M. K. (1977). Imitation of facial and manual gestures by human neonates. *Science, 198,* 75–78.

Meltzoff, A. N., & Moore, M. K. (1983). Newborn infants imitate adult facial gestures. *Child Development, 54,* 702–709.

Merckelbach, H., Arntz, A., & de Jong, P. (1991). Conditioning experiences in spider phobics. *Behavioral Research and Therapy, 29,* 333–335.

Meuret, A. E., Wilhelm, F. H., & Roth, W. T. (2004). Respiratory feedback for treating panic disorder. *Journal of Clinical Psychology, 60,* 197–207.

Meyer, E. A., Hagopian, L. P., & Paclawskyj, T. R. (1999). A function-based treatment for school refusal behavior using shaping and fading. *Research in Developmental Disabilities, 20,* 401–410.

Middleton, M. B., & Cartledge, G. (1995). The effects of social skills instruction and parental involvement on the aggressive behaviors of African American males. *Behavior Modification, 19,* 192–210.

Miles, H. L. (1999). Symbolic communication with and by great apes. In S. Parker, R. W. Mitchell, & H. L. Miles (Eds.), *The mentalities of gorillas and orangutans: Comparative perspectives* (pp. 197–210). New York: Cambridge University Press.

Milgrom, P., Mancl, L., King, B., & Weinstein, P. (1995). Origins of childhood dental fear. *Behavior Research and Therapy, 33,* 313–319.

Mill, J. (1829). *Analysis of the phenomena of the human mind.* London: Baldwin & Cradock.

Mill, J. S. (1843). *A system of logic, ratiocinative and inductive, being a connected view of the principles of evidence, and the methods of scientific investigation.* London: J. W. Parker.

Miller, G. A. (1956). The magical number seven, plus or minus two. *Psychological Review, 63,* 81–97.

Miller, H. C., Rayburn-Reeves, R., & Zentall, T. R. (2009). What do dogs know about hidden objects? *Behavioural Processes, 81,* 439–446.

Miller, H. L. (1976). Matching-based hedonic scaling in the pigeon. *Journal of the Experimental Analysis of Behavior, 26,* 335–347.

Miller, J. S., Jagielo, J. A., & Spear, N. E. (1993). The influence of retention interval on the US preexposure effect: Changes in contextual blocking over time. *Learning and Motivation, 24,* 376–394.

Miller, N. E. (1948). Studies of fear as an acquirable drive: I. Fear as motivation and fear-reduction as reinforcement in the learning of new responses. *Journal of Experimental Psychology, 38,* 89–101.

Miller, N. E. (1951). Learnable drives and rewards. In S. S. Stevens (Ed.), *Handbook of experimental psychology.* New York: Wiley.

Miller, N. E. (1959). Liberalization of basic S-R concepts: Extensions to conflict behavior, motivation, and social learning. In S. Koch (Ed.), *Psychology: A study of a science* (Vol. 2). New York: McGraw-Hill, 196–292.

Miller, N. E. (1985). The value of behavioral research with animals. *American Psychologist, 40,* 423–440.

Miller, N. E., & DiCara, L. (1967). Instrumental learning of heart rate changes in curarized rats: Shaping, and specificity to discriminative stimulus. *Journal of Comparative and Physiological Psychology, 63,* 12–19.

Miller, N. E., & Dollard, J. (1941). *Social learning and imitation.* New Haven, CT: Yale University Press.

Miller, N. E., & Dworkin, B. R. (1974). Visceral learning: Recent difficulties with curarized rats and significant problems for human research. In P. A. Obrist, A. H. Black, J. Brener, & L. V. DiCara (Eds.), *Cardiovascular psychophysiology.* Chicago, IL: Aldine, 312–331.

Miller, R. R., & Schachtman, T. R. (1985). The several roles of context at the time of retrieval. In P. D. Balsam & A. Tomie (Eds.), *Context and learning*. Hillsdale, NJ: Erlbaum, 167–194.

Miller, R. R., & Spear, N. E. (Eds.). (1985). *Information processing in animals: Conditioned inhibition*. Hillsdale, NJ: Erlbaum.

Miller, W. S., & Armus, H. L. (1999). Directed forgetting: Short-term memory or conditioned response? *Psychological Record, 49,* 211–220.

Millin, P. M., & Riccio, D. C. (2004). Is the context shift effect a case of retrieval failure? The effects of retrieval enhancing treatments on forgetting under altered stimulus conditions in rats. *Journal of Experimental Psychology: Animal Behavior Processes, 30,* 325–334.

Milmine, M., Watanabe, A., & Colombo, M. (2008). Neural correlates of directed forgetting in the avian prefrontal cortex. *Behavioral Neuroscience, 122,* 199–209.

Milo, J. S., Mace, F. C., & Nevin, J. A. (2010). The effects of constant versus varied reinforcers on preference and resistance to change. *Journal of the Experimental Analysis of Behavior, 93,* 385–394.

Miltenberger, R. G. (2011). *Behavior modification: Principles and procedures* (5th ed.). Pacific Grove, CA: Wadsworth.

Mineka, S., Davidson, M., Cook, M., & Kerr, R. (1984). Observational conditioning of snake fear in rhesus monkeys. *Journal of Abnormal Psychology, 93,* 355–372.

Mineka, S., & Sutton, J. (2006). Contemporary learning theory perspectives on the etiology of fears and phobias. In M. G. Craske, D. Hermans, D. Vansteenwegen, M. G. Craske, D. Hermans, & D. Vansteenwegen (Eds.), *Fear and learning: From basic processes to clinical implications* (pp. 75–97). Washington, DC: American Psychological Association.

Mintz, D. E., Mourer, D. J., & Gofseyeff, M. (1967). Sequential effects in fixed-ratio postreinforcement pause duration. *Psychonomic Science, 9,* 387–388.

Miranda, A., & Presentacion, M. J. (2000). Efficacy of cognitive-behavioral therapy in the treatment of children with ADHD, with and without aggressiveness. *Psychology in the Schools, 37,* 169–182.

Mischel, W. (1966). Theory and research on the antecedents of self-imposed delay of reward. *Progress in Experimental Personality Research, 3,* 85–132.

Mischel, W. (1981). Objective and subjective rules for delay of gratification. In G. D'Ydewalle & W. Lens (Eds.), *Cognition in human motivation and learning*. Hillsdale, NJ: Erlbaum, 33–58.

Mischel, W. (1983). Delay of gratification as process and as person variable in development. In D. Magnusson & V. L. Allen (Eds.), *Human development*. New York: Academic Press, 149–165.

Mischel, W., & Ebbesen, E. B. (1970). Attention in delay of gratification. *Journal of Personality and Social Psychology, 16,* 329–337.

Mischel, W., Ebbesen, E. B., & Zeiss, A. R. (1972). Cognitive and attentional mechanisms in delay of gratification. *Journal of Personality and Social Psychology, 21,* 204–218.

Mischel, W., Shoda, Y., & Rodriguez, M. L. (1989). Delay of gratification in children. *Science, 244,* 933–938.

Mitchell, C. J., Lovibond, P. F., Minard, E., & Lavis, Y. (2006). Forward blocking in human learning sometimes reflects the failure to encode a cue-outcome relationship. *Quarterly Journal of Experimental Psychology, 59,* 830–844.

Mitchell, S. H. (1999). Measures of impulsivity in cigarette smokers and non-smokers. *Psychopharmacology, 146,* 455–464.

Modaresi, H. A. (1990). The avoidance barpress problem: Effects of enhanced reinforcement and an SSDR-congruent lever. *Learning and Motivation, 21,* 199–220.

Molchan, S. E., Sunderland, T., McIntosh, A. R., Herscovitch, P., & Schreurs, B. G. (1994). A functional anatomical study of associative learning in humans. *Proceedings of the National*

Academy of Sciences United States of America, 91, 8122–8126.

Moon, J., & Lee, J. (2009). Cue exposure treatment in a virtual environment to reduce nicotine craving: A functional MRI study. *CyberPsychology & Behavior, 12,* 43–45.

Moore, B. R. (1973). The role of directed Pavlovian reactions in simple instrumental learning in the pigeon. In R. A. Hinde & J. Stevenson-Hinde (Eds.), *Constraints on learning.* New York: Academic Press, 159–188.

Moreno, J., Avila, F., Damas, J., Garcia, J. A., Luis, V., Reina, R., et al. (2003). Contextual interference in learning precision skills. *Perceptual and Motor Skills, 97,* 121–128.

Morgan, C. L. (1894). *An introduction to comparative psychology.* London: W. Scott.

Morgan, C. L. (1896). *Habit and instinct.* London: E. Arnold.

Morganstern, K. P. (1973). Implosive therapy and flooding procedures: A critical review. *Psychological Bulletin, 79,* 318–334.

Mowrer, O. H. (1947). On the dual nature of learning—a reinterpretation of "conditioning" and "problem solving." *Harvard Educational Review, 17,* 102–148.

Mowrer, O. H., & Jones, H. (1945). Habit strength as a function of the pattern of reinforcement. *Journal of Experimental Psychology, 35,* 293–311.

Mowrer, O. H., & Mowrer, W. M. (1938). Enuresis: A method for its study and treatment. *American Journal of Orthopsychiatry, 8,* 436–459.

Mueller, M. M., & Palkovic, C. M. (2007). Errorless learning: Review and practical application for teaching children with pervasive developmental disorders. *Psychology in the Schools, 44,* 691–700.

Mulder, T., & Hulstijn, W. (1985a). Delayed sensory feedback in the learning of a novel motor task. *Psychological Research, 47,* 203–209.

Mulder, T., & Hulstijn, W. (1985b). Sensory feedback in the learning of a novel motor task. *Journal of Motor Behavior, 17,* 110–128.

Mulick, J. A., & Butler, E. M. (2002). Educational advocacy for children with autism. *Behavioral Interventions, 17,* 57–74.

Muller, M. D., & Fountain, S. B. (2010). Concurrent cognitive processes in rat serial pattern learning: Item memory, serial position, and pattern structure. *Learning and Motivation, 41,* 252–272.

Murphy, J. G., MacKillop, J., Skidmore, J. R., & Pederson, A. A. (2009). Reliability and validity of a demand curve measure of alcohol reinforcement. *Experimental and Clinical Psychopharmacology, 17,* 396–404.

Murray, J. P. (2008). Media violence: The effects are both real and strong. *American Behavioral Scientist, 51,* 1212–1230.

Myers, D. L., & Myers, L. E. (1977). Undermatching: A reappraisal of performance on concurrent variable-interval schedules of reinforcement. *Journal of the Experimental Analysis of Behavior, 27,* 203–214.

Nabeyama, B., & Sturmey, P. (2010). Using behavioral skills training to promote safe and correct staff guarding and ambulation distance of students with multiple physical disabilities. *Journal of Applied Behavior Analysis, 43,* 341–345.

Nagaishi, T., & Nakajima, S. (2010). Overshadowing of running-based taste aversion learning by another taste cue. *Behavioural Processes, 83,* 134–136.

Nagin, D. S., & Pogarsky, G. (2004). Time and punishment: Delayed consequences and criminal behavior. *Journal of Quantitative Criminology, 20,* 295–317.

Nakagawa, E. (1999). Acquired equivalence of discriminative stimuli following two concurrent discrimination learning tasks as a function of overtraining in rats. *Psychological Record, 49,* 327–348.

Nakao, M., Nomura, S., Shimosawa, T., Fujita, T., & Kuboki, T. (2000). Blood pressure biofeed-back treatment of white-coat hypertension. *Journal of Psychosomatic Research, 48,* 161–169.

Navakatikyan, M. A. (2007). A model for residence time in concurrent variable interval performance.

Journal of the Experimental Analysis of Behavior, 87(1), 121–141.

Navakatikyan, M. A., & Davison, M. (2010). The dynamics of the law of effect: A comparison of models. *Journal of the Experimental Analysis of Behavior, 93,* 91–127.

Neef, N. A., Bill-Harvey, D., Shade, D., Iezzi, M., & DeLorenzo, T. (1995). Exercise participation with videotaped modeling: Effects on balance and gait in elderly residents of care facilities. *Behavior Therapy, 26,* 135–151.

Neef, N. A., Mace, F. C., Shea, M. C., & Shade, D. (1992). Effects of reinforcer rate and reinforcer quality on time allocation: Extensions of matching theory to educational settings. *Journal of Applied Behavior Analysis, 25,* 691–699.

Neef, N. A., Shade, D., & Miller, M. S. (1994). Assessing influential dimensions of reinforcers on choice in students with serious emotional disturbances. *Journal of Applied Behavior Analysis, 27,* 575–583.

Nestoriuc, Y., & Martin, A. (2007). Efficacy of biofeedback for migraine: A meta-analysis. *Pain, 128,* 111–127.

Nestoriuc, Y., Martin, A., Rief, W., & Andrasik, F. (2008). Biofeedback treatment for headache disorders: A comprehensive efficacy review. *Applied Psychophysiology and Biofeedback, 33,* 125–140.

Neuman, S. B. (1988). The displacement effect: Assessing the relation between television viewing and reading performance. *Reading Research Quarterly, 23,* 414–440.

Neuringer, A. J. (1970). Superstitious key pecking after three peck-produced reinforcements. *Journal of the Experimental Analysis of Behavior, 13,* 127–134.

Nevin, J. A. (1969). Interval reinforcement of choice behavior in discrete trials. *Journal of the Experimental Analysis of Behavior, 12,* 875–885.

Nevin, J. A. (1974). Response strength in multiple schedules. *Journal of the Experimental Analysis of Behavior, 21,* 389–408.

Nevin, J. A. (1979). Overall matching versus momentary maximizing: Nevin (1969) revisited. *Journal of Experimental Psychology: Animal Behavior Processes, 5,* 300–306.

Nevin, J. A. (1992). An integrative model for the study of behavioral momentum. *Journal of the Experimental Analysis of Behavior, 57,* 301–316.

Nevin, J. A. (1998). Choice and behavior momentum. In W. O'Donohue (Ed.), *Learning and behavior therapy.* New York: Allyn & Bacon, 230–251.

Nevin, J. A., & Grace, R. C. (2000). Behavioral momentum and the law of effect. *Behavioral and Brain Sciences, 23,* 73–130.

Newell, K. M. (1974). Knowledge of results and motor learning. *Journal of Motor Behavior, 6,* 235–244.

Newton, T. F., Kalechstein, A. D., Tervo, K. E., & Ling, W. (2003). Irritability following abstinence from cocaine predicts euphoric effects of cocaine administration. *Addictive Behaviors, 28,* 817–821.

Nicholas, J. M. (1984). Lessons from the history of science. *Behavioral and Brain Sciences, 7,* 530–531.

Nichols, D. F., Betts, L. R., & Wilson, H. R. (2010). Decoding of faces and face components in face-sensitive human visual cortex. *Frontiers in Perception Science, 1*(29), 1–13.

Nikopoulous, C. K., & Keenan, M. (2004). Effects of video modeling on social initiations by children with autism. *Journal of Applied Behavior Analysis, 37,* 93–96.

North, M. M., North, S. M., & Coble, J. R. (2002). Virtual reality therapy: An effective treatment for psychological disorders. In K. M. Stanney (Ed.), *Handbook of virtual environments: Design, implementation, and applications.* Mahwah, NJ: Erlbaum, 1065–1078.

Nottebohm, F. (1970). The ontogeny of birdsong. *Science, 167,* 950–956.

Nower, L., & Blaszczynski, A. (2010). Gambling motivations, money-limiting strategies, and precommitment preferences of problem versus non-problem gamblers. *Journal of Gambling Studies, 26,* 361–372.

Oberman, L. M., & Ramachandran, V. S. (2009). Reflections on the mirror neuron system: Their evolutionary functions beyond motor representation. In J. A. Pineda (Ed.), *Mirror neuron systems: The role of mirroring processes in social cognition* (pp. 39–59). Totowa, NJ: Humana Press.

O'Connor, R. D. (1969). Modification of social withdrawal through symbolic modeling. *Journal of Applied Behavior Analysis, 2,* 15–22.

Odum, A. L., & Baumann, A. L. (2010). Delay discounting: State and trait variable. In G. J. Madden & W. K. Bickel (Eds.), *Impulsivity: The behavioral and neurological science of discounting* (pp. 39–65). Washington, DC: American Psychological Association.

Odum, A. L., & Rainaud, C. P. (2003). Discounting of delayed hypothetical money, alcohol, and food. *Behavioural Processes, 64,* 305–313.

Öhman, A., Dimberg, U., & Ost, L. G. (1985). Animal and social phobias: Biological constraints on learned fear responses. In S. Reiss & R. R. Bootzin (Eds.), *Theoretical issues in behavior therapy.* New York: Academic Press, 123–178.

Öhman, A., Flykt, A., & Esteves, F. (2001). Emotion drives attention: Detecting the snake in the grass. *Journal of Experimental Psychology: General, 130,* 466–478.

Öhman, A., & Mineka, S. (2001). Fears, phobias, and preparedness: Toward an evolved module of fear and fear learning. *Psychological Review, 108,* 483–522.

Okouchi, H. (2003). Stimulus generalization of behavioral history. *Journal of the Experimental Analysis of Behavior, 80,* 173–186.

Okouchi, H., & Lattal, K. A. (2006). An analysis of reinforcement history effects. *Journal of the Experimental Analysis of Behavior, 86,* 31–42.

Olds, J., & Milner, P. (1954). Positive reinforcement produced by electrical stimulation of septal area and other regions of rat brain. *Journal of Comparative and Physiological Psychology, 47,* 419–427.

O'Leary, K. D., Kaufman, K. F., Kass, R. E., & Drabman, R. S. (1970). The effects of loud and soft reprimands on the behavior of disruptive students. *Exceptional Children, 37,* 145–155.

Oliveira-Castro, J. M. (2003). Effects of base price upon search behavior of consumers in a supermarket: An operant analysis. *Journal of Economic Psychology, 24,* 637–652.

Ollendick, T. H., & King, N. J. (1998). Empirically supported treatments for children with phobic and anxiety disorders: Current status. *Journal of Clinical Child Psychology, 27,* 156–167.

Oller, D. K., & Eilers, R. E. (1988). The role of audition in infant babbling. *Child Development, 59,* 441–449.

Olson, S. L., Bates, J. E., & Bayles, K. (1990). Early antecedents of childhood impulsivity: The role of parent-child interaction, cognitive competence, and temperament. *Journal of Abnormal Child Psychology, 18,* 317–334.

Olton, D. S. (1978). Characteristics of spatial memory. In S. H. Hulse, H. Fowler, & W. K. Honig (Eds.), *Cognitive processes in animal behavior.* Hillsdale, NJ: Erlbaum, 341–373.

Olton, D. S., Collison, C., & Werz, W. A. (1977). Spatial memory and radial arm maze performance by rats. *Learning and Motivation, 8,* 289–314.

Osgood, C. E. (1949). The similarity paradox in human learning: A resolution. *Psychological Review, 56,* 132–143.

Pace, G. M., Iwata, B. A., Cowdery, G. E., Andree, P. J., & McIntyre, T. (1993). Stimulus (instructional) fading during extinction of self-injurious escape behavior. *Journal of Applied Behavior Analysis, 26,* 205–212.

Packer, J. S., Clark, B. M., Bond, N. W., & Siddle, D. A. (1991). Conditioning with facial expression of emotion: A comparison of aversive and non-aversive unconditioned stimuli. *Journal of Psychophysiology, 5,* 79–88.

Page, H. A., & Hall, J. F. (1953). Experimental extinction as a function of the prevention of a response. *Journal of Comparative and Physiological Psychology, 46,* 33–34.

Paletta, M. S., & Wagner, A. R. (1986). Development of context-specific tolerance to morphine: Support for a dual-process interpretation. *Behavioral Neuroscience, 100,* 611–623.

Palmer, C., & Meyer, R. K. (2000). Conceptual and motor learning in music performance. *Psychological Science, 11,* 63–68.

Palya, W. L., & Allan, R. W. (2003). Dynamical concurrent schedules. *Journal of the Experimental Analysis of Behavior, 79,* 1–20.

Papastergiou, M. (2009). Exploring the potential of computer and video games for health and physical education: A literature review. *Computers & Education, 53,* 603–622.

Patterson, F. G. (1978). The gestures of a gorilla: Language acquisition in another pongid. *Brain and Language, 5,* 72–97.

Patterson, F. G., & Linden, E. (1981). *The education of Koko.* New York: Holt, Rinehart & Winston.

Patterson, G. R., Chamberlain, P., & Reid, J. B. (1982). A comparative evaluation of a parent-training program. *Behavior Therapy, 13,* 638–650.

Paul, E. F., & Paul, J. (Eds.). (2001). *Why animal experimentation matters: The use of animals in medical research.* New Brunswick, NJ: Transaction Publishers.

Paul, G. L. (1969). Outcome of systematic desensitization: II. Controlled investigations of individual treatment, technique variations, and current status. In C. M. Franks (Ed.), *Behavior therapy: Appraisal and status.* New York: McGraw-Hill, 105–159.

Paulsen, K., Rimm, D. C., Woodburn, L. T., & Rimm, S. (1977). A self-control approach to inefficient spending. *Journal of Consulting and Clinical Psychology, 45,* 433–435.

Pavlov, I. P. (1927). *Conditioned reflexes.* Oxford: Oxford University Press.

Pavlov, I. P. (1928). *Lectures on conditioned reflexes.* New York: International Publishers.

Pearce, J. M. (1989). The acquisition of an artificial category by pigeons. *Quarterly Journal of Experimental Psychology, 41B,* 381–406.

Pearce, J. M., & Hall, G. (1980). A model for Pavlovian learning: Variations in the effectiveness of conditioned but not unconditioned stimuli. *Psychological Review, 87,* 532–552.

Peissig, J. J., & Tarr, M. J. (2007). Visual object recognition: Do we know more now than we did 20 years ago. *Annual Review of Psychology, 58,* 75–96.

Penfield, W. (1959). The interpretive cortex. *Science, 129,* 1719–1725.

Pepperberg, I. M. (1987). Evidence for conceptual quantitative abilities in the African parrot: Labeling of cardinal sets. *Ethology, 75,* 37–61.

Pepperberg, I. M. (1999). *The Alex studies: Cognitive and communicative abilities of Grey parrots.* Cambridge, MA: Harvard University Press.

Pepperberg, I. M. (2010). Vocal learning in Grey parrots: A brief review of perception, production, and cross-species comparisons. *Brain and Language, 115,* 81–91.

Pepperberg, I. M., & Funk, M. S. (1990). Object permanence in four species of psittacine birds: An African Grey parrot (*Psittacus erithacus*), an Illiger mini macaw (*Ara maracana*), a parakeet (*Melopsittacus undulatus*), and a cockatiel (*Nymphicus hollandicus*). *Animal Learning and Behavior, 18,* 97–108.

Perrins, R., & Weiss, K. R. (1996). A cerebral central pattern generation in *Aplysia* and its connections with buccal feeding circuitry. *Journal of Neuroscience, 16,* 7030–7045.

Peterson, C., Maier, S. F., & Seligman, M. E. P. (1993). *Learned helplessness: A theory for the age of personal control.* New York: Oxford University Press.

Peterson, G. B., Ackil, J. E., Frommer, G. P., & Hearst, E. S. (1972). Conditioned approach and contact behavior towards signals for food or brain-stimulation reinforcement. *Science, 177,* 1009–1011.

Peterson, L. R., & Peterson, M. J. (1959). Short-term retention of individual verbal items. *Journal of Experimental Psychology, 58,* 193–198.

Petrinovich, L. F. (1999). *Darwinian dominion: Animal welfare and human interests.* Cambridge, MA: MIT Press.

Petscher, E. S., Rey, C., & Bailey, J. S. (2009). A review of empirical support for differential reinforcement of alternative behavior. *Research in Developmental Disabilities, 30,* 409–425.

Pfautz, P. L., Donegan, N. H., & Wagner, A. R. (1978). Sensory preconditioning versus protection from habituation. *Journal of Experimental Psychology: Animal Behavior Processes, 4,* 286–295.

Phillips, D. P. (1982). The impact of fictional television stories on U.S. adult fatalities: New evidence on the effect of the mass media on violence. *American Journal of Sociology, 87,* 1340–1359.

Phillips, E. L. (1968). Achievement place: Token reinforcement procedures in a home-style rehabilitation setting for "pre-delinquent" boys. *Journal of Applied Behavior Analysis, 1,* 213–223.

Phillips, R. G., & LeDoux, J. E. (1992). Differential contribution of amygdala and hippocampus to cued and contextual fear conditioning. *Behavioral Neuroscience, 106,* 274–285.

Piaget, J. (1926). *The language and thought of the child* (M. Gabain, Trans.). London: Routledge and Kegan Paul.

Piazza, C. C., Patel, M. R., Gulotta, C. S., Sevin, B. M., & Layer, S. A. (2003). On the relative contributions of positive reinforcement and escape extinction in the treatment of food refusal. *Journal of Applied Behavior Analysis, 36,* 309–324.

Pietras, C. J., Brandt, A. E., & Searcy, G. D. (2010). Human responding on random-interval schedules of response-cost punishment: The role of reduced reinforcement density. *Journal of the Experimental Analysis of Behavior, 93,* 5–26.

Pietras, C. J., Locey, M. L., & Hackenberg, T. D. (2003). Human risky choice under temporal constraints: Tests of an energy-budget model. *Journal of the Experimental Analysis of Behavior, 80,* 59–75.

Pietras, C. J., Searcy, G. D., Huitema, B. E., & Brandt, A. E. (2008). Effects of monetary reserves and rate of gain on human risky choice under budget constraints. *Behavioural Processes, 78,* 358–373.

Pinker, S. (2002). *The blank slate.* New York: Viking.

Platt, J. (1973). Social traps. *American Psychologist, 28,* 641–651.

Platt, J. R. (1973). Percentile reinforcement: Paradigms for experimental analysis of response shaping. In G. H. Bower (Ed.),*The psychology of learning and motivation: Vol 7. Advances in theory and research.* New York: Academic Press, 271–296.

Platt, J. R. (1979). Interresponse-time shaping by variable-interval-like interresponse-time reinforcement contingencies. *Journal of the Experimental Analysis of Behavior, 31,* 3–14.

Podlesnik, C. A., & Shahan, T. A. (2010). Extinction, relapse, and behavioral momentum. *Behavioural Processes, 84,* 400–410.

Polka, L., Rvachew, S., & Molnar, M. (2008). Speech perception by 6- to 8-month-olds in the presence of distracting sounds. *Infancy, 13,* 421–439.

Polman, H., de Castro, B., & van Aken, M. G. (2008). Experimental study of the differential effects of playing versus watching violent video games on children's aggressive behavior. *Aggressive Behavior, 34,* 256–264.

Portier, S. J., Van Galen, G. P., & Meulenbroek, R. G. (1990). Practice and the dynamics of handwriting performance: Evidence for a shift of motor programming load. *Journal of Motor Behavior, 22,* 474–492.

Postman, L. (1947). The history and present status of the law of effect. *Psychological Review, 44,* 489–563.

Pouthas, V., Droit, S., Jacquet, A. Y., & Wearden, J. H. (1990). Temporal differentiation of response duration in children of different ages: Developmental changes in relations between verbal and nonverbal behavior. *Journal of the Experimental Analysis of Behavior, 53,* 21–31.

Powell, R. W. (1969). The effect of reinforcement magnitude upon responding under fixed-ratio schedules. *Journal of the Experimental Analysis of Behavior, 12,* 605–608.

Prather, J. F., Peters, S. S., Nowicki, S. S., & Mooney, R. R. (2008). Precise auditory-vocal mirroring in neurons for learned vocal communication. *Nature, 451,* 305–310.

Premack, D. (1959). Toward empirical behavioral laws: I. Positive reinforcement. *Psychological Review, 66,* 219–233.

Premack, D. (1963). Rate differential reinforcement in monkey manipulation. *Journal of the Experimental Analysis of Behavior, 6,* 81–89.

Premack, D. (1965). Reinforcement theory. In D. Levine (Ed.), *Nebraska symposium on motivation.* Lincoln, NE: University of Nebraska Press, 123–180.

Premack, D. (1971a). Catching up with common sense or two sides of a generalization: Reinforcement and punishment. In R. Glaser (Ed.), *The nature of reinforcement.* New York: Academic Press, 121–150.

Premack, D. (1971b). Language in chimpanzee. *Science, 172,* 808–822.

Premack, D. (1983). The codes of man and beasts. *Behavioral and Brain Sciences, 6,* 125–167.

Premack, D. (1986). *Gavagai!* Cambridge, MA: MIT Press.

Preston, K. L., Umbricht, A., Wong, C. J., & Epstein, D. H. (2001). Shaping cocaine abstinence by successive approximation. *Journal of Consulting and Clinical Psychology, 69,* 643–654.

Prochaska, J., Smith, N., Marzilli, R., Colby, J., & Donovan, W. (1974). Remote-control aversive stimulation in the treatment of head-banging in a retarded child. *Journal of Behavior Therapy and Experimental Psychiatry, 5,* 285–289.

Provine, R. R. (1989). Faces as releasers of contagious yawning: An approach to face detection using normal human subjects. *Bulletin of the Psychonomic Society, 27,* 211–214.

Purkis, H. M., & Lipp, O. V. (2009). Are snakes and spiders special? Acquisition of negative valence and modified attentional processing by non-fear-relevant animal stimuli. *Cognition and Emotion, 23,* 430–452.

Quinlan, C. K., Taylor, T. L., & Fawcett, J. M. (2010). Directed forgetting: Comparing pictures and words. *Canadian Journal of Experimental Psychology/ Revue canadienne de psychologie expérimentale, 64,* 41–46.

Rachlin, H. (1969). Autoshaping of key pecking in pigeons with negative reinforcement. *Journal of the Experimental Analysis of Behavior, 12,* 521–531.

Rachlin, H. (1970). *Introduction to modern behaviorism.* San Francisco, CA: W. H. Freeman.

Rachlin, H. (1974). Self-control. *Behaviorism, 2,* 94–107.

Rachlin, H. (1976). *Behavior and learning.* San Francisco, CA: W. H. Freeman.

Rachlin, H. (1990). Why do people gamble and keep gambling despite heavy losses. *Psychological Science, 1,* 294–297.

Rachlin, H., & Green, L. (1972). Commitment, choice, and self-control. *Journal of the Experimental Analysis of Behavior, 17,* 15–22.

Rachlin, H., Green, L., Kagel, J. H., & Battalio, R. C. (1976). *Economic demand theory and psychological studies of choice.* In G. H. Bower (Ed.), *The psychology of learning and motivation* (Vol. 10, pp. 129–154). New York: Academic Press.

Rachman, S. (1977). The conditioning theory of fear-acquisition: A critical examination. *Brain Research and Therapy, 15,* 375–387.

Rainer, G., Rao, S. C., & Miller, E. K. (1999). Prospective coding for objects in primate prefrontal cortex. *Journal of Neuroscience, 19,* 5493–5505.

Range, F., Aust, U., Steurer, M., & Huber, L. (2008). Visual categorization of natural stimuli by domestic dogs. *Animal Cognition, 11,* 339–347.

Rashotte, M. E., Griffin, R. W., & Sisk, C. L. (1977). Second-order conditioning of the pigeon's keypeck. *Animal Learning and Behavior, 5,* 25–38.

Rasmussen, E. B., & Newland, M. C. (2008). Asymmetry of reinforcement and punishment in human choice. *Journal of the Experimental Analysis of Behavior, 89,* 157–167.

Ratelle, C. F., Larose, S., Guay, F., & Senécal, C. (2005). Perceptions of parental involvement and support as predictors of college students' persistence in a science curriculum. *Journal of Family Psychology, 19,* 286–293.

Rauhut, A. S., McPhee, J., DiPietro, N. T., & Ayres, J. J. B. (2000). Conditioned inhibition training of the competing cue after compound conditioning does not reduce cue competition. *Animal Learning and Behavior, 28,* 92–108.

Redmon, W. K., & Lockwood, K. (1986). The matching law and organizational behavior. *Journal of Organizational Behavior Management, 8,* 57–72.

Reese, E. S. (1963). The behavioral mechanisms underlying shell selection by hermit crabs. *Behaviour, 21,* 78–126.

Regan, T. (1983). *The case for animal rights.* Berkeley, CA: University of California Press.

Rehfeldt, R. A., & Chambers, M. R. (2003). Functional analysis and treatment of verbal perseverations displayed by an adult with autism. *Journal of Applied Behavior Analysis, 36,* 259–261.

Reid, J., Patterson, G., & Snyder, J. (Eds.). (2002). *Antisocial behavior in children and adolescents: A developmental analysis and model for intervention.* Washington, DC: American Psychological Association.

Reilly, S., & Schachtman, T. R. (2009). *Conditioned taste aversion: Behavioral and neural processes.* New York: Oxford University Press.

Reisel, W. D., & Kopelman, R. E. (1995). The effects of failure on subsequent group performance in a professional sports setting. *Journal of Psychology, 129,* 103–113.

Rescorla, R. A. (1966). Predictability and number of pairings in Pavlovian fear conditioning. *Psychonomic Science, 4,* 383–384.

Rescorla, R. A. (1968). Probability of shock in the presence and absence of CS in fear conditioning. *Journal of Comparative and Physiological Psychology, 66,* 1–5.

Rescorla, R. A. (1969). Pavlovian conditioned inhibition. *Psychological Bulletin, 72,* 77–94.

Rescorla, R. A. (1973). Second order conditioning: Implications for theories of learning. In F. J. McGuigan & D. B. Lumsden (Eds.), *Contemporary approaches to conditioning and learning.* New York: Wiley, 127–150.

Rescorla, R. A. (1982). Simultaneous second-order conditioning produces S-S learning in conditioned suppression. *Journal of Experimental Psychology: Animal Behavior Processes, 8,* 23–32.

Rescorla, R. A. (2003). More rapid associative change with retraining than with initial training. *Journal of Experimental Psychology: Animal Behavior Processes, 29,* 251–260.

Rescorla, R. A., Durlach, P. J., & Grau, J. W. (1985). Contextual learning in Pavlovian conditioning. In P. D. Balsam & A. Tomie (Eds.), *Context and learning.* Hillsdale, NJ: Erlbaum, 23–46.

Rescorla, R. A., & LoLordo, V. M. (1965). Inhibition of avoidance behavior. *Journal of Comparative and Physiological Psychology, 59,* 406–412.

Rescorla, R. A., & Wagner, A. R. (1972). A theory of Pavlovian conditioning: Variations in the effectiveness of reinforcement and nonreinforcement. In A. H. Black & W. F. Prokasy (Eds.), *Classical conditioning II: Current research and theory.* New York: Appleton-Century-Crofts, 64–99.

Revusky, S. (2009). Chemical aversion treatment of alcoholism. In T. R. Schachtman & S. Reilly (Eds.), *Conditioned taste aversion: Behavioral and neural processes* (pp. 445–472). New York: Oxford University Press.

Reynolds, G. S. (1961). An analysis of interactions in a multiple schedule. *Journal of the Experimental Analysis of Behavior, 4,* 107–117.

Ricciardi, J. N., Luiselli, J. K., & Camare, M. (2006). Shaping approach responses as intervention for specific phobia in a child with autism. *Journal of Applied Behavior Analysis, 39,* 445–448.

Rice, M. L., Huston, A. C., Truglio, R., & Wright, J. (1990). Words from "Sesame Street": Learning vocabulary while viewing. *Developmental Psychology, 26,* 421–428.

Richards, C. S. (1981). Improving college students' study behaviors through self-control techniques: A brief review. *Behavioral Counseling Quarterly, 1,* 159–175.

Richards, J. B., Sabol, K. E., & Seiden, L. S. (1993). DRL interresponse-time distributions: Quantification by peak deviation analysis. *Journal of the Experimental Analysis of Behavior, 60,* 361–385.

Rider, R. A., & Abdulahad, D. T. (1991). Effects of massed versus distributed practice on gross and fine motor proficiency of educable mentally handicapped adolescents. *Perceptual and Motor Skills, 73,* 219–224.

Riley, W. T., Mihm, P., Behar, A., & Morin, C. M. (2010). A computer device to deliver behavioral interventions for insomnia. *Behavioral Sleep Medicine, 8,* 2–15.

Rivera, D. M., & Smith, D. D. (1987). Influence of modeling on acquisition and generalization of computational skills: A summary of research findings from three sites. *Learning Disability Quarterly, 10,* 69–80.

Rizzolatti, G., Craighero, L., & Fadiga, L. (2002). The mirror system in humans. In M. I. Stamenov, V. Gallese, M. I. Stamenov, & V. Gallese (Eds.), *Mirror neurons and the evolution of brain and language* (pp. 37–59). Amsterdam, Netherlands: John Benjamins Publishing Company.

Robbins, S. J. (1990). Mechanisms underlying spontaneous recovery in autoshaping. *Journal of Experimental Psychology: Animal Behavior Processes, 16,* 235–249.

Robert, M. (1990). Observational learning in fish, birds, and mammals: A classified bibliography spanning over 100 years of research. *Psychological Record, 40,* 289–311.

Roberts, D. F., Christenson, P. G., & Gentile, D. A. (2003). The effects of violent music on children and adolescents. In D. A. Gentile (Ed.), *Media violence and children.* Westport, CT: Praeger.

Roberts, S. (1981). Isolation of an internal clock. *Journal of Experimental Psychology: Animal Behavior Processes, 7,* 242–268.

Roberts, S. (1982). Cross modal use of an internal clock. *Journal of Experimental Psychology: Animal Behavior Processes, 8,* 2–22.

Roberts, S. (1983). Properties and function of an internal clock. In R. L. Mellgren (Ed.), *Animal cognition and behavior.* Amsterdam, Netherlands: North-Holland, 345–397.

Roberts, W. A. (2006). The questions of temporal and spatial displacement in animal cognition. In E. A. Wasserman & T. R. Zentall (Eds.), *Comparative cognition: Experimental explorations of animal intelligence* (pp. 145–163). New York: Oxford University Press.

Roberts, W. A., & Mazmanian, D. S. (1988). Concept learning at different levels of abstraction by pigeons, monkeys, and people. *Journal of Experimental Psychology: Animal Behavior Processes, 14,* 247–260.

Roberts, W. A., Mazmanian, D. S., & Kraemer, P. J. (1984). Directed forgetting in monkeys. *Animal Learning and Behavior, 12,* 29–40.

Robinson, S., Druks, J., Hodges, J., & Garrard, P. (2009). The treatment of object naming, definition, and object use in semantic dementia: The effectiveness of errorless learning. *Aphasiology, 23,* 749–775.

Rodgers, W., & Rozin, P. (1966). Novel food preferences in thiamine-deficient rats. *Journal of Comparative and Physiological Psychology, 61,* 1–4.

Roitblat, H. L. (1980). Codes and coding processes in pigeon short-term memory. *Animal Learning and Behavior, 8,* 341–351.

Roitblat, H. L., Pologe, B., & Scopatz, R. A. (1983). The representation of items in serial position. *Animal Learning and Behavior, 11,* 489–498.

Rolider, A., & Van Houten, R. (1985). Suppressing tantrum behavior in public places through the use of delayed punishment mediated by audio recordings. *Behavior Therapy, 16,* 181–194.

Romanowich, P., Bourret, J., & Vollmer, T. R. (2007). Further analysis of the matching law to describe two- and three-point shot allocation by professional basketball players. *Journal of Applied Behavior Analysis, 40,* 311–315.

Roper, K. L., & Zentall, T. R. (1993). Directed forgetting in animals. *Psychological Bulletin, 113,* 513–532.

Rosch, E. (1973). On the internal structure of perceptual and semantic categories. In T. E. Moore (Ed.), *Cognitive development and the acquisition of language.* New York: Academic Press, 111–144.

Rosch, E. (1975). Cognitive representations of semantic categories. *Journal of Experimental Psychology: General, 104,* 192–233.

Rosch, E. (1977). Human categorization. In N. Warren (Ed.), *Advances in cross-cultural psychology* (Vol. 1). London: Academic Press, 3–49

Rosenberg, D., Depp, C. A., Vahia, I. V., Reichstadt, J., Palmer, B. W., Kerr, J., et al. (2010). Exergames for subsyndromal depression in older adults: A pilot study of a novel intervention. *American Journal of Geriatric Psychiatry, 18,* 221–226.

Rosenthal, T. L., & Zimmerman, B. J. (1972). Modeling by exemplification and instruction in training conservation. *Developmental Psychology, 6,* 392–401.

Rosenthal, T. L., & Zimmerman, B. J. (1978). *Social learning and cognition.* New York: Academic Press.

Rosenzweig, M. R. (1966). Environmental complexity, cerebral change, and behavior. *American Psychologist, 21,* 321–332.

Rosenzweig, M. R. (1984). Experience and the brain. *American Psychologist, 39,* 365–376.

Rosenzweig, M. R., Mollgaard, K., Diamond, M. C., & Bennet, T. E. L. (1972). Negative as well as positive synaptic changes may store memory. *Psychological Review, 79,* 93–96.

Ross, J. A. (1974). The use of contingency contracting in controlling adult nailbiting. *Journal of Behavior Therapy and Experimental Psychiatry, 5,* 105–106.

Ross, R. T., & Holland, P. C. (1981). Conditioning of simultaneous and serial feature-positive discriminations. *Animal Learning and Behavior, 9,* 293–303.

Rowan, J. D., Fountain, S. B., Kundey, S. A., & Miner, C. L. (2001). A multiple species approach to sequential learning: Are you a man or a mouse? *Behavior Research Methods, Instruments & Computers, 33,* 435–439.

Rowland, W. J. (1989). Mate choice and the supernormality effect in female sticklebacks (*Gasterosteus aculeatus*). *Behavioral Ecology and Sociobiology, 24,* 433–438.

Rozin, P., & Kalat, J. W. (1971). Specific hungers and poison avoidance as adaptive specializations of learning. *Psychological Review, 78,* 459–486.

Rozin, P., Reff, D., Mack, M., & Schull, J. (1984). Conditioned opponent responses in human tolerance to caffeine. *Bulletin of the Psychonomic Society, 22,* 117–120.

Rudolph, R. L., Honig, W. K., & Gerry, J. E. (1969). Effects of monochromatic rearing on the acquisition of stimulus control. *Journal of Comparative and Physiological Psychology, 67,* 50–57.

Rumbaugh, D. M., Savage-Rumbaugh, E. S., & Sevcik, R. A. (1994). Biobehavioral roots of language: A comparative perspective of chimpanzee, child, and culture. In R. W. Wrangham, W. C. McGrew, F. B. M. de Waal, & P. G. Heltne (Eds.), *Chimpanzee cultures.* Cambridge, MA: Harvard University Press, 257–274.

Rushford, N. B., Burnett, A., & Maynard, R. (1963). Behavior in Hydra: Contraction responses of *Hydra pirardi* to mechanical and light stimuli. *Science, 139,* 760–761.

Russek, M., & Pina, S. (1962). Conditioning of adrenalin anorexia. *Nature, 193,* 1296–1297.

Russell, C., & Grealy, M. A. (2010). Avoidant instructions induce ironic and overcompensatory movement errors differently between and within individuals. *Quarterly Journal of Experimental Psychology, 63,* 1671–1682.

Russell, D. M., & Newell, K. M. (2007). On No-KR tests in motor learning, retention and transfer. *Human Movement Science, 26,* 155–173.

Sachs, D. A., & Mayhall, B. (1971). Behavioral control of spasms using aversive conditioning with a cerebral palsied adult. *Journal of Nervous and Mental Disorders, 152,* 362–363.

Sahoo, F. M., & Tripathy, S. (1990). Learned helplessness in industrial employees: A study on non-contingency, satisfaction and motivational deficits. *Psychological Studies, 35,* 79–87.

Sakagami, T., Hursh, S. R., Christensen, J., & Silberberg, A. (1989). Income maximizing in concurrent interval-ratio schedules. *Journal of the Experimental Analysis of Behavior, 52,* 41–46.

Salmoni, A. W., Schmidt, R. A., & Walter, C. B. (1984). Knowledge of results and motor learning: A review and critical reappraisal. *Psychological Bulletin, 95,* 355–386.

Sauter, D. A., Eisner, F., Ekman, P., & Scott, S. K. (2010). Cross-cultural recognition of basic emotions through nonverbal emotional vocalizations. *PNAS Proceedings of the National Academy of Sciences of the United States of America, 107,* 2408–2412.

Savage-Rumbaugh, E. S. (1984). Acquisition of functional symbol usage in apes and children. In H. L. Roitblat, T. G. Bever, & H. S. Terrace (Eds.), *Animal cognition.* Hillsdale, NJ: Erlbaum.

Savage-Rumbaugh, E. S. (1986). *Ape language: From conditioned response to symbol.* New York: Columbia University Press, 291–310.

Savage-Rumbaugh, E. S., McDonald, K., Sevcik, R. A., Hopkins, W. D., & Rubert, E. (1986). Spontaneous symbol acquisition and communicative use by pygmy chimpanzees (*Pan paniscus*). *Journal of Experimental Psychology: General, 115,* 211–235.

Savage-Rumbaugh, E. S., Shanker, S. G., & Taylor, T. J. (1998). *Apes, language, and the human mind.* New York: Oxford University Press.

Savastano, H. I., & Fantino, E. (1994). Human choice in concurrent ratio-interval schedules of reinforcement. *Journal of the Experimental Analysis of Behavior, 61,* 453–463.

Scalera, G., & Bavieri, M. (2009). Role of conditioned taste aversion on the side effects of chemotherapy in cancer patients. In T. R. Schachtman & S. Reilly (Eds.), *Conditioned taste aversion: Behavioral and neural processes* (pp. 513–541). New York: Oxford University Press.

Scarpa, A., Haden, S., & Abercromby, J. M. (2010). Pathways linking child physical abuse, depression, and aggressiveness across genders. *Journal of Aggression, Maltreatment & Trauma, 19,* 757–776.

Schachtman, T. R., Ramsey, A., & Pineño, O. (2009). Postconditioning event manipulations on processing of the target conditioned stimulus in conditioned taste aversion. In T. R. Schachtman & S. Reilly (Eds.), *Conditioned taste aversion: Behavioral and neural processes* (pp. 134–158). New York: Oxford University Press.

Schaefer, H. H., & Martin, P. L. (1966). Behavioral therapy for "apathy" of schizophrenics. *Psychological Reports, 19,* 1147–1158.

Scharff, L., Marcus, D. A., & Masek, B. J. (2002). A controlled study of minimal-contact thermal biofeedback treatment in children with migraine. *Journal of Pediatric Psychology, 27,* 109–119.

Schedlowski, M., & Pacheco-López, G. (2010). The learned immune response: Pavlov and beyond. *Brain, Behavior, and Immunity, 24,* 176–185.

Schell, A. M., Dawson, M. E., & Marinkovic, K. (1991). Effects of potentially phobic conditioned stimuli on retention, reconditioning, and extinction of the conditioned skin conductance response. *Psychophysiology, 28,* 140–153.

Schilder, M. B. H., & van der Borg, J. A. M. (2004). Training dogs with help of the shock collar: Short and long term behavioural effects. *Applied Animal Behaviour Science, 85,* 319–334.

Schmajuk, N. A. (2010). *Mechanisms in classical conditioning: A computational approach.* New York: Cambridge University Press.

Schmajuk, N. A., & Larrauri, J. A. (2006). Experimental challenges to theories of classical conditioning: Application of an attentional model of storage and retrieval. *Journal of Experimental Psychology: Animal Behavior Processes, 32,* 1–20.

Schmidt, R. A. (1975). A schema theory of discrete motor skill learning. *Psychological Review, 82,* 225–260.

Schmidt, R. A. (1988). *Motor control and learning: A behavioral emphasis* (2nd ed.). Champagne, IL: Human Kinetics.

Schmidt, R. A. (2003). Motor schema theory after 27 years: Reflections and implications for a new theory. *Research Quarterly for Exercise and Sport, 74,* 366–379.

Schmidtke, K. A., Katz, J. S., & Wright, A. A. (2010). Differential outcomes facilitate same/different concept learning. *Animal Cognition, 13,* 583–589.

Schneider, S. M., & Lickliter, R. (2010). Choice in quail neonates: The origins of generalized matching. *Journal of the Experimental Analysis of Behavior, 94,* 315–326.

Schneiderman, N., McCabe, P. M., Haselton, J. R., Ellenberger, H. H., Jarrell, T. W., & Gentile, C. G. (1987). Neurobiological bases of conditioned bradycardia in rabbits. In I. Gormezano, W. F. Prokasy, & R. F. Thompson (Eds.), *Classical conditioning* (3rd ed.). Hillsdale, NJ: Erlbaum, 37–63.

Schneirla, T. C. (1933). Some important features of ant learning. *Zeitschrift für Vergleichenden Physiologie, 19,* 439–452.

Schoenfeld, W. N. (1950). An experimental approach to anxiety, escape, and avoidance behavior. In P. H. Hoch & J. Zubin (Eds.), *Anxiety.* New York: Grune and Stratton, 70–101.

Schrier, A. M., & Brady, P. M. (1987). Categorization of natural stimuli by monkeys (*Macaca mulatta*): Effects of stimulus set size and modification of exemplars. *Journal of Experimental Psychology: Animal Behavior Processes, 13,* 136–143.

Schull, J. (1979). A conditioned opponent theory of Pavlovian conditioning and habituation. In G. H. Bower (Ed.), *The psychology of learning and motivation* (Vol. 13). New York: Academic Press, 57–90.

Schuster, R. (1969). A functional analysis of conditioned reinforcement. In D. P. Hendry (Ed.), *Conditioned reinforcement.* Homewood, IL: Dorsey Press, 192–234.

Schuster, R., & Rachlin, H. (1968). Indifference between punishment and free shock: Evidence for the negative law of effect. *Journal of the Experimental Analysis of Behavior, 11,* 777–786.

Schusterman, R. J., & Krieger, K. (1984). California sea lions are capable of semantic comprehension. *Psychological Record, 34,* 3–23.

Schwab, C., Bugnyar, T., Schloegl, C., & Kotrschal, K. (2008). Enhanced social learning between siblings in common ravens, Corvus corax. *Animal Behaviour, 75,* 501–508.

Schwartz, M. S., & Andrasik, F. (2003). *Biofeedback: A practitioner's guide* (3rd ed.). New York: Guilford Press.

Schwartz, S. P., Taylor, A. E., Scharff, L., & Blanchard, E. B. (1990). Behaviorally treated irritable bowel syndrome patients: A four-year follow-up. *Behavioral Research and Therapy, 28,* 331–335.

Schweitzer, J. B., & Sulzer-Azaroff, B. (1988). Self-control: Teaching tolerance for delay in impulsive children. *Journal of the Experimental Analysis of Behavior, 50,* 173–186.

Scott, D., Scott, L. M., & Goldwater, B. (1997). A performance improvement program for an international-level track and field athlete. *Journal of Applied Behavior Analysis, 30,* 573–575.

Scott, L. S., Shannon, R. W., & Nelson, C. A. (2006). Neural correlates of human and monkey face processing in 9-month-old infants. *Infancy, 10,* 171–186.

Segerdahl, P., Fields, W., & Savage-Rumbaugh, S. (Eds.). (2005). *Kanzi's primal language: The cultural initiation of primates into language.* New York: Palgrave.

Seligman, M. E. P. (1970). On the generality of the laws of learning. *Psychological Review, 77,* 406–418.

Seligman, M. E. P. (1975). *Helplessness: On depression, development, and death.* San Francisco, CA: W. H. Freeman.

Seligman, M. E. P. (2006). *Learned optimism: How to change your mind and your life.* New York: Vintage Books.

Seligman, M. E. P., & Hager, J. L. (1972). *Biological boundaries of learning.* New York: Appleton-Century-Crofts.

Seligman, M. E. P., & Johnston, J. C. (1973). A cognitive theory of avoidance learning. In F. J. McGuigan & D. B. Lumsden (Eds.), *Contemporary approaches to conditioning and learning.* Washington, DC: Winston-Wiley, 69–110.

Seligman, M. E. P., Schulman, P., & Tryon, A. M. (2007). Group prevention of depression and anxiety symptoms. *Behaviour Research and Therapy, 45,* 1111–1126.

Shaffer, L. H. (1978). Timing in the motor programming of typing. *Quarterly Journal of Experimental Psychology, 30,* 333–345.

Shah, K., Bradshaw, C. M., & Szabadi, E. (1989). Performance of humans in concurrent variable-ratio variable-ratio schedules of monetary reinforcement. *Psychological Reports, 65,* 515–520.

Shahan, T. A. (2010). Conditioned reinforcement and response strength. *Journal of the Experimental Analysis of Behavior, 93,* 269–289.

Shahan, T. A., Bickel, W. K., Madden, G. J., & Badger, G. J. (1999). Comparing the reinforcing efficacy of nicotine containing and de-nicotinized cigarettes: A behavioral economic analysis. *Psychopharmacology, 147,* 210–216.

Shapiro, D. C., Zernicke, R. F., Gregor, R. J., & Diestel, J. D. (1981). Evidence for generalized motor programs using gait pattern analysis. *Journal of Motor Behavior, 13,* 33–47.

Shea, C. H., Lai, Q., Black, C., & Park, J. C. (2000). Spacing practice sessions across days benefits the learning of motor skills. *Human Movement Science, 19,* 737–760.

Shea, C. H., Wright, D. L., Wulf, G., & Whitacre, C. (2000). Physical and observational practice afford unique learning opportunities. *Journal of Motor Behavior, 32,* 27–36.

Shea, C. H., & Wulf, G. (2005). Schema theory: A critical appraisal and reevaluation. *Journal of Motor Behavior, 37,* 85–101.

Shea, J. B., & Morgan, R. L. (1979). Contextual interference effects on the acquisition, retention, and transfer of a motor skill. *Journal of Experimental Psychology: Human Learning and Memory, 5,* 179–187.

Sheffield, F. D. (1948). Avoidance training and the contiguity principle. *Journal of Comparative and Physiological Psychology, 41,* 165–177.

Sheffield, F. D., Wulff, J. J., & Backer, R. (1951). Reward value of copulation without sex drive reduction. *Journal of Comparative and Physiological Psychology, 44,* 3–8.

Shepard, R. N. (1967). Recognition memory for words, sentences, and pictures. *Journal of Verbal Learning and Verbal Behavior, 6,* 156–163.

Shettleworth, S. J. (1983). Function and mechanism in learning. In M. D. Zeiler & P. Harzem (Eds.), *Advances in analysis of behavior: Vol. 3. Biological factors in learning.* New York: Wiley, 1–39.

Shields, W. E., Smith, J., Guttmannova, K., & Washburn, D. A. (2005). Confidence judgments by humans and rhesus monkeys. *Journal of General Psychology, 132,* 165–186.

Shimoyama, M., & Sonoyama, S. (2010). Treatment of severe self-injurious behavior by curricular modification and differential reinforcement of alternative behavior using precursor behavior. *Japanese Journal of Behavior Analysis, 25,* 30–41.

Shimp, C. P. (1966). Probabilistically reinforced choice behavior in pigeons. *Journal of the Experimental Analysis of Behavior, 9,* 443–455.

Shimp, C. P. (1968). Magnitude and frequency of reinforcement and frequencies of interresponse times. *Journal of the Experimental Analysis of Behavior, 11,* 525–535.

Shimp, C. P. (1969). Optimal behavior in free-operant experiments. *Psychological Review, 76,* 97–112.

Shimp, C. P. (1973). Synthetic variable-interval schedules of reinforcement. *Journal of the Experimental Analysis of Behavior, 19,* 311–330.

Shukla-Mehta, S., Miller, T., & Callahan, K. J. (2010). Evaluating the effectiveness of video instruction on social and communication skills training for children with autism spectrum disorders: A review of the literature. *Focus on Autism and Other Developmental Disabilities, 25,* 23–36.

Sidman, M. (1953). Two temporal parameters of the maintenance of avoidance behavior by the white rat. *Journal of Comparative and Physiological Psychology, 46,* 253–261.

Sidman, M., Rauzin, R., Lazar, R., Cunningham, S., Tailby, W., & Carrigan, P. (1982). A search for symmetry in the conditional discriminations of rhesus monkeys, baboons and children. *Journal of the Experimental Analysis of Behavior, 43,* 21–42.

Sidman, M., & Tailby, W. (1982). Conditional discrimination versus matching to sample: An extension of the testing paradigm. *Journal of the Experimental Analysis of Behavior, 37,* 5–22.

Siegel, S. (1975). Evidence from rats that morphine tolerance is a learned response. *Journal of Comparative and Physiological Psychology, 89,* 498–506.

Siegel, S. (1982). Pharmacological habituation and learning. In M. L. Commons, R. J. Herrnstein, & A. R. Wagner (Eds.), *Quantitative analyses of behavior: Vol. 3. Acquisition.* Cambridge, MA: Ballinger, 195–217.

Siegel, S. (2005). Drug tolerance, drug addiction, and drug anticipation. *Current Directions in Psychological Science, 14,* 296–300.

Siegel, S., & Domjan, M. (1971). Backward conditioning as an inhibitory procedure. *Learning and Motivation, 2,* 1–11.

Siegel, S., Hinson, R. E., Krank, M. D., & McCully, J. (1982). Heroin "overdose" death: The contribution of drug-associated environmental cues. *Science, 216,* 436–437.

Siegel, S., & Ramons, B. M. C. (2002). Applying laboratory research: Drug anticipation and the treatment of drug addiction. *Experimental and Clinical Psychopharmacology, 10,* 162–183.

Siegel, S., Sherman, J. E., & Mitchell, D. (1980). Extinction of morphine analgesic tolerance. *Learning and Motivation, 11,* 289–301.

Silberberg, A., Bauman, R., & Hursh, S. (1993). Stock optimizing: Maximizing reinforcers per session on a variable-interval schedule. *Journal of the Experimental Analysis of Behavior, 59,* 389–399.

Silberberg, A., Hamilton, B., Ziriax, J. M., & Casey, J. (1978). The structure of choice. *Journal of Experimental Psychology: Animal Behavior Processes, 4,* 368–398.

Silberberg, A., Thomas, J. R., & Berendzen, N. (1991). Human choice on concurrent variable-interval, variable-ratio schedules. *Journal of the Experimental Analysis of Behavior, 56,* 575–584.

Silva, K. M., & Timberlake, W. (2000). A clarification of the nature of backward excitatory conditioning. *Learning and Motivation, 31,* 67–80.

Silverman, I. W., & Ragusa, D. M. (1990). Child and maternal correlates of impulse control in 24-month-old children. *Genetic, Social, and General Psychology Monographs, 116,* 435–473.

Sisson, L. A., Hersen, M., & Van Hasselt, V. B. (1993). Improving the performance of youth with dual sensory impairment: Analyses and social validation of procedures to reduce maladaptive responding in vocational and leisure settings. *Behavior Therapy, 24,* 553–571.

Skinner, B. F. (1938). *The behavior of organisms.* New York: Appleton-Century-Crofts.

Skinner, B. F. (1948). "Superstition" in the pigeon. *Journal of Experimental Psychology, 38,* 168–172.

Skinner, B. F. (1950). Are theories of learning necessary? *Psychological Review, 57,* 193–216.

Skinner, B. F. (1956a). A case history in scientific method. *American Psychologist, 11,* 221–233.

Skinner, B. F. (1956b). What is psychotic behavior? In F. Gildea (Ed.), *Theory and treatment of the psychoses: Some newer aspects.* St. Louis, MO: Washington University Press.

Skinner, B. F. (1958). Teaching machines. *Science, 128,* 969–977.

Skinner, B. F. (1966). The phylogeny and ontogeny of behavior. *Science, 11,* 159–166.

Skinner, B. F. (1969). *Contingencies of reinforcement: A theoretical analysis.* Upper Saddle River, NJ: Prentice Hall.

Skinner, B. F. (1977). Herrnstein and the evolution of behaviorism. *American Psychologist, 32,* 1006–1012.

Skinner, B. F. (1985). Cognitive science and behaviourism. *British Journal of Psychology, 76,* 291–301.

Slifer, K. J., & Amari, A. (2009). Behavior management for children and adolescents with acquired brain injury. *Developmental Disabilities Research Reviews, 15,* 144–151.

Smith, J., Redford, J. S., Haas, S. M., Coutinho, M. C., & Couchman, J. J. (2008). The comparative psychology of same-different judgments by humans (*Homo sapiens*) and monkeys (*Macaca mulatta*). *Journal of Experimental Psychology: Animal Behavior Processes, 34,* 361–374.

Smith, J. D. (2009). The study of animal metacognition. *Trends in Cognitive Sciences, 13,* 389–396.

Smith, J. W., & Frawley, P. J. (1990). Long-term abstinence from alcohol in patients receiving aversion therapy as part of a multimodal inpatient program. *Journal of Substance Abuse Treatment, 7,* 77–82.

Smith, K. U. (1962). *Delayed sensory feedback and behavior.* Philadelphia, PA: Saunders.

Smith, M. C., & Gormezano, I. (1965). *Conditioning of the nictitating membrane response of the rabbit as a function of backward, simultaneous and forward CS–UCS intervals.* Paper presented at the meeting of the Psychonomic Society, Chicago, IL.

Smith, O. A., Astley, C. A., DeVito, J. L., Stein, J. M., & Walsh, K. E. (1980). Functional analysis of hypothalamic control of the cardiovascular responses accompanying emotional behavior. *Federation Proceedings, 39,* 2487–2494.

Smith, R. G., Russo, L., & Le, D. D. (1999). Distinguishing between extinction and punishment effects of response blocking: A replication. *Journal of Applied Behavior Analysis, 32,* 367–370.

Smith, S. M., & Vela, E. (2001). Environmental context-dependent memory: A review and meta-analysis. *Psychonomic Bulletin & Review, 8,* 203–220.

Sokolowska, M., Siegel, S., & Kim, J. A. (2002). Intraadministration associations: Conditional hyperalgesia elicited by morphine onset cues. *Journal of Experimental Psychology: Animal Behavior Processes, 28,* 309–320.

Solomon, P. R. (1977). Role of the hippocampus in blocking and conditioned inhibition of the rabbit's nictitating membrane response. *Journal of Comparative and Physiological Psychology, 91,* 407–417.

Solomon, P. R., Blanchard, S., Levine, E., Velazquez, E., & Groccia-Ellison, M. (1991). Attenuation of age-related conditioning deficits in humans by extension of the interstimulus interval. *Psychology and Aging, 6,* 36–42.

Solomon, R. L. (1980). The opponent process theory of acquired motivation. *American Psychologist, 35,* 691–712.

Solomon, R. L., & Corbit, J. D. (1974). An opponent-process theory of motivation: I. Temporal dynamics of affect. *Psychological Review, 81,* 119–145.

Solomon, R. L., Kamin, L. J., & Wynne, L. C. (1953). Traumatic avoidance learning: The outcomes of several extinction procedures with dogs. *Journal of Abnormal and Social Psychology, 48,* 291–302.

Solomon, R. L., & Wynne, L. C. (1953). Traumatic avoidance learning: Acquisition in normal dogs. *Psychological Monographs, 67,* 354.

Solomon, R. L., & Wynne, L. C. (1954). Traumatic avoidance learning: The principles of anxiety conservation and partial irreversibility. *Psychological Review, 61,* 353–385.

Solvason, H. B., Ghanata, V., & Hiramoto, R. H. (1988). Conditioned augmentation of natural killer cell activity: Independence from nociceptive effects and dependence on interferon-B. *Journal of Immunology, 140,* 661–665.

Spalding, T. L., & Ross, B. H. (2000). Concept learning and feature interpretation. *Memory & Cognition, 28,* 439–451.

Sparrow, W. A., & Summers, J. J. (1992). Performance on trials without knowledge of results (KR) in reduced relative frequency presentations of KR. *Journal of Motor Behavior, 24,* 197–209.

Spear, N. E. (1971). Forgetting as retrieval failure. In W. K. Honig & P. H. R. James (Eds.), *Animal memory.* New York: Academic Press, 45–109.

Spence, K. W. (1937). The differential response in animals to stimuli varying within a single dimension. *Psychological Review, 44,* 430–444.

Spetch, M. L. (1995). Overshadowing in landmark learning: Touch-screen studies with pigeons and humans. *Journal of Experimental Psychology: Animal Behavior Processes, 21,* 166–181.

Spetch, M. L., & Cheng, K. (1998). A step function in pigeons' temporal generalization in the peak shift task. *Animal Learning and Behavior, 26,* 103–118.

Spinelli, D. H., Jensen, F. E., & DiPrisco, G. V. (1980). Early experience effect on dendritic branching in normally reared kittens. *Experimental Neurology, 62,* 1–11.

Staats, S., & Pierfelice, L. (2003). Travel: A long-range goal of retired women. *Journal of Psychology, 137,* 483–494.

Staddon, J. E. R., & Simmelhag, V. L. (1971). The "superstition" experiment: A reexamination of its implications for the principles of adaptive behavior. *Psychological Review, 78,* 3–43.

Starek, J., & McCullagh, P. (1999). The effect of self-modeling on the performance of beginning swimmers. *Sport Psychologist, 13,* 269–287.

Starr, M. D., & Mineka, S. (1977). Determinants of fear over the cause of avoidance learning. *Learning and Motivation, 8,* 332–350.

Stasiewicz, P. R., Brandon, T. H., & Bradizza, C. M. (2007). Effects of extinction context and retrieval cues on renewal of alcohol-cue reactivity among alcohol-dependent outpatients. *Psychology of Addictive Behaviors, 21,* 244–248.

Staub, E. (1968). Duration of stimulus-exposure as determinant of the efficacy of flooding procedures in the elimination of fear. *Behavior Research and Therapy, 6,* 131–132.

Steinmetz, J. E. (1999). A renewed interest in human classical eyeblink conditioning. *Psychological Science, 10,* 24–25.

Stilling, S. T., & Critchfield, T. S. (2010). The matching relation and situation-specific bias modulation in professional football play selection. *Journal of the Experimental Analysis of Behavior, 93,* 435–454.

Stoops, W. W., Dallery, J., Fields, N. M., Nuzzo, P. A., Schoenberg, N. E., Martin, C. A., et al. (2009). An internet-based abstinence reinforcement smoking cessation intervention in rural smokers. *Drug and Alcohol Dependence, 105,* 56–62.

Stout, S. C., & Miller, R. R. (2007). Sometimes-competing retrieval (SOCR): A formalization of the comparator hypothesis. *Psychological Review, 114,* 759–783.

St. Peter Pipkin, C., & Vollmer, T. (2009). Applied implications of reinforcement history effects. *Journal of Applied Behavior Analysis, 42,* 83–103.

Stuart, R. B. (1971). A three-dimensional program for the treatment of obesity. *Behaviour Research and Therapy, 9,* 177–186.

Stubbs, A. (1968). The discrimination of stimulus duration by pigeons. *Journal of the Experimental Analysis of Behavior, 11,* 223–238.

Sturges, J. W., & Sturges, L. V. (1998). In vivo systematic desensitization in a single-session treatment of an 11-year-old girl's elevator phobia. *Child & Family Behavior Therapy, 20,* 55–62.

Suge, R., & Okanoya, K. (2010). Perceptual chunking in the self-produced songs of Bengalese finches (*Lonchura striata var. domestica*). *Animal Cognition, 13,* 515–523.

Sulzer-Azaroff, B., Loafman, B., Merante, R. J., & Hlavacek, A. C. (1990). Improving occupational safety in a large industrial plant: A systematic replication. *Journal of Organizational Behavior Management, 11,* 99–120.

Summers, J. J. (1981). Motor programs. In D. Holding (Ed.), *Human skills.* New York: Wiley, 49–69.

Suri, R., Long, M., & Monroe, K. B. (2003). The impact of the Internet and consumer motivation on evaluation of prices. *Journal of Business Research, 56,* 379–390.

Sutton, N. P., Grace, R. C., McLean, A. P., & Baum, W. M. (2008). Comparing the generalized matching law and contingency discriminability model as accounts of concurrent schedule performance using residual meta-analysis. *Behavioural Processes, 78,* 224–230.

Swan, J. A., & Pearce, J. M. (1987). The influence of predictive accuracy on serial autoshaping: Evidence of orienting responses. *Journal of Experimental Psychology: Animal Behavior Processes, 13,* 407–417.

Swinnen, S. P. (1990). Interpolated activities during the knowledge-of-results delay and post-knowledge-of-results interval: Effects on performance and learning. *Journal of Experimental Psychology: Learning, Memory, and Cognition, 16,* 692–705.

Swinnen, S. P., Schmidt, R. A., Nicholson, D. E., & Shapiro, D. C. (1990). Information feedback for skill acquisition: Instantaneous knowledge of results degrades learning. *Journal of Experimental Psychology: Learning, Memory, and Cognition, 16,* 706–716.

Tait, D. S., & Brown, V. J. (2007). Difficulty overcoming learned non-reward during reversal learning in rats with ibotenic acid lesions of orbital prefrontal cortex. *Annals of the New York Academy of Sciences, 1121,* 407–420.

Taktek, K., & Hochman, J. (2004). Ahsen's triple code model as a solution to some persistent problems within Adams' closed loop theory and Schmidt's motor schema theory. *Journal of Mental Imagery, 28,* 115–158.

Tanno, T., & Sakagami, T. (2008). On the primacy of molecular processes in determining response rates under variable-ratio and variable-interval schedules. *Journal of the Experimental Analysis of Behavior, 89,* 5–14.

Tarbox, J., & Hayes, L. (2005). Verbal behavior and behavioral contrast in human subjects. *Psychological Record, 55,* 419–437.

Tarbox, J., Schiff, A., & Najdowski, A. C. (2010). Parent-implemented procedural modification of escape extinction in the treatment of food selectivity in a young child with autism. *Education and Treatment of Children, 33,* 223–234.

Taub, E., & Berman, A. J. (1968). Movement and learning in the absence of sensory feedback. In S. J. Freedman (Ed.), *The neuro-psychology of spatially oriented behavior.* Homewood, IL: Dorsey Press, 172–193.

Taylor, D. J., & Roane, B. M. (2010). Treatment of insomnia in adults and children: A practice-friendly review of research. *Journal of Clinical Psychology, 66,* 1137–1147.

Terrace, H. S. (1963). Errorless transfer of a discrimination across two continua. *Journal of the Experimental Analysis of Behavior, 6,* 223–232.

Terrace, H. S. (1966). Stimulus control. In W. K. Honig (Ed.), *Operant conditioning: Areas of research and application.* Upper Saddle River, NJ: Prentice Hall, 271–344.

Terrace, H. S. (1979). *Nim*. New York: Knopf.

Terrace, H. S. (1985). On the nature of animal thinking. *Neuroscience & Biobehavioral Reviews, 9*, 643–652.

Terrace, H. S. (1991). Chunking during serial learning by a pigeon: I. Basic evidence. *Journal of Experimental Psychology: Animal Behavior Processes, 17*, 81–93.

Terrace, H. S., & Chen, S. (1991). Chunking during serial learning by a pigeon: II. Integrity of a chunk on a new list. *Journal of Experimental Psychology: Animal Behavior Processes, 17*, 94–106.

Thompson, R. F., McCormick, D. A., & Lavond, D. G. (1986). Localization of the essential memory-trace system for a basic form of associative learning in the mammalian brain. In S. H. Hulse & B. F. Green, Jr. (Eds.), *One hundred years of psychological research in America*. Baltimore, MD: Johns Hopkins University Press, 125–171.

Thompson, R. F., & Spencer, W. A. (1966). Habituation: A model phenomenon for the study of neuronal substrates of behavior. *Psychological Review, 73*, 16–43.

Thompson, R. H., Iwata, B. A., Conners, J., & Roscoe, E. M. (1999). Effects of reinforcement for alternative behavior during punishment of self-injury. *Journal of Applied Behavior Analysis, 32*, 317–328.

Thorndike, E. L. (1898). Animal intelligence: An experimental study of the associative processes in animals. *Psychological Review Monograph Supplement, 2*, 8.

Thorndike, E. L. (1911). *Animal intelligence*. New York: Macmillan.

Thorndike, E. L. (1927). The law of effect. *American Journal of Psychology, 39*, 212–222.

Thorndike, E. L. (1946). Expectation. *Psychological Review, 53*, 277–281.

Till, B. D., & Priluck, R. L. (2000). Stimulus generalization in classical conditioning: An initial investigation and extension. *Psychology and Marketing, 17*, 55–72.

Timberlake, W. (1983). Rats' responses to a moving object related to food or water: A behavior-systems analysis. *Animal Learning and Behavior, 11*, 309–320.

Timberlake, W. (1993). Behavior systems and reinforcement: An integrative approach. *Journal of the Experimental Analysis of Behavior, 60*, 105–128.

Timberlake, W. (2001). Motivational modes in behavior systems. In R. R. Mowrer & S. B. Klein (Eds.), *Handbook of contemporary learning theories*. Mahwah, NJ: Erlbaum, 155–209.

Timberlake, W., & Allison, J. (1974). Response deprivation: An empirical approach to instrumental performance. *Psychological Review, 81*, 146–164.

Timberlake, W., & Farmer-Dougan, V. A. (1991). Reinforcement in applied settings: Figuring out ahead of time what will work. *Psychological Bulletin, 110*, 379–391.

Timberlake, W., & Grant, D. L. (1975). Autoshaping in rats to the presentation of another rat predicting food. *Science, 190*, 690–692.

Timberlake, W., & Lucas, G. A. (1985). The basis of superstitious behavior: Chance contingency, stimulus substitution, or appetitive behavior. *Journal of the Experimental Analysis of Behavior, 44*, 279–299.

Timberlake, W., & Lucas, G. A. (1989). Behavior systems and learning: From misbehavior to general principles. In S. B. Klein & R. R. Mowrer (Eds.), *Contemporary learning theories: Instrumental conditioning theories and the impact of biological constraints on learning*. Hillsdale, NJ: Erlbaum, 237–275.

Timmann, D., Musso, C., Kolb, F. P., Rijntjes, M., Jüptner, M., Müller, S. P., et al. (1998). Involvement of the human cerebellum during habituation of the acoustic startle response: A PET study. *Journal of Neurology, Neurosurgery & Psychiatry, 65*, 771–773.

Tinbergen, N. (1951). *The study of instinct*. Oxford: Oxford University Press.

Tinklepaugh, O. L. (1928). An experimental study of representative factors in monkeys. *Journal of Comparative Psychology, 8*, 197–236.

Todrank, J., Byrnes, D., Wrzesniewski, A., & Rozin, P. (1995). Odors can change preferences for people in photographs: A cross-modal evaluative conditioning study with olfactory USs and visual CSs. *Learning and Motivation, 26,* 116–140.

Tolman, E. C. (1932). *Purposive behavior in animals and men.* New York: Appleton-Century-Crofts.

Tolman, E. C. (1951). *Collected papers in psychology.* Berkeley, CA: University of California Press.

Tolman, E. C. (1959). Principles of purposive behavior. In S. Koch (Ed.), *Psychology: A study of a science* (Vol. 2). New York: McGraw-Hill, 92–157.

Tolman, E. C., & Honzik, C. H. (1930). Introduction and removal of reward, and maze performance in rats. *University of California Publications in Psychology, 4,* 257–275.

Tomie, A., Grimes, K. L., & Pohorecky, L. A. (2008). Behavioral characteristics and neurobiological substrates shared by Pavlovian sign-tracking and drug abuse. *Brain Research Reviews, 58,* 121–135.

Toth, N., Schich, K. D., Savage-Rumbaugh, E. S., Sevcik, R. A., & Rumbaugh, D. M. (1993). Pan the tool-maker: Investigations into the stone tool-making and tool-using capabilities of a Bonobo (*Pan paniscus*). *Journal of Archaeological Science, 20,* 81–91.

Toussaint, K. A., & Tiger, J. H. (2010). Teaching early braille literacy skills within a stimulus equivalence paradigm to children with degenerative visual impairments. *Journal of Applied Behavior Analysis, 43,* 181–194.

Tracy, W. K. (1970). Wavelength generalization and preference in monochromatically reared ducklings. *Journal of the Experimental Analysis of Behavior, 13,* 163–178.

Troje, N. F., Huber, L., Loidolt, M., Aust, U., & Fieder, M. (1999). Categorical learning in pigeons: The role of texture and shape in complex static stimuli. *Vision Research, 39,* 353–366.

Trowbridge, M. H., & Cason, H. (1932). An experimental test of Thorndike's theory of learning. *Journal of General Psychology, 7,* 245–260.

Turnbull, O. H., Evans, C. Y., Kemish, K., Park, S., & Bowman, C. H. (2006). A novel set-shifting modification of the Iowa gambling task: Flexible emotion-based learning in schizophrenia. *Neuropsychology, 20,* 290–298.

Turney, T. H. (1982). The association of visual concepts and imitative vocalization in the mynah (*Gracula religiosa*). *Bulletin of the Psychonomic Society, 19,* 59–62.

Ulrich, R., Giray, M., & Schaffer, R. (1990). Is it possible to prepare the second component of a movement before the first one. *Journal of Motor Behavior, 22,* 125–148.

Ulrich, R. E., & Azrin, N. H. (1962). Reflexive fighting in response to aversive stimulation. *Journal of the Experimental Analysis of Behavior, 5,* 511–520.

Urcelay, G. P., & Miller, R. R. (2008). Counteraction between two kinds of conditioned inhibition training. *Psychonomic Bulletin & Review, 15,* 103–107.

Urcelay, G. P., Perelmuter, O., & Miller, R. R. (2008). Pavlovian backward conditioned inhibition in humans: Summation and retardation tests. *Behavioural Processes, 77,* 299–305.

Urcuioli, P. J. (2006). Responses and acquired equivalence classes. In E. A. Wasserman & T. R. Zentall (Eds.), *Comparative cognition: Experimental explorations of animal intelligence* (pp. 405–421). New York: Oxford University Press.

Urcuioli, P. J. (2008). Associative symmetry, antisymmetry, and a theory of pigeons' equivalence-class formation. *Journal of the Experimental Analysis of Behavior, 90,* 257–282.

Urcuioli, P. J., & Zentall, T. R. (1986). Retrospective coding in pigeons' delayed matching-to-sample. *Journal of Experimental Psychology: Animal Behavior Processes, 12,* 69–77.

Vander Wall, S. B. (1982). An experimental analysis of cache recovery by Clark's nutcracker. *Animal Behaviour, 30,* 84–94.

Vangheluwe, S., Suy, E., Wenderoth, N., & Swinnen, S. P. (2006). Learning and transfer of bimanual multifrequency patterns:

Effector-independent and effector-specific levels of movement representation. *Experimental Brain Research, 170,* 543–554.

Van Gucht, D., Vansteenwegen, D., Beckers, T., Hermans, D., Baeyens, F., & Van den Bergh, O. (2008). Repeated cue exposure effects on subjective and physiological indices of chocolate craving. *Appetite, 50,* 19–24.

Vargas-Perez, H., Ting-A-Kee, R. A., Heinmiller, A., Sturgess, J. E., & van der Kooy, D. (2007). A test of the opponent-process theory of motivation using lesions that selectively block morphine reward. *European Journal of Neuroscience, 25,* 3713–3718.

Vasconcelos, M. (2008). Transitive inference in non-human animals: An empirical and theoretical analysis. *Behavioural Processes, 78,* 313–334.

Vaughan, W. (1981). Melioration, matching, and maximization. *Journal of the Experimental Analysis of Behavior, 36,* 141–149.

Vaughan, W. (1985). Choice: A local analysis. *Journal of the Experimental Analysis of Behavior, 43,* 383–405.

Vaughan, W. (1987). Dissociation of value and response strength. *Journal of the Experimental Analysis of Behavior, 48,* 367–381.

Vaughan, W. (1988). Formation of equivalence sets in pigeons. *Journal of Experimental Psychology: Animal Behavior Processes, 14,* 36–42.

Vaughan, W., & Greene, S. L. (1983). Acquisition of absolute discriminations in pigeons. In M. L. Commons, A. R. Wagner, & R. J. Herrnstein (Eds.), *Quantitative analyses of behavior: Vol. 4. Discrimination processes.* Cambridge, MA: Ballinger, 231–238.

Vaughan, W., & Greene, S. L. (1984). Pigeon visual memory capacity. *Journal of Experimental Psychology: Animal Behavior Processes, 10,* 256–271.

Vedeniapin, A., Cheng, L., & George, M. S. (2010). Feasibility of simultaneous cognitive behavioral therapy and left prefrontal rTMS for treatment resistant depression. *Brain Stimulation, 3,* 207–210.

Ventis, W. L., Higbee, G., & Murdock, S. A. (2001). Using humor in systematic desensitization to reduce fear. *Journal of General Psychology, 128,* 241–253.

Vera, J. G., & Montilla, M. M. (2003). Practice schedule and acquisition, retention, and transfer of a throwing task in 6-yr-old children. *Perceptual and Motor Skills, 96,* 1015–1024.

Voegtlin, W. L. (1940). The treatment of alcoholism by establishing a conditioned reflex. *American Journal of Medical Science, 199,* 802–810.

Vollmer, T. R. (2002). Punishment happens: Some comments on Lerman and Vorndran's review. *Journal of Applied Behavior Analysis, 35,* 469–473.

Vonk, J., & MacDonald, S. E. (2004). Levels of abstraction in orangutan (*Pongo abelii*) categorization. *Journal of Comparative Psychology, 118,* 3–13.

Vuchinich, R. E. (1999). Behavioral economics as a framework for organizing the expanded range of substance abuse interventions. In J. A. Tucker, D. M. Donovan, & G. A. Marlatt (Eds.), *Changing addictive behavior: Bridging clinical and public health strategies.* New York: Guilford Press, 191–218.

Vyse, S. A., & Belke, T. W. (1992). Maximizing versus matching on concurrent variable-interval schedules. *Journal of the Experimental Analysis of Behavior, 58,* 325–334.

Wagner, A. R. (1978). Expectancies and the priming of STM. In S. H. Hulse, H. Fowler, & W. K. Honig (Eds.), *Cognitive aspects of animal behavior.* Hillsdale, NJ: Erlbaum.

Wagner, A. R. (1981). SOP: A model of automatic memory processing in animal behavior. In N. E. Spear & R. R. Miller (Eds.), *Information processing in animals: Memory mechanisms.* Hillsdale, NJ: Erlbaum, 5–48.

Wagner, A. R., Rudy, J. W., & Whitlow, J. W. (1973). Rehearsal in animal conditioning. *Journal of Experimental Psychology, 97,* 407–426.

Wagner, G. A., & Morris, E. K. (1987). "Superstitious" behavior in children. *Psychological Record, 37,* 471–488.

Waldrep, D., & Waits, W. (2002). Returning to the Pentagon: The use of mass desensitization following the September 11, 2001 attack. *Military Medicine, 167,* 58–59.

Waldron, F. A., Wiegmann, D. D., & Wiegmann, D. A. (2005). Negative incentive contrast induces economic choice behavior by bumble bees. *International Journal of Comparative Psychology, 18,* 358–371.

Walker, L. E. A. (2009). *The battered woman syndrome* (3rd ed.). New York: Springer.

Wallin, J. A., & Johnson, R. D. (1976). The positive reinforcement approach to controlling employee absenteeism. *Personnel Journal, 55,* 390–392.

Walton, D. (1960). The application of learning theory to the treatment of a case of neurodermatitis. In H. J. Eysenck (Ed.), *Behavior therapy and the neuroses.* Oxford: Pergamon Press, 272–274.

Wanchisen, B. A., Tatham, T. A., & Mooney, S. E. (1989). Variable-ratio conditioning history produces high- and low-rate fixed-interval performance in rats. *Journal of the Experimental Analysis of Behavior, 52,* 167–179.

Wang, S.-H., & Morris, R. G. M. (2010). Hippocampal-neocortical interactions in memory formation, consolidation, and reconsolidation. *Annual Review of Psychology, 61,* 49–79.

Warren, J. M. (1965). Primate learning in comparative perspective. In A. M. Schrier, H. F. Harlow, & F. Stollnitz (Eds.), *Behavior of nonhuman primates* (Vol. 1). New York: Academic Press, 249–282.

Wasserman, E. A. (1973). Pavlovian conditioning with heat reinforcement produces stimulus-directed pecking in chicks. *Science, 81,* 875–877.

Watanabe, S., Kirino, Y., & Gelperin, A. (2008). Neural and molecular mechanisms of micro-cognition in Limax. *Learning & Memory, 15,* 633–642.

Watanabe, S., Sakamoto, J., & Wakita, M. (1995). Pigeons' discrimination of paintings by Monet and Picasso. *Journal of the Experimental Analysis of Behavior, 63,* 165–174.

Watson, D. L., & Tharp, R. G. (1997). *Self-directed behavior: Self-modification for personal adjustment* (7th ed.). Belmont, CA: Brooks/Cole.

Watson, J. B. (1919). *Psychology from the standpoint of a behaviorist.* Philadelphia, PA: Lippincott.

Watson, J. B. (1925). *Behaviorism.* New York: Norton.

Watson, J. B., & Rayner, R. (1921). Studies in infant psychology. *Scientific Monthly, 13,* 493–515.

Watson, T. S., Ray, K. P., Turner, H. S., & Logan, P. (1999). Teacher-implemented functional analysis and treatment: A method for linking assessment to intervention. *School Psychology Review, 28,* 292–302.

Wearden, J. H. (1988). Some neglected problems in the analysis of human behavior. In G. Davey & C. Cullen (Eds.), *Human operant conditioning and behavior modification.* Chichester, England: Wiley, 197–224.

Weaver, M. T., & McGrady, A. (1995). A provisional model to predict blood pressure response to biofeedback-assisted relaxation. *Biofeedback and Self-Regulation, 20,* 229–239.

Wegner, D. M. (1997). When the antidote is the poison: Ironic mental control processes. *Psychological Science, 8,* 148–150.

Wegner, D. M., Ansfield, M., & Pilloff, D. (1998). The putt and the pendulum: Ironic effects of the mental control of action. *Psychological Science, 9,* 196–199.

Weiner, H. (1964). Conditioning history and human fixed-interval performance. *Journal of the Experimental Analysis of Behavior, 7,* 383–385.

Weir, A. A. S., Chappell, J., & Kacelnik, A. (2002). Shaping of hooks in New Caledonian crows. *Science, 297,* 981.

Werner, G. A. (1992). Employee recognition: A procedure to reinforce work attendance. *Behavioral Residential Treatment, 7,* 199–204.

Werner, G. E., & Hall, D. J. (1974). Optimal foraging and size selection of prey by the bluegill sunfish (*Lepomis macrochirus*). *Ecology, 55,* 1042–1052.

West, R. E., & Young, R. J. (2002). Do domestic dogs show any evidence of being able to count. *Animal Cognition, 5,* 183–186.

Wheeler, J. J., & Richey, D. D. (2009). *Principles and practices of positive behavioral supports.* Upper Saddle River, NJ: Prentice Hall.

Whitacre, C. A., & Shea, C. H. (2000). Performance and learning of generalized motor programs: Relative (GMP) and absolute (parameter) errors. *Journal of Motor Behavior, 32,* 163–175.

White, A. G., & Bailey, J. S. (1990). Reducing disruptive behaviors of elementary physical education students with sit and watch. *Journal of Applied Behavior Analysis, 23,* 353–359.

White, K., & Davey, G. C. L. (1989). Sensory preconditioning and UCS inflation in human "fear" conditioning. *Behaviour Research and Therapy, 27,* 161–166.

White, K. G., Parkinson, A. E., Brown, G. S., & Wixted, J. T. (2004). Local proactive interference in delayed matching to sample: The role of reinforcement. *Journal of Experimental Psychology: Animal Behavior Processes, 30,* 83–95.

Whiten, A., & Ham, R. (1992). On the nature and evolution of imitation in the animal kingdom: Reappraisal of a century of research. In P. J. B. Slater, J. S. Rosenblatt, C. Beer, & M. Milinski (Eds.), *Advances in the study of behavior* (Vol. 21). New York: Academic Press, 239–283.

Wickelgren, W. A. (1979). Chunking and consolidation: A theoretical synthesis of semantic networks, configuring in conditioning, S-R versus cognitive learning, normal forgetting, the amnesiac syndrome, and the hippocampal arousal system. *Psychological Review, 86,* 44–60.

Wilcoxon, H. C., Dragoin, W. B., & Kral, P. A. (1971). Illness-induced aversions in rat and quail: Relative salience of visual and gustatory cues. *Science, 171,* 826–828.

Wilder, D. A., Austin, J., & Casella, S. (2009). Applying behavior analysis in organizations: Organizational behavior management. *Psychological Services, 6,* 202–211.

Wilder, D. A., White, H., & Yu, M. L. (2003). Functional analysis and treatment of bizarre vocalizations exhibited by an adult with schizophrenia: A replication and extension. *Behavioral Interventions, 18,* 43–52.

Wilkie, D. M., & Slobin, P. (1983). Gerbils in space: Performance on the 17-arm radial maze. *Journal of the Experimental Analysis of Behavior, 40,* 301–312.

Williams, B. A. (1994). Conditioned reinforcement: Neglected or outmoded explanatory construct? *Psychonomic Bulletin & Review, 1,* 457–475.

Williams, B. A. (2002). Behavioral contrast redux. *Animal Learning and Behavior, 30,* 1–20.

Williams, B. A., & Dunn, R. (1991). Preference for conditioned reinforcement. *Journal of the Experimental Analysis of Behavior, 55,* 37–46.

Williams, D. A., Johns, K. W., & Brindas, M. (2008). Timing during inhibitory conditioning. *Journal of Experimental Psychology: Animal Behavior Processes, 34,* 237–246.

Williams, D. A., MacKenzie, H. K., & Johns, K. W. (2010). Intertrial unconditioned stimuli preferentially interfere with delay conditioning. *Journal of Experimental Psychology: Animal Behavior Processes, 36,* 232–242.

Williams, D. R., & Williams, H. (1969). Automaintenance in the pigeon: Sustained pecking despite contingent non-reinforcement. *Journal of the Experimental Analysis of Behavior, 12,* 511–520.

Williams, H., & Staples, K. (1992). Syllable chunking in zebra finch (*Taeniopygia guttata*) song. *Journal of Comparative Psychology, 106,* 278–286.

Williams, J. L., & Lierle, D. M. (1986). Effects of stress controllability, immunization, and therapy on the subsequent defeat of colony intruders. *Animal Learning and Behavior, 14,* 305–314.

Wilson, A., Brooks, D. C., & Bouton, M. E. (1995). The role of the rat hippocampal system in several effects of context in extinction. *Behavioral Neuroscience, 109,* 828–836.

Wilson, P. H., Thomas, P. R., & Maruff, P. (2002). Motor imagery training ameliorates motor clumsiness in children. *Journal of Child Neurology, 17,* 491–498.

Windle, M. (2000). Parental, sibling, and peer influences on adolescent substance use and alcohol problems. *Applied Developmental Science, 4,* 98–110.

Winnick, W. A., & Hunt, J. McV. (1951). The effect of an extra stimulus upon strength of response during acquisition and extinction. *Journal of Experimental Psychology, 41,* 205–215.

Winstein, C. J., & Schmidt, R. A. (1990). Reduced frequency of knowledge of results enhances motor skill learning. *Journal of Experimental Psychology: Learning, Memory, and Cognition, 16,* 677–691.

Winterbauer, N. E., & Bouton, M. E. (2010). Mechanisms of resurgence of an extinguished instrumental behavior. *Journal of Experimental Psychology: Animal Behavior Processes, 36,* 343–353.

Wixted, J. (2004). The psychology and neuroscience of forgetting. *Annual Review of Psychology, 55,* 235–269.

Wolfe, J. B. (1936). Effectiveness of token rewards for chimpanzees. *Comparative Psychology Monographs, 12,* 1–72.

Wolpe, J. (1958). *Psychotherapy by reciprocal inhibition.* Stanford, CA: Stanford University Press.

Wood, D. C. (1973). Stimulus specific habituation in a protozoan. *Physiology and Behavior, 11,* 349–354.

Woodruff-Pak, D. S., & Disterhoft, J. F. (2008). Where is the trace in trace conditioning. *Trends in Neurosciences, 31,* 105–112.

Wright, A. A. (2006). Memory processing. In E. A. Wasserman & T. R. Zentall (Eds.), *Comparative cognition: Experimental explorations of animal intelligence* (pp. 164–185). New York: Oxford University Press.

Wright, A. A., & Lickteig, M. T. (2010). What is learned when concept learning fails?—a theory of restricted-domain relational learning. *Learning and Motivation, 41,* 273–286.

Wulf, G., Shea, C., & Lewthwaite, R. (2010). Motor skill learning and performance: A review of influential factors. *Medical Education, 44,* 75–84.

Wulf, G., & Shea, C. H. (2004). Understanding the role of augmented feedback: The good, the bad, and the ugly. In A. M. Williams & N. J. Hodges (Eds.), *Skill acquisition in sport: Research, theory, and practice* (pp. 121–144). New York: Routledge.

Yamadori, A., & Albert, M. L. (1973). Word category aphasia. *Cortex, 9,* 112–125.

Yell, M. L. (1994). Timeout and students with behavior disorders: A legal analysis. *Education and Treatment of Children, 17,* 293–301.

Yerkes, R. M., & Morgulis, S. (1909). The method of Pavlov in animal psychology. *Psychological Bulletin, 6,* 257–273.

Yin, H., Barnet, R. C., & Miller, R. R. (1994). Trial spacing and trial distribution effects in Pavlovian conditioning: Contributions of a comparator mechanism. *Journal of Experimental Psychology: Animal Behavior Processes, 20,* 123–134.

Young, G. C., & Morgan, R. T. (1972). Overlearning in the conditioning treatment of enuresis: A long-term follow-up study. *Behavior Research and Therapy, 10,* 419–420.

Yule, W., Sacks, B., & Hersov, L. (1974). Successful flooding treatment of a noise phobia in an eleven-year-old. *Journal of Behavior Therapy and Experimental Psychiatry, 5,* 209–211.

Zalstein-Orda, N., & Lubow, R. E. (1995). Context control of negative transfer induced by preexposure to irrelevant stimuli: Latent inhibition in humans. *Learning and Motivation, 26,* 11–28.

Zeldin, R. K., & Olton, D. S. (1986). Rats acquire spatial learning sets. *Journal of Experimental Psychology: Animal Behavior Processes, 12,* 412–419.

Zener, K. (1937). The significance of behavior accompanying conditioned salivary secretion for theories of the conditioned response. *American Journal of Psychology, 50,* 384–403.

Zentall, T. R. (2004). Action imitation in birds. *Learning and Behavior, 32,* 15–23.

Zentall, T. R. (2010). Coding of stimuli by animals: Retrospection, prospection, episodic memory and future planning. *Learning and Motivation, 41,* 225–240.

Zhou, S., Hou, Z., & Bai, R. (2008). Effect of group assertiveness training on university students' assertive competence. *Chinese Journal of Clinical Psychology, 16,* 665–667.

Zhuikov, A. Y., Couvillon, P. A., & Bitterman, M. E. (1994). Quantitative two-process analysis of avoidance conditioning in goldfish. *Journal of Experimental Psychology: Animal Behavior Processes, 20,* 32–43.

Zimmerman, B. J., & Blom, D. E. (1983). Toward an empirical test of the role of cognitive conflict in learning. *Developmental Review, 3,* 18–38.

Zoefel, B., Huster, R. J., & Herrmann, C. S. (2011). Neurofeedback training of the upper alpha frequency band in EEG improves cognitive performance. *NeuroImage, 54,* 1427–1431.

Zoellner, L. A., Abramowitz, J., Moore, S. A., & Slagle, D. M. (2009). Flooding. In W. T. O'Donohue & J. E. Fisher (Eds.), *General principles and empirically supported techniques of cognitive behavior therapy* (pp. 300–308). Hoboken, NJ: Wiley.

ADDITIONAL ACKNOWLEDGMENTS

FIGURE 4-11A: An adaptation of Figure 3 on page 1034 from Baron, A., Kaufman, A., & Fazzini, D. (1969). Density and delay of punishment of free-operant avoidance. *Journal of the Experimental Analysis of Behavior, 12,* 1029–1037. Copyright 1969 by the Society for the Experimental Analysis of Behavior, Inc. Reprinted by permission of the publisher.

FIGURE 4-11B: An adaptation of Figure 1 on page 288 from Andrews, E. A., & Braveman, N. S. (1975). The combined effects of dosage level and interstimulus interval on the formation of one-trial poison-based aversions in rats. *Animal Learning & Behavior, 3,* 287–289. Copyright 1975 by the Psychonomic Society.

FIGURE 5-3: Record of cat B on page 46 from Guthrie, E. R., & Horton, G. P. (1946). *Cats in a puzzle box.* New York: Rinehart & Company. Copyright 1946 by Edwin R. Guthrie and George P. Horton.

FIGURE 5-4: Record of cat G on page 52 from Guthrie, E. R., & Horton, G. P. (1946). *Cats in a puzzle box.* New York: Rinehart & Company. Copyright 1946 by Edwin R. Guthrie and George P. Horton.

FIGURE 8-1: An adaptation of Figure 4 on page 267 from Tolman, E. C., & Honzik, C. H. (1930). Introduction and removal of reward, and maze performance in rats. *University of California Publications in Psychology, 4,* 257–275. Copyright 1930 by the University of California Press.

FIGURE 10-2A: An adaptation of Figure 1 on page 210 from Grant, D. S. (1975). Proactive interference in pigeon short-term memory. *Journal of Experimental Psychology: Animal Behavior Processes, 1,* 207–220. Copyright 1975 by the American Psychological Association. Adapted by permission.

FIGURE 10-2B: An adaptation of Figure 1 on page 329 from D'Amato, M. R., and O'Neill, W., Effect of delay-interval illumination on matching behavior in the capuchin monkey. *Journal of the Experimental Analysis of Behavior, 15,* 327–333. Copyright 1971 by the Society for the Experimental Analysis of Behavior, Inc. Reprinted by permission of the publisher.

FIGURE 10-9: Reprinted from Miller, H. C., Rayburn-Reeves, R., & Zentall, T. R. (2009). What do dogs know about hidden objects? *Behavioural Processes, 81,* 439–446. Copyright 2009, with permission from Elsevier.

ADDITIONAL TEXT CREDITS

Chapter 1, page 43, excerpted text from Church, LoLordo, and Overmeir, et al.: Reprinted from *Journal of Comparative and Physiological Psychology, 62*(1), Church, Lolordo, and Overmeir, "Cardiac response to shock in curarized dogs," pages 1–7, copyright ©1966, American Psychological Association. Reprinted with permission; chapter 5, page 106, excerpted text from Skinner: " 'Superstition' in the pigeon," *Journal of Experimental Psychology: General*, 1948, ©American Psychological Association. Reprinted with permission; chapter 5, page 117: excerpted text from Shahan: From Shahan, "Conditioned reinforcement and response strength," *Journal of the Experimental Analysis of Behavior, Vol. 93*(2), 2010, pages 269–289. Copyright 2010 by the Society for the Experimental Analysis of Behavior, Inc.; chapter 6, page 145, excerpted text from Hackenburg: From Hackenburg, "Token reinforcement: A review and analysis," *Journal of the Experimental Analysis of Behavior, 91*(2), pages 557–586. Copyright 2009 by the Society for the Experimental Analysis of Behavior, Inc.; chapter 7, page 159, excerpted text from Bolles: Bolles, "Species-specific defense reactions and avoidance learning," *Psychological Review, 77*(1), Jan 1970, 32–48, ©American Psychological Association. Reprinted with permission; chapter 10, page 241, excerpted text from Capaldi and Miller: Capaldi and Miller, "Counting in rats: Its functional significance and the independent cognitive processes that constitute it," *Journal of Experimental Psychology: Animal Behavior and Processes, 14*(1), Jan 1988, 3–17, ©American Psychological Association. Reprinted with permission; chapter 11, page 273, excerpted text from Meichenbaum and Goodman: Meichenbaum, D.H. and Goodman, J., "Training impulsive children to talk to themselves: A means of developing self-control," *Journal of Abnormal Psychology, 77*(2) April 1971, 115–126, ©American Psychological Association. Reprinted with permission; chapter 13, page 314, excerpts from Olson, Bates, and Bayles: From Olson, Bates, and Bayles, "Early Antecedents of Childhood Impulsivity: The Role of Parent–Child Interaction, Cognitive Competence, and Temperament," *Journal of Abnormal Child Psychology, 18*(3), 1990, reprinted with kind permission from Spring Science + Business Media B.V.

AUTHOR INDEX

A

Abdulahad, D. T., 279
Abercromby, J. M., 261
Abramowitz, A. J., 166
Abramowitz, J., 161
Abravanel, E., 252
Acebes, F., 77
Ackil, J. E., 122
Adams, C. D., 173
Adams, J. A., 279, 281–287, 294
Adelinis, J. D., 193
Ader, R., 67
Adler, C. S., 183
Adornetto, M., 315
Aeschleman, S. R., 108
Ahearn, W. H., 136
Ainslie, G., 311–313, 315–316
Akins, C. K., 254
Albert, M., 63, 96, 238
Albert, M. L., 23
Alberts, E., 206
Albiach-Serrano, A., 246
Albright, T. D., 20
Alferink, L. A., 299
Allan, R. W., 297
Allen, J. D., 125
Allison, J., 192
Alterson, C. J., 174
Altus, D. E., 146–147
Alvero, A. M., 149
Amari, A., 111, 190
Amundson, J. C., 234
Anderson, C. A., 263–264
Anderson, D. I., 277
Andrasik, F., 184
Andree, P. J., 174
Andrews, E. A., 91
Andrews, J. A., 265
Anger, D., 141
Anger, W. K., 148
Ansfield, M., 282
Antonov, I., 39
Aparicio, C. F., 308–309
Arantes, J., 237
Arcediano, F., 63
Ariely, D., 316
Aristotle, 4, 5, 24

Armsworth, C. G., 30
Armus, H. L., 231
Arntz, A., 264
Asahina, K., 206
Ash, D. W., 118
Ashenden, B., 144
Aslin, R. N., 38
Astley, C. A., 97
Athens, E. S., 111
Aust, U., 217–218
Austin, J., 148–149
Ayllon, T., 174–175
Ayres, J. J. B., 63, 83, 96
Azrin, N. H., 164–169, 191

B

Babb, S. J., 229
Backer, R., 187
Baddeley, A., 226
Badets, A., 284
Badger, G. J., 198
Baer, D. M., 256
Baeyens, F., 66, 158
Bagshaw, M., 136
Bai, R., 267
Bailey, C. H., 97
Bailey, J. S., 173, 175
Baker, M., 34
Baker, T. B., 45–46
Balaban, M. T., 168
Balaz, M. A., 82
Baldwin, E., 12
Balleine, B. W., 181
Balsam, P. D., 84, 124
Bandettini, P. A., 97
Bandura, A., 251–252, 255–262, 264, 267–269, 272
Barlow, H. B., 20
Barnes, D., 132
Barnet, R. C., 83
Barth, J., 246
Baron, A., 91, 132, 140
Bates, J. E., 314
Batsell, W. R., 85
Batson, J. D., 85
Battalio, R. C., 142, 305
Battig, W. F., 216, 287–288
Baum, M., 158

SUBJECT INDEX